# SUDDEN UNEXPECTED DEATH IN EPILEPSY

Mechanisms and New Methods for Analyzing Risks

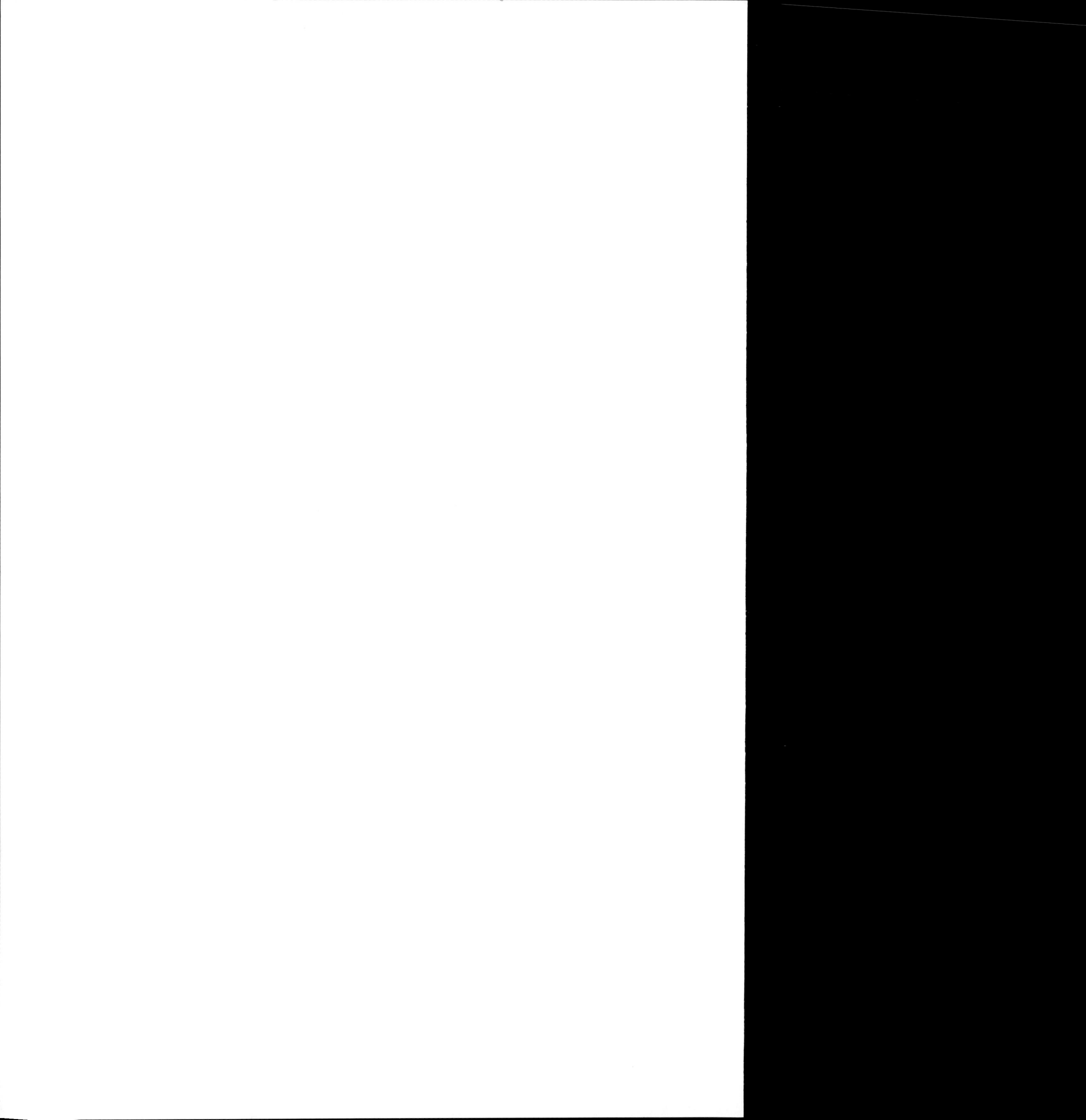

# SUDDEN UNEXPECTED DEATH IN EPILEPSY

Mechanisms and New Methods for Analyzing Risks

Edited by
Claire M. Lathers
Paul L. Schraeder
Jan E. Leestma
Braxton B. Wannamaker
Richard L. Verrier
Steven C. Schachter

**CRC Press**
Taylor & Francis Group
Boca Raton  London  New York

CRC Press is an imprint of the
Taylor & Francis Group, an **informa** business

CRC Press
Taylor & Francis Group
6000 Broken Sound Parkway NW, Suite 300
Boca Raton, FL 33487-2742

First issued in paperback 2021

© 2015 by Taylor & Francis Group, LLC
CRC Press is an imprint of Taylor & Francis Group, an Informa business

No claim to original U.S. Government works

Version Date: 20150211

ISBN 13: 978-0-367-77844-6 (pbk)
ISBN 13: 978-1-4822-2385-9 (hbk)

**Visit the Taylor & Francis Web site at**
**http://www.taylorandfrancis.com**

**and the CRC Press Web site at**
**http://www.crcpress.com**

# Dedications

*To (DS), a 4-year-old boy with a history of nocturnal seizures who found hidden Christmas presents, including the one he wanted most of all, a remote control car, 2 weeks before Christmas. The next morning, he was found dead in bed. He and other victims of SUDEP challenge all of us to find preventive measures as quickly as possible.*

*To Marcel J. Lajoy and Camille Lajoie and to Richard S. Lathers for their love, support, and words of wisdom while completing this endeavor. To the memory of Schuyler W. and Carol F. Lathers, who provided the engineering and liberal arts backgrounds and education to support me as a scientist with an interest in autonomic questions related to epilepsy, sudden death, cardiovascular pharmacology, and space flight.*

**Claire M. Lathers**

*To the lasting memory of my older brothers, "Boyd" (Robert Boyd Wannamaker) and "Tommy" (Thomas Elliott Wannamaker, Jr.). Boyd and Tommy courageously lived their lives with refractory epilepsy. Their lives ended too soon and because of epilepsy, Boyd at 20 years by accident and Tommy at 31 years by SUDEP.*

**Braxton B. Wannamaker**

*To individuals with epilepsy, whose bravery challenges us all and inspires our best work to address the SUDEP enigma.*

**Richard L. Verrier**

*To my patients who lost their lives to SUDEP and their families.*

**Steven C. Schachter**

# Contents

## SECTION I  Forensics of SUDEP and Cluster Risk Factor Identification

## SECTION II  SUDEP Animal Models: Mechanisms of Risks

## SECTION III  SUDEP Risk Mechanisms: Animal Models and Clinical Studies

Contents

# Foreword by Michael W. Bungo

The determination of Claire Lathers has ensured the timely completion of this book and has sustained her professional legacy as an advocate for people with epilepsy who are at risk of SUDEP.

"Sudden Death." The words get your attention immediately. Even in the sporting world, sudden death conveys an unpredictable finality that seems to circumvent any preparation. In the clinical world, the ramifications for the person and the families hold a much more significant outcome. Couple this now with a somewhat perplexing diagnosis of a disorder called epilepsy, a usually young patient, and an as yet incomplete scientific understanding of the phenomena, and "sudden unexpected death in epileptic patients" (SUDEP) has emotional impact even beyond its monumental consequences.

Incidence of the problem per 1000 patient-years has been described to occur between 0.09 and 2.65 in a community population or up to 9.3 when a high-risk cohort was examined (Devinsky 2011). In 1990, Drs. Lathers and Schraeder, realizing the need to involve the scientific and medical community more in this dreadful diagnosis, put together an excellent book (*Epilepsy and Sudden Death*), lighting the path forward to the many issues that confront the patients and caregivers in this realm. It was a full 21 years later (2011) that what can be described as a second edition (*Sudden Death in Epilepsy: Forensic and Clinical Issues*) was published. With this 2011 publication, new editors were added, the knowledge base of SUDEP was reviewed, and the cutting-edge investigatory needs and results were presented. A multidisciplinary approach to basic science, clinical science, and practical applications was the hallmark of that volume. In spite of the two decade hiatus, much still needed to be said about SUDEP and even more needed to be done. With no proved preventive strategy for SUDEP, education, investigation, collaboration, and review continue to be paramount in meeting the challenge for current and future patients.

Now, 3 or 4 years later, this book, *Sudden Unexpected Death in Epilepsy: Mechanisms and New Methods for Analyzing Risks* expands the work begun by the earlier volumes. New editors and new chapters examine everything from clinical case studies, patient investigation and management, and risk factors to animal studies, mechanistic proposals, predictive models, and potential therapies. With these enlightenments, we step closer to offering hope that practical and effective solutions are within reach.

**Michael W. Bungo**
*Professor of Medicine in Cardiology*
*University of Texas Health Science Center*
*Houston, Texas*

## REFERENCE

Devinsky O. Sudden, unexpected death in epilepsy. *New Engl J Med* 2011;365:1801–11.

# Foreword by Steven A. Koehler

Our understanding of sudden unexpected death in epilepsy (SUDEP) has been limited, in part, due to a lack of information. One of the most overlooked and underutilized sources of information and available biological samples relating to SUDEP is the medical examiners' and coroners' offices around the country and the world. Having over 20 years of experience in the forensic community, I understand first-hand the wealth of information collected during the forensic investigation and the biological material that is collected and available for research during the course of a forensic autopsy.

By definition, all deaths via SUDEP are sudden and unexpected and, therefore, by local and/or state statutes governing death investigations must undergo a complete forensic death investigation. The forensic investigation is composed of three main phases: the death scene investigation, an autopsy, and a toxicological analysis. Each of these three phases can provide unique information about SUDEP and will ultimately assist in a greater understanding of SUDEP.

The forensic death scene investigation is the first phase of the investigation. During this phase, death investigators from the medical examiners' or coroners' office collect information about the victim and the circumstances leading to the death by interviewing next of kin, family members, and witnesses. In addition, they collect the victim's past medical history (PMH), past and current medications, and recent life-changing events in the victim's life. The information collected during this early phase of investigation is very important because it sets the tone and direction for the rest of the forensic investigation. Death investigators must become familiar with the features of SUDEP, and the key questions to ask that might indicate whether the death may be a SUDEP-related death. They must ask questions relating to a history of epilepsy, seizure history, current medications, specificity of antiepileptic drugs (AEDs), recent changes in AED medication or dosage levels, and the victim's compliance history. The victim's primary care physician must be contacted to ascertain the diagnosis of epilepsy and the form of epilepsy. In addition to the normal data collected as part of a standard death investigation, medical examiners' and coroners' offices must have a standard SUDEP questionnaire protocol in place for cases with a PMH of epilepsy who had died suddenly and unexpectedly. This will ensure a standardized method of information collection. The information collected should include the following: a complete medical history of the epilepsy, age of onset of seizures, a history of the AED medications by type and dosage, any changes in medication and dosage, and life-changing events around the time of the death. In addition, the questionnaire should inquire about a history of heart disease, arrhythmia, or sudden death in the

victim's family. To ensure that information is collected in a complete and meaningful manner, the investigative staff in medical examiners'/coroners' offices must receive education about SUDEP, the risk factors, and the type of information that needs to be collected on each death. The standard collection of epidemiological, anatomical, and forensic data has played a key role in sudden infant death syndrome. Analysis of the data helped in identifying risk factors and modifiable risky behaviors and allowed for a better understanding of the syndrome, which would not have been possible without the systemic collection of forensic data.

The second phase of the death investigation is forensic autopsy of the body, typically conducted by a forensic pathologist. A forensic autopsy involves examination of all the internal organs and documentation of their weights, stage of disease, and pathology. In addition, each organ undergoes a microscopic examination. A standard forensic protocol should be developed and used when a death is identified as a possible SUDEP death. This protocol will ensure that large sections of the heart, containing the cardiac system; large sections of the lungs, and respective sections of the brain are preserved to be used in future examinations and research. During the autopsy, blood, bile, urine, and eye fluid are collected and sent for toxicological analysis. The forensic pathologist plays an important role in advancing our understanding of SUDEP. To ensure that key SUDEP data are collected during the postmortem examination and that samples are preserved, medical examiners, coroners, and forensic pathologists must receive education about current theories relating to the mechanism of SUDEP and the importance of information that needs to be collected for each death.

The third phase is toxicological analysis of the body fluids collected during the autopsy and is conducted by a forensic toxicologist. The analysis provides a list of the detected compounds and corresponding concentrations. It is unrealistic and extremely expensive to test for every compound. Therefore, cases of suspected SUDEP should undergo a special drug panel designed to detect AED medications. Forensic toxicologists must undergo education about the risks of SUDEP and the role that AED medication plays in these types of deaths. In addition, they should be provided with a current list of AED medications and their therapeutic levels. The forensic toxicologist should initiate the collection and storage of blood samples from all suspected cases of SUDEP that can be used in future genetic research.

*Sudden Unexpected Death in Epilepsy: Mechanisms and New Methods for Analyzing Risks* is a great reference book for forensic pathologists, medical examiners, coroners, death scene investigators, and forensic toxicologists. This textbook provides a detailed discussion of the theories of SUDEP risk factors and the current level of understanding of the mechanism of SUDEP and highlights the key types of information that need to be collected to gain a better understanding of SUDEP. In addition, this book underscores the importance that forensic science plays in the investigation of sudden death and the major role it plays in the ultimate goal of a better understanding of the risk factors, triggers, mechanisms, and the roles of AEDs in SUDEP deaths.

**Steven A. Koehler, Forensic Epidemiologist**
*Director of Forensic Medical Investigations, LLC*
*Associate Professor, Graduate School of Public Health*
*Department of Epidemiology, University of Pittsburgh*
*Former Chief Forensic Epidemiologist*
*Allegheny County Medical Examiner Office*
*Pittsburgh, Pennsylvania*

# Foreword by Steven C. Schachter

If sudden death in epilepsy is the most feared and serious consequence of epilepsy, why does it continue to be under-discussed and substantially underresearched?

Problems identified in the last edition of this book have largely continued—inadequate animal models and basic understanding, lack of clinical recognition from treating physicians and medical examiners, inability to completely eliminate the possibility of sudden death in the nearly one in three patients with drug-resistant epilepsy, and reluctance among medical professionals to discuss sudden death with patient and their families. Compounding these issues is the silo-style infrastructure of academic medicine, which creates intrinsic barriers for clinical and research collaborations across disciplines relevant to sudden death in epilepsy, such as epidemiology, neurology, cardiology, and pulmonology, as well as specialties among the applied sciences, such as electrical and computer engineering.

Yet, there are reasons to be encouraged. National and international epilepsy foundations and organizations are breaking down silos and have committed substantial advocacy and research funding to the prevention of SUDEP, as have passionate researchers who are studying SUDEP from the bench to the bedside. Numerous patient advocacy groups and survivors are talking openly about sudden death in epilepsy at conferences and on websites and providing support for research projects and inspiration to the entire community.

This book represents another reason for hope. Identification of specific groupings, or clusters, of historical, demographic, clinical, and epilepsy-related factors that may combine together to significantly increase the risk of SUDEP should help facilitate our focus for collaborative research in the laboratory and the clinic, which could bring us closer to effective SUDEP prevention strategies. Until then, as physicians caring for patients with epilepsy we must accept the imperfect state of knowledge and inform our patients in a meaningful and compassionate way about sudden death and work as much as possible to reduce their risks.

**Steven C. Schachter**
*Departments of Neurology, Beth Israel Deaconess
Medical Center, Massachusetts General Hospital and
Harvard Medical School
Chief Academic Officer, Center for Integration of Medicine
and Innovative Technology
Boston, Massachusetts*

# Preface

This is our third book focused on the clinical problem of sudden unexpected death in epilepsy (SUDEP). We explore and highlight our new SUDEP Classification System and present a new method called "SUDEP Risk Factor Cluster ID" in this book. Our method evaluates likely mechanisms of and risk factors for premature death in individuals with epilepsy. SUDEP is thought to be a heterogeneous syndrome with multiple causes and mechanisms, including central and peripheral roles for the brain, heart and arrhythmias, respiratory system with both central and obstructive apnea, as well as unknown mechanisms. Different mechanisms of SUDEP may apply to different patients, implying that their risk factors will differ. The ultimate goal of our approach is a better ability to individualize risk for SUDEP and therefore better individual patient management, such as selection of AEDs and other preventive strategies.

Case histories of SUDEP, definite or probable, as well as near miss cases are included in the book with illustrative SUDEP Cluster IDs. One chapter addresses how to use self-learning techniques and apply this new method to patients with epilepsy. Patient management is discussed. A number of other chapters demonstrate how to use our new method of SUDEP Risk Factor analysis, which will allow neurologists, emergency room physicians, and attending physicians to identify individuals at risk for SUDEP and hopefully lessen the chance of occurrence. Our book can therefore be used to teach the public, professionals, and students about the risk factors for SUDEP.

Our SUDEP Risk Factor Classification and Cluster ID method and its use to evaluate 115 cases of SUDEP are presented. We have begun to develop an international database of human cases and animal models of SUDEP. We demonstrate how medical examiners' and coroners' offices can provide information about SUDEP victims to strengthen the foundation of the database. It is our hope that physicians will use our SUDEP database to determine the level of risk of patients with similar Cluster IDs.

We present related clinical and animal studies needed to classify risk factors for SUDEP victims.

Further clinical, epidemiological, genetic, and many other studies are needed to identify underlying pathophysiologic mechanisms. All of our collaborators and coauthors are working on related clinical or animal studies to classify risk factors for SUDEP for use with our Risk Factor Cluster IDs. We are building the new SUDEP classification system and SUDEP Risk Factor Cluster IDs in the hope that they will transform the care of patients who are at risk for SUDEP.

Our involvement with SUDEP through research and books spans 25 years, from 1990 to 2014. Previous books discussed animal data and models with relevance to the problem of SUDEP as well as clinical SUDEP data and studies. Multiple institutions, multiple disciplines, and many coauthors nationally and internationally have participated to address known risk factors for SUDEP and identify gaps in our knowledge to resolve the mystery of SUDEP.

Dr. Lathers' first medical book was *Cardiovascular Therapeutics in Clinical Practice*, published by John Wiley & Sons, New York, in 1984 (Frankl et al. 1984). Coeditors were William S. Frankl, MD; Jay Roberts, PhD, FCP; and Claire M. Lathers, PhD, FCP. This book was a culmination of collaborative work initiated in 1972 and fostered multidisciplinary cardiology, clinical pharmacology, and pharmacology. Eventually, this collaboration between basic scientists and clinicians evolved to encompass cardiovascular pharmacology, clinical pharmacology, and neurology/epilepsy as Lathers and Schraeder began to collaborate on animal studies of SUDEP in 1979.

Lathers and Schraeder were the coeditors of our first medical book on SUDEP entitled *Epilepsy and Sudden Death* published by Marcel Dekker, New York, in 1990 to discuss original animal studies of Lathers and Schraeder, which were designed to shed light on the problem of SUDEP. Clinical updates on the current status of SUDEP were also included.

In 2011, coeditors Claire M. Lathers, PhD, emeritus fellow clinical pharmacology; Paul L. Schraeder, MD, Drexel University Medical School; Michael W. Bungo, MD, University of Texas; and Jan Leestma, MD, a forensic pathologist, published our 1000-page, second medical book *Sudden Death in Epilepsy: Forensic and Clinical Issues* with CRC Press, Taylor & Francis Group, Boca Raton, Florida, owner of publisher Marcel Dekker. We collaborated with 86 international contributors working in government, private industry, and/or academia. Subsequently, in December 2011 coauthors Claire M. Lathers, Steven A. Koehler, Cyril H. Wecht, and Paul L. Schraeder published a research paper titled "Forensic Antiepileptic Drug Levels in Autopsy Cases of Sudden Death in Epilepsy" (Lathers et al. 2011), analyzing forensic autopsy data for Allegheny County, Pennsylvania, in *Epilepsy & Behavior*, chief editor Steven C. Schachter, MD. These data became the foundation for our new SUDEP Classification and Risk Factor Cluster ID method and were expanded after publishing our preliminary data by Dr. Koehler et al. in Chapter 9 of our 2011 book on SUDEP.

Thus, the books, research studies, and reviews of Lathers, Schraeder, et al. (Lathers and Schraeder 1990; Lathers et al. 2008; Lathers, Schraeder et al. 2011; and Lathers et al. 2014) began to address and identify possible mechanisms and risk factors for SUDEP. This book explores the interactions among the central and peripheral autonomic nervous systems and the cardiopulmonary systems. Speculations about potential preventive measures to minimize the risk of SUDEP are presented. This current book has begun a new approach for addressing patient management for people with epilepsy and the best preventive measures. Answers are long overdue. The new SUDEP Classification System and Risk Factor Cluster ID method, developed over the last 2 years, will help to address gaps in our knowledge about causes and preventions of SUDEP.

**Claire M. Lathers**

**Paul L. Schraeder**

**Jan E. Leestma**

**Braxton B. Wannamaker**

**Richard L. Verrier**

**Steven C. Schachter**

## REFERENCES

Frankl WS, Roberts J, Lathers, CM (Coeditors). *Cardiovascular therapeutics in clinical practice*. New York, NY: John Wiley; 1984, pp. 1–339.

Lathers CM, Koehler SA, Wecht CH, Schraeder PL. Forensic antiepileptic drug levels in autopsy cases of epilepsy. *Epilepsy Behav* 2011;22(4):778–85.

Lathers CM, Schraeder PL (Coeditors). *Epilepsy and sudden death*. New York, NY: Marcel Dekker; 1990, pp. 1–531.

Lathers CM, Schraeder PL, Bungo MW. The mystery of sudden death: mechanisms for risks. *Epilepsy Behav* 2008;12(1):3–24.

Lathers, CM, Schraeder PL, Bungo MW, Leestma JE (Coeditors). *Sudden death in epilepsy: Forensic and clinical issues*. Boca Raton, FL: CRC Press/Taylor & Francis Group; 2011, pp. 1–1011.

Lathers CM, Schraeder PL, Leestma JE, Wannamaker BB, Verrier RL, Schachter SC (Coeditors). *Sudden death in epilepsy: Risk analyses SUDEP cluster risk factor classification and identifications*. Boca Raton, FL: CRC Press/Taylor & Francis Group; 2014.

# Acknowledgments

*I want to acknowledge the motivation, dedication, and hard work of Claire M. Lathers to move our book along.*

**Paul L. Schraeder**

# Editors

**Claire M. Lathers**, PhD, Emeritus FCP, served as President Clinton's lead person on the Food Safety Program at the U.S. Food and Drug Administration (FDA). She has received acknowledgment of her service to the nation for her efforts from both President Bill Clinton and President Barack Obama. Dr. Lathers has been credentialed as a Senior Biomedical Research Scientist by the FDA for international recognition of her work in the two areas of cardiovascular autonomic dysfunction associated with sudden death in persons with epilepsy and with space flight and for her professional management experience in drug development, the business world, and clinical pharmacology. The primary focus of her international cardiovascular pharmacology research career has centered on autonomic peripheral and central mechanisms involved in the control and regulation of blood pressure, heart rate and rhythm, and electroencephalogram.

Dr. Lathers and Dr. Schraeder have collaborated and published numerous studies and three books focused on epilepsy and sudden unexplained death. Dr. Lathers served the FDA for a total of 11 years, including 4 years as the Senior Advisor for Science to the Director in the Center for Veterinary Medicine and Director of the Office of New Animal Drug Evaluation and 5 years in the Center for Drug Evaluation and Research as a Pharmacology Reviewer. Claire also served the FDA as a Special Government Expert for 2 years. At the FDA, Dr. Lathers worked with multiple risk experts and risk analyses to evaluate the effect of antibiotic use in food animals on efficacy of antibiotics in humans. She wrote papers on risk analyses, risk methods, data outcome, and risk management. This experience provided the foundation for Claire to serve as the lead clinical pharmacologist, working with coeditors and authors, to develop the new method to classify Cluster SUDEP risk factors and mechanisms described in this book. The ultimate goal is to better understand and manage risk, prediction, and prevention of SUDEP. Dr. Lathers and coauthors are currently collaborating with a number of academicians on basic and clinical studies of risk factors for and mechanisms of SUDEP. Previously, she conducted a multi-institutional effort focused on the nexus between human and veterinary medicine and clinical pharmacology, antimicrobial resistance, and food safety. Dr. Lathers has worked more than 14 years as a visiting scientist at National Aeronautics and Space Administration/ Universities Space Research Association, collecting data from subjects in ground-based studies and from astronauts and cosmonauts before, during, and after space flight.

Dr. Lathers earned a BS in pharmacy from Albany College of Pharmacy, Union University, and her PhD in pharmacology from the State University of New York at Buffalo School of Medicine. She completed a National Institute of Health–funded 2-year postdoctoral fellowship at the Medical College of Pennsylvania. Her academic faculty experience includes working at the Medical College of Pennsylvania (15 years), Albany College of Pharmacy (2 years as President, Dean, and tenured Professor), Uniformed Services University of the Health Sciences (3 years part-time), and Gwynedd Mercy College (11 years part-time.). In addition to her academic and government service, Dr. Lathers has worked in the pharmaceutical industry. She served as Chief Scientific Officer of Barr Pharmaceuticals for 3 years and worked part-time with four other pharmaceutical companies during a 15-year period. Dr. Lathers, working with her students and collaborators, has authored or coauthored over 300 publications, including research studies, reviews, book chapters, and abstracts; edited four books; and presented data at over 140 international meetings. She is an Emeritus Fellow, an Honorary Member of the Board of Regents, and a Past President of the American College of Clinical Pharmacology, having served as Regent, Treasurer, President-Elect, and President. Dr. Lathers also served as the Section Editor of the educational series entitled "Innovative Teaching Methods in Clinical Pharmacology" for the *Journal of Clinical Pharmacology* for 17 years. Claire served as a member of the Board of the Annapolis Center, charged with evaluating risk assessments, and worked on the Epidemiology, Toxicology, and Food Safety Workshops and Accords. In recognition of her work, Dr. Lathers has been the recipient of numerous awards and honors.

**Paul L. Schraeder**, MD, FAAN, is Professor Emeritus of neurology at Drexel University College of Medicine; former Chief of Neurology at the Medical College of Pennsylvania Hospital, Philadelphia, Pennsylvania; former Professor of Medicine and Neurology at the Robert Wood Johnson School of Medicine, Camden, New Jersey; and head of the Division of Neurology at Cooper Hospital/University Medical Center, Camden; and former Associate Professor of Neurology at the Medical College of Pennsylvania. He is a member of the Philadelphia Neurological Society and the American Epilepsy Society and a fellow of the American Academy of Neurology. He has served on the Professional Advisory Board of the Epilepsy Foundation of Southeastern Pennsylvania and the Epilepsy Foundation of America and as Medical Advisor to Epilepsy Bereaved, a support organization for surviving friends and family of victims of sudden unexplained death in epileptic persons (SUDEP) in the United Kingdom. Dr. Lathers and Dr. Schraeder coedited the first book addressing the topic of epilepsy and sudden death (Marcel Dekker, 1990). Dr. Lathers and Dr. Schraeder have collaborated for over three decades studying and investigating the mystery of SUDEP and developed the first experimental animal models of this fatal phenomenon. Dr. Schraeder organized a collaborative nationwide survey of how coroners and medical examiners evaluate the deaths of persons with a history of epilepsy. Dr. Schraeder earned the AB degree from

Bucknell University, Lewisburg, Pennsylvania, and MD from Jefferson Medical College, Philadelphia. He completed his residency in neurology and fellowship in electroencephalography and experimental epilepsy at the University of Wisconsin.

**Jan E. Leestma**, MD, MBA, is a pathologist residing in Chicago, Illinois. Dr. Leestma is licensed as a physician in the states of Illinois and Michigan and certified by the American Board of Pathology in both Anatomic Pathology and Neuropathology (1970). He is a graduate of the University of Michigan School of Medicine (1964). Dr. Leestma earned his pathology training at the University of Colorado School of Medicine, Denver, Colorado (1964–1966, anatomic pathology; 1966–1967, neuropathology), and at the Albert Einstein College of Medicine, Bronx, New York (1967–1968, neuropathology). He served in the U.S. Air Force Medical Corps (USAF MC), 1968–1971, and was stationed at the Armed Forces Institute of Pathology in Washington, DC. He was honorably discharged in 1971 with the rank of major, USAF MC. Dr. Leestma was Chief of Neuropathology first as an Assistant Professor and later an Associate Professor (with tenure) in the Department of Pathology and Neurology, Northwestern University School of Medicine (1971–1985). He was an Assistant Medical Examiner and consultant in neuropathology at the Cook County Medical Examiner's Office, 1977–1988. He attended the JL Kellogg Graduate School of Management at Northwestern University and earned a masters of management (MBA) degree in 1986. Dr. Leestma served as Professor of Pathology and Neurology and Associate Dean for the Division of the Biological Sciences and the Pritzker School of Medicine, University of Chicago, 1986–1987. He was Associate Medical Director and Neuropathologist for the Chicago Institute of Neurosurgery and Neuroresearch, Columbus Hospital, Chicago, 1987–2001, and served as interim Neuropathologist at the Children's Memorial Hospital, Northwestern University Medical Center, 2003–2005 (previously he was Chief of Neuropathology at Children's Memorial, 1982–1985). Dr. Leestma has been retired from institutional and hospital practice of medicine since 2005. His areas of expertise and publication history include sudden unexpected death in epilepsy, viral infections of the central nervous system, and forensic neuropathology. He is currently employed by Brainworks, LLC engaging in consultations involving forensic neuropathology. Dr. Leestma is the author of *Forensic Neuropathology* (in three editions: 1988, 2009, and 2014), Taylor & Francis, Boca Raton, FL.

**Braxton B. Wannamaker**, MD, FAAN, serves with pleasure as a coeditor and contributing author to this book. He is currently Clinical Professor of Neurology at the Medical University of South Carolina (MUSC). He was awarded in 1962 a BS degree in chemical engineering from Clemson University and in 1966 an MD from the MUSC. This was followed by an internship, a neurology residency, and a fellowship (neurochemistry) at the University of Wisconsin. Dr. Wannamaker returned to South Carolina in 1973 and joined the faculty at MUSC for 10 years. In 1983, he organized for Dr. Harold E. Booker, the then President of

the American Epilepsy Society, the first symposium for epileptologists on the topic of sudden unexpected death in epilepsy. Collaborators included Drs. Claire M. Lathers, Jan E. Leestma, Paul L. Schraeder, C. F. Terrence, and the late John Annegers. During a 20-year tenure of private practice from 1984 to 2004, he established in 1986 the Roper Hospital Seizure Unit for inpatient monitoring and epilepsy surgery. Dr. Wannamaker also contributed to prior books by Dr. Lathers and Dr. Schraeder, *Epilepsy and Sudden Death* (Marcel Dekker, 1990) and *Sudden Death in Epilepsy: Forensic and Clinical Issues* (CRC Press, Taylor & Francis Group, 2011). In 2004, Dr. Wannamaker began a long-term collaboration with Dr. Anbesaw Selassie at MUSC investigating South Carolina epidemiology of epilepsy including mortality. In his long career devoted to comprehensive care of persons with epilepsy, Dr. Wannamaker has served as a member of the NINDS Epilepsy Advisory Committee, as a board member of the Epilepsy Foundation of America, and as president (1991) of the American Epilepsy Society.

**Richard L. Verrier**, PhD, FACC, is Associate Professor of medicine, Harvard Medical School, Beth Israel Deaconess Medical Center, Boston, Massachusetts, and has investigated autonomic factors in sudden cardiac death for over 25 years in both clinical and experimental studies. He demonstrated that the phenomenon of T-wave alternans (TWA) is strongly correlated with ventricular fibrillation, the arrhythmia responsible for sudden cardiac death, in patients with cardiovascular disease and headed basic science investigations of its mechanisms in the settings of myocardial ischemia and reperfusion and its abrogation with pharmacological therapy. He also participated in clinical studies of TWA in the settings of the exercise stress laboratory and ambulatory electrocardiogram monitoring that demonstrated its capacity to stratify risk for lethal ventricular arrhythmias. He is lead author of a clinical consensus guideline statement on the utility of TWA that is endorsed by several cardiology societies. Recently, in collaboration with Dr. Steven Schachter and colleagues, he found that vagus nerve stimulation reduces the heightened levels of TWA found in patients with epilepsy.

**Steven C. Schachter**, MD, is Professor of Neurology at Harvard Medical School; Chief Academic Officer and Director of Neurotechnology for the Center for Integration of Medicine and Innovative Technology in Boston, Massachusetts; and Senior Neurologist at Beth Israel Deaconess Medical Center, Boston. He is past president of the American Epilepsy Society and Past Chair of the Professional Advisory Board of the Epilepsy Foundation and serves on the Epilepsy Foundation board of directors. He has directed over 70 research projects involving antiepileptic therapies and published over 200 articles and chapters. He compiled the six-volume *Brainstorms* series, which has been distributed to over 150,000 patients and families worldwide, and edited or wrote 23 other books on epilepsy and behavior. Dr. Schachter is the founding editor and editor in chief of *Epilepsy & Behavior* and *Epilepsy & Behavior Case Reports*.

# Contributors

**Karim Alkadhi**
Department of Pharmacological and
    Pharmaceutical Sciences
College of Pharmacy
University of Houston
Houston, Texas

**Karem Alzoubi**
Faculty of Pharmacy
Jordan University of Science and Technology
Irbid, Jordan

**Anne Anderson**
Department of Pediatrics
Baylor College of Medicine
Houston, Texas

**Steven L. Bealer**
Department of Pharmacology and Toxicology
College of Pharmacy
University of Utah
Salt Lake City, Utah

**Amy Brewster**
Department of Pediatrics
Baylor College of Medicine
Houston, Texas

**Esper A. Cavalheiro**
Department of Experimental Neurology
Paulista School of Medicine/Federal University of
    São Paulo
São Paulo, Brazil

**H. Gregg Claycamp**
Risk Analysis and Decision Analysis
FDA Office of New Animal Drug Evaluation,
    Office of Foods, Center for Veterinary
    Medicine
Rockville, Maryland

**Roberta M. Cysneiros**
Graduate Program in Disorders
Center for Development of Biological Sciences and Health
Mackenzie Presbyterian University
Sãn Paulo, Brazil

**Antonio-Carlos G. de Almeida**
Experimental Neuroscience Laboratory and Computational
    Biosystems Engineering Department
Federal University of São João del Rei
Minas Gerais, Brazil

**Jeffrey M. Dodd-O**
Department of Pharmacology
Eastern Pennsylvania Psychiatric Institute
Medical College of Pennsylvania
Philadelphia, Pennsylvania

**Carl L. Faingold**
Departments of Pharmacology and Neurology
Southern Illinois University School of Medicine
Springfield, Illinois

**Jane Hanna**
Epilepsy Bereaved
Wantage, United Kingdom

**John D. Hughes**
National Institutes of Neurological Disorders and Stroke
National Institutes of Health
Bethesda, Maryland

**Joon Kang**
Jefferson Comprehensive Epilepsy Center
Philadelphia, Pennsylvania

**Steven A. Koehler**
Forensic Epidemiologist
Forensic Medical Investigations
and
University of Pittsburgh Graduate School of
    Public Health
Pittsburgh, Pennsylvania

**Srinivasa P. Kommajosyula**
Departments of Pharmacology and Neurology
Southern Illinois University School of Medicine
Springfield, Illinois

**Claire M. Lathers**
Emeritus Fellow Clinical Pharmacology (FCP)
Claire M. Lathers, LLC
Albany, New York

**Jan E. Leestma**
Brainworks, LLC
Chicago, Illinois

**Jason G. Little**
Department of Pharmacology and Toxicology
College of Pharmacy
University of Utah
Salt Lake City, Utah

**Xiaoyan Long**
Departments of Pharmacology and Neurology
Southern Illinois University School of Medicine
Springfield, Illinois

**Angela M. Malek**
Department of Neurosciences
Department of Public Health Sciences
Medical University of South Carolina
Charleston, South Carolina

**Cameron S. Metcalf**
Department of Pharmacology and Toxicology
College of Pharmacy
University of Utah
Salt Lake City, Utah

**Isaac Naggar**
Departments of Physiology & Pharmacology and Neurology
State University of New York Downstate Medical Center
Brooklyn, New York

**Lina Nashef**
Department of Clinical Neuroscience
King's College Hospital
London, United Kingdom

**Maromi Nei**
Clinical Neurophysiology Fellowship Program
Jefferson Comprehensive Epilepsy Center
Philadelphia, Pennsylvania

**Mariana B. Nejm**
Department of Experimental Neurology
Paulista School of Medicine
Federal University of São Paulo
São Paulo, Brazil

**Daniel K. O'Rourke**
Department of Pharmacology
Eastern Pennsylvania Psychiatric Institute
Medical College of Pennsylvania
Philadelphia, Pennsylvania

**Rosemary Panelli**
Research Fellow
Department of Medicine
Royal Melbourne Hospital
University of Melbourne
Victoria, Australia

**Steven Poelzing**
Department of Bioengineering
and
The Cardiovascular Research Training Institute
University of Utah
Salt Lake City, Utah

**Marc Randall**
Departments of Pharmacology and Neurology
Southern Illinois University School of Medicine
Springfield, Illinois

**Philippe Ryvlin**
Department of Functional Neurology and
    Epileptology
Hospices Civils de Lyon
and
Lyon's Neuroscience Research Centre
Lyon, France

**Susumu Sato**
National Institutes of Neurological
    Disorders and Stroke
National Institutes of Health
Bethesda, Maryland

**Steven C. Schachter**
Department of Neurology
Harvard Medical School
Beth Israel Deaconess Medical Center
and
Center for Integration of Medicine and Innovative
    Technology
Boston, Massachusetts

**Paul L. Schraeder**
Department of Neurology
Drexel University Medical School
Philadelphia, Pennsylvania

**Carla A. Scorza**
Department of Experimental Neurology
Paulista School of Medicine
Federal University of São Paulo
São Paulo, Brazil

**Fulvio A. Scorza**
Department of Neurology and Neurosurgery
Undergraduate Program in Neurology/Neuroscience
and
Department of Neuroscience
and
Research Laboratory of Sudden Unexpected Death
    in Epilepsy
Paulista School of Medicine
Federal University of São Paulo
São Paulo, Brazil

**Jeremy D. Slater**
Department of Neurology
and
Texas Comprehensive Epilepsy Program
Mischer Neuroscience Institute
University of Texas Health Science Center at
    Houston
Houston, Texas

**W. Henry Smithson**
Professor of General Practice
School of Medicine
University College Cork
Cork, Ireland

**Amy Z. Stauffer**
Department of Pharmacology
Eastern Pennsylvania Psychiatric Institute
Medical College of Pennsylvania
Philadelphia, Pennsylvania

**Mark Stewart**
Departments of Physiology & Pharmacology and
    Neurology
State University of New York Downstate
    Medical Center
Brooklyn, New York

**Torbjörn Tomson**
Department of Neurology
Karolinska University Hospital
Stockholm, Sweden

**Srinivasan Tupal**
Departments of Pharmacology and Neurology
Southern Illinois University School of
    Medicine
Springfield, Illinois

**Victor V. Uteshev**
Departments of Pharmacology and
    Neurology
Southern Illinois University School of
    Medicine
Springfield, Illinois

**Richard L. Verrier**
Harvard Medical School
and
Beth Israel Deaconess Medical Center
Boston, Massachusetts

**Braxton B. Wannamaker**
Department of Neurosciences
Medical University of South Carolina
Charleston, South Carolina

# Section I

*Forensics of SUDEP and Cluster
Risk Factor Identification*

# 1 Mechanistic Mystery
## Risk Factors in SUDEP

*Claire M. Lathers, Steven C. Schachter, Jan E. Leestma, Steven A. Koehler, H. Gregg Claycamp, Braxton B. Wannamaker, and Paul L. Schraeder*

## CONTENTS

How do we identify those patients with epilepsy who are at greatest risk of sudden unexpected death and prevent them from dying prematurely? How do we unravel the mystery of SUDEP?

Most likely, different mechanisms and/or a different combination of mechanisms are responsible for death in people with epilepsy (Lathers et al. 2011, ch. 1). A global, comprehensive approach is needed to resolve the risk factors for and mechanisms of epilepsy and SUDEP (Lathers 2009). Accordingly, in this book we describe the rationale and details for a new and unique method of research for studying the risk factors and mechanisms underlying SUDEP and introduce our approach in this chapter. Our hope is that discussions and strategies described here and throughout this book will be applied to help unravel the mystery of SUDEP.

## THE MYSTERIES OF SUDEP

Lathers et al. conducted a retrospective examination of SUDEP forensic autopsy cases in the 2001 records of the Allegheny County coroner (Lathers et al. 2011, Epilepsy & Behavior). The findings of that study as well as the following quotes emphasize the problems associated with the mechanistic mystery of SUDEP and further emphasize the need for a new approach to unraveling the mysteries of SUDEP.

> SUDEP is a heterogeneous syndrome with multiple causes and cardiac arrhythmia is thought to be one cause. Further clinical, epidemiological, and genetic studies are needed to delve deeply into its underlying pathophysiologic mechanisms.
>
> **Herreros (2011)**

> Clearly there are different mechanisms of SUDEP involved in different patients. ...Mechanisms of SUDEP are various...

and include central and obstructive apnea and cardiovascular, including cardiac arrhythmias. ... In some victims, SUDEP has been attributed to a mechanism of cardiac arrhythmia. In some cases, the arrhythmias may be triggered by cerebral events." .... "...both respiratory and cardiac changes do occur in people with epilepsy. The timing of events such as seizures, respiratory and/or laryngospasm and cardiac ECG changes does vary in different patients. The physician must consider risk factors for a given individual patient and protective procedures to prescribe to protect the person from future unwanted events that may result in SUDEP.

> **Lathers (2011, ch. 44)**

It is likely that SUDEP is a syndrome with several if not many potential underlying mechanisms. We propose to group the data into specific related clusters, much as has now been done with epilepsy syndromes using factors of incidence, risk factors, supportive animal data and clinical features.

> **Schachter (2012)**

Understanding risk factors for sudden unexpected death in epilepsy (SUDEP) is important for both research-oriented and practical reasons. Current thinking regarding the pathophysiology and prevention of SUDEP remains largely speculative. Defining circumstances surrounding SUDEP and the patient and epilepsy characteristics associated with SUDEP could help direct investigations of pathophysiology. Risk factors can sometimes be modified and could offer an approach to prevention though we must remember that additional prospective studies with active intervention are necessary to demonstrate that modifying risk factors is effective. More practically, a consistent set of risk factors could define a population that may be especially prone to SUDEP. This group can then be targeted for more detailed discussion of SUDEP and for any potential interventions.

> **Walczak (2011, ch. 12)**

To identify the people with epilepsy who are at risk for SUDEP and to use all available preventive medical and lifestyle measures, it will be necessary to glean as much information as possible about SUDEP victims by talking with the medical examiners and coroners, reviewing autopsy reports (Schraeder et al. 2006, 2009, 2011), and obtaining verbal autopsy information from family members and close friends of the victims. The latter technique will help to fill in details missing from the physical autopsy or when no autopsy is performed (Lathers and Schraeder 2009).

## CLUES TO THE CAUSES OF SUDEP: THE NEED FOR ACCURATE DIAGNOSES AND THOROUGH FORENSIC EXAMINATION

From the application of the cluster identification method described elsewhere in this book, and during a literature search of the medical literature, we note that although both cardiac and respiratory effects of seizure are well known and can contribute to SUDEP, there is continued controversy over the etiology of some SUDEP cases. For example, not all cases of supposed SUDEP are in fact epilepsy-related, because those patients may have been misdiagnosed. In a series of 74 patients diagnosed with epilepsy, 31 (41.9%) were found to have cardiac disorders rather than epilepsy (Zaidi et al. 2000). Misdiagnosis of cardiovascular disorders as epilepsy has been reported in long QT syndrome (Stollberger and Finsterer 2004; Rossenbacker et al. 2007; Johnson et al. 2009), catecholaminergic polymorphic ventricular tachycardia (Johnson et al. 2010), idiopathic cardiac asystole (Venkataraman et al. 2001) and syncope (Linzer et al. 1994). An 18-year old female with anti-epileptic therapy and sudden cardiac death suffered from repeated syncopes misdiagnosed as epileptic seizures and emphasizes the need to evaluate whether the brain or the heart is the primary problem, as further discussed in Chapter 14 (Witzenbichler et al. 2003).

Investigating the brain, heart, and lungs in autopsies of people with epilepsy who died suddenly is critically important to the understanding of SUDEP. Microscopic brain findings including neuronal clusters, increased perivascular oligodendroglia, gliosis, cystic gliotic lesions, decreased myelin, cerebellar Bergmann's glosis, and folial atrophy were found to be present in a higher percentage of the brains of SUDEP victims when compared to brains from age- and sex-matched control subjects (Shields et al. 2002; Lathers et al. 2011, ch. 8). Cardiac pathology reports in SUDEP findings at autopsy include mild to moderate cardiac hypertrophy, mild to moderate coronary stenosis, and similar degrees of coronary narrowing but no myocardial hypertrophy (Lathers et al. 2011, ch. 8). In another study, weights of hearts were above the expected weight, after adjusting for body weight and sex. Left ventricle hypertrophy occurred in two cases (Koehler et al. 2011, ch. 9). SUDEP victims have increased lung weights compared to controls (Leestma et al. 1984; Leestma 1990a,b), findings that suggest the possible mechanistic role of seizure-induced or related neurogenic pulmonary edema

in SUDEP, which is further supported by animal models of epilepsy.

Clinical studies that focus on the contribution of cardiac autonomic dysfunction and/or antiepileptic drugs (AEDs), with or without other drugs, to the development of cardiac abnormalities have contributed to understanding the mechanisms of death in people with epilepsy (Lathers and Schraeder 1982) but postmortem correlates are not well characterized. The occurrence of seizures is often associated with changes in myocardial substrate and cardiac conduction and rhythm. Chin et al. (2004) reported myocardial infarction following brief convulsive seizures. They (Chin et al. 2005) later described the occurrence of postictal neurogenic stunned myocardium resulting from seizures. Natelson et al. (1998) described irreversible pathological changes in the form of subendocardial perivascular and interstitial fibrosis in four of seven people with epilepsy who died suddenly and unexpectedly. Such evidence of cardiac changes in SUDEP cases emphasizes the need to educate the coroner's and medical examiners' staffs about the importance of obtaining cardiac and pulmonary autopsy information in people with a history of epilepsy inasmuch as additional autopsy results are needed to clarify the role of cardiac changes in SUDEP victims. Likewise, disturbed function of the autonomic nervous system may contribute to SUDEP but the pathways are unknown (Lathers et al. 2008) as are related postmortem findings.

## IS SUDEP CARDIAC OR RESPIRATORY? THE ANSWER MAY BE BOTH

The ongoing discussion of the differential role of cardiac versus respiratory mechanisms as operant in SUDEP has, to some degree, resulted in an "either/or" discussion (Jay and Leestma 1981; Simon et al. 1982; Nashef 1997; Lathers and Schraeder 2011, ch. 61). The fallacy of such a dichotomous approach is that it diminishes the likelihood of interactive relationships.

*Pulmonarymechanisms.* Epilepsy may disturb respiratory regulation, and apnea may be central nervous system (CNS)-mediated (Johnston et al. 1997; So et al. 2000). Neurogenic pulmonary edema is seen in association with seizures and is a common finding on autopsy of SUDEP victims (Terrence et al. 1981; Leestma et al. 1989; Sedy et al. 2008). Acute pulmonary edema may develop during a clinical seizure. Lung weights are known to be increased in animal studies of seizure (Lathers and Schraeder 1982; Carnel et al. 1985) and in victims of SUDEP (Koehler et al. 2011, ch. 9). Simon et al. (1982) and Johnston et al. (1995, 1997) demonstrated that seizure induction in a sheep model produced acute pulmonary edema and a neurogenically induced increase in pulmonary microvascular pressure with accompanying prolonged change in endothelial conductance to protein. In some animals, the neurogenic pulmonary edema associated with seizures led to CNS-induced apnea. Thus, acute hypoxemia associated with the occurrence of neurogenic pulmonary edema and/or associated central apnea may trigger sudden death. The role of acute hypoxia as a risk factor for SUDEP has been recently reviewed (Lathers et al. 2008; Lathers et al. 2011, ch. 1; Lathers et al. 2011, ch. 4; Mameli and Cario 2011, ch. 37).

*Cardiac mechanisms.* Occurrence of tachyarrhythmias, bradyarrhythmias/asystole, and cardiac conduction changes has been reported in association with seizures (Brugada et al. 2003; Aurlien et al. 2009). Though it is known that the greater the sensitivity to beta-adrenergic agonists, whether from hormones, exercise, or genetics, the greater the level of arrhythmia and mortality (Billman et al. 1997, 2006; Du et al. 2000; Houle et al. 2001; Lujan et al. 2007), and that beta-adrenergic blocking agents can counteract these effects, applications of this work to patients with epilepsy are needed.

Although SUDEP may occur from (1) seizure-related central apnea plus neurogenic pulmonary edema leading to a respiratory death, (2) centrally provoked cardiac arrhythmia, and (3) psychological stress in susceptible individuals (Schraeder and Lathers 2011, ch. 59), a combination of these factors and perhaps others may also be operative. Although epileptic seizures may be associated with arrhythmogenic actions, in some patients, the mechanism of marked central suppression of respiratory activity and/or apnea after seizures is involved and may result in sudden death (Lathers 2011, ch. 44). As the possible mechanisms of SUDEP are multiple and include central and obstructive apnea and cardiovascular abnormalities, including cardiac arrhythmias, caution must be exerted when concluding respiratory changes alone are the primary mechanism of death. At the first onset of the clinical problem, cardiac arrhythmias may be felt by the patient but may not be visually detected by a witness. "Invisible" cardiac arrhythmias may be initiated and then followed by "visible" respiratory distress. Therefore, in addition to repositioning of the patient to ensure ease of respiration and/or stimulation of respiration, it is important, if possible, also to monitor and medically support cardiac rate and rhythm. The answer to the questions, "Which is the cart and which is the horse?" or "Which is the egg and which is the chicken?" will vary from patient to patient depending on the type of initiating clinical event. Furthermore, postictal laryngospasm may be one potential mechanism for SUDEP. Activation of laryngeal mucosa results in apnea mediated through, and elicited via, electrical stimulation of the superior laryngeal nerve. In some SUDEP victims, mechanisms may interrelate via a sequence in which seizures and/or subconvulsant interictal activity trigger cardiac arrhythmias and then subsequent pulmonary complications and failure leading to death. In addition, cardiac–brain interactions are altered by stress via interactions in the central and peripheral autonomic nervous systems, resulting in changes in left ventricular contractile function, ischemia, and/or cardiac arrhythmias including ventricular fibrillation. Myocardial infarction or plaque rupture or coronary thrombosis may occur. Factors triggering emotion-associated seizure activation may include activation of neural networks, sleep deprivation, noncompliance, alcohol use, use of pharmacological drugs that may lower the seizure threshold, and hyperventilation (Lathers and Schraeder 2006, 2011, ch. 17).

## APPROACHES FOR SOLUTIONS TO UNDERSTANDING SUDEP: FROM BEDSIDE TO BENCH

To improve prediction and prevention of SUDEP, both mechanistic studies in animals and interventional studies in humans are required, guided by clinical observations.

*The bedside.* The observation of autonomic dysfunction in association with seizures argues in favor of a role for autonomically mediated acute disturbances in SUDEP (Schraeder and Lathers 2011, ch. 59). For example, Hilz et al. (2002) found cardiac SPECT evidence of decreased norepinephrine uptake in cardiac sympathetic nerves during seizures. Opherk et al. (2002) described increased ictal heart rate, ST-depression, and T-wave inversion in association with seizures. Rugg-Gunn et al. (2004), using prolonged implanted EKG monitoring, observed ictal bradycardia, with 4/19 refractory epileptic patients who required pacemaker implantation. Other instances of ictal bradycardia are well documented (Rocamora et al. 2003). Autonomic changes consequent to cortical stimulation in people with epilepsy have been documented for over half a century. Penfield and Jasper (1954), who undertook systematic stimulation of multiple cortical areas in people undergoing surgery for epilepsy while awake and under local anesthesia, documented a variety of autonomic responses to cortical stimulation. These included salivation with suprasylvian stimulation; gastrointestinal activation with nausea, abdominal discomfort, boborygmi, and a desire to defecate during insula stimulation and apnea with maintained voluntary ability to breathe during anterior and inferior cingulate stimulation. Interestingly, the sensation of breathlessness without impairment of breathing also occurs in some patients as a side effect of vagus nerve stimulation. Irresistible apnea, i.e., inability to overcome apnea with voluntary effort, was reported during rolandic or uncal region stimulation; abdominal sensations, increased heart rate, flushing and pupillary changes were noted during stimulation of the supplementary motor area.

Ictal tachycardia is commonly observed during generalized tonic-clonic seizures (Marshall et al. 1983), and ictal tachycardia and premature ventricular contractions occur in association with complex partial seizures. Nei et al. (2004) reported increased ictal heart rates in people who subsequently became victims of SUDEP and implicated increased autonomic activity with repolarization and rhythm abnormalities, especially during sleep. Ictal related bradyarrhythmias seem to be associated most often with insular, cingulate, pyriform cortex, or amygdale activation. Of interest is the observation of associated episodes of apnea (Penfield and Jasper 1954; Leung et al. 2006). The association of cerebral discharges and disturbances of the normal balance between cardiac autonomic neural discharges has been reported. This is illustrated by the lock step phenomenon (Lathers, Schraeder, and Weiner 1987; Lathers and Schraeder 2011, ch. 28).

The lock step phenomenon provides evidence of a direct relationship between ictal, and even interictal discharges, and disturbance of cardiac sympathetic and parasympathetic neural discharges involved in controlling normal cardiac conduction and rhythm. Although the potential for adverse autonomic effects were alluded to above, few investigations have been conducted since Lathers and Schraeder (1982, 1983, 1990; Lathers et al. 1987), and Mameli et al. (1988) reported in animal experiments that interictal discharges resulted in sinus arrest, supraventricular extrasystoles, bradycardia, junctional rhythms, and associated drop in blood pressure. These investigators also observed a very short latency period that existed between epileptiform discharges and the cardiovascular changes, implying that these were indeed neurogenic, and not neurohumoral, events. The changes persisted beyond the duration of the interictal events.

Seizure-related central apnea can occur concurrently or independently of the acute pulmonary changes (Johnston et al. 1995, 1997). The occurrence of central apnea in these series of experiments supports the reports by Penfield and Jasper (1954) and Bonvallet and Bobo (1972), as discussed earlier. However, determination of whether any seizure-related observations are concomitant occurrences, potential risk factors, or potential mechanisms requires further investigation.

When possible, risk factors and all supporting medical information must be obtained from people with epilepsy who are thought to be at risk for sudden death (Lathers 2011, ch. 25, p. 386). Clinicians have a key role in this strategy by thoroughly gathering information from their patients' medical and neurological/epilepsy histories and family history to aid scientists in developing more focused preventive strategies for particular causes of SUDEP. As described in greater detail elsewhere in this book (Chapters 4 through 17), a number of clinical variables could be included in cluster analyses to identify patients at increased risk of SUDEP, such as type and frequency of seizures, AEDs taken, biomarkers (e.g., EKG, EEG), compliance with AED use as measured by blood level profile, onset age of seizures, history of any EKG conduction abnormalities in patient and family members, family history of unexplained deaths, localized versus generalized EEG epileptic discharges (and if localized, the location and frequency of discharges interictally), nature and location of static brain pathology on MRI, genetic profiling of epilepsy patients and family members for inherited conduction abnormalities or channelopathies, routine neuropsychological testing for stress/anxiety/depression followed by ongoing appropriate therapeutic intervention, testing at-risk patients for non-prescribed/illicit drug and excess alcohol use, possible role of SSRIs, and/or beta blockers in reducing risk. (See the entire list of SUDEP risk factors in Table 5.1 in Chapter 5). A risk factor for SUDEP centers on changes in the role of serotonin in brainstem respiratory centers. One question from the bedside deals with the role of medullary serotonergic abnormalities in sudden infant death syndrome (SIDS), which has implications in SUDEP and serves as a focus for SUDEP research at the bench. As suggested by Paterson (2011): "Given the similarities in the defining characteristics of SIDS and SUDEP and the evidence implicating serotonin dysfunction in seizure genesis and cardiorespiratory failure underlies the pathogenesis of SUDEP. Thus the

brain stem and other studies done for SIDS suggest a possible direction for SUDEP research and may provide novel insight into the pathogenesis of this disease." At the bench level, Faingold et al. (2011 a,b) have a mouse model of respiratory arrest-mediated SUDEP that allows examination of the role of serotonin as a neurotransmitter in brainstem respiratory centers known to control normal respiration and to enhance respiratory rate in response to elevated carbon dioxide levels.

Once a categorical risk factor or factors have been identified in a given patient, an individualized prevention plan specific to the risk cluster could be formulated. However, in view of the lack of "hard" data, we first need more research on intervention strategies based on the cluster data results, which in turn can be informed by animal studies.

*The bench.* Animal models have the potential to shed light on mechanisms of SUDEP. For example, stimulation of the sympathetic ventrolateral cardiac nerve produces a shift in the origin of the pacemaker and tachyarrhythmias because the nerve is not uniformly distributed to the various regions of the heart but rather is localized to the atrioventricular junction and ventricular regions (Randall 1978). Such nonuniform distribution of sympathetic nerves also contributes to initiation of arrhythmia as a nonuniform neural discharge occurs. Although sympathetic innervation and its role in normal and abnormal cardiac function require further investigation (Lathers et al. 1977a, b, 1978), application of this animal model to studies of epileptogenic activity and sudden death has examined the physiology and pharmacology of sympathetic innervation associated with nonuniform autonomic discharge, cardiac arrhythmias, and sudden death (Lathers and Schraeder 1982; Schraeder and Lathers 1983; Lathers et al. 1987, 1988, 1990; Stauffer et al. 1989).

Use of this animal model has allowed questions to be raised such as whether epilepsy alters the function of this neural discharge and if the sympathetic postganglionic neural discharge represents one site of action for pharmacological agents to act by preventing the nonuniform neural discharge (Lathers et al. 1977a, b, 1978; Lathers and Schraeder 1982; Schraeder and Lathers 1983). A postmortem study of postganglionic cardiac sympathetic innervation in patients with chronic temporal lobe epilepsy (Druschky et al. 2001) found sympathetic dysfunction in the form of altered postganglionic cardiac sympathetic innervation, confirming translational work (Lathers et al. 1977a,b, 1978, 1982; Lathers 1980) suggesting that altered postganglionic cardiac sympathetic innervation may increase the risk of cardiac abnormalities and/or SUDEP. Nonetheless, the exact role of innervation in arrhythmogenesis and developmental and regulatory mechanisms determining density and pattern of cardiac sympathetic innervation remain unclear.

Likewise, early ouabain toxicity and coronary occlusion studies (Lathers et al. 1977a,b, 1978) and subsequent SUDEP studies (Lathers and Schraeder 1982; Ieda et al. 2008) provide evidence that dysregulation of cardiac nerves contributes significantly to sudden cardiac death. Innervation density is high in the subepicardium and the central conduction system. In diseased hearts, cardiac innervation density varies, a condition that may lead to sudden cardiac death.

After myocardial infarction, sympathetic denervation is followed by reinnervation within the heart, leading to unbalanced neural activation and lethal arrhythmia (Lathers et al. 1986b, 1988a, 1990).

Molecular mechanisms underlying innervation density are under investigation. Ieda et al. (2008) demonstrated that cardiac sympathetic innervation is determined by the balance of neural chemoattraction and chemorepulsion, both of which occur in the heart. Nerve growth factor, a potent chemoattractant, is synthesized by cardiomyocytes and is induced by endothelin-1 upregulation in the heart. In contrast, Sema3a, a neural chemorepellent that is expressed strongly in the trabecular layer in early stage embryos and at a lower level after birth, causes an epicardial-to-endocardial transmural sympathetic innervation pattern. Cardiac nerve growth factor downregulation is a cause or consequence of diabetic neuropathy, and nerve growth factor supplementation rescues silent myocardial ischemia in diabetic neuropathy. Both Sema3a-deficient and Sema3a-overexpressing mice showed sudden death or lethal arrhythmias due to disruption of innervation patterning (Ieda et al. 2007).

With regard to the autonomic nervous system, stimulus of the amygdala (Bonvallet and Bobo 1972) in animals activates neuronal groupings responsible for cardiac or respiratory control. Within the amygdala, stimulation of one grouping of neurons resulted in bradycardia together with respiratory deactivation, whereas stimulation of a different, nearby group resulted in tachycardia in association with respiratory activation. The complex interconnections between various cortical and subcortical structures, including the amygdala, hypothalamus, and cardiovascular/respiratory control centers in the brainstem would give credence to the possibility of intertwined seizure-related potentially fatal cardiovascular and/or respiratory disruption contributing to the risk of SUDEP (Stollberger and Finsterer 2004).

The clinical correlates of these findings in patients with epilepsy remain to be determined.

## POTENTIAL ROLE OF PSYCHOLOGICAL FACTORS IN SUDEP

Perhaps the least studied risk factor in SUDEP is psychological morbidity. This state of affairs is in marked contrast with the longstanding acknowledgment of the association of psychological factors with sudden death in people with cardiac disease (Lathers and Schraeder 2006, 2011, ch. 17).

The investigational scotoma related to the question of what role adverse psychological circumstances may have in SUDEP is difficult to explain. It is well known that people with epilepsy are more likely to suffer from depression and anxiety than those with other disorders (Mendez et al. 1986), and that these disorders are multifactorial in origin.

## CONCLUSIONS AND NEXT STEPS

Patients with epilepsy and at possible risk of SUDEP can be managed in a number of ways, one of which is the use of

the Cluster Risk Factor Identifiers. Physicians should collect and evaluate data relating to family history of sudden cardiac death, myocardial infarction, exercise-induced cardiac changes, or other factors associated with SUDEP. They should also collect and evaluate indirect evidence channelopathies in the family history. Forensic international SUDEP databases should be reviewed to evaluate known risk factors for SUDEP and to be cognizant of gaps in our knowledge of risk factors. A review of background information on SUDEP is helpful (Schraeder and Lathers 2011, ch. 59; Lathers and Schraeder 2011, ch. 60 and 61). Multicenter autopsy studies are needed with particular attention to detailed microscopic examination of the brain, autonomic nervous system tissue, and the heart and lungs at autopsy to determine the profile of people at risk for SUDEP (Schraeder et al. 2006, 2009, 2011). These studies should be augmented by detailed interviews of witnesses, family members, and health-care providers (Lathers and Schraeder 2009) in the search for environmental, medical, genetic, and psychological risk related data. A potential link between the genetic cardiac channelopathies and risk of SUDEP should be investigated with detailed cardiac history, EKGs, and genetic screening for channelopathy genes in surviving family members. Finally, animal models should address gaps in our knowledge and test whether there is simultaneous occurrence of seizure-related cardiovascular autonomic and respiratory dysfunction.

As further clues to potential causes of SUDEP are identified, possible preventive interventions should be considered including prophylactic use of antiarrhythmic or beta-adrenergic blocking drugs, use of SSRIs to stimulate postictal respiration, methods for improving patient compliance with prescribed AEDs, and stress management protocols for people with epilepsy (Schraeder and Lathers 2011, ch. 59).

Research in the lab, the clinic, and the morgue, and identification of potential preventive measures will all be enhanced by building a large database to identify clusters of SUDEP risk factors (see Chapters 4 through 17), which will eventually be used to ascertain a given patient's type of SUDEP Syndrome Cluster category and risk of SUDEP.

## REFERENCES

Aurlien D, Leren TP, Tauboll E, Gjerstad L. New SCN5A mutation in a SUDEP victim with idiopathic epilepsy. *Seizure* 2009;18(2):158–60.

Billman GE, Castillo LC, Hensley J, Hohl CM, Altschuld RA. Beta2-adrenergic receptor antagonists protect against ventricular fibrillation: In vivo and in vitro evidence for enhanced sensitivity to beta2-adrenergic stimulation in animals susceptible to sudden death. *Circulation.* 1997;96(6):1914–22.

Bonvallet M, Bobo EG. Changes in phrenic activity and heart rate elicited by localized stimulation of amygdala and adjacent structures. *Electroencephalogr Clin Neurophysiol.* 1972;32(1):1–16.

Brugada J, Brugada R, Brugada P. Determinants of sudden cardiac death in individuals with the electrocardiographic pattern of Brugada syndrome and no previous cardiac arrest. *Circulation.* 2003;108(25):3092–6.

Carnel SB, Schraeder PL, Lathers CM. Effect of Phenobarbital pretreatment on cardiac neural discharge and pentylenetetrazol-induced epileptogenic activity in the cat. *Pharmacology* 1985;30(4):225–40.

Chin PS, Branch KR, Becker KJ. Myocardial infarction following brief convulsive seizures. *Neurology* 2004;63:2453–4.

Chin PS, Branch KR, Becker KJ. Postictal neurogenic stunned myocardium. *Neurology* 2005;64(11):1977–8.

Druschky A, Hiltz MJ, Hopp P, Platsch G, Radespiel-Tröger M, Druschky K, Kuwert T, Stefan H, Neundörfer B. Interictal cardiac autonomic dysfunction in temporal lobe epilepsy demonstrated by [ (123) I]meta iodobenzylguanidine-SPECT. *Brain* 2001;124(Pt 12):372–82.

Du XJ, Gao XM, Jennings GL, Dart AM, Woodcock EA. Preserved ventricular contractility in infarcted mouse heart overexpressing beta 2 adrenergic receptors. *Am J Physiol Heart Circ Physiol* 2000;279(5):H2456–63.

Faingold CL, Tupal S, Mhaskar Y, Uteshev VV. DBA mice as models of sudden unexpected death in epilepsy. Chapter 41 In: Lathers CM, Schraeder PL, Bungo MW, Leestma JE, eds. *Sudden Death in Epilepsy: Forensic and Clinical Issues.* Boca Raton, FL: CRC Press/Taylor & Francis; 2011a, pp. 659–78.

Faingold CL, Tupal S, Randall M. Prevention of seizure-induced sudden death in a chronic SUDEP model by semichronic administration of a selective serotonin reuptake inhibitor. *Epilepsy Behav* 2011b;22(2):186–90.

Herreros B. Cardiac channelopathies and sudden death. In: Lathers CM, Schraeder PL, Bungo MW, Leestma JE, eds. *Sudden Death in Epilepsy: Forensic and Clinical Issues.* Boca Raton, FL: CRC Press/Taylor & Francis; 2011, pp. 285–302.

Hilz MJ, Devinsky O, Doyle W, Mauerer A, Dutsch M. Decrease of sympathetic cardiovascular modulation after temporal lobe epilepsy surgery. *Brain* 2002;125(Pt. 5):985–95.

Houle MS, Altschuld RA, Billman GE. Enhanced in vivo and in vitro contractile responses to beta (2)-adrenergic receptor stimulation in dogs susceptible to lethal arrhythmias. *J Appl Physiol* (1985) 2001;91(4):1627–37.

Ieda M, Kanazawa H, Kimura K, Hattori F, Ieda Y, Taniguchi M, Lee JK et al.. Sema3a maintains normal heart rhythm through sympathetic innervation patterning. *Nat Med* 2007;13(5):604–12.

Ieda M, Kimura K, Kanazawa H, Fukuda K. Regulation of cardiac nerves. A new paradigm in the management of sudden cardiac death? *Curr Med Chem* 2008;15:1731–6.

Jay GW, Leestma JE. Sudden death in epilepsy: A comprehensive review of the literature and proposed mechanisms. *Acta Neurol Scand* Suppl 1981;82:S1–66.

Johnson, Hofman N, Haglund CM, Cascino GD, Wilde AAM, Ackerman MJ. Identification of a possible pathogenic link between congenital long QT syndrome and epilepsy. *Neurology* 2009; 72(3): 224–31.

Johnson JN, Tester DJ, Bass NE, Ackerman MJ. Cardiac channel molecular autopsy for sudden unexpected death in epilepsy. *J Child Neurol* 2010;25(7):916–21.

Johnston SC, Horn JK, Valente J, Simon RP. The role of hypoventilation in a sheep model of epileptic sudden death. *Ann Neurol* 1995;37(4):531–7.

Johnston SC, Seidenberg R, Min JK, Jerome EH, Laxer KD. Central apnea and acute cardiac ischemia in a sheep model of epileptic sudden death. *Ann Neurol* 1997;42(4):588–94.

Koehler SA, Schraeder PL, Lathers CM, Wecht CH. One-year post-mortem forensic analysis of deaths in persons with epilepsy. In: Lathers CM, Schraeder PL, Bungo MW, Leestma JE, eds. *Sudden Death in Epilepsy: Forensic and Clinical Issues.* Boca Raton, FL: CRC Press/Taylor & Francis; 2011, pp. 145–59.

Langan Y. Sudden unexpected death in epilepsy (SUDEP): Risk factors and case control studies. *Seizure*. 2000 Apr;9(3):179–83.

Lathers CM. Arrhythmogenic, respiratory, and psychological risk factors for sudden unexpected death and epilepsy: Case histories. Chapter 44 In: Lathers CM, Schraeder PL, Bungo MW, Leestma JE, Eds. *Sudden Death in Epilepsy: Forensic and Clinical Issues.* Boca Raton, FL: CRC Press/Taylor & Francis; 2011, pp. 713–4.

Lathers CM. Effect of timolol on autonomic neural discharge associated with ouabain-induced arrhythmia. *Eur J Pharmacol.* 1980;64(2–3):95–106.

Lathers CM. Sudden death animal models to examine nervous system sites of action for disease and pharmacological intervention. Chapter 25 In: Lathers CM, Schraeder PL, Bungo MW, Leestma JE, eds. *Sudden Death in Epilepsy: Forensic and Clinical Issues.* Boca Raton, FL: CRC Press/Taylor & Francis; 2011, pp. 363–94.

Lathers CM. Sudden death. Personal reflections global call for action. *Epi Behav* 2009;15 (3):269-77.

Lathers CM, Kelliher GJ, Roberts J, Beasley AB. Nonuniform cardiac sympathetic nerve discharge: Mechanism for coronary occlusion and digitalis-induced arrhythmia. *Circulation* 1978;57(6):1058–65. Young Investigator Award, American College of Cardiology, February 24, 1976.

Lathers CM, Kelliher G, Roberts J, Beasley, AB. Role of the adrenergic nervous system in arrhythmia produced by acute coronary artery occlusion. Myocardial Ischemia Symposium, Philadelphia Physiological Society, May 6, 1976. In: A Lefer, G Kelliher, M Rovetto eds. *Pathophysiology and Therapeutics of Myocardial Ischemia.* New York, NY: Spectrum Publications; 1977b, pp. 123–47.

Lathers CM, Koehler SA, Wecht CH, Schraeder PL. Forensic antiepileptic drug levels in autopsy cases of epilepsy. *Epilepsy Behav* 2011;22(4):778–85.

Lathers CM, Roberts J, Kelliher GJ. Correlation of ouabain-induced arrhythmia and nonuniformity in the histamine-evoked discharge of cardiac sympathetic nerves. *J Pharmacol Exp Ther* 1977a;203(2):467–79.

Lathers CM, Schraeder PL. Animal model for sudden unexpected death in persons with epilepsy. Chapter 28 In: Lathers CM, Schraeder PL, Bungo MW, Leestma JE, eds. *Sudden Death in Epilepsy: Forensic and Clinical Issues.* Boca Raton, FL: CRC Press/Taylor & Francis; 2011, pp. 437–64.

Lathers CM, Schraeder PL. Autonomic dysfunction in epilepsy: Characterization of autonomic cardiac neural discharge associated with pentylenetetrazol-induced epileptogenic activity. *Epilepsia* 1982;23(6):633–47.

Lathers CM, Schraeder PL, eds. *Epilepsy and Sudden Death.* New York, NY: Marcel Dekker, 1990.

Lathers CM, Schraeder PL. Epilepsy and SUDEP. Lessons learned: Scientific and clinical experience. Chapter 60 In: Lathers CM, Schraeder PL, Bungo MW, Leestma JE, eds. *Sudden Death in Epilepsy: Forensic and Clinical Issues.* Boca Raton, FL: CRC Press/Taylor & Francis Group; 2011, pp. 953–66.

Lathers CM, Schraeder PL. Stress and SUDEP. Chapter 17 In: Lathers CM, Schraeder PL, Bungo MW, Leestma JE, eds. *Sudden Death in Epilepsy: Forensic and Clinical Issues.* Boca Raton, FL: CRC Press/Taylor & Francis Group; 2011, pp. 253–67.

Lathers CM, Schraeder PL. Stress and sudden death. Epilepsy Behav 2006 9;(2):236–42.

Lathers CM, Schraeder PL. SUDEP: A mystery yet to be solved. Chapter 60 In: Lathers CM, Schraeder PL, Bungo MW, Leestma JE, eds. *Sudden Death in Epilepsy: Forensic and Clinical Issues.* Boca Raton, FL: CRC Press/Taylor & Francis Group; 2011, pp. 953–966.

Lathers CM, Schraeder PL. SUDEP: Mastery yet to be solved. Chapter 61 In: Lathers CM, Schraeder PL, Bungo, MW, Leestma JE, eds. *Sudden Death in Epilepsy: Forensic and Clinical Factors.* Boca Raton, FL: CRC Press/Taylor & Francis Group; 2011, pp. 967–72.

Lathers CM, Schraeder PL. Verbal autopsies and SUDEP. Epilepsy Behav 2009;14:573–6.

Lathers CM, Schraeder PL, Bungo MW. The mystery of sudden death: Mechanisms for risks. *Epilepsy Behav* 2008;12:3–24.

Lathers CM, Schraeder PL, Bungo MW. Neurocardiologic mechanistic risk factors in sudden unexpected death in epilepsy. Chapter 1 In: Lathers CM, Schraeder PL, Bungo MW, Leestma JE, eds. *Sudden Death in Epilepsy: Forensic and Clinical Issues.* Boca Raton, FL: CRC Press/Taylor & Francis Group; 2011, pp. 1–36.

Lathers CM, Schraeder PL, Bungo MW. Unanswered questions: SUDEP studies needed. Chapter 4 In: Lathers CM, Schraeder PL, Bungo, MW, Leestma JE, eds. *Sudden Death in Epilepsy: Forensic and Clinical Issues.* Boca Raton, FL: CRC Press/Taylor & Francis Group; 2011, pp. 67–76.

Lathers CM, Schraeder PL, Bungo MW, Leestma JE, eds. *Sudden Death in Epilepsy.* Boca Raton, FL: CRC Press/Taylor & Francis Group; 2011.

Lathers CM, Schraeder PL, Koehler SA, Wecht CH. Forensic postmortem examination of victims of SUDEP. Chapter 8 In: Lathers CM, Schraeder PL, Bungo, MW, Leestma JE, eds. *Sudden Death in Epilepsy: Forensic and Clinical Issues.* Boca Raton: CRC Press/Taylor & Francis Group; 2011, pp. 131–43.

Lathers CM, Schraeder PL, Weiner FL. Synchronization of cardiac autonomic neural discharge with epileptogenic activity: The lockstep phenomenon. *Electroencephalogr Clin Neurophysiol* 1987;67(3):247–59.

Lathers CM, Spivey WH, Levin RM. The effect of chronic timolol in an animal model for myocardial infarction. *J Clin Pharmacol* 1988;28:736–45.

Lathers CM, Spivey WH, Levin RM, Tumer N. The effect of dilevalol on cardiac autonomic neural discharge, plasma catecholamines, and myocardial beta receptor density associated with coronary occlusion. *J Clin Pharmacol* 1990;30(3):241–53.

Lathers CM, Spivey WH, Suter LE, Lerner JP, Tumer N, Levin RM. The effect of acute and chronic administration of timolol on cardiac sympathetic neural discharge, arrhythmia, and beta adrenergic receptor density associated with coronary occlusion in the cat. *Life Sci* 1986;39(22):2121–41.

Leestma, JE. Natural history of epilepsy. In: Lathers CM, Schraeder PL, eds. *Epilepsy and Sudden Death.* New York, NY: Marcel Dekker; 1990a, pp. 1–26.

Leestma, JE. Sudden unexpected death associated with seizures: A pathological review. In: Lathers CM, Schraeder PL, eds. *Epilepsy and Sudden Death.* New York, NY: Marcel Dekker;1990b, pp. 61–88.

Leestma JE, Kalelkar MB, Teas S, Jay GW, Hughes JR. Sudden unexpected death associated with seizures: Analysis of 66 cases. *Epilepsia* 1984;25:84–8.

Leestma JE, Walczak T, Hughes JR, Kalelkar MB, Teas SS. A prospective study on sudden unexpected death in epilepsy. *Ann Neurol* 1989;26(2):195–203.

Leung H, Kwan P, Elger CE. Finding the missing link between ictal bradyarrhythmia, ictal asystole, and sudden unexpected death in epilepsy. *Epilepsy Behav* 2006;9(1):19–30.

Linzer M, Grubb BP, Ho S, Ramakrishnan L, Bromfield E, Estes NA. Cardiovascular causes of loss of consciousness in patients with presumed epilepsy: A cause of the increased sudden death rate in people with epilepsy? *Am J Med* 1994;96(2):146–54.

Lujan HL, Kramer VJ, DiCarlo SC. Sex influences the susceptibility to reperfusion-induced sustained ventricular tachycardia and beta adrenergic receptor blockade in conscious rats. *Am J Physiol Heart Circ Physiol* 2007; 293(5):H2799–808.

Mameli O, Caria MA. Sudden epileptic death in experimental animal models. Chapter 37 In: Lathers CM, Schraeder PL, Bungo, MW, Leestma JE, eds. *Sudden Death in Epilepsy: Forensic and Clinical Issues.* Boca Raton, FL: CRC Press/ Taylor & Francis Group; 2011, pp. 1–1000.

Mameli P, Mameli O, Tulu E, Padua G, Giraud D, Caria MA, Melisa F. Neurogenic myocardial arrhythmias in experimental focal epilepsy. *Epilepsia.* 1988;29(1):74–82.

Marshall DW, Westmoreland BF, Sharbrough FW. Ictal tachycardia during temporal lobe seizures. *Mayo Clin Proc* 1983;58(7):443–6.

Mendez MF, Cummings JL, Benson DF. Depression in epilepsy. Significance and phenomenology. *Arch Neurol* 1986;43(8):766–70.

Nashef L. Sudden unexplained death in epilepsy: Terminology and definitions. *Epilepsia* 1997;38(11 Suppl):S6–8.

Natelson BH, Suarez RV, Terrence CF, Turizo R. Patients with epilepsy who die suddenly have cardiac disease. *Arch Neurol* 1998;55(6):857–60.

Nei M, Ho RT, Abou-Khalil BW, Drislane FW, Liporace J, Romeo A, Sperling MR. EEG and ECG in sudden unexplained death in epilepsy. *Epilepsia* 2004;45(4):338–45.

Opherk C, Coromilas J, Hirsch LJ. Heart rate and EKG changes in 102 seizures: Analysis of influencing factors. *Epilepsy Res* 2002;52(2):117–27.

Paterson DS. Medullary serotonergic abnormalities in sudden infant death syndrome: Implications in sudden unexplained death in epilepsy. In: Lathers CM, Schraeder PL, Bungo MW, Leestma JE, eds. *Sudden Death in Epilepsy: Forensic and Clinical Issues.* Boca Raton, FL: CRC Press/Taylor & Francis Group; 2011, pp. 77–94.

Penfield W, Jasper H. Summary of clinical analysis and seizure patterns. In: Jasper H, Penfield W, eds. *Epilepsy and the Functional Anatomy of the Human Brain.* Boston, MA: Little, Brown; 1954;pp. 830–1.

Randall WC, Thomas JX, Euler DE, Rozanski GJ. Cardiac dysrhythmias associated with autonomic nervous system imbalance in the conscious dog. In: Schwartz PJ, Brown AM, Malliani A, Zanchetti A, eds. *Perspectives in Cardiovascular Research vol 2, Neural Mechanisms in Cardiac Arrhythmias.* New York, NY: Raven Press; 1978, pp. 123–38.

Rocamora R, Kurthen M, Lickfett L, Von Oertzen J, Elger CE. Cardiac asystole in epilepsy: Clinical and neurophysiologic features. *Epilepsia* 2003;44(2):179–85.

Rossenbacker T, Nuyens D, Van Paesschen W, Heidbuchel H. Epilepsy? Video monitoring of long QT syndrome-related aborted sudden death. *Heart Rhythm* 2007;4(10):1366–7.

Rugg-Gunn FJ, Simister RJ, Squirrell M, Holdright DR, Duncan JS. Cardiac arrhythmias in focal epilepsy: A prospective long-term study. *Lancet* 2004;364(9452):2212–9.

Schraeder PL, Delin K, McClelland RL, So EL. Coroner and medical examiner documentation of SUDEP. *Epilepsy Res* 2006;68:137–43.

Schraeder PL, Delin K, McClelland RL, So EL. A nationwide survey of the extent of autopsy examination in SUDEP, *Am J Forensic Med Path* 2009;30:123–6.

Schraeder PL, Lathers CM. Cardiac neural discharge and epileptogenic activity in the cat: An animal model for unexplained death. *Life Sci* 1983;32:1371–82.

Schraeder PL, Lathers CM. SUDEP: A clinical and communicative conundrum. Chapter 59 In: Lathers CM, Schraeder PL, Bungo, MW, Leestma JE, eds. *Sudden Death in Epilepsy: Forensic and Clinical Issues*. Boca Raton, FL: CRC Press/ Taylor & Francis Group; 2011, pp. 943–52.

Schraeder PL, So EL, Lathers CM. Forensic case identification. Chapter 6 In: Lathers CM, Schraeder PL, Bungo MW, Leestma JE, eds. *Sudden Death in Epilepsy: Forensic and Clinical Issues*. Boca Raton, FL: CRC Press/Taylor & Francis Group; 2011, pp. 95–108.

Schachter SC, personal communication, August 12, 2012.

Sedý J, Zicha J, Kunes J, Jendelová P, Syková E. Mechanisms of neurogenic pulmonary edema development. *Physiol Res* 2008;57(4):499–506.

Shields LB, Hunsaker DM, III, Hunsaker JC, Parker JC Jr. Sudden unexpected death in epilepsy: Neuropathologic findings. *Am J Forensic Med Pathol* 2002;23(4):307–14.

Simon RP, Bayne LL, Tranbaugh RF, Lewis FR. Elevated pulmonary lymph flow and protein content during status epilepticus in sheep. *J Appl Physiol Respir Environ Exerc Physiol* 1982;52(1):91–5.

So EL, Sam MC, Lagerlund TL. Postictal central apnea as a cause of SUDEP: Evidence of near-SUDEP incidence. *Epilepsia* 2000; 41(11):1494–7.

Stauffer AZ, Dodd-O JM, Lathers CM. The relationship of the lockstep phenomenon and precipitous changes in mean arterial blood pressure. *Electroencephalogr Clin Neurophysiol* 1989;72(4):340–5.

Stöllberger C, Finsterer J. Brain or heart—that is the question. Regarding the article "18-year old patient with antiepileptic therapy and sudden cardiac death." *Z Kardiol* 2004;93(4):322–3.

Terrence CE, Rao GR, Perper JA. Neurogenic pulmonary edema in unexpected, unexplained death in epileptic patients. *Neurol* 1981;25:594–5.

Venkataraman V, Wheless JW, Willmore LJ, Motookal H. Idiopathic cardiac asystole presenting as an intractable adult onset partial seizure disorder. *Seizure* 2001;10(5):359–64.

Walczak TS. Risk factors for sudden death in epilepsy. In: Lathers CM, Schraeder PL, Bungo MW, Leestma J, eds. *Sudden Death in Epilepsy: Forensic and Clinical Issues*. Boca Raton, FL: CRC Press/Taylor & Francis; 2011, pp. 187–201.

Witzenbichler B, Schulze-Bahr E, Haverkamp W, Breithardt G, Sticherling C, Behrens S, Shultheiss HP. 18-year old patient with antiepileptic therapy and sudden cardiac death. *Z Kardiol* 2003;92(9):747–53.

Zaidi A, Clough P, Cooper P, Scheepers B, Fitzpatrick AP. Misdiagnosis of epilepsy: Many seizure-like attacks have a cardiovascular cause. *J Am Coll Cardiol* 2000;36:181–4.

# 2 SUDEP
## A Syndrome with Several If Not Many Potential Underlying Mechanisms

*Claire M. Lathers, Steven C. Schachter, Jan E. Leestma, Steven A. Koehler, H. Gregg Claycamp, Braxton B. Wannamaker, and Paul L. Schraeder*

## CONTENTS

We developed a forensic sudden unexpected death in epilepsy (SUDEP) syndrome cluster risk identification method to unravel the SUDEP mystery. The collaborative goal for basic scientists to unravel the mystery of SUDEP should be to develop and conduct animal studies designed to identify mechanisms of SUDEP, autonomic status, and associated risk factors using different animal models; examine the roles of different neurotransmitters; and study possible protective/preventive pharmacological agents such as β-adrenergic blocking agents, serotonin-related drugs, and others. The same pharmacological agents should be examined in two or three different animal models and in different species to gain a broader perspective. Identified risk factors found in our new innovative SUDEP Mechanistic and Risk Factor Classification and ID method by Lathers, Leestma, Schachter, Koehler, Claycamp, Wannamaker, and Schraeder (Chapters 4 and 5) will be used in our new risk factor model to direct the data gathering in animal studies. Additionally, data mining of studies conducted in scientists' laboratories will further build our animal database with cluster IDs. The study of multiple animal models will help to define different SUDEP risk mechanisms and potential combinations thereof across a spectrum of patients with epilepsy.

Classification of seizures and epilepsy syndromes is being currently pursued (Nashef 1997, 2007; Edwards 2001; Engel 2006; Seino 2006; Valentin et al. 2007; Helbig et al. 2008; Tuxhorn and Kotagal 2008; Beghi 2009; Zara and Bianchi 2009; Durá-Travé et al. 2009; Medina 2010; Gomez and Bellas-Lumas 2011; Camfield 2012; Christensen and Sidenius 2012; Noachtar and Remi 2012; Panayiotopoulos 2012; Zhang et al. 2012). Cluster Risk Factor and Mechanism ID method is based on the understanding that SUDEP is a syndrome with many potential underlying mechanisms. We used published human and animal data to develop a SUDEP syndrome-related cluster risk identification classification using SUDEP risk factors and categories. A SUDEP syndrome cluster identifier (cluster ID was defined as a combination of all known risk factors, as well as seizure-related therapeutic, clinical, and environmental circumstances, for a given individual. The person may be alive, with a diagnosis of epilepsy and considered to be a potential victim for SUDEP, or deceased and deemed to be a SUDEP victim. The SUDEP Syndrome Cluster Chart (Tables 5.1 through 5.7) in Chapter 5 includes proposed SUDEP risk factors and subcategories of risk factors and other (therapeutic, clinical, and environmental) factors to form related clusters of SUDEP risk factors; account for the incidence of SUDEP and clinical features, if available; and provide supportive animal data for the suspected underlying mechanism of death. As other possible risk factor categories are determined, they will be added. Results for both human and animal data and patient management using our SUDEP Cluster Risk Factor ID are found in Chapters 6 through 17.

Our research strategy to solve the mechanistic mystery of SUDEP uses two approaches. First, we will utilize this innovative SUDEP cluster method to analyze the mechanisms and risk factor data collected in human and animal studies to fill in data gaps in our method presented in Chapters 4 and 5 and to obtain a larger incidence for statistical analysis. Then, we will use our SUDEP Cluster Risk Factor method to identify patients at risk for SUDEP and pursue strategies designed to prevent its occurrence.

## SUDEP MECHANISMS AND RISK FACTORS

The evolution of our thinking about SUDEP risk factors demonstrates the challenges in this arena. Risk factors first discussed in by Lathers et al. (2008) noted that there are at least four categories of factors that may be operative in the mechanisms for SUDEP: (1) cardiac arrhythmogenicity due to changes in autonomic neural and cardiac function, (2) respiratory impairment and hypoxia, (3) central mechanisms including the direct effects of seizures, and (4) psychological stress. Each of these main risk factor categories in all likelihood includes many subcategories. For example, the cardiac arrhythmogenic category includes pharmacological drug effects, genetically determined ion channelopathies, and acquired heart disease. The psychological risk factors include stress, anxiety, and depression states. This list of primary areas of mechanism for SUDEP was expanded to include eight topics in our 2011 SUDEP book (Lathers et al. 2011), including (1) pathophysiological mechanisms: Brain and cardio/autonomic; (2) respiratory/autonomic factors and hypoxia; (3) syncope; (4) genetic/structural mechanistic factors; (5) risk factors for SUDEP: Number of seizures, behavioral, position, and so on; (6) therapies: Increased or decreased risk; (7) psychological factors; and (8) unusual factors possibly modifying risk.

### Pathophysiological Mechanisms

Pathophysiological mechanisms of SUDEP are not fully identified. In terms of cardiac mechanisms, it is well recognized that the sympathetic component of cardiac innervation is involved in the production of potentially fatal tachyarrhythmias. Postganglionic cardiac sympathetic innervation is altered in association with temporal lobe epilepsy and may be a pathophysiological risk factor for SUDEP (Druschky et al. 2001). These clinical data confirm animal studies that reported epileptiform discharge-related postganglionic cardiac sympathetic abnormalities associated with cardiac conduction disturbances and arrhythmias (Lathers and Schraeder 1982, 1987; Schraeder and Lathers 1983, 1989; Lathers et al. 1984, 1986a,b, 1987, 1988a,b, 1989a,b, 1990, 1993, 2008; Carnel et al. 1985; Lathers and Spivey 1987; Lathers 2011, chs. 25, 44). In addition to the risk of neurogenically induced arrhythmias, neurogenic apnea could be associated with SUDEP. Table 5.1 summarizes the SUDEP risk factors of respiratory/autonomic changes and hypoxia. Rare clinical case reports describe incidences of apnea associated with epileptiform activity (So et al. 2000). In addition, experiments using a well-known sheep model of epilepsy (Simon et al. 1982; Johnston et al.1995, 1997) showed that although neurogenic pulmonary edema was commonly observed, the mechanism of death in the animals was central neurogenic hypoventilation. Likewise, syncope is recognized as a factor in our new SUDEP Cluster Risk Factor ID.

Multiple risk factors likely contribute to SUDEP discussions of risk factors and are found in this book and our 2011 SUDEP book by Lathers et al. and include arrhythmias, lockstep phenomenon (LSP), respiratory factors, syncope, genetics, stress, therapies, unusual factors that may modify SUDEP risk, and others. There is general agreement that central and peripheral autonomic nervous systems and cardiorespiratory interactions may result in arrhythmias and apnea.

Complicating the nervous system–cardiac relationship are relatively recent discoveries of genetically determined predispositions to arrhythmias that may result in seizure-like events at the time of acute cardiac dysfunction. How these genetic cardiac predispositions interact with the central and autonomic nervous systems is not yet understood. It is generally accepted that certain associated clinical features (e.g., male sex, poorly controlled generalized tonic-clonic seizures, use of multiple antiepileptic drugs, changing doses and drugs, withdrawal of antiepileptic drugs, and poor compliance with antiepileptic drug use) are associated with an increased risk of SUDEP.

### Psychological Risk Factors

There has been minimum effort to determine the role of stress as a risk factor for SUDEP. The stress response involves acute or chronic increases in sympathetic neural activity. Scorza and colleagues have identified unusual environmental factors that may modify the risk for SUDEP such as ambient temperature, lunar phases of the moon, and other factors (Table 5.1). The likelihood that a risk factor for SUDEP is related to centrally initiated peripheral autonomic dysfunction in association with epileptiform discharges and stress requires investigation. Issues that need resolution include a better understanding of the individual risks, mechanisms of cardiac arrhythmia and arrest in people without a previously identified structural heart disease, a definition of abnormal interactions between the central nervous system and the heart, the role of neurogenic pulmonary edema and central apnea in combination with cardiac autonomic neural and subtle anatomic and genetic factors as risk for SUDEP, and development of primary and secondary preventive measures along with educational programs to disseminate essential information to physicians, patients, and families. Hanna and Panelli (2011, ch. 57) discuss how to educate people with epilepsy about their risk factors and how to help families and survivors of SUDEP deal with the unexpected deaths. In our 2014 innovative method, the risk factors and subcategories presented in the 2011 book have been greatly expanded.

## SUDEP ANIMAL MODELS

The importance of using many different animal models to study SUDEP to glean insights into the various mechanisms of risks and their contribution to the initiation of the death event is discussed by Lathers (2011). Some emphasize the significance of using audiogenic seizure mice to study postictal respiratory arrest induced by serotonin receptor inhibition and prevented by selective serotonin reuptake inhibitors. The possible role of serotonin in SUDEP must be examined in future animal studies (Faingold et al. 2011, ch. 41). The firing pattern of cardiac parasympathetic neurons, as well as cardiac sympathetic postganglionic nerves, during an epileptic seizure has been shown to change and has been termed the LSP (Lathers et al. 1987; Stauffer et al. 1989, 2011; Dodd-O and Lathers 2011; O'Rourke and Lathers 2011). The observation that autonomic neural discharges were time locked to cortical epileptiform is evidence that epileptogenic activation of cardiac parasympathetic nerves, revealed by ictal bradyarrhythmias or cardiac asystole, may contribute to SUDEP. Likewise, epileptogenic activation of cardiac sympathetic nerves may be another contributing cause of SUDEP. In addition, an imbalance between the two systems, i.e., the cardiac parasympathetic and the cardiac sympathetic neural discharge patterns, may contribute to SUDEP (Lathers and Schraeder 1982, 1987; Schraeder and Lathers 1983, 1989). Wang et al. (2006) provided supporting data for the LSP finding. They examined blockade of inhibitory neurotransmission-evoked seizure-like firing of cardiac parasympathetic neurons in brain stem slices of newborn rats. Specifically, blockade of GABAergic and glycinergic receptors in medulla slices evoked intermittent seizure-like firing of cardiac parasympathetic neurons, suggesting that the seizure-like pattern of firing during an epileptic seizure may cause neurogenic ictal bradyarrhythmias, cardiac asystole, or even SUDEP.

## AUTONOMIC SYMPATHETIC NEURAL CONTRIBUTION TO ARRHYTHMIAS

Nonuniform autonomic cardiac postganglionic neural discharges are associated with coronary occlusion of left anterior descending coronary artery and/or ouabain toxicity in cats (Lathers et al. 1974, 1977, 1978, 1981; Lathers 1980). Nonuniform (increases, decreases, and/or no change) autonomic neural postganglionic cardiac sympathetic discharges traveling through the stellate ganglia may cause cardiac arrhythmias, ventricular fibrillation, and/or sudden cardiac death in the manner described by Han and Moe (1964), i.e., nonuniform recovery of excitability in ventricular muscle. It was suggested that the modification of neural discharge is a way for drugs to modify the occurrence of arrhythmia and death (Lathers et al. 1974, 1977, 1978, 1981; Lathers 1980; Han and Moe 1964). Nonuniform autonomic cardiac postganglionic neural discharge was also found to be associated with pentylenetetrazol-induced interictal epileptogenic activity in cats. Nonuniform autonomic neural discharges leading to autonomic neural imbalance of postganglionic cardiac sympathetic and vagal discharge may lead to fatal cardiac arrhythmias, ventricular fibrillation, asystole, and/or SUDEP. Regional differences in β-adrenoceptor densities reflect differences in postganglionic cardiac sympathetic innervation of the myocardium (Randall 1977, 1984; Randall et al. 1978). These site differences will vary the release of norepinephrine in various sympathetic nerve terminals and sites in the heart to modify cardiac contractile function and may trigger development of fatal arrhythmias and/or sudden death. Innervation density of β-adrenoceptor densities is high in the subepicardium and central conduction system. Nonuniform postganglionic cardiac sympathetic cardiac innervation is related to the nonuniform β-adrenergic receptor locations in heart and affects cardiac contractility and development of fatal arrhythmias and/or death. In diseased hearts, cardiac innervation density varies and may lead to sudden cardiac death (Lathers et al. 1985, 1986a,b, 1988b, 1990, 1993, 2011).

Since tachyarrhythmias are common during epileptic seizures, whereas bradyarrhythmias or asystole occur less frequently, Kerling et al. (2008) evaluated cardiac postganglionic denervation in patients with epilepsy to determine its association with ictal asystole. I(123)-metaiodobenzylguanidine was used as a marker of postganglionic cardiac norepinephrine uptake, using single photon emission computed tomography. They concluded that pronounced reduction in cardiac single photon emission computed tomography uptake in patients with asystole indicates postganglionic cardiac catecholamine disturbance. Impaired sympathetic cardiac innervation limits adjustment and heart rate modulation and may increase the risk of asystole and eventually SUDEP. These data support the aforementioned finding of Lathers and colleagues. Lathers and Levin (2011) examined nonuniform sympathetic innervation and β-adrenergic receptor location and their potential effects on cardiac contractility and the development of fatal cardiac arrhythmias and/or sudden death.

*Cerebral ischemia* is associated with neuron degeneration. Accumulation of excess excitatory amino acids in the synaptic cleft, activation of excitatory amino acid receptors, and influx of calcium into neurons are involved in the development of ischemia-induced neuronal death. Schwartz et al. (1995) hypothesized that neuroprotection may occur if inhibitory transmission via γ-aminobutyric acid (GABA) is enhanced to offset excitation. They studied diazepam, a drug known to increase GABA-induced chloride channel opening, in rats after hippocampal GABA levels had returned to basal levels post transient global ischemia and concluded delayed enhancement of GABAergic neurotransmission directly at the site of vulnerability after an ischemic event protects vulnerable neurons from death. This model could be adapted to an animal model of seizure activity to study the effect of diazepam on GABA-mediated effects that may prevent ischemia-induced neuronal death and ultimately the worsening of central neuronal communication due to epileptogenic activity, thereby contributing a protective central nervous system effect that lessens risk for SUDEP. The potential of neuronal death to predispose to SUDEP requires further investigation.

## POSTMORTEM PULMONARY FINDINGS

Multiple areas of hemorrhages and large areas of gross hemorrhage and edema have been observed in animals dying after inducing epileptogenic activity, asystole, or ventricular fibrillation (Lathers and Schraeder 1982; Schraeder and Lathers 1983; Lathers et al. 1984; Carnel et al.1985). Tissue hypoxia and hypercarbia and alterations in acid–base balance may have contributed to these results (Lathers and

Schraeder 1982, 1987; Schraeder and Lathers 1983, 1989; Carnel et al. 1985; Stauffer et al. 1989, 2011). Changes in cardiac function alter cerebral blood flow, which in turn produces central hypoxia that then results in epileptogenic activity. Some patients exhibit changes in cardiovascular status preceding the onset of convulsions (Schott et al. 1977; Schraeder et al. 1983). So (2008) emphasized that risk factors of postictal apnea and hypoxia, with or without pulmonary congestion in combination with generalized tonic-clonic seizures and to a lesser degree with complex partial seizures, can produce respiratory arrest to cause SUDEP. So et al. (2000) also noted that although epileptic seizures may be associated with arrhythmogenic actions at the heart, in their patient the mechanism of marked central suppression of respiratory activity after seizures was clearly involved and almost resulted in sudden death. Schraeder et al. (1983) also highlighted the occurrence of both respiratory and cardiac changes in people with epilepsy. The timing of events such as seizures, respiratory problems and/or laryngospasm, and cardiac EKG changes may vary in different patients.

Ryvlin et al. (2009) noted that postictal central or obstructive apnea is one likely mechanism of SUDEP. Recently, Ryvlin et al. (2013) reported that SUDEP in epilepsy monitoring units primarily follows an early postictal, centrally mediated, and severe alteration of respiratory and cardiac function induced by generalized tonic-clonic seizures, leading to immediate death or a short period of partly restored cardiorespiratory function followed by terminal apnea and then cardiac arrest. Improved supervision is warranted in epilepsy monitoring units, in particular during nighttime.

Lathers (2011) prompted awareness of potential for ongoing cardiac arrhythmias: "Caution must be exerted when concluding respiratory changes alone are the primary mechanism of death. At the first onset of the clinical problem cardiac arrhythmias may be underway but may not be visually detected by a witness. 'Invisible' cardiac arrhythmias may be initiated and then followed by 'visible' respiratory distress. Therefore, in addition to repositioning of the patient to ensure ease of respiration and/or stimulation of respiration, it is important, if possible, also to simultaneously monitor and medically support cardiac rate and rhythm."

Case histories focused on arrhythmogenic, respiratory, and brain and psychological risk factors are summarized in Chapter 8 and in our preliminary data of 115 SUDEP cases included in Chapters 6 through 11.

Finally, Helmstaedter et al. 2014 noted that the prevalence of neurobehavioral abnormalities such as cognitive and mood disorders, autism spectrum disorder, and attention deficit and hyperactivity disorder is significantly higher among patients with epilepsy than in the general population. A long-held view that comorbidities of epilepsy represent mere epiphenomena of seizures has undergone substantial transformation during the past decade, as emerging clinical evidence and experimental evidence suggest the involvement of specific neurobiological mechanisms in the evolution of neurobehavioral deficits in patients with epilepsy.

## SUMMARY: SOME MECHANISMS/SITES ASSOCIATED WITH SUDEP (LATHERS 2009)

1. Autonomic postganglionic cardiac sympathetic neural discharge was nonuniform just prior to the development of arrhythmias with interictal and ictal activity.
2. Examination of the distribution of cardiac β-adrenergic receptors revealed a correlation with the release of norepinephrine at sympathetic nerve terminals in the heart in a manner that produced arrhythmia. Innervation density is high in the subepicardium and the central conduction system. Nonuniform postganglionic sympathetic cardiac innervation is related to the nonuniform β-adrenergic receptor locations in the heart, and these two areas affect cardiac contractility and development of fatal cardiac arrhythmias. In diseased hearts, cardiac innervation density varies and this may lead to sudden cardiac death. After myocardial infarction, sympathetic denervation is followed by reinnervation within the heart, leading to unbalanced neural activation and lethal arrhythmia (Lathers 1980; Lathers et al. 1986a; Lathers et al. 1988a; Lathers et al. 1990; Lathers and Levin 2011, ch. 33; Spivey and Lathers 1985; Lathers, Spivey et al. 1986b; Lathers and Spivey 1987).
3. Autonomic parasympathetic neural discharge was increased or decreased and often accompanied by a respective decrease or increase in sympathetic neural discharge and epileptogenic activity.
4. Autonomic imbalance between sympathetic and parasympathetic discharges occurred in association with epileptogenic activity. Variability, as indicated by the large standard deviations of the mean, occurred in both divisions of the autonomic nervous system, but the timing differed.
5. Autonomic cardiac arrhythmias may induce ventricular fibrillation or asystole. Both sympathetic and parasympathetic autonomic components via combinations of central and peripheral mechanisms have been demonstrated to occur with epileptogenic activity. In man, asystole at the time of an observed seizure is thought to be mediated via a massive vagal discharge (Van Buren 1958; Hahn 1960; Van Buren and Ajmone-Marsan 1960; Johnson and Davidoff 1964).
6. Dysfunction between the autonomically controlled parameters of heart rate and blood pressure occurred prior to the development of interictal discharges and continued with ictal discharges.
7. LSP was discovered and characterized. Cardiac postganglionic sympathetic and vagus nerve discharges have been correlated with interictal and

ictal discharges. Autonomic cardiac neural discharges were intermittently synchronized 1:1 with the epileptogenic discharge, an observation that was designated the LSP. The occurrence of LSP was not observed in the control period (Lathers and Schraeder 2011, ch. 28).

8. Epileptogenic activity may alter autonomic central or peripheral autonomic release of catecholamines, including those from the adrenal medulla.

9. In the lungs, multiple areas of punctuate hemorrhages and large areas of gross hemorrhage and edema were observed in animals that died after induced epileptogenic activity, asystole, or ventricular fibrillation.

10. Tissue hypoxia and hypercarbia and alterations in acid–base balance may have contributed to the results in this model. Acid–base balance was maintained within physiological range prior to the initiation of epileptogenic activity.

11. Changes in cardiac function were observed to alter cerebral blood flow, which in turn can produce central hypoxia resulting in epileptogenic activity. Some patients exhibit changes in cardiovascular status preceding the onset of convulsions.

12. Modulation of presynaptic aminobutyric acid GABA by prostaglandin E2 may be the basis for epileptogenic activity and dysfunction in autonomic cardiac neural discharge leading to arrhythmias.

13. GABA, the major inhibitory neurotransmitter in the central nervous system, has a prominent role in maintaining control over neuronal excitability. Compounds that inhibit GABA synthesis (3-mercaptopropionic acid and isoniazid) and receptor antagonists that block GABA recognition sites (bicucullinine) or the chloride channel directly (picrotoxin and pentylenetetrazol) have the potential to induce seizures. Mechanisms for interference of GABA neurotransmission may lead to initiation of arrhythmias and/or epileptogenic activity in people with epilepsy. This chain of events may produce sudden death.

14. Cerebral intraventricular D-ala2-methionine enkephalinamide affects cardiovascular parameters in the cat. It is unknown if it plays a role in the origin of arrhythmia and SUDEP.

15. Investigation of autonomic dysfunction in association with epileptogenic activity produced by injecting penicillin into the hippocampus of the cat provided evidence that epileptogenic activity spread to left and right hippocampi and cerebral cortices and was associated with autonomic dysfunction in the parameters of blood pressure and the ECG.

16. β-Adrenergic blocking agents exhibited anticonvulsant activity whether administered via the intraosseous route or intravenously (Jim et al. 1988, 1989).

## RESEARCH STRATEGY FOR OUR NEW SUDEP CLUSTER RISK FACTOR AND MECHANISTIC IDs

The background for the development of the Cluster Risk Factor approach dates from 1973 with numerous studies of arrhythmic digitalis toxicity, sudden cardiac death, and SUDEP in collaboration with Drs. Jay Roberts, Paul L. Schraeder, John B. Charles, Michael W. Bungo, John Sarvey, Raymond J. Lipicky, and many others (Lathers 2009).

To unravel the mystery of SUDEP, Lathers published the following suggestions in 2009:

1. Many different relevant animal models for SUDEP are still needed to understand the pathophysiology of SUDEP, hypothesize about effective treatments, develop small pilot studies in people with epilepsy, and finally conduct confirmatory large-scale clinical trials.

2. Researchers should "think outside of the box" when evaluating an established animal model with potential for modifications to be used to address questions about the mechanisms of SUDEP.

3. The field of pharmacology/clinical pharmacology has much to offer as we work to improve compliance and develop new antiepileptic drugs (AEDs) and/or apply new categories of drugs, such as β-adrenergic blockers and selective serotonin reuptake inhibitors, to prevent and resolve the mystery of SUDEP. Different routes should be considered for AED administration, such as the intraosseous and endotracheal routes, and during emergency situations that may evolve into an unwanted SUDEP if not corrected immediately.

4. Collaboration is needed among different multidisciplinary professionals working in clinical settings and/or within a laboratory, among laboratories within the United States, and in laboratories located around the world to solve the global mystery of SUDEP.

5. Ambulatory simultaneous ECG and EEG telemetry along with respiratory monitoring patients thought to be at risk for sudden death will help to identify the interrelationship of cardiac, respiratory, and brain activity.

6. Academic fellowships and competitions for medical students and postdoctoral fellows/residents and faculty will attract medical and graduate students and faculty to work in the field of SUDEP.

7. Establishing the true incidence of SUDEP by correct use of the term SUDEP on autopsy reports and/or the use of verbal autopsies postmortem should create new and large markets for the pharmaceutical industry. The expectation would be for new antiepileptic and/or other new drugs in different categories to treat SUDEP. The Food and Drug Administration category of orphan drug development should be considered if necessary.

8. Grant funding is essential to move the SUDEP knowledge base forward. Academic administrative

leaders are not interested in faculty and investigators addressing a problem that is not well funded at the national/international level.

9. Leadership foundations of vision, knowledge, and courage are essential to address the global mystery of SUDEP. A leadership philosophy foundation should be used that provides strength primarily for research and teaching programs from faculty members and students and, secondarily, for the administration that must provide the innovative vision and approaches, facilities, and monies to support the needs of faculty and students. The interaction of teaching and research is essential. The components of teaching, including excellent communication and writing skills, coupled with patience, form the foundation for communicating the findings of research to the academic and research communities and to funding agencies. Today's medical and graduate programs will not be able to train each student for each and every advance that will develop in his or her selected profession, including a focus on SUDEP. Therefore, the program must help today's student understand the basic approach to survival in a rapidly changing technological, academic, and political environment. The best prepared student for the challenges of tomorrow will be one trained to be flexible, possessing the basic knowledge and tools and courage to adapt to the different career twists and turns encountered as modern technology rushes to the forefront with numerous new techniques, understandings, and thoughts foreign to us at this time in our lives. Today's medial and graduate leadership must have the vision to provide a fertile and proper environment for teachers to work with academic freedom to teach today's students how to become the self-learning student of tomorrow. While addressing issues of SUDEP, teach our students of today to become self-learners and leaders in the field for tomorrow's solutions.

## CONCLUSIONS

SUDEP issues continue to form the focus of our professional interests. A new risk factor method and related clinical studies to classify risk factors for SUDEP victims were begun. We began with the concept that SUDEP is probably a heterogeneous syndrome with multiple causes and that basic science, clinical, epidemiological, and genetic studies are needed to identify underlying pathophysiologic mechanisms. Clearly, different mechanisms of SUDEP are operative in different patients. Mechanisms of SUDEP include central and peripheral roles for the brain, heart, and respiratory system, with both central and obstructive apnea. The ultimate goal will be to improve individual patient management via better understanding of the relative risk of death in SUDEP and evaluation of new AEDs and other preventives while minimizing

stress in a given patient (Lathers and Schraeder 2006). This new model and method are presented in Chapters 4 and 5, respectively, and their use in the evaluation of 115 cases of epilepsy and SUDEP is found in Chapters 6 through 11.

## REFERENCES

Beghi E. The concept of the epilepsy syndrome: How useful is it in clinical practice? *Epilepsia* 2009;50 (Suppl 5):4–10.

Camfield P. Issues in epilepsy classification for population studies. *Epilepsia* 2012;53 (Suppl 2):10–3.

Carnel SB, Schaeder PL, Lathers CM. Effect of phenobarbital pretreatment on cardiac neural discharge and pentylenetetrazol-induced epileptogenic activity in the cat. *Pharmacology* 1985;30(4):225–40.

Christensen J, Sidenius P. Epidemiology of epilepsy in adults: Implementing the ILAE classification and terminology into population-based epidemiologic studies. *Epilepsia* 2012; (Suppl 2):14–7.

Dodd-O JM, Lathers CM. Characterization of lock step phenomenon. Chapter 29 In: Lathers CM, Schraeder PL, Bungo MW, Leestma JE, eds. *Sudden Death in Epilepsy: Forensic and Clinical Issues.* Boca Raton, FL: CRC Press/Taylor & Francis Group; 2011, pp. 465–80.

Druschky A, Hiltz MJ, Hopp P, Platsch G, Radespiel-Tröger M, Druschky K, Kuwert T, Stefan H, Neundörfer B. Interictal cardiac autonomic dysfunction in temporal lobe epilepsy demonstrated by [ (123) I]meta iodobenzylguanidine-SPECT. *Brain* 2001;124(Pt 12):372–82.

Durá-Travé T, Yoldi-Petri ME, Hualde-Olascoga J, Etoya-Etoya V. Epilepsy and epileptic syndromes during the first year of life. *Neurol* 2009;48(6):281–4.

Edwards JC. Seizure types, epilepsy syndromes, etiology, and diagnosis. *CNS Spectr* 2001;6:750–5.

Engel J, Jr. ILAE classification of epilepsy syndromes. *Epilepsy Res* 2006;70 (Suppl 1):S5–10.

Faingold CL, Tupal S, Mhaskar Y, Uteshev VV. DBA mice as models of sudden unexpected death in epilepsy. Chapter 41 In: Lathers CM, Schraeder PL, Bungo MW, Leestma JE, eds. *Sudden Death in Epilepsy: Forensic and Clinical Issues.* Boca Raton, FL: CRC Press/Taylor & Francis Group; 2011, pp. 659–78.

Gomez-AJ, Bellas-Lumas P. The new International League against Epilepsy (ILAE) classification of epilepsies: A step in the wrong direction? *Rev Neurol* 2011;52:541–7.

Hahn F. Analeptics. *Pharm Rev* 1960;12:447–530.

Han J, Moe GK. Nonuniform recovery of excitability in ventricular muscle. *Circ Res* 1964;14:44–60.

Hanna J, Panelli R. Challenges in overcoming ethical, legal, and communication barriers. Chapter 57 In: Lathers CM, Schraeder PL, Bungo MW, Leestma JE, eds. *Sudden Death in Epilepsy: Forensic and Clinical Issues.* Boca Raton, FL: CRC Press/Taylor & Francis Group; 2011, pp. 915–36.

Helbig I, Scheffer IE, Mulley JC, Berkovic SF. Navigating the channels and beyond: Unraveling the genetics of the epilepsies. *Lancet Neurol* 2008;7(3):231–45.

Helmstaedter C, Aldenkamp AP, Baker GA, Mazarati A, Ryvlin P, Sankar R. Disentangling the relationship between epilepsy and its behavioral comorbidities: The need for prospective studies in new-onset epilepsies. *Epilepsy Behav* 2014;31:43–7.

Jim KF, Lathers CM, Farris VL, Pratt LF, Spivey WH. Suppression of pentylenetetrazol-elicited seizure activity by intraosseous lorazepam in pigs. *Epilepsia* 1989;30(4):480–6.

Jim KF, Lathers CM, Spivey WH, Matthews WD, Kahn C, Dolce K. Suppression of pentylenetetrazol-elicited seizure activity by intraosseous propranolol in pigs. *J Clin Pharmacol* 1988;28(12):1106–11.

Johnson LC, Davidoff RA. Autonomic changes during paroxysmal EEG activity. *Neurophysiol* 1964;17:25–35.

Johnston SC, Horn JK, Valente J, Simon RP. The role of hypoventilation in a sheep model of epileptic sudden death. *Ann Neurol* 1995;37:531–7.

Johnston SC, Siedenberg R, Min JK, Jerome EH, Laxer KD. Central apnea and acute cardiac ischemia in a sheep model of epileptic sudden death. *Ann Neurol* 1997;42:588–94.

Kerling F, Blümcke I, Stefan H. Pitfalls in diagnosing limbic encephalitis—a case report. *Acta Neurol Scand* 2008;118(5):339–42.

Lathers CM. Arrhythmogenic, respiratory and psychological risk factors for sudden unexpected death in epilepsy: Case histories. Chapter 44 In: Lathers CM, Schraeder PL, Bungo MW, Leestma JE, eds. *Sudden Death in Epilepsy: Forensic and Clinical Issues*. Boca Raton, FL: CRC Press/Taylor & Francis Group; 2011a, pp. 713–4.

Lathers CM. Effect of timolol on autonomic neural discharge associated with ouabain-induced arrhythmia. *Eur J Pharmacol* 1980;64(2–3):95–106.

Lathers CM. Sudden death: Animal models to examine nervous system sites of action for disease and pharmacological intervention. Chapter 25 In: Lathers CM, Schraeder PL, Bungo MW, Leestma JE, eds. *Sudden Death in Epilepsy: Forensic and Clinical Issues*. Boca Raton, FL: CRC Press/Taylor & Francis Group; 2011b, pp. 363–94.

Lathers CM. Sudden death. Personal reflections global call for action. *Epi Behav* 2009;15(3):269–77.

Lathers CM, Gerard-Ciminera JL, Baskin SI, Krusz JC, Kelliher GJ, Roberts J. The action of reserpine, 6-hydroxydopamine, and bretylium on digitalis-induced cardiotoxicity. *Europ J Pharmacol* 1981;76:371–9.

Lathers CM, Jim KF, Spivey WH. A comparison of intra osseous and intravenous routes of administration for antiseizure agents. *Epilepsia* 1989a;30(4):472–9.

Lathers CM, Kelliher GJ, Roberts J, Beasley AB. Nonuniform cardiac sympathetic nerve discharge: Mechanism for coronary occlusion and digitalis-induced arrhythmia. *Circulation* 1978;57(6):1058–65.

Lathers CM, Levin RM. Animal model for sudden cardiac death. Sympathetic innervations and myocardial beta-receptor densities. Chapter 33 In: Lathers CM, Schraeder PL, Bungo MW, Leestma JE, eds. *Sudden Death in Epilepsy: Forensic and Clinical Issues*. Boca Raton, FL: CRC Press/Taylor & Francis Group; 2011, pp. 539–49.

Lathers CM, Levin RM, Spivey WH. Regional distribution of myocardial beta receptors in the cat. *Europ J Pharmacol* 1986a;130:111–17.

Lathers CM, Roberts J, Kelliher GJ. Correlation of ouabain-induced arrhythmia and nonuniformity in the histamine-evoked discharge of cardiac sympathetic nerves. *J Pharmacol Exp Ther* 1977;203(2):467–79.

Lathers CM, Roberts J, Kelliher GJ. Relationship between the effect of ouabain on arrhythmia and interspike intervals (ISI) of cardiac accelerator nerves. *Pharmacologist* 1974;16:201.

Lathers CM, Schraeder PL. Animal model for sudden unexpected death in people with epilepsy. Chapter 28 In: Lathers CM, Schraeder PL, Bungo MW, Leestma JE, eds. *Sudden Death in Epilepsy: Forensic and Clinical Issues*. Boca Raton, FL: CRC Press/Taylor & Francis Group; 2011, pp. 437–64.

Lathers CM, Schraeder PL. Autonomic dysfunction in epilepsy: Characterization of autonomic cardiac neural discharge associated with pentylenetetrazol-induced epileptogenic activity. *Epilepsia* 1982;23(6):633–47.

Lathers CM, Schraeder, PL. Review of autonomic dysfunction, cardiac arrhythmias, and epileptogenic activity. *J. Clin Pharmacol* 1987;27:346–56.

Lathers CM, Schraeder PL. Stress and sudden death. *Epilepsy Behav* 2006;9(2):236–42.

Lathers CM, Schraeder PL, Bungo MW. The mystery of sudden death: Mechanisms for risks. *Epilepsy Behav* 2008;12(1):3–24.

Lathers CM, Schraeder PL, Bungo MW, Leestma JE, eds. *Sudden Death in Epilepsy: Forensic and Clinical Issues*. Boca Raton, FL: CRC Press/Taylor & Francis Group, CRC Press. Francis Taylor; 2011.

Lathers CM, Schraeder PL, Carnel SB. Neural mechanisms in cardiac arrhythmias associated with epileptogenic activity: The effect of phenobarbital. *Life Sci* 1984;34(20):1919–36.

Lathers CM, Schraeder PL, Tumer N. The effect of phenobarbital upon autonomic function and epileptogenic activity induced by the hippocampal injection of penicillin in cats. *J Clin Pharmacol* 1993;33(9):837–44.

Lathers CM, Schraeder PL, Weiner FL. Synchronization of cardiac autonomic neural discharge with epileptogenic activity: The lock step phenomenon. *Electroencephalogr Clin Neurophysiol* 1987;67(3):247–59.

Lathers, CM, Spivey WH, Levin RM. The effect of 1, 2, and 8 weeks timolol pretreatment on beta receptor density and cardiac neural discharge associatged with coronary occlusion in cats. *J Clin Pharmacol* 1985;25:466.

Lathers CM, Spivey WH. The effect of timolol, metoprolol, and practolol on postganglionic cardiac neural discharge associated with acute coronary occlusion-induced arrhythmia. *J. Clin Pharmacol* 1987;27:582–92.

Lathers CM, Spivey WH, Levin RM. The effect of beta blockers on cardiac neural discharge associated with coronary occlusion in the cat. *J Clin Pharmacol* 1988a;28(8):736–45.

Lathers CM, Spivey WH, Levin RM, Tumer N. The effect of dilevalol on cardiac autonomic neural discharge, plasma catecholamines, and myocardial beta receptor density associated with coronary occlusion. *J Clin Pharmacol* 1990;30(3):241–53.

Lathers CM, Spivey WH, Suter LE, Lerner JP, Tumer N, Levin RM. The effect of acute and chronic administration of timolol on cardiac sympathetic neural discharge, arrhythmia, and beta receptor density associated with coronary occlusion in the cat. *Life Sci* 1986b;39:2121–41.

Lathers CM, Spivey WH, Tumer N. The effect of timolol given five minutes post coronary occlusion on plasma catecholamines. *J. Clin Pharmacol* 1988b;28(4):289–99.

Lathers CM, Stauffer AZ, Tumer N, Kraras CM, Goldman BD. Anticonvulsant and antiarrthymic actions of the beta blocking agent timolol. *Epilepsy Res* 1989b;4(1):42–54.

Medina-MC. Epilepsy: Classification for a diagnostic approach based on etiology and complexities. Santafe de Bogota, Colombia. *Rev Neurol* 2010;50 (Suppl 3):S25–30.

Nashef L. Sudden unexplained death in epilepsy: Terminology and definitions. *Epilepsia* 1997;38:S6–8.

Nashef L. Idiopathic generalized epilepsy with absences: Syndrome classification. *Epilepsia* 2007;48:2187–90.

Noachtar S, Remi J. Classification of epileptic seizures and syndromes. *Nervevarzt* 2012;83:156–61.

O'Rourke D, Lathers CM. Interspike interval histogram characterization of synchronized cardiac sympathetic neural discharge and epileptogenic activity in electrocorticogram of cat. Chapter 31 In: Lathers CM, Schraeder PL, Bungo MW, Leestma JE, eds. *Sudden Death in Epilepsy: Forensic and Clinical Issues*. Boca Raton, FL: CRC Press/Taylor & Francis Group; 2011, pp. 495–512.

Panayiotopoulos CP. The new ILAE on terminology and concepts for the organizations of epilepsies: Critical review and contribution. *Epilepsia* 2012;5:399–404.

Randall WC. Neural regulation of the heart. New York, NY: Oxford University Press; 1977.

Randall WC. *Nervous Control of Cardiovascular Function*. New York, NY: Oxford University Press; 1984.

Randall WC, Thomas JX, Euler DE, Rozanski GJ. Cardiac dysrhythmias associated with autonomic nervous system imbalance in the conscious dog. In: Schwartz PJ, Brown AM, Malliani A, Zanchetti A, eds. *Perspectives in Cardiovascular Research, vol 2, Neural Mechanisms in Cardiac Arrhythmias*. New York, NY: Raven Press; 1978, pp. 123–38.

Ryvlin P, Nashef L, Lhatoo SD, Bateman LM, Bird J, Bleasel A, Boon P et al. Incidence and mechanisms of cardiorespiratory arrests in epilepsy monitoring units (MORTEMUS): A retrospective study. *Lancet Neurol* 2013;12(10):966–77.

Ryvlin P, Tomson T, Montavont A. Excess mortality and sudden unexpected death in epilepsy. *Presse Med* 2009;38(6):905–10.

Schott GD, McLeod AA, Jewitt DE. Cardiac arrhythmias that masquerade as epilepsy. *Br Med J* 1977;1(6074):1454–7.

Schraeder PL, Lathers CM. Cardiac neural discharge and epileptogenic activity in the cat: An animal model for unexplained death. *Life Sci* 1983;32(12):1371–82.

Schraeder PL, Lathers CM. Paroxysmal autonomic dysfunction, epileptogenic activity and sudden death. *Epilepsy Res* 1989;3(1):55–62.

Schraeder PL, Pontzer R, Engel TR. A case of being scared to death. *Arch Intern Med* 1983;143:1793–4.

Schwartz PJ, Priori SG, Locati EH, Napolitano C, Cantù F, Towbin JA, Keating MT, Hammoude H, Brown AM, Chen LS. Long QT syndrome patients with mutations of the SCN5A and HERG genes have differential responses to Na⁺ channel blockade and to increases in heart rate. Implications for gene-specific therapy. *Circulation* 1995;92(12):3381–6.

Seino M. Classification criteria of epileptic seizures and syndromes. *Epilepsy Res* 2006;70 (Suppl 1):S27–33.

Simon RP, Bayne LL, Tranbaugh RF, Lewis FR. Elevated pulmonary lymph flow and protein content during status epilepticus in sheep. *J Appl Physiol Respir Environ Exerc Physiol* 1982;52(1):91–5.

So EL. What is known about the mechanisms underlying SUDEP? *Epilepsia* 2008;49 (Suppl 9):93–8.

So EL, Sam MC, Lagerlund TL. Postictal central apnea as a cause of SUDEP: Evidence from near-SUDEP incident. *Epilepsia* 2000;41(11):1494–7.

Spivey WH, Lathers CM. Effect of timolol on the sympathetic nervous system in coronary occlusion in cats. *Ann Emerg Med* 1985;14(10):939–44.

Stauffer AZ, Dodd-O JM, Lathers CM. The relationship of the lock step phenomenon and precipitous changes in mean arterial blood pressure. *Electroencephalogr Clin Neurophysiol* 1989;72(4):340–5.

Stauffer AZ, Dodd-O JM, Lathers CM. Relationship of lock step phenomenon and precipitous changes in blood pressure. Chapter 30 In: Lathers CM, Schraeder PL, Bungo MW, Leestma JE, eds. *Sudden Death in Epilepsy: Forensic and Clinical Issues*. Boca Raton, FL: CRC Press/Taylor & Francis Group; 2011, pp. 481–94.

Tuxhorn I, Kotagal P. Classification. *Seminar Neurol* 2008;28:277–88.

Valentin A, Hindocha N, Osei-Lah A, Fisniku L, McCormick D, Asherson P, Moran N, Makoff A, Nashef L. Idiopathic generalized epilepsy with absences: Syndrome classification. *Epilepsia* 2007;48:2187–90.

Van Buren JM. Some autonomic concomitants of ictal automatism. *Brain* 1958;81:505–28.

Van Buren JM, Ajmone-Marsan C. A correlation of autonomic EEG components in temporal lobe epilepsy. *Arch Neurol* 1960;3:683–703.

Wang J, Chen Y, Li K, Hou L. Blockade of inhibitory neurotransmission evoked seizure-like firing of cardiac parasympathetic neurons in brainstem slices of newborn rats: Implications for sudden deaths in patients of epilepsy. *Epilepsy Res* 2006;70:172–83.

Zara F, Bianchi A. Impact of genetics on the classification of epilepsy syndromes. *Epilepsia* 2009;50:(Suppl 5):11–4.

Zhang GQ, Sahoo SS, Lhatoo SD. From classification to epilepsy ontology and informatics. *Epilepsia* 2012;(Suppl 2):28–32.

# 3 Unraveling the Global Mystery of SUDEP

*Claire M. Lathers, Steven C. Schachter, Jan E. Leestma, Steven A. Koehler, H. Gregg Claycamp, Braxton B. Wannamaker, and Paul L. Schraeder*

## CONTENTS

## AUTONOMIC AND OTHER RISK FACTORS FOR SUDEP

We will apply a new method of research for studying the risk factors and mechanism(s) underlying SUDEP by identifying risk factors to characterize a given individual's health status and, thereby, risk of SUDEP. Individual risk IDs will define central and peripheral changes relevant to SUDEP. Related clusters will identify the degree of risk for individuals and risk cluster IDs will allow better medical management of patients with epilepsy. Our innovative risk factor method of classification and identification will be applied to SUDEP issues to assess, predict, prevent, or minimize the risks for its occurrence and to develop new pharmacological therapies and other preventive strategies. SUDEP is a syndrome with several potential underlying mechanisms. Available human and animal data were reviewed to develop a SUDEP Syndrome Related Cluster Risk Identification Classification using SUDEP Risk Factors and Categories. SUDEP Syndrome Cluster identifier (Cluster ID) was defined as a combination of all known risk factors for a given person (Lathers 2009; Koehler et al. 2011, ch. 9; Lathers et al. 2011, ch. 1; Lathers et al. 2011). A mechanistic model (Chapter 4) was developed comprising pharmacological, physiological, genetic, environmental, location of death, age at death, and other variables in Chapter 5 to address the goal of improving individual patient management via better understanding of SUDEP risk factors. Individual Risk IDs define risk factors, including central and peripheral autonomic nervous system changes, for SUDEP. Related or similar clusters will identify the types of risk factors for people with similar risk Cluster IDs. Related clusters will identify the degree of risk for patients, and risk cluster IDs will allow better medical management.

Control data for parameters monitored in living individuals for statistical analysis of the Cluster IDs will be extracted in a retrospective study of NASA databases, which will be mined for parameters of astronaut controls, during space flight, parabolic flight, and/or bed rest. Control data will be used to build Cluster Risk Factors for 115 SUDEP or epilepsy cases and for 100 astronauts/subjects. Larger enrollments will provide stronger risk cluster identifications and more robust statistical analyses. Data mining of de-identified archived space, parabolic flight, and bed rest data for astronauts or subjects in data bases at NASA or NASA's Life Sciences Data Archive (LSDA), working with the life science archived holdings (LSAH) Life Science Ad Hoc Advisory Board approval, will be performed to establish "Parameters" of EEG (normal or aberrant), measurements of intracranial and intraocular pressure, optic nerve and visual status, blood pressure, cardiac rate and rhythm including arrhythmias, and pulmonary function. Other variables of interest are age; gender; race; ethnicity; smoking status; legal or nonlegal drug use (if known); diseases of brain, heart, or lung; syncope status; genetic structural channelopathies if known; diagnosed diseases; psychological status, environmental circumstances, including posture and sleep wake cycle, collected during human studies in epilepsy, sleep, clinical pharmacology or bed rest units. Data mining may also be performed using retrospective analyses in healthy humans, patients with epilepsy, and/or victims of SUDEP. Prospective human studies will be conducted by our international and national Co-PIs to collect data for human risk factors to be used to fill gaps in our databases to complete the SUDEP Cluster Risk Factor IDs.

## PRIMARY APPROACHES OF STUDIES

1. Use retrospective data mining methods to identify risk parameters to classify a de-identified person with epilepsy. The determination will be based on central and peripheral neurological assessments, electroencephalography, and cardiovascular and pulmonary measurements obtained in supine and seated positions. All risk factors, including

autonomic risk factors, will be used to compare and evaluate risk of a given patient as a candidate for SUDEP.

   a. Status epilepticus produces chronic alterations in cardiac sympathovagal balance which may increase cardiac risk and mortality (Metcalf et al. 2009; Goldstein 2013).

   b. Identification of specific autonomic triggers in different arrhythmias suggests one may medically modulate autonomic activities for both prevention and treatment of these arrhythmias (Shen and Zipes 2014).

   c. Not all patients responded identically to changes in autonomic function induced by epileptic seizures nor was the change in a given individual always the same (Eggleston et al. 2014).

   d. Persons with well-controlled versus intractable epilepsy may present different autonomic responses (Mukherjee et al. 2009).

   e. We will use the technique of Poh et al. (2012) to evaluate persons with well-controlled versus intractable epilepsy to compare SUDEP Risk Factor Cluster IDs for both groups to determine if the two groups do present with different autonomic responses.

   f. We will compare the effect of yoga in persons with well-controlled versus intractable epilepsy to determine if they present different autonomic responses as evidenced by SUDEP Risk Factor Cluster IDs (Streeter et al. 2012).

2. Use prospective human studies to measure and collect data parameters to fill in risk factor gaps in our Cluster Risk Factor Method to classify a de-identified person with epilepsy.

3. Identify all known risk factors for each de-identified person.

4. Construct individual Cluster ID of risk factors for a given de-identified person.

5. Group parameters in related groups and/or multiple subgroup clusters.

6. Use related clusters of risk factors to identify the risk of SUDEP in newly diagnosed patients with epilepsy or to determine their risk of side effects, including autonomic side effects, whether physiological, such as syncopal, orthostatic hypotension, asystolic, or pharmacological, with antiepileptic drugs (AEDs), or environmental and/or other such as death site. See Table 5.1 in Chapter 5.

7. Develop databases for experimental animal models, cases of epilepsy, and SUDEP cases with risk factor classification and Individual Cluster IDs.

8. Additional variables may be chosen as scientific concepts evolve. Examples: risk factors for SUDEP include death due to respiratory changes and our cluster risk method will separate risks from cardiac versus respiratory, brain versus cardiac, etc. Intracranial pressure will be added as a risk factor.

It is hypothesized that Cluster Risk Factor Identification for individuals will lead to testable interventions designed to protect patients with epilepsy from SUDEP and to decrease unwanted side effects, including autonomic changes, during seizures. The potential to identify patients with heightened risk for SUDEP and to improve medical management are paramount.

## AUTONOMIC NERVOUS SYSTEM, AUTONOMIC TONE, SEIZURES, ARRHYTHMIAS, AND SUDEP

The designation "autonomic nervous system" suggests a single entity but in reality it has functional and neurochemical components that respond differentially to stressors and pathophysiologic events (Goldstein 2013). Seizures, a stressor, may change the autonomic nervous system. The laboratory of Bealer (Metcalf et al. 2009) reported status epilepticus activates the autonomic nervous system with a chronic shift in sympathovagal balance favoring sympathetic dominance due to decreased parasympathetic activity and decreased baroreflex sensitivity, assumed to be due to decreased vagal activation. The autonomic nervous system modifies cardiac electrophysiology and arrhythmogenesis, and "identification of specific autonomic triggers in different arrhythmias may be a site to modulate prevention and treatment" (Shen and Zipes 2014). Seizures and the associated ictal tachycardia and actual heart rate exhibited variability in magnitude (Eggleston et al. 2014). "Not all patients responded identically nor was the change in a given individual always reproduced again." Mukherjee et al. (2009) discussed the autonomic imbalance of sympathetic and parasympathetic activity thought to contribute to SUDEP and suggested that "persons with well-controlled versus intractable epilepsy may present different autonomic responses." Additional evidence supporting the suggestion that autonomic imbalance of sympathetic and parasympathetic activity may contribute to SUDEP was provided by Poh et al. (2012). They studied autonomic dysfunction, seizures, and postictal EEG suppression and refractory epilepsy. Findings demonstrated the size of sympathetic activation and parasympathetic suppression increased with duration of EEG suppression after tonic-clonic seizures. Resistant cases of epilepsy and depression treatment include vagal nerve stimulation to reverse parasympathetic suppression. Streeter et al. (2012) theorize that yoga may correct disorders exacerbated by stress, including imbalance of the autonomic nervous system, and perhaps decreased activity of the inhibitory gamma aminobutyric acid neurotransmitter. Full discussion of these topics is in Chapter 12, Risk Predictor: Individual SUDEP Risk Factor Cluster IDs.

## SUDEP: ADDRESSING THE GAPS

NASA databases will be mined for de-identified astronaut and test subject healthy control data values and values obtained during space flight, parabolic flight, and/or bed rest. Control values will then be used in a SUDEP risk cluster identification methodology to characterize the risk for SUDEP. No such control data exist for patients with epilepsy. Data will also be used to compare and evaluate risk factors for a given patient as a candidate for SUDEP. A given individual will be scored using risk factors A–W and all subcategories in Table 5.1. Use of the Forensic SUDEP Syndrome Clusters carries the promise of better medical management of patients with epilepsy and identifying degrees of risk. The risk cluster guide is designed to allow physicians to determine how each patient with epilepsy is categorized using the SUDEP Syndrome Cluster ID and to ascertain this patient's risk of SUDEP using the risk/incidence data in the related cluster ID's to improve selection of medical treatment and patient management. This approach constitutes a new physiological and pharmacological perspective. This innovative method develops a new risk factor classification system. Physicians and neurologists can use this system of risk factor classification to identify patients at high or highest risk of SUDEP. The system can also educate professionals in medical examiners' and coroners' offices, as well as forensic pathologists. This methodology will also allow patients with epilepsy to be graded at low, medium, or high risk of sudden death.

The incidence of SUDEP requires more accurate monitoring. The diagnosis of SUDEP is underutilized in the United States and the term is not standard on death certificates. Worldwide, SUDEP has been found to be more prevalent than assumed (Schraeder et al. 2006, 2009, 2011). Our method of SUDEP risk factors will address this deficiency since it will report incidence rate of SUDEP. Related clusters will identify the degree of risk on an individual patient basis and risk cluster IDs will allow better medical management before, during, after seizures. Risk IDs define central/peripheral autonomic status and all risk factors A–W as they relate to the risk of SUDEP.

## CONCLUSION

Our research goals are to develop a method of SUDEP Risk Factor Classification and Cluster Identifications (IDs). We will build a Forensic International Database of human and experimental animal model risk factor data containing our new unique SUDEP Risk Factor Classification and Cluster Identifications (IDs). We will develop and test new AEDs and/or combinations of AEDs and medical regimens based on risk IDs. Cluster membership identifies degree of risk for future newly diagnosed patients with epilepsy. Risk cluster IDs will provide better information for medical management before, during, after seizure activity, or interictal discharges, allow future individual evaluations to find their unique Risk Factor Cluster Identifier for epilepsy and identify the best medical treatments for a given individual to provide a low risk of potential side effects problems, including a, smallest risk of SUDEP and a higher performance on AEDs and the best AED for prevention. The overarching goal for our animal experimental studies is to identify mechanisms of

SUDEP, autonomic status and all associated risk factors using different animal models, examine the role of different neurotransmitters, and study possible protective/preventive pharmacological agents such as beta blockers, serotonin-related drugs, cholinergic drugs, and others (details are found in Lathers 2011, ch. 25 and Chapter 18 of this book). If possible, we will examine the same pharmacological agents in two or three different animal models and different species to gain a broader perspective. The study of multiple animal models will help identify the different SUDEP risk mechanisms and possible combinations thereof in humans, such as those in the study of Leestma et al. 1984. These data will be used to interpret the SUDEP Risk Factors for humans, such as those in the study of Leestma et al. 1984, to be utilized in our new SUDEP Cluster Risk Factor Method for people with epilepsy.

## REFERENCES

Eggleston KS, Olin BD, Fisher RS. Ictal tachycardia: The head-heart connection. *Seizure* 2014; p. ii: S1059–1311.

Goldstein DS. Differential responses of components of the autonomic nervous system. *Handb Clin Neurol* 2013;117:13–22.

Koehler SA, Schraeder PL, Lathers CM, Wecht CH. One-year postmortem forensic analysis of deaths in persons with epilepsy. Chapter 9 In: Lathers CM, Schraeder PL, Bungo MW, Leestma JE, eds. *Sudden Death in Epilepsy: Forensic and Clinical Issues.* Boca Raton, FL: CRC Press/Taylor & Francis Group; 2011, p. 145–59.

Lathers CM. Sudden death. Personal reflections global call for action. *Epi Behav* 2009;15(3):269–77.

Lathers CM. Sudden death animal models to examine nervous system sites of action for disease and pharmacological intervention. Chapter 25 In: Lathers CM, Schraeder PL, Bungo MW, Leestma JE, eds. *Sudden Death in Epilepsy: Forensic and Clinical Issues.* Boca Raton, FL: CRC Press/Taylor & Francis Group; 2011, p. 363–94.

Lathers CM, Koehler SA, Wecht CH, Schraeder PL. Forensic antiepileptic drug levels in autopsy cases of epilepsy. *Epi Behav* 2011; 22(4);778–85.

Lathers CM, Schraeder PL, Bungo MW. Neurocardiologic mechanistic risk factors in sudden unexpected death in epilepsy. Chapter 1 In: Lathers CM, Schraeder PL, Bungo MW, Leestma JE, eds. *Sudden Death in Epilepsy: Forensic and Clinical Issues.* Boca Raton, FL: CRC Press/Taylor & Francis Group; 2011, p. 1–36.

Leestma JE, Kalelkar MB, Teas S, Jay GW, Hughes JR. Sudden unexpected death associated with seizures: Analysis of 66 cases. *Epilepsia* 1984;25:84–8.

Metcalf CS, Radwanski PB, Bealer SL. Status epilepticus produces chronic alterations in cardiac sympathovagal balance. *Epilepsia* 2009;50(4):747–54.

Mukherjee S1, Tripathi M, Chandra PS, Yadav R, Choudhary N, Sagar R, Bhore R, Pandey RM, Deepak KK. Cardiovascular autonomic functions in well-controlled and intractable partial epilepsies. *Epilepsy Res* 2009;85(2–3):261–9.

Poh MZ, Loddenkemper T, Reinsberger C, Swenson NC, Goyal S, Madsen JR, Picard RW. Autonomic changes with seizures correlate with postictal EEG suppression. *Neurology* 2012 5;78(23):1868–76.

Schraeder PL, Delin K, McClelland RL, So EL. Coroner and medical examiner documentation of SUDEP. *Epilepsy Res* 2006 68:137–43.

Schraeder PL, Delin K, McClelland RL, So EL. A nationwide survey of the extent of autopsy examination in SUDEP. *Am J Forensic Med Path* 2009;30:123–6.

Schraeder PL, So EL, Lathers CM. Forensic case identification In: Lathers CM, Schraeder PL, Bungo MW, Leestma JE, eds. *Sudden Death in Epilepsy: Forensic and Clinical Issues*. Boca Raton, FL: CRC Press/Taylor & Francis Group; 2011, p. 95–108.

Shen MJ1, Zipes DP. Role of the autonomic nervous system in modulating cardiac arrhythmias. *Circ Res* 2014;114(6):1004–21.

Streeter CC1, Gerbarg PL, Saper RB, Ciraulo DA, Brown RP. Effects of yoga on the autonomic nervous system, gamma-aminobutyric-acid, and allostasis in epilepsy, depression, and post-traumatic stress disorder. *Med Hypotheses* 2012;78(5):571–9.

# 4 Decision Analysis and Classification Methods for SUDEP Risk Factor Identification

*H. Gregg Claycamp, Claire M. Lathers, Paul L. Schraeder, and Braxton B. Wannamaker*

## CONTENTS

A common conclusion from published research on risk factor identification and predictive modeling for sudden unexpected death in epilepsy (SUDEP) is that complex multifactorial interactions limit the predictive value of predictive modeling from population studies and clinical series. In addition, the sample size of confirmed, "true" SUDEP cases in studies is typically small. Most epidemiologic studies have relied on parametric methods to identify risk factors and to estimate the relative risks (RRs), hazard ratios (HRs), or standardized mortality ratios (SMRs) for factors taken one at a time (Lhatoo et al. 2001). Finally, lacking a "gold standard" diagnosis for either epilepsy or SUDEP, some of the key risk factors for epilepsy rely on linguistic categorical variables, such as "confirmed," "probable," "likely," or "possible" (Nilsson et al. 1999; Lhatoo et al. 2001).

The combination of numerous factors with interactions and small numbers of observations creates two significant challenges for SUDEP research. First, small numbers of observations ($n$) in the face of relatively large numbers of parameters ($p$) or risk factors might exceed the practical limits of parametric modeling techniques (National Research Council 2001). Second, the absence of an incontrovertible "gold standard" diagnosis based on attributes of the risk factors adds to uncertainty in the performance of predictive and prognostic models.

This chapter discusses a new approach to modeling SUDEP from a mixture of SUDEP datasets. Here, we suggest that decision analytic and machine learning tools can be applied to SUDEP forensic and population-based research to possibly improve the positive predictive value of SUDEP models.

## RISK FACTOR IDENTIFICATION AND CLUSTERING USING MACHINE LEARNING

Machine learning is a major focus of artificial intelligence in which computational tools are designed to "learn" from the data without assuming specific distributions and sometimes model structure. Whereas classical distribution-based statistics are used mainly for descriptive analysis, hypothesis testing and inference, machine learning focuses on representation and generalization. Representation generally finds patterns among the data analogously to descriptive statistics, although a single parametric equation as a result of modeling might be difficult to achieve for some machine learning algorithms. Generalization is the ability of a "learning machine" to perform accurate predictions from unseen observations after learning on a known set of observations. Generalization with machine learning algorithms is mapping the inputs to the outputs by recognizing patterns and similarities among the examples.

There are a variety of algorithm types that are considered to be machine learning. Most important for our research on SUDEP are those characterized as "supervised" or "unsupervised" learning algorithms. The former refers to training the algorithm on a known set of exemplars—a "training set." The algorithm is left to generalize predictions with iterative cycles with or without human decisions about the desired performance or degree of model convergence. Unsupervised learning, such as cluster analysis, uses examples of unknown outcomes to look for patterns and similarities among the data, not measures of prediction. For example, so-called "-omics" studies often model hundreds or thousands of genes or proteins (as $k$) to create complex dendritic trees in which the length of the branches represent the similarity among the $k$s—genes, DNA fragments, or proteins.

Although machine learning often excels in situations in which the number of parameters ($p$) might even exceed the number of observations ($n$), it is also useful for identifying risk factors (e.g., predictors) and generating testable hypotheses about complex interactions among the risk factors when $p$ and $n$ are more balanced.

Such applications of machine learning are "unsupervised" explorations of the data that might feed iteratively into a supervised learning method. In $p \ll n$ designs, machine learning also has a long history in prognostication (Nativ et al. 1988). There are nearly limitless ways to combine machine learning methods, with or without classical statistics, to describe and generalize the prediction of outcomes from observations. The choice of modeling tools depends not only on the characteristic of the tools but also on the research groups' knowledge and preference for particular methods.

## DECISION ANALYSIS WITH RECURSIVE PARTITIONING

Clinical and forensic studies on syndromes, having complex etiologies and manifestations, often report similar, but not identical, notions of "true" cases and controls. Even within a single study, expert clinicians and scientists are likely to debate the relative importance of diverse risk factors, attribute scales, and the category definitions within a given risk factor. Ultimately, a consensus definition of cases and controls is necessary to use machine learning or inferential statistical tools in a supervised learning mode such that a predictive model can be developed. Research groups are increasingly turning to decision analytical tools for structured methods that can aggregate expert judgments into a unique model definition.

The past several decades have witnessed an exponential growth in the application of prescriptive decision analysis to areas including scientific research. Decision analysis calls for purposefully confronting the subjectivities among decision makers and the uncertainties in the outcomes for the decision alternatives (Keeney 2004; Claycamp 2010) and it is useful for situations in which multiobjective decisions are made by multiple decision makers (Keeney 2013). Multicriteria decision analysis (MCDA) is a group of techniques increasingly applied to complex medical and public health decision making (Linkov et al. 2006; Nutt et al. 2010). MCDA has its origins in subjective probability of the 1950s and the seminal work by Keeney and Raiffa on multiobjective decision making (Keeney and Raiffa 1976). More recently, MCDA has been applied to pharmaceutical benefit-risk decision making, particularly in the United Kingdom and EU communities (Nutt et al. 2010; Neely et al. 2011).

The role that MCDA has in our SUDEP risk factor and cluster analysis research is to develop a standardized data instrument and use the instrument to classify cases and controls for the modeling, respectively. Although developing a standardized data extraction instrument is a basic step in general

epidemiological method, the use of MCDA as part of the supervised machine learning process is believed to be novel.

It is generally accepted that domain experts, with the possible exception of meteorologists, are poor or "no-better-than-random" at prognostication from complex, multivariable information (Silver 2012). Here, we are viewing diagnosis *per se* as a classification problem in which the diagnostician scores an observation under dichotomous "diseased" or "normal" groups by either qualitative or quantitative similarities with the defined diseased or normal groups. Our prediction problems call for expert judgments for the identity and relative importance of predictors (risk factors) from among a broad set of candidate risk factors. The process of expert elicitation is used to correct and iteratively fine-tune experts' judgments of probabilities associated with the risk factors and their attributes (Cooke 1991; Ayyub 2002; O'Hagan et al. 2006). Here, our expert team has identified risk factors and groupings of risk factors that can be tested iteratively against new sets of forensic observations of SUDEP.

There are numerous ways to approach building structural models, data extraction tools for meta-analytical studies, and predictive models. We believe the method described here is one which the expertise of clinicians in forensic and prognostic diagnoses can be combined sequentially with a machine learning approach. The principles of expert elicitation used in MCDA can guide the creation of a data extraction instrument. Once data are extracted from one or many published or current sources, then the data set can be submitted to the machine learning algorithm of recursive partitioning.*

Recursive partitioning is a basic nonparametric approach for grouping observations in a study population by similarity among the responses. Recursive partitioning has been implemented in numerous software packages, such as the trademarked, "classification and regression trees" (CART™) (Breiman et al. 1983) and "recursive partitioning" (RPART) (Therneau and Atkinson 1997) in the statistical software, R (R Development Core Team 2011). The result of a recursive partitioning is a "classification tree" if the outcome is dichotomous or categorical and a "regression tree" if the outcome is continuous. The basic process generally "grows" a tree from the data in which each branching point (node) of the tree represents a splitting rule (Figure 4.3). For example, "if *age ≥ 15 years* then *branch left*, else *branch right*" might split a data set into two groups due to an underlying bimodal distribution of ages. Theoretically, the partitioning process can split the data for each $k$ (risk factor) in the data set as long as there are at least two different observations for the risk factor. Of course, the ability to mathematically split data might be nonsense, scientifically speaking. Thus, modelers typically monitor machine learning to prune branches from trees or aggregate branches under a higher branch (level) in hierarchical models. A number of diagnostic statistics can be applied to a tree to monitor (and supervise) convergence of

---

* Recursive partitioning is a generalized term. The more precise name, "classification and regression trees" or CART®, has been trademarked by Salford Systems, http://www.salford-systems.com/company/the-company.

the model calculations or to find an optimal solution; however, the best measure of a tree's optimality is typically its ability to correctly classify new cases and controls. If a "gold standard" diagnostic instrument is known for a "training set" having observations of known outcomes, then measures such as sensitivity, specificity, and the area under the receiver-operator characteristic (ROC) curve can be used to build a predictive classifier (Weiss and Kulikowski 1991).

A candidate predictive model derived from observations of presumptive cases and controls is typically subjected to one or more validation exercises. The measurement of model validity usually relies on comparison with a "gold standard" set of data or diagnostic test. Machine learning-based models are generally validated by splitting the observations into "learning" and "testing" sets, both of which have known outcomes. The tool "learns" patterns from the learning set by measuring how predictive outcomes perform against the known outcomes. In order to prevent over-fitting, the learned classification tree is run on a testing set or multiples of testing sets generated randomly performance is measured in terms of sensitivity, specificity, and the receiver-operator characteristic curve. In brief, the overall method includes the following general steps:

1. *Develop a hierarchical model for SUDEP.* Use MCDA principles to elicit risk factor identities, hierarchies, and probabilities from SUDEP experts (Figure 4.1).
2. *Define a data extraction instrument from the hierarchical model.* The data extraction instrument will define systematic constrain attribute data for the risk factors (see Chapter 5).
3. *Create a set of well-defined SUDEP cases and similar controls.* The data set is split into learning and testing subsets for supervised learning. It is more important to build the set to be representative of the outcome space of SUDEP rather than to, for example, seek a large sample.
4. *Perform recursive portioning on the learning and testing sets of observations.* Using diagnostic criteria for tree generation, iteratively train and test classification trees for an optimal tree. Calculate performance parameters in the fully validated tree(s) (Figures 4.2 and 4.3).
5. *Use cutting-edge methods for increasing the signal-to-noise of the candidate trees.* If necessary, use boot-strap aggregation ("bagging," below) of trees

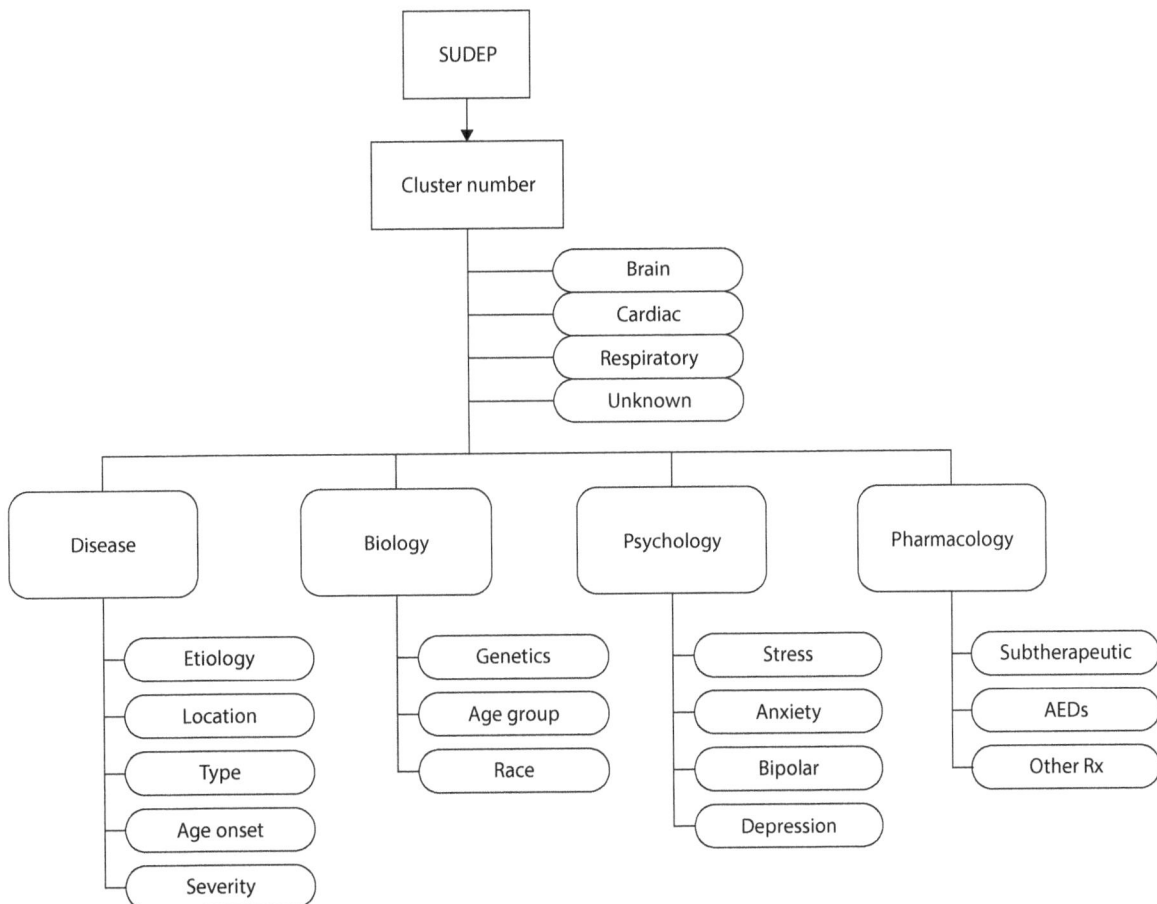

**FIGURE 4.1** Notional and incomplete view of a possible SUDEP hierarchy. A number of variables and blocking factors (e.g., decomposition status in postmortem examination) are not shown for clarity of presentation. Classification tree modeling will be used to elucidate the branch probabilities, given the database of cases and controls. The relative weighting and position that experts place on nodes in the hierarchy informs design of the data extraction tool.

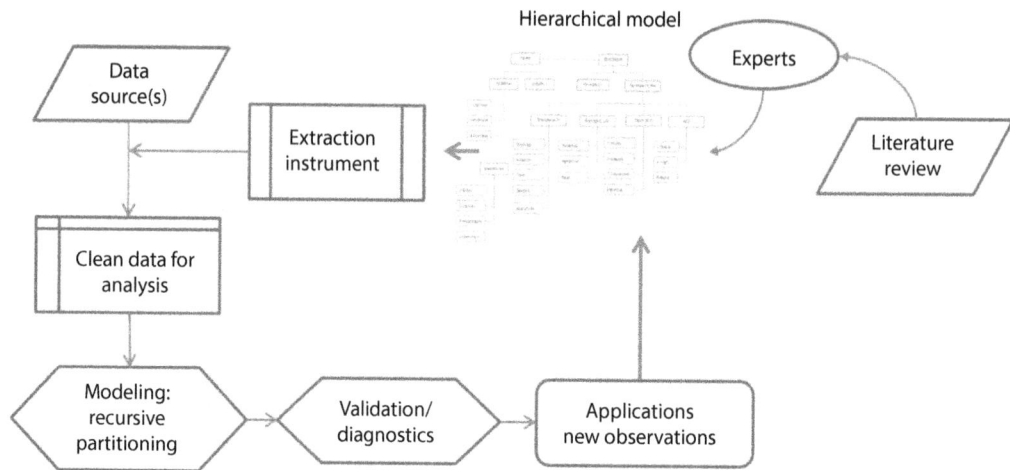

**FIGURE 4.2**  High-level view of the modeling process. The assembled team of experts creates a hierarchical model or view of SUDEP risk factors as shown in detail in Figure 4.1. From the model, a data extraction instrument is created for use with new data sources to build a more complete and balanced sampling of SUDEP cases and controls. Once a model is built using recursive partitioning and related tools, the hierarchical model is tested against the original assumptions about SUDEP risk factors. A "tuned" model can be applied predictively to new potential cases.

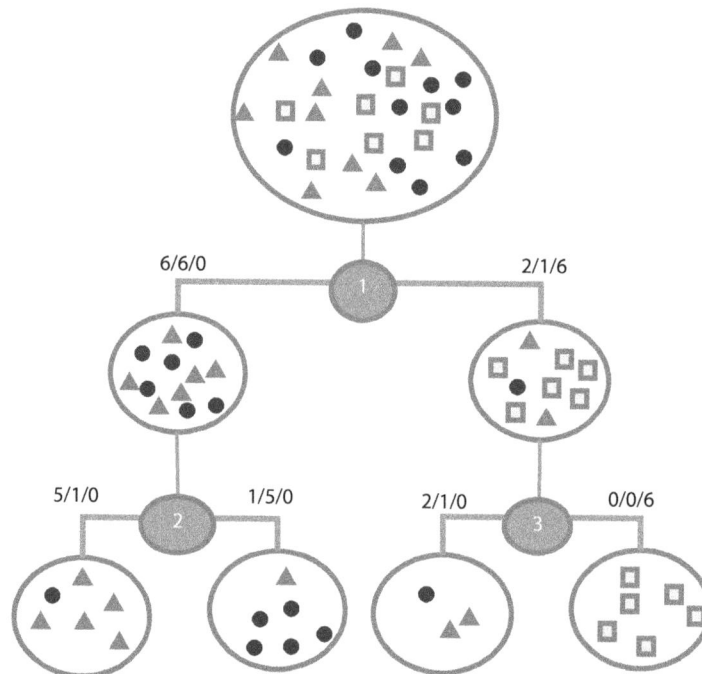

**FIGURE 4.3**  Schematic for a recursive partitioning classifier. The true class membership of a subject is given by the shape: triangles, circles, and squares. The risk factor is given by the nodes (1, 2, and 3). The classification process generated rules for the risk factors: e.g., Risk Factor 1 (node 1), "squares go right, triangles and circles go left." Node 1 mis-classified 2 triangles and 1 circle as predicted "squares." Given the numerical values represented by the shapes, node 3 correctly classified the squares into the right terminal node. Note that the triangles and circle on the left arm of node 3 remain misclassified—If the classifier were perfect, these shapes would have gone left at node.

or random selection of possible branches in trees ("random forests," below) to improve tree performance (Figure 4.4).

6. *Use the resulting decision tree to classify new and alternate data sets.* Apply the developed decision tree to data sets from the literature or otherwise that have not been used in the training process.

7. *Re-train and re-test with alternative validation strategies or as new information can update the model.*

Many enhancements of the basic classification and regression algorithm have been added since the original work by Breiman et al. including "bagging" or bootstrap aggregation of trees (Breiman 1996), "boosting" (Schapire 1990) and "random forests" (Breiman 2001). Bagging calls for bootstrap sampling (with replacement) of the learning set as a means of reducing variance and limiting the prospect of over fitting the model. Boosting is a meta-analytical process for boosting the signal from weak classifiers (or learning

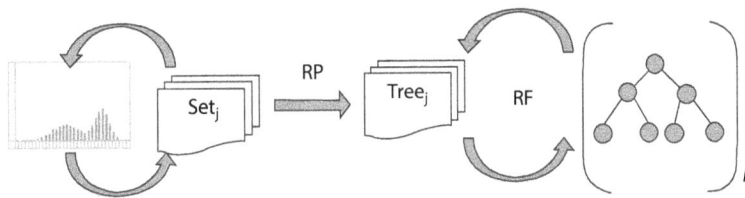

**FIGURE 4.4** Classification trees: Bagging and random forest schematic. The bootstrap aggregation (bagging) process constructs an average classification tree by randomly sampling (with replacement) the original learning set of data for recursive partitioning (RP). Multiple candidate (bagged) trees can also be sampled by selecting variables within the trees in order to create a "random forest" of trees (RF). The mode (e.g., most probable) tree, measured using performance measures against a testing set of data, can be saved as the "final" classification tree.

machines in general). Boosting classification trees involves growing multiple trees from random samples of the learning set and summing the candidate models. Node weighting and exemplar weighting schemes might then be used to improve the predictivity of the final, "boosted" tree. Finally, "random forest" is another meta-model or "ensemble learning" approach that generates numerous random trees, including the random selection of factors. Random forests is essentially "bagging trees" instead of resampling only the exemplars (Figure 4.3).

## ALGORITHM DEVELOPMENT AND TESTING

The application of machine learning to new research problems and supporting datasets is seldom reducible to a simple "off-the-shelf" software solution. Rather, researchers typically find optimal solutions by linking together various algorithms as needed to improve prediction or case identification within their specific problem area. Fortunately, the machine learning and statistical computing communities have a long-standing practice of sharing research results in open-source formats. This practice enables not only the peer-review of published methods but also a means for "standardized" testing of de novo algorithms or software implementation. For example, there are numerous diverse collections of data sets in online data repositories at sites ranging from universities, such as University of California, Irvine and Carnegie Mellon University, to cloud service innovators, such as Amazon.com Cloud Services (Bache and Lichman 2013; Amazon Web Services 2014; CMU 2014). The public data sets include an array of modeling problems encountered including some that have relatively high factor numbers compared to sample size and overlapping sets of factors. Such known, problematic data sets can be used to develop robust modeling approaches for SUDEP.

## LIMITATIONS OF THE METHODS

A casual review of recursive partitioning and machine learning generally might suggest that these approaches are relatively free of assumptions about underlying population measures when compared to parametric statistical methods. In fact, there are judgments about probability and scale definitions—Assumptions and expert judgments

about the expected values that might be observed in a study population. As a result, expert-generated interval scales and defined categories might not adequately capture the real world of observations. For instance, an ordinal scale given to a variable might misrepresent the underlying signal in terms of its intensity. Perhaps the "true" value of the variable follows logarithmic scale (e.g., 1, 10, 100...). In addition, interval scales are often derived for human convenience, while the natural intervals provide richer information about the attribute. Essentially, intervals are handled in calculations no differently from ordinal-scaled variables; thus, intervals that are [1–10; 11–100] or [1–5; 6–10] will both be represented as "1" and "2" in calculations unless the interval is weighted by the relative scale width or a midpoint value. Finally, true for any modeling approach is the fact that reducing a continuous variable to categorical "bins" removes some of the information that might otherwise be represented by the attribute.

## SUMMARY AND CONCLUSION

An application of decision analytic methods can be used to hone the complex array of published or newly identified risk factors for SUDEP into testable, hierarchical models. Some of the factors might occur in overlapping clusters. The MCDA process can lead into application or recursive partitioning (classification and regression trees) to find robust decision trees for predictions of SUDEP among published data sets and possible prognostic application in real time. Advanced machine learning methods, such as bagging and random forests, might also be employed to develop optimal decision trees. In conclusion, novel uses of machine learning tools offer a path to development and testing new models of SUDEP risk factor identification and prediction.

## REFERENCES

Amazon Web Services. Public Data Sets on AWS, 2014.
Ayyub BM. *Elicitation of Expert Opinions for Uncertainty and Risks.* Boca Raton, FL: CRC Press, 2002.
Bache K and Lichman M. *UCI Machine Learning Repository.* Irvine, CA: University of California, School of Information and Computer Science, 2013.

Breiman L. Bagging predictors. *Machine Learning* 1996;24:123–140.

Breiman L. Random forests. *Machine Learning* 2001;45(1):5–32.

Breiman L, Friedman J, Olshen R, and Stone C. *Classification and Regression Trees*. Belmont, CA: Wadsworth, 1983.

Claycamp H. Decision analysis and risk management. In: Lathers CM, Bungo MW, and Leetsma JE, eds., *Sudden Death in Epilepsy: Forensic and Clinical Issues*. Boca Raton, FL: CRC Press/Taylor & Francis; 2010, pp. 887–904.

CMU. StatLib—CMU Datasets Archive, 2014.

Cooke R. *Experts in Uncertainty: Opinion and Subjective Probability in Science*. Oxford, UK: Oxford Universtiy Press, 1991.

Keeney R. Making better decision makers. *Decision Analysis* 2004;1(4):93–204.

Keeney R. Foundations for group decision analysis. *Decision Analysis* 2013;10:103–120.

Keeney R and Raiffa H. *Decisions With Multiple Objectives. Preferences and Value Tradeoffs*. New York, NY: John Wiley, 1976. Reprinted Cambridge University Press, 1993.

Lhatoo S, Johnson A, Goodridge D, MacDonald B, Sander J, and Shorvon S. Mortality in epilepsy in the first 11 to 14 years after diagnosis: Multivariate analysis of a long-term, prospective, population-based cohort. *Annals of Neurology* 2001;49:336–344.

Linkov I, Satterstrom FK, Kiker G, Batchelor C, Bridges T, and Ferguson E. From comparative risk assessment to multicriteria decision analysis and adaptive management: Recent developments and applications. *Environment international* 2006;32(8):1072–1093.

National Research Council. *Small Clinical Trials: Issues and Challenges*. Washington, DC: National Academy of Sciences, National Academy Press, 2001.

Nativ O, Raz Y, Winkler H, Hosaka Y, Boyle E, Therneau T, Farrow G, Meyers R, Zincke H, and Lieber M. Prognostic value of flow cytometric nuclear DNA analysis in stage C prostate carcinoma. *Surgical Forum* 1988;685–687.

Neely T, Walsh-Mason B, Russell P, Van Der Horst A, O'Hagan S, and Lahorkar P. A multi-criteria decision analysis model to assess the safety of botanicals utilizing data on history of use. *Toxicology international* 2011;18(Suppl 1):S20–S29.

Nilsson L, Farahmand B, Persson P-G, Thiblin I, and Tomson T. 1999. Risk factors for sudden unexpected death in epilepsy: A case-control study. *Lancet* 353:888–893.

Nutt D, King L, and Phillips L. Drug harms in the UK: A multicriteria decision analysis. *Lancet* 2010;376:1558–1565.

O'Hagan A, Buck C, Daneshkhah A, Eiser J, Garthwaite P, Jenkinson D, Oakley J, and Rakow T. *Uncertain Judgements. Eliciting Experts' Probabilities*. Chichester, England: Wiley, 2006.

R Development Core Team. *R: A Language and Environment for Statistical Computing*. Vienna, Austria: R Foundation for Statistical Computing, 2011.

Schapire R. The strength of weak learnability. *Machine Learning* 1990;5:197–227.

Silver N. *The Signal and the Noise: Why So Many Predictions Fail—But Some Don't*. New York, NY: Penguin Group, 2012.

Therneau T and Atkinson E. An introduction to recursive partitioning using the RPART routines. Technical Report 61, Rochester, NY: Mayo Clinic; 1997.

Weiss S and Kulikowski C. *Computer Systems That Learn: Classification and Prediction Methods from Statistics, Neural Nets, Machine Learning and Expert Systems*. San Francisco, CA: Morgan Kaufmann Publishers, 1991.

# 5 Forensic SUDEP Cluster Risk Factor Identifier Method

*Claire M. Lathers, Jan E. Leestma, Steven C. Schachter, Steven A. Koehler, H. Gregg Claycamp, Braxton B. Wannamaker, and Paul L. Schraeder*

## CONTENTS

## SUDEP RISK FACTORS

There are multiple contributing risk factors that, in combinations including environmental circumstances for any given individual with epilepsy, may result in death. Although at the present time the scientific understanding of SUDEP favors the notion that it is "unexpected" and thus unpredictable, we believe SUDEP might be predictable and potentially avoidable based on the presence or absence of risk factors. In-depth discussions of SUDEP risk factors are found in the following references: All 1000 pages of the SUDEP book by Lathers et al. (2011) and especially chapter 1, chapter 12 by Walczak, chapter 24 by Wannamaker, and chapter 37 by Mameli and Alessandro; Jay and Leestma (1981); and Leestma et al. (1989). Detailed discussions of some SUDEP Risk Factors and Mechanisms for and relevant author citations are listed below

1. Cardiac arrhythmias: Lathers and Schraeder 1982, 1987; Lathers et al. 1987; Tester and Ackerman, 2006, 2007; Aurlien et al. 2007; Alkadhi and Alzoubi 2011, ch. 26; Bealer et al. 2011, ch. 38
2. Lock step phenomenon mechanism: Lathers and Schraeder 1983, 1989 and students Stauffer et al. 1989 and 2011; O'Rourke and Lathers, 2011; Dodd-O and Lathers 2011
3. Respiratory and hypoxia pathology: Lathers and Schraeder 1982; Carnel et al. 1985; Simon et al. 1982; Sedy et al. 2008; So et al. 2000; Stewart 2011; Terrence et al. 1981; Johnston et al. 1995, 1997
4. Cardiac and respiratory: All above references and Scorza et al. 2007; Finsterer and Stollesburg 2011, ch. 42; Koehler et al. 2011, ch. 9
5. Syncope: Lathers et al. 2011, chapters 1 and 22
6. Genetic: Tester and Ackerman, 2006, 2007; Herreros 2011, ch. 19
7. Stress: Lathers and Schraeder 2006; Alkadhi and Alzoubi 2011, ch. 26
8. Therapies: Lathers and Schraeder 2002, ch. 47; Lathers and Schraeder 2011; Lathers et al. 2003, odds ratios; Ryvlin et al. 2009; Tomson 2011
9. Sleep/wake cycle and lock step phenomenon: Hughes and Sato 2011, ch. 23
10. Unusual factors that may modify SUDEP risk: Scorza et al. 2007, winter temperatures, 2008, protective omega 3 fatty acids, 2011, ch. 3; Calderazzo et al. 2009, climate fluctuations; Terra-Bustamante et al., 2009 lunar phase
11. See Tables in this Chapter for expansion of risk factors discussion.

There is agreement that the central and peripheral autonomic nervous system and the resulting brain and cardiorespiratory interactions include arrhythmias and apnea and are involved in SUDEP. Confounding the effect of the nervous system/cardiac relationship are relatively recent discoveries of genetically determined predispositions to arrhythmias that may result in seizure-like events at the time of the acute cardiac dysfunction. How these genetic cardiac predispositions interact with the central and autonomic nervous systems is not yet understood. It is generally accepted that certain associated clinical circumstances (e.g., male sex, poorly controlled generalized tonic-clonic seizures, use of multiple antiepileptic drugs [AEDs], changing doses and drugs, withdrawal of AEDs, and poor compliance with AED use) are associated with an increased risk of SUDEP. All references discuss risk factors *for* and mechanisms *of* SUDEP. Decision analysis and risk management are important approaches that can help prioritize risk factors for risk management strategies designed to reduce and/or to prevent the occurrence of SUDEP (Claycamp 2011, ch. 55).

## RESEARCH METHOD

We will use our new method of Risk Factor Classification and Cluster Identifiers (IDs) for SUDEP to evaluate AEDs, regimens of AEDs and preventives using retrospective and prospective data. We are using two methods to develop control values for our SUDEP Cluster IDs. First, a retrospective study of NASA and other databases to mine parameters from normal subject controls will be performed. Control data will be used to build Cluster Risk Factor IDs for 115 SUDEP/ epilepsy cases that can serve as learning and testing sets against SUDEP cases. Larger denominators provide greater signal-to-noise for risk cluster identifications and more robust modeling for predictive clusters. AEDs are included in our method and will be examined in Risk Factor Clusters. For a second source of control data, Dr. Wannamaker will use data from approximately 3000 epileptic patients who are alive in his practice and/or those who have died from non-SUDEP causes to develop a method to use their data as controls to score our SUDEP cases.

## SUDEP CLUSTER RISK FACTOR METHOD

Parameters in published SUDEP cases, our own SUDEP cases, NASA and other databases will be entered into a Method Table to develop Control Cluster Risk Factor classification and IDs for SUDEP and individual autonomic IDs described in Step1 #1–5. SUDEP Cluster ID has seven categories (Table 5.1). Four categories for each victim death are SUDEP Definite, W1; SUDEP Probable, W2; SUDEP Possible, W3; and Non-SUDEP, W5. Three categories are used if a person is alive. One category is for a person with epilepsy who is alive and includes those with an unwanted medical event but SUDEP was Prevented, W4. Another category includes Alive Patients diagnosed with epilepsy who

have not had a medical event but will benefit from knowledge gained of Cluster IDs, their individual degree of risk and the best medical regimen to prevent SUDEP in the future, W6. The last category of alive people includes a Survivor who did not have epilepsy, W7, that is, a person with an unwanted medical event who survived but did not have epilepsy. Mechanistic risk categories for death via SUDEP are based on pathophysiological mechanisms occurring in brain, cardiac, or respiratory sites with assigned numbers of 1, 2, or 3, respectively, or category 4—Unknown mechanism. In Table 5.2 through 5.6 SUDEP Cluster Chart, subsets of epilepsy risk factor identifiers are labeled A through W. These Risk Factors must be evaluated for each victim and people with epilepsy at risk for SUDEP. Subcategories include Risk Factors of A–E (etiology, origin, type, severity of seizures, and age of onset of epilepsy), F (cardiac autonomic arrhythmogenic findings such as ventricular fibrillation or asystole), G (cardiac function), H (respiratory and hypoxia pathology), I (syncope), J (genetics), Q (age group), and so on. Cluster Identifier K for subcategory of AEDs, if determined, indicates if levels were found to be therapeutic, sub-therapeutic, above the therapeutic range, or absent. Question: Is risk related to the AED used or tapering of AED and is increased risk related to the number of AEDs, types of co-medications, and/or alcohol (L1a4) or illicit drug (L1a5) use? Variable *M* is concomitant diagnosed diseases, whether contributory to cause of death, progressive pathology such as tumor, which contributed to death in a person with epilepsy but not SUDEP Mc2, and Mc14 are variables of intracranial and intraocular pressures, vision, and optic nerve. Psychological diseases N, with subcategories of stress N1, anxiety N2, depression N3, and bipolar disease N4 are included. Unusual factors of climate, temperature, omega 3 fatty acids, lunar phase, time of year, traffic, and so on are in cluster identifier O. Gender is Cluster Identifier P, age at time of death is Q, R indicates if a person was a smoker while S is incidence/occurrence of SUDEP as reported or determined for a given study, if known, S1 U.S. states/counties of death and S2 foreign countries. Cluster Identifier T1 indicates human data and T2 animal, U is race/ethnicity, and V ID is postmortem examination.

---

**TABLE 5.1**

**SUDEP Syndrome Cluster Risk Identification. Seven Categories of SUDEP Victims, Near-Miss SUDEP, Epilepsy Patients Who May Be Future SUDEP Victims, Non Epileptic Survivors**

W1 SUDEP definite with postmortem

W2 SUDEP probable with or without postmortem

W3 SUDEP possible

W4 SUDEP prevented, near-miss SUDEP who survived

W5 Non-SUDEP victims who were thought to have epilepsy but did not have the diagnosis of epilepsy or those who were correctly diagnosed with epilepsy but died of another cause such as a glial brain tumor

W6 A patient who is alive and diagnosed with epilepsy and must be medically evaluated to determine what preventive actions should be taken in the day-to-day events to protect the person from becoming a victim of SUDEP at some time in the future

W7 Survivor, Not epilepsy

**TABLE 5.2**

**SUDEP Syndrome Cluster Identifiers. Related Clusters of Incidence, Risk Factors, Supportive Animal Data and Clinical Features (If Available) Based on the Suspected Underlying Mechanism of Death**

Brain: Postictal seizure = flat line EEG final result — Epilepsy Syndrome or Categories — Cluster Number 1

Category columns: M / Mnp / Mc = Cardiac 2 · N = Respiratory & Hypoxia 3 · O = Unknown 4

| Cluster Identifier A–E | F–G | H | I | J | K–L | M Mnp Mc (Cardiac 2) | N (Respiratory & Hypoxia 3) | O (Unknown 4) | P | Q | R | S | T/U | V | V | V Post |
|---|---|---|---|---|---|---|---|---|---|---|---|---|---|---|---|---|
| A. Brain epilepsy syndrome or categories | Cardiac arrhythmogenic includes subcategories | H. Respiratory & hypoxia | I. Syncope | J. Genetic structural channelopathies | K. AEDs | M. Mnp normal postmortem path | N. Psychological | O. Unusual, other, Environment Circumstances | S | Q. AGE | R. | S. | T1 | V Postmortem exam | V | V1a. External exam only |
| | | | | | K1. AEDS prescribed prescriptions. | Mnp3 Heart | | O1. Climate | EX | Q1.<10 | S | I | H | | | V |
| | | H1. Central apnea | | | Benzodiazepines BENZO K1a1. Yes. K1a2-No, K1a3-Unknown | Mnp4 Lung | N1. Stress +/- | O2. Temperature | P1M | Q2.10-20 | M | N | U | | | V |
| | | H1a. Laryngospasm | | | Carbamazepine CBZ K1b1[a] | Mnp5 Brain | N2. Anxiety | O3. Omega 3 FA | P2 | Q3.21-30 | O | C | M | | | 1 |
| A1-10. | F. ANA[b] Neural F1. Sym[b] | H1b. Lung | | J1. Epileptic syndromes | Clonazepine CLZ K1c1[a] | Mnp6 Liver | N3. Depression | O4. Month of death[a] | F | Q4.31-40 | K | I | A | | | b. |
| A11 EEG origin | F1a. Fibrillation | Edema | | J1a-n. Different mutations in genes encoding alpha subunits of neuronal Na+ channels J1d. (SCN 1A and J1c. SCN 2A) or J1e. | Diazepam DZP K1d1[a] | Mnp7 Brain vascular | N4. Bipolar | O5. Day of week[a] | | Q5.41-50 | E | D | N | | | Autopsy |
| A11a L hemisphere | F1b cardiac defibrillator implanted | H1c. Obstructive apnea | | Beta subunit (SCN 1B) neuronal isoforms Na+ channel | Felbamate FELB K1e1[a] | Mp. Postmortem pathology | N5. Psychiatric drugs | O6. Year of death[a] | | Q6.51-60 | R | E | T2 | | | V1c. No autopsy |
| A11a1 Temporal | F1b seizure free | H1d. Ictal hypoxemia, hypercapnia | | J1n. Dysfunction K+ channels | Gaba penta neurontin? GPN K1f1[a] | Mp3b Cardiomegally, Mp3c Microscopic Myocardial Fibrosis, Mp3d Conduction System abnormality, Mp3e Unknown | N5a. Anti psychotics | O7. Site fatal event[a] | | Q7.61-70 | Y | N | A | | | V2 |

(Continued)

**TABLE 5.2  (Continued)**

**SUDEP Syndrome Cluster Identifiers. Related Clusters of Incidence, Risk Factors, Supportive Animal Data and Clinical Features (If Available) Based on the Suspected Underlying Mechanism of Death**

| Cluster Identifier A–E | F–G | H | I | J | K–L | M / Mnp / Mc | N | O | P | Q | R | S | T U | V | V Post genetics |
|---|---|---|---|---|---|---|---|---|---|---|---|---|---|---|---|
| A11a2 Frontal | F2. PNS[b] | H2. Successful resuscitation | | J1e. Epileptic and cardiac | Lamotrigine LAMO K1g1[a] | Mp4 Lung Pathology: | N5b. Antidepressants | O8. Location pronounced dead | Q8.>71 | R1 | C | N | | | genetics |
| A11b R | F2a. Asystolic | | | Beta subunit SCN 1B. common for both cardiac and neuronal isoforms Na+ channel | Levetiracetam LEVE K1h1[a] | Mp4b COPD, Mp4c Other, Mp4d Unknown, Mp4e congestion/ increased wt, Mp4f Pneumonia, | N5b1 SSRIs | O8a. Residence | | N | E | I | | | |
| A11b1 Temporal | F2a1 Pacemaker implanted 9 mon seizure free | | | J2. Cardiac: | Neurontin NEURO K1f[a] | Mp5 Brain, non epilepsy related disease | N5b1. Other antidepressants. | O8b. Outdoors | | R2 | | M | | | |
| A11b2 Frontal | F2b. Ictal bradycardia and | | | J2a12. Brugada S. & J2a3. LQT3 mutation gene SCN 5A, encodes alpha subunit cardiac Na+ channel | Oxyazepam OZP K1j1[a] | Mp5b Edema, Mp5c Benign Tumor, Mp5d Malignant tumor, Mp5e Mesial temporal stenosis, Mp5f Other, Mp5g Unknown | N5c. antianxiety meds | O8c. Hospital | | UKR | | A | | | |
| A11b3 Other | | | | | Phenobarbital PB K1k1[a] | Mp6 Liver, Mp6b Fatty, Mp6c Fibrosis, Mp6d Cirrhosis, Mp6e Tumor, Mp6f unknown | N6. Other medications. Prinavil, ACE Inhibitor antihypertensive | 08d. Work | | 3 | | L | | | |
| Hemisphere | G. Cardiac | | | J1e. Beta subunit (SCN 1B) cardiac isoforms Na+ channel | Phenytoin PHT K1L1[a] | Mp7 Brain Vascular, Mp7aStroke, Mp7b Intracerebral hemorrhage, Mp7c Subarachnoid hemorrhage | N7. Other psychological factors | O8e. Traffic, | | | | U | | | |

(Continued)

| Race U1-6/Eth-nicity U7 | O8f. Criminal, / O8g. Restraint, / O8h. Sleep-wake circadian cycle, / O8i. Other / O8j. Unknown / O9. Posture | Mp8. Post traumatic changes (scar tissue) / Mp9. Pathology unknown / Mp10. Other / Mc. Clinical/premortem disease / Mc1c. Premortem static brain pathology: Likely etiology of seizures, M1c1. Developmental/perinatal, Mc1c2. vascular, Mc1c3. Static benign tumor, Mc1c4. Post traumatic brain injury, Mc1c4 Other, Mc1c5 Negative imaging studies, Mc1c6 Pathology Unknown / Mc2. Premortem progressive pathology: Possible contributory cause of death. Mc2a History of Epilepsy. Mc2b Cardiac. Mc2d Postictal Generalized EEG Suppression (PGES) Mc2a Epilepsy, Mc2b Cardiac Disease, Mc2c Pulmonary Disease. Mc2e Other. | Tegretol TGL K1b1[a] / Topiramate TOP K1n1[a] / Trazodone TZD K1o1[a] / Valproic Acid VPA K1p1[a] / Primidone K1r1[a] / Tiagabine TGBK1s[a] | G1/Function, Long QT / Torsades de Pointes, AV block / G2. Microscopic cardiac lesions, / G3. Postictal increase in T-wave alternans G3a. Post generalized tonic–clonic seizures | A11cNon Lateralized / A11d Multifocal / A11e Generalized including epilepsy / B. Refractory epilepsy |
| --- | --- | --- | --- | --- | --- |

**TABLE 5.2**  (*Continued*)

SUDEP Syndrome Cluster Identifiers. Related Clusters of Incidence, Risk Factors, Supportive Animal Data and Clinical Features (If Available) Based on the Suspected Underlying Mechanism of Death

| Cluster Identifier A–E | F–G | H | I | J | K–L | M / Mnp / Mc | N | O | P | Q | R | S | T / U | V | V Post |
|---|---|---|---|---|---|---|---|---|---|---|---|---|---|---|---|
| C. Epileptogenic activity | G3b. Sudden cardiac | | | | Vigabatrin VB K1t[a] | Mc11. Negative imaging studies | | O9a. Prone | | | | | | | |
| Distribution Type & Duration sz | Death | | | | Zonisamide ZNA K1u[a] | Mc12. Hypertension | | O9b. Supine | | | | | | | |
| C1. Interictal activity = sub convulsant/ | G3b1. MI | | | | OtherK1v[a] | Mc13. Diabetes | | | | | | | | | |
| C2. Brief ictal | | | | | K2. AEDS detected by postmortem toxicology analysis. K2a-K2v. | Mc14. Intracranial pressure, intraocular pressure, optic nerve, vision | | | | | | | | | |
| C3. Ictal | | | | | Benzodiazepines BENZO K2a1-Therapeutic, K2a2-Subtherapeutic, K2a3-Undetected. K2a4-No sample available[a] see below K3. Number of AEDs prescribed by physician. K3a-None | | | | | | | | | | |
| C4. EEG source see | | | | | | | | | | | | | | | |
| C4a. Clinical; C4b. ICU; C4c. EMU | | | | | | | | | | | | | | | |
| C5. Temporal lobe origin–not lateralized | | | | | K3b-1 | | | | | | | | | | |
| C6. Frontal lobe origin–not lateralized | | | | | K3c-2 | | | | | | | | | | |
| C7. Other origin–not lateralized | | | | | K3d-3 | | | | | | | | | | |
| C8. Post ictal generalized EEG suppression (PGES) | | | | | K3e->3 | | | | | | | | | | |

C9. Aureas

C91. Fear

C92. Palpitations

C93. Epigastric changes

C94. Pupil changes

C95. Disconnected feelings

C96. Illusions

C97. Anxiety

C98 Other

ANA symptoms

Normal EEG

D. Age at Onset

D1. Full term neonate <24h – 28 days; preterm neonates

D2. 1–3 months

D3. 3.1–12 months

D4. 12.1 mon-10 years

D5. 11–20 years

D6. 21–30 years

D7. 31–40 years

D8. 41–50 years

D9. 51–60 years

D10. 61–70 years

D99. Unknown

K3f. Unknown

K4. Number of AEDs detected postmortem.

K4a-None

K4b-1

K4c-2

K4d-3

K4e->3

K5. AEDS

K5a. Blank was therapeutic

K5b. Blank was subtherapeutic

K5c. Blank was no AED level

K5d. Compliant

K5e. Too high levels

K5e1. No change in RX

K5e2. Change in RX

K5e3. No documentation

K5f. Toxic

K5g. Tapering & process changing

K6. AEDs withdrawn

K7. AEDs unknown

K8. No postmortem

L1. Premortem

L1a. Non AEDs

(Continued)

**TABLE 5.2  (Continued)**

**SUDEP Syndrome Cluster Identifiers. Related Clusters of Incidence, Risk Factors, Supportive Animal Data and Clinical Features (If Available) Based on the Suspected Underlying Mechanism of Death**

| Cluster Identifier A–E | F–G | H | I | J | K–L | M Mnp Mc | N | O | P | Q | R | S | U (T) | V | V Post |
|---|---|---|---|---|---|---|---|---|---|---|---|---|---|---|---|
| E1. Frequency of seizures before or near time of death | | | | | L1a1. Psychotropic drug | | | | | | | | | | |
| E1a. | | | | | | | | | | | | | | | |
| Seizure-free | | | | | L1a2. Antidepressants, SSRI celexa | | | | | | | | | | |
| E1b. ≤1/mon | | | | | L1a3. Antianxiety | | | | | | | | | | |
| E1c. 2/mon | | | | | L1a4. Alcohol | | | | | | | | | | |
| E1d. 3/mon | | | | | L1a5. Illicit Drugs | | | | | | | | | | |
| E1e. >3/mon | | | | | L1a6. Narcotics | | | | | | | | | | |
| E1f. <1/year | | | | | L1a7. Antihistamines | | | | | | | | | | |
| E1g. Seizure just prior to death | | | | | L1a8. NSAIDS | | | | | | | | | | |
| E1x. Unknown | | | | | L1a8a. Non aspirin | | | | | | | | | | |
| E2. Average yearly frequency of seizures | | | | | L1a8b. N-acetylslicyclic acid (ASA) | | | | | | | | | | |
| E2a. <one | | | | | L2. Premortem | | | | | | | | | | |
| E2b. One | | | | | L2a. Non AEDs | | | | | | | | | | |
| E2c. Two | | | | | L2a1. Psychotropic drug | | | | | | | | | | |
| E2d. Three or more | | | | | L2a2. Antidepressants | | | | | | | | | | |
| E2e. Unknown | | | | | L2a3. Antianxiety | | | | | | | | | | |
| | | | | | L2a4. Alcohol | | | | | | | | | | |
| | | | | | L2a5. Illicit Drugs | | | | | | | | | | |
| | | | | | L2a6. Narcotics | | | | | | | | | | |
| | | | | | L2a7. Antihistamines | | | | | | | | | | |
| | | | | | L2a8. NSAIDS | | | | | | | | | | |
| | | | | | L2a8a. Non Aspirin | | | | | | | | | | |
| | | | | | L2a8b. N-acetylslicyclic acid (ASA) | | | | | | | | | | |

[a] See rest of Cluster ID category in Tables 5.3 through 5.7.

[b] ANA, Autonomic nervous system; Sym, Sympathetic nervous system; PNS, Parasympathetic nervous system.

**TABLE 5.3**

**SUDEP Syndrome Cluster Identifiers A1–10 and J1a–m. Genes Found to Be Factors in Epilepsy**

| SUDEP Syndrome Cluster ID A1–10 Monogenic Epilepsies | Cluster ID Ja–mGene | Reference |
|---|---|---|
| A1 Benign familial neonatal seizure | *KCNQ2* J1a | Singh et al. 1998 |
| | *KCNQ3* J1b | Charlier et al. 1998 |
| A2 Benign familial neonatal-infantile seizures | *SCN2A* J1c | Heron et al. 2002 |
| | | Striano et al. 2006 |
| A3 GEFS+; SMEI; FS | *SCN1A* J1d | Claes et al. 2001 |
| | | Escayg et al. 2000 |
| A4 GEFS+ | *SCN1B* J1e | Wallace et al. 1998 |
| A5 GEFS+; SMEI; FS | *GABRG2* J1f | Harkin et al. 2002 |
| A6 Absence epilepsy and FS | *GABRG2* J1g | Baulac et al. 2001 |
| A7 IGE | *CLCN2* J1h | Haug et al. 2003 |
| A8 JME | *GABRA1* J1i | Cossette et al. 2002 |
| A9 Autosomal dominant lateral temporal lobe epilepsy | *LGI1* J1j | Kalachikov et al. 2002 |
| A10 Autosomal dominant nocturnal frontal lobe epilepsy | *CHRNA4* J1k | Steinlein et al. 1995 |
| | *CHRNB2* J1l | De Fusco et al. 2000 |
| | *CHRNA2* J1m | Aridon et al. 2006 |

*Source:* Modified from Ghali and Nashef, ch. 18 in Lathers CM, et al., *Sudden Death in Epilepsy: Forensic and Clinical Factors*, Boca Raton, FL: CRC Press/Taylor & Francis, 2011. p.268.

*Notes:* GEFS+, generalized epilepsy with febrile seizures plus; SMEI, severe myoclonic epilepsy of infancy; FS, febrile seizures; IGE, idiopathic generalized epilepsy; JME, juvenile myoclonic epilepsy.

**TABLE 5.4**

**SUDEP Syndrome Cluster Identifiers A11, A12, C4, D-I**

A. Epilepsy Localization Categories Continued

  A1–10.

  A11. EEG Origin:

  A11a. Left hemisphere

  A11a1- Temporal

  A11a2- Frontal

  A11b. Right Hemisphere

  A11b1- Temporal

  A11b2- Frontal

  A11c. Both Hemisphere

  A11c1- Multi Focal L hemisphere

  A11c2- Multi Focal R hemisphere

  A11c3. Generalized

  A11c4. Multifocal bilateral

  A11c5. Undetermined

  A12a. Idiopathic: Generally genetic

  A12b. Cryptogenic: Underlying causes suspected, but etiology remains undetected

  A12c. Symptomatic: Is an underlying structural cause or major metabolic derangement

 B1. Refractory

 B99. Unknown

 C4. Epileptogenic Activity EEG Source continued

  C4a. Clinical

  C4b. ICU

  C4c. EMU

 C5. Temporal lobe origin-not lateralized

 C6. Frontal lobe origin-not lateralized

*(Continued)*

**TABLE 5.4** (*Continued*)

## SUDEP Syndrome Cluster Identifiers A11, A12, C4, D-I

C7. Other origin-not lateralized

C8. Postictal generalized EEG suppression (PGES)

C9. Aureas

C91. Fear

C92. Palpitations

C93. Epigastric changes

C94. Pupil changes

C95. Disconnected feelings

C96. Illusions

C97. Anxiety

C98. Olfactory

C99. Unknown

C100 Gustatory

D. Age of onset. See p 240 in Neville et al. (2009), for discussion of physiologic changes in metabolic, drug distribution site, renal function; and GI function in neonates, infants, children and adolescents that effect clinical pharmacology of AED and other drugs in a given person

    D1. Full term neonate <24 hours–28 days; could include preterm neonates here

    D2. 1–3 months

    D3. 3.1–12 months

    D4. 1 (12.1 mon)–10 years

    D5. 11–20 years

    D6. 21–30 years

    D7. 31–40 years

    D8. 41–50 years

    D9. 51–60 years

    D10. 61–70 years

    D99. Unknown

E1. Frequency of seizures before and near to the time of death

    E1a. Seizure free

    E1b. ≤1/mon

    E1c. 2/mon

    E1d. 3/mon

    E1e. >3/mon

    E1f. <1/year

    E1g. Seizure just before death

    E1x. Unknown

E2. Average yearly frequency of seizures

    E2a. <one

    E2b. One

    E2c. Two

    E2d. Three or more

F. Cardiac arrhythmogenic, includes following subcategory

    F. Autonomic (ANA) Neural

    F1. Sympathetic (Sym)

    F1a- Fibrillation

    F1b- Cardiodefibrillator implanted

    F1c- Seizure free

    F1d. Autonomic sym ganglia 5-HT3 mechanism

    F2. Parasympathetic (PNS)

    F2a. Asystolic

    F2a1. Pace maker implant 9 months seizure free

    F2b. Ictal bradycardia

    F2c. Multiple PVCs, premature ventricular beats

    F99. Unknown

**TABLE 5.4    (*Continued*)**
**SUDEP Syndrome Cluster Identifiers A11, A12, C4, D-I**

G. Cardiac:

G1. Function, long QT, Torsades de Pointes, AV block

G2. Microscopic cardiac lesions, including epilepsy

G3. Postictal increase in T-wave alternant

G3a. Post generalize tonic-clonic seizures

G3b. Cardiac sudden death

G3b1. Myocardial infarction

G99. Unknown

H. Respiratory and hypoxia pathology

H1. Central apnea

H1a. Laryngospasm serotonin mechanism

H1b. Lung edema

H1c. Obstructive apnea

H1d. Ictal hypoxemia, hypercapnia

H1e. Respiratory arrest. 5-HT2c, 5-HT3, 5-HT4, 5-HT2b

H2. Successful resuscitation

I. Syncope

I.99. Unknown

**TABLE 5.5**
**SUDEP Syndrome Cluster Identifiers J2a1–J2a18. J1a–m Table 1a. Genetic Structural Channelopathies. Genes Involved in Arrhythmogenic Cardiac Channelopathies Related to SCD**

| Syndrome | Subtype | Gene | Protein | Effect |
|---|---|---|---|---|
| Long QT syndrome J2a1 | LQT1 | *KCNQ1* | $I_{Ks}$ K⁺ channel α subunit | $I_{Ks}$ loss of function |
| J2a2 | LQT2 | *KCNH2* | $I_{Kr}$ K⁺ channel α subunit | $I_{Kr}$ loss of function |
| J2a3 | LQT3 | *SCN5A* | Na⁺ channel α subunit | $I_{Na}$ gain of function |
| J2a4 | LQT4 | *ANK2* | Anchoring protein ankyrin B | Reduction of several ionic currents |
| J2a5 | LQT5 | *KCNE1* | $I_{Ks}$ K⁺ channel β subunit | $I_{Ks}$ loss of function |
| J2a6 | LQT6 | *KCNE2* | $I_{Kr}$ K⁺ channel β subunit | $I_{Kr}$ loss of function |
| J2a7 | LQT7 | *KCNJ2* | $I_{K1}$ K⁺ channel α subunit | $I_{K1}$ loss of function |
| J2a8 | LQT8 | *CACNA1c* | $I_{Ca,L}$ Ca⁺⁺ channel α subunit | $I_{Ca,L}$ gain of function |
| J2a9 | LQT9 | *CAV3* | Caveolin 3 | $I_{Na}$ gain of function |
| J2a10 | LQT10 | *SCN4B* | Na⁺ channel β4 subunit | $I_{Na}$ gain of function |
| J2a11 | LQT11 | *AKAP9* | Yotiao (A-kinase anchoring protein) | $I_{Ks}$ loss of function |
| Brugada syndrome J2a12 | BrS1 | *SCN5A* | Na⁺ channel α subunit | $I_{Na}$ loss of function |
| J2a13 | BrS2 | *GPD1L* | Glycerol-3-P dehydrogenase 1 like protein | $I_{Na}$ loss of function |
| Catecholaminergic VT J2a14 | CPVT1 | *RyR2* | Cardiac ryanodine receptor | Cytoplasmic Ca⁺⁺ overload |
| J2a15 | CPVT2 | *CASQ2* | Cardiac calsequestrin | Cytoplasmic Ca⁺⁺ overload |
| Short QT syndrome J2a16 | SQT1 | *KCNH2* | $I_{Kr}$ K⁺ channel α subunit | $I_{Kr}$ gain of function |
| J2a17 | SQT2 | *KCNQ1* | $I_{Ks}$ K⁺ channel α subunit | $I_{Ks}$ gain of function |
| J2a18 | SQT3 | *KCNJ2* | $I_{K1}$ K⁺ channel α subunit | $I_{K1}$ gain of function |

J.99 unknown

*Sources:*    Modified Herreros, B, Cardiac channelopathies and sudden death, ch. 19 In: Lathers CM, Schraeder PL, Bungo MW, Leestma JE, eds. *Sudden Death in Epilepsy: Forensic and Clinical Issues*, p 289, CRC Press/Taylor & Francis, Boca Raton, FL, 2011; Chromosome numbers are indicated in Dhillon and Behr 2011, ch. 45, p. 727. The congenital long QT syndrome: Subtypes, their genetic basis and frequencies.

*Notes:*    $I_{Ks}$, slow rectifying potassium current; $I_{Kr}$, rapid rectifying potassium current; $I_{Na}$, inward sodium current; $I_{K1}$, Kir 2.1 inward rectifying current; Ca$_v$1.2, L-type calcium channel current (Splawski et al. 2000; Tester et al. 2005; Chen et al. 2007; Hofman et al. 2007; Ueda et al. 2008). Gene mutations associated with Brugada syndrome: $I_{Na}$, inward sodium current; $I_{Ks}$, slow rectifying potassium current; $I_{to}$, transient outward potassium current; $I_{Ca}$, L-type calcium channel current (Hedley et al. 2009). Ref. citations from Dhillon and Behr, 2011, ch. 45.

## TABLE 5.6
## SUDEP Syndrome Cluster Identifiers K-W

**K1. AEDS prescribed prescriptions:**

| | |
|---|---|
| Benzodiazepines BENZO: | K1a1-Yes. K1a2-No, K1a3-Unknown |
| Carbamazepine CBZ Tegretol TGL: | K1b1-Yes. K1b2-No, K1b3-Unknown |
| Clonazepine CLZ: | K1c1-Yes. K1c2-No, K1c3-Unknown |
| Diazepam DZP: | K1d1-Yes. K1d2-No, K1d3-Unknown |
| Felbamate FELB: | K1e1-Yes. K1e2-No, K1e3-Unknown |
| Gaba penta GPN Neurontin NEURO: | K1f1-Yes. K1f2-No, K1f3-Unknown |
| Lamotrigine LAMO: | K1g1-Yes. K1g2-No, K1g3-Unknown |
| Levetiracetan LEVE: | K1h1-Yes. K1h1-No, K1h3-Unknown |
| Blank deleted K1i: | K1i1-Yes. K1i2-No, K1i3-Unknown |
| Oxyazepam OZP: | K1j1-Yes. K1j2-No, K1j3-Unknown |
| Phenobarbital PB: | K1k1-Yes. K1k2-No, K1k3-Unknown |
| Phenytoin PHT: | K1L1-Yes. K1l2-No, K1l3-Unknown |
| Mephenytoin: | K1m1-Yes. K1m2-No, K1m3-Unknown |
| Topiramate TOP: | K1n1-Yes. K1n2-No, K1n3-Unknown |
| Trazodone TZD: | K1o1-Yes. K1o2-No, K1o3-Unknown |
| Valproic Acid VPA: | K1p1-Yes. K1p2-No, K1p3-Unknown |
| Blank | |
|   Primidone PRM: | K1r1-Yes. K1r2-No, K1r3-Unknown |
|   Tiagabine TGB | K1s-Yes. K1s2-No, K1s3-Unknown |
| Vigabatrin VBT | K1t-Yes. K1t2-No, K1t3-Unknown |
| Zonisamide ZNA | K1u-Yes. K1u2-No, K1u3-Unknown |
| Other | K1v-Yes. K1v2-No, K1v3-Unknown |

**K2b1-K2v1. AEDs detected by postmortem toxicology analysis. K2a5 Toxic add category for all drugs = K5f.**

| | |
|---|---|
| Benzodiazepines BENZO | K2a1-Therapeutic, K2a2-Subtherapeutic, K2a3Undetected, K2a4-No sample available |
| Carbamazepine CBZ tegretol TGL | K2b1-Therapeutic, K2b2-Subtherapeutic, K2b3-Undetected, K2b4-No sample available |
| Clonazepine CLZ | K2c1-Therapeutic, K2c2Subtherapeutic, K2c3-Undetected, K2c4-No sample available |
| Diazepam DZP | K2d1-Therapeutic, K2d2-Subtherapeutic, K2d3-Undetected, K2d4-No sample available |
| Felbamate FELB | K2e1-Therapeutic, K2e2-Subtherapeutic, K2e3-Undetected, K2e4-No sample available |
| Gaba penta GPN neurontin Neuro | K2f1-Therapeutic, K2f2-Subtherapeutic, K2f3-Undetected, K2f4-No sample available |
| Lamotrigine LAMO | K2g1-Therapeutic, K2g2-Subtherapeutic, K2g3-Undetected, K2g4-No sample available |
| Levetiracetan LEVE | K2h1-Therapeutic, K2h2-Subtherapeutic, K2h3-Undetected, K2h4-No sample available |
| Blank deleted | K2i K2i1-Therapeutic, K2i2-Subtherapeutic, K2i3-Undetected, K2i4-No sample available |
| Oxyazepam OZP | K2j1-Therapeutic, K2j2-Subtherapeutic, K2j3-Undetected, K2j4-No sample available |
| Phenobarbital PB | K2k1-Therapeutic, K2k2-Subtherapeutic, K2k3-Undetected, K2k4-No sample available |
| Phenytoin PHT | K2L1-Therapeutic, K2L2-Subtherapeutic, K2L3-Undetected, K2L4-No sample available |
| Mephenytoin | K2m1-Therapeutic, K2m2-Subtherapeutic, K2m3-Undetected, K2m4-No sample available |
| Topiramate TOP | K2n1-Therapeutic, K2n2-Subtherapeutic, K2n3-Undetected, K2n4-No sample available |
| Trazodone TZD | K2o1-Therapeutic, K2o2-Subtherapeutic, K2o3-Undetected, Ko4-No sample available |
| Valproic Acid VPA | K2p1-Therapeutic, K2p2-Subtherapeutic, K2p3-Undetected, K2p4-No sample available |
| Blank | |
|   Primidone PRM: | K2r1-Therapeutic, K2r2-Subtherapeutic, K2r3-Undetected, K2r4-No sample available |
|   Tiagabine TGB | K2s1-Therapeutic, K2s2-Subtherapeutic, K2s3-Undetected, K2s4-No sample available |
|   Vigabatrin VBT | K2t1-Therapeutic, K2t2-Subtherapeutic, K2t3-Undetected, K2t4-No sample available |
|   Zonisamide ZNA | K2u1-Therapeutic, K2u2-Subtherapeutic, K2u3-Undetected, K2u4-No sample available |
| Other | K2v1-Therapeutic, K2v2-Subtherapeutic, K2v3-Undetected, K2v4-No sample available |

K3. Number of AEDs prescribed by physician.

  K3a-None

  K3b-1

  K3c-2

  K3d-3

  K3e->3

  K3f unknown

K4. Number of AEDs detected postmortem.

  K4a-None

  K4b-1

**TABLE 5.6    (*Continued*)**
**SUDEP Syndrome Cluster Identifiers K-W**

K4c-2
K4d-3
K4e->3
K5. AEDs
   K5a. Blank (was Therapeutic)
   K5b. Blank (was Subtherapeutic)
   K5c. Blank (was No AED level)
   K5d. Compliant
   K5d1 Non compliant
   K5e. Too high levels
      K5e1. No change in RX
      K5e2. Change in RX
      K5e3. No documentation
   K5f. Toxic
   K5g. Tapering & process changing
K6. AEDs withdrawn
K7. AEDs unknown
K8. No postmortem

L1. Premortem
L1a. Non AEDs
L1a1. Psychotropic drug
L1a2. Antidepressants, SSRI Celexa, Trazodone, Venlfaxine
L1a3. Antianxiety
L1a4. Alcohol
L1a5. Illicit Drugs
L1a6. Narcotics
L1a7. Antihistamines
L1a8. NSAIDS
L1a8a. Non Aspirin
L1a8b. *N*-acetylsalicylic acid (ASA)
L2. Postmortem
L2a. Non AEDs
L2a1. Psychotropic drug
L2a2. Antidepressants SSRI Celexa, Trazodone, Venlfaxine
   Venlfaxine VENL:         L1q1-Yes. K1q2-No, K1q3-Unknown
   Venlfaxine VENL:         L2q1-Therapeutic, K2q2-Subtherapeutic, K2q3-Undetected, K2q4-No sample available
L2a3. Antianxiety
L2a4. Alcohol
L2a4n. None Present
L2a5. Illicit Drugs
L2a6. Narcotics
L2a7. Antihistamines
L2a8. NSAIDS
L2a8a. Non Aspirin
L2a8b. *N*-acetylsalicylic acid (ASA)

Mnp. Normal postmortem path
Mnp3. Heart
Mnp4. Lung
Mnp5. Brain
Mnp6. Liver
Mnp7. Brain vascular

Mp. Postmortem pathology
Mp3b. Cardiomegally, Mp3c Microscopic myocardial fibrosis, Mp3d Conduction system abnormality, Mp3e Unknown

(*Continued*)

**TABLE 5.6**    (*Continued*)

## SUDEP Syndrome Cluster Identifiers K-W

Mp4. Lung pathology:

Mp4b. COPD, Mp4c Other, Mp4d Unknown, Mp4e Congestion/increased wt, Mp4f Pneumonia,

Mp5. Brain, non-epilepsy-related disease

Mp5b. Edema, Mp5c Benign tumor, Mp5d Malignant tumor, Mp5e Mesial temporal stenosis, Mp5f Other, Mp5g Unknown

Mp6. Liver, Mp6b Fatty, Mp6c Fibrosis, Mp6d Cirrhosis, Mp6e Tumor, Mp6f Unknown

Mp7. Brain vascular, Mp7aStroke, Mp7b Intracerebral hemorrhage, Mp7c Subarachnoid hemorrhage

Mp8. Posttraumatic changes (scar tissue)

Mp9. Pathology unknown

Mp10. Other

Mc. Clinical/premortem disease

Mc1c. Premortem static brain pathology: Likely etiology of seizures, M1c1. Developmental/perinatal, Mc1c2. Vascular, Mc1c3. Static benign tumor,
  Mc1c4. Posttraumatic brain injury, Mc1c4 Other, Mc1c5 Negative imaging studies, Mc1c6 Pathology unknown

Mc2. Premortem Progressive pathology: Possible contributory cause of death. Mc2a History of epilepsy, Mc2b Cardiac, Mc2d Postictal generalized EEG
  suppression (PGES) Mc2a Epilepsy, Mc2b Cardiac disease, Mc2c Pulmonary disease, Mc2e Other

Mc11. Negative imaging studies

Mc12. Hypertension

Mc13. Diabetes

Mc14. Intracranial pressure, intraocular pressure, optic nerve, vision

N. Psychological subcategories

| N1. | Stress ±/- |
| N2. | Anxiety |
| N3. | Depression |
| N4. | Bipolar |

N5. Psychiatric drugs.

N5a. Antipsychotics

N5b. Antidepressants

N5b1. SSRIs

N5b1. Other antidepressants. SNRIs, etc.

N5c. Antianxiety meds

N6. Other medications. Prinavil, ACE inhibitor antihypertensive

N7. Other psychological factors

N99. Unknown

O. Unusual, others, environment/circumstances at time of death.

O1. Climate

O2. Temperature

O3. Omega 3 FA

O4. Month of death:

O4a1-Jan, O4a2-Feb, O4a3-March, O4a4-April, O4a5-May, O4a6-June, O4a7-July, O4a8-Aug, O4a9-Sept, O4a10-Oct, O4a11-Nov, O4a12-Dec,
  o4a99 unknown

O5. Day of week:

O5a1-Monday, O5a2-Tues, O5a3-Wed, O5a4-Thur, O5a5-Fri, O5a6-Sat, O5a7Sunday, O5a99 unknown.

O6. Year of death: Actual year of death.

O7. Site of fatal event.

O7a-Home, O7b-Work, O7c-Outdoors, O7d-Driving, O7e-Phyical activity, O7f-Other

O8. Location pronounced dead.

O8a-Residence, O8b-Outdoors scene, O8c-Hospital, 08d Work, O8e Traffic, O8f. Criminal, O8g. Restraint,

O8h. Sleep–wake circadian cycle, O8i. Other, O8j.-Unknown

O9. Posture

  O9a. Prone

  O9b. Supine

  O9c. Sitting

P. Gender.

  P1-Male

  P2-Female

**TABLE 5.6   (Continued)**
**SUDEP Syndrome Cluster Identifiers K-W**

Q. Age at death.

| | |
|---|---|
| Q1. | <10 years old |
| Q2. | 10–20 |
| Q3. | 21–30 |
| Q4. | 31–40 |
| Q5. | 41–50 |
| Q6 . | 51–60 |
| Q7. | 61–70 |
| Q8. | >71 |

QS. Age at event, survive.

| | |
|---|---|
| QS1. | <10 years old |
| QS2. | 10–20 |
| QS3. | 21–30 |
| QS4. | 31–40 |
| QS5. | 41–50 |
| QS6. | 51–60 |
| QS7. | 61–70 |
| QS8. | >71 |

R. Smoking history. R1 yes, R2 no, R3 unknown

S1. Incidence of SUDEP: Report definite SUDEP and an incidence for the combination of definite SUDEP and possible SUDEP, etc. Obviously, the incidence cannot be given for just one case. When a study, such as the retrospective SUDEP study of Lathers et al. 2001 data from Allegheny County, PA, includes cases obtained from 1 geographical area (County, U.S. State, or Country) or when the author gives us the incidence, the data should be included in the Cluster ID. The incidence number will also include cases/categories of definite, probable, possible SUDEP, etc. W1–W7 and should be noted in our classification chart. In Dr. Wannamakers' study, where cases have been collected over many years, an incidence may be given, along with the number of years studied for SUDEP victims in a given practice in a given region.

See S1b. List of countries

S2. Country, states, or counties where deaths occurred

S2a. U.S. State

S2.1-Alabama
S2.2-Alaska
S2.3-Arizona
S2.4-Arkansas
S2.5-California
S2.6-Colorado
S2.7-Connecticut
S2.8-Delaware
S2.9-Florida
S2.10-Georgia
S2.11-Hawaii
S2.12-Idaho
S2.13-Illinois
S2.14-Indiana
S2.15-Iowa
S2.16-Kansas
S2.17-Kentucky
S2.18-Louisiana
S2.19-Maine
S2.20-Maryland
S2.21-Massachusetts
S2.22-Michigan
S2.23-Minnesota
S2.24-Mississippi
S2.25-Missouri

(Continued)

**TABLE 5.6    (*Continued*)**
## SUDEP Syndrome Cluster Identifiers K-W

S2.26-Montana
S2.27-Nebraska
S2.28-Nevada
S2.29-New Hampshire
S2.30-New Jersey
S2.31-New Mexico
S2.32-New York
S2.33-North Carolina
S2.34-North Dakota
S2.35-Ohio
S2.36-Oklahoman
S2.37-Orego
S2.38-Pennsylvania
S2.39-Rhode Island
S2.40-South Carolina
S2.41-South Dakota
S2.42-Tennessee
S2.43-Texas
S2.44-Utah
S2.45-Vermont
S2.46-Virginia
S2.47-Washington
S2.48-West Virginia
S2.49-Wisconsin
S2.50-Wyoming

T. Subject
T1. Human data
T2. Animal data

U. Race U1-6/Ethnicity U7
U1. Unknown
U2. Caucasian
U3. Black of African–American
U4. American Indian or Alaska Native
U5. Native Hawaiian or Other South Pacific Islander
U6. Asian
U7. Ethnicity Hispanic or Latino

V. Postmortem Examination.
V1a-Non-decomposed body: Complete external and internal postmortem autopsy with toxicological analysis
V1b-Non-decomposed body: Complete external, internal postmortem autopsy without toxicological analysis
V2a-Non-decomposed body: External examination only with toxicological analysis
V2b-Non-decomposed body: External examination only without toxicological analysis
V3a-Decomposed body: Complete external and internal postmortem autopsy with toxicological analysis
V3b-Decomposed body: Complete external and internal postmortem autopsy without toxicological analysis
V4 was V2. Genetic screen

## S1b: List of Countries

| | | | |
|---|---|---|---|
| S1b-1 Afghanistan | S1b-76 Ethiopia | S1b-151 Mauritania | S1b-226 Tajikistan |
| S1b-2 Akrotiri | S1b-77 Europa Island | S1b-152 Mauritius | S1b-227 Tanzania |
| S1b-3 Albania | S1b-78 Falkland Islands (Islas Malvinas) | S1b-153 Mayotte | S1b-228 Thailand |
| S1b-4 Algeria | S1b-79 Faroe Islands | S1b-154 Mexico | S1b-229 Timor-Leste |
| S1b-5 American Samoa | S1b-80 Fiji | S1b-155 Micronesia, Federated States of | S1b-230 Togo |

**TABLE 5.6** (*Continued*)
**S1b: List of Countries**

| | | | |
|---|---|---|---|
| S1b-6 Andorra | S1b-81 Finland | S1b-156 Moldova | S1b-231 Tokelau |
| S1b-7 Angola | S1b-82 France | S1b-157 Monaco | S1b-232 Tonga |
| S1b-8 Anguilla | S1b-83 French Guiana | S1b-158 Mongolia | S1b-233 Trinidad and Tobago |
| S1b-9 Antarctica | S1b-84 French Polynesia | S1b-159 Montserrat | S1b-234 Tromelin Island |
| S1b-10 Antigua & Barbuda | S1b-85 French Southern and Antarctic Lands | S1b-160 Morocco | S1b-235 Tunisia |
| S1b-11 Argentina | S1b-86 Gabon | S1b-161 Mozambique | S1b-236 Turkey |
| S1b-12 Armenia | S1b-87 Gambia, The | S1b-162 Namibia | S1b-237 Turkmenistan |
| S1b-13 Aruba | S1b-88 Gaza Strip | S1b-163 Nauru | S1b-238 Turks and Caicos Islands |
| S1b-14 Ashmore & Cartier Islands | S1b-89 Georgia | S1b-164 Navassa Island | S1b-239 Tuvalu |
| S1b-15 Australia | S1b-90 Germany | S1b-165 Nepal | S1b-240 Uganda |
| S1b-16 Austria | S1b-91 Ghana | S1b-166 Netherlands | S1b-241 Ukraine |
| S1b-17 Azerbaijan | S1b-92 Gibraltar | S1b-167 Netherlands Antilles | S1b-242 United Arab Emirates |
| S1b-18 Bahamas, The | S1b-93 Glorioso Islands | S1b-168 New Caledonia | S1b-243 United Kingdom |
| S1b-19 Bahrain | S1b-94 Greece | S1b-169 New Zealand | S1b-244 United States Note: Used only if the specific state where the case can from is unknown |
| S1b-20 Bangladesh | S1b-95 Greenland | S1b-170 Nicaragua | S1b-245 Uruguay |
| | | | S1b-246 Uzbekistan |
| S1b-21 Barbados | S1b-96 Grenada | S1b-171 Niger | S1b-247 Vanuatu |
| S1b-22 Bassas da India | S1b-97 Guadeloupe | S1b-172 Nigeria | S1b-248 Venezuela |
| S1b-23 Belarus | S1b-98 Guam | S1b-173 Niue | S1b-249 Vietnam |
| S1b-24 Belgium | S1b-99 Guatemala | S1b-174 Norfolk Island | S1b-250 Virgin Islands |
| S1b-25 Belize | S1b-100 Guernsey | S1b-175 Northern Mariana Islands | S1b-251 Wake Island |
| S1b-26 Benin | S1b-101 Guinea | S1b-176 Norway | S1b-252 Wallis and Futuna |
| S1b-27 Bermuda | S1b-102 Guinea-Bissau | S1b-177 Oman | S1b-253 West Bank |
| S1b-28 Bhutan | S1b-103 Guyana | S1b-178 Pakistan | S1b-254 Western Sahara |
| S1b-29 Bolivia | S1b-104 Haiti | S1b-179 Palau | S1b-255 Yemen |
| S1b-30 Bosnia & Herzegovina | S1b-105 Heard Island and McDonald Islands | S1b-180 Panama | S1b-256 Zambia |
| S1b-31 Botswana | S1b-106 Holy See (Vatican City) | S1b-181 Papua New Guinea | S1b-257 Zimbabwe |
| S1b-32 Bouvet Island | S1b-107 Honduras | S1b-182 Paracel Islands | |
| S1b-33 Brazil | S1b-108 Hong Kong | S1b-183 Paraguay | |
| S1b-34 British Indian Ocean Territory | S1b-109 Hungary | S1b-184 Peru | |
| S1b-35 British Virgin Islands | S1b-110 Iceland | S1b-185 Philippines | |
| S1b-36 Brunei | S1b-111 India | S1b-186 Pitcairn Islands | |
| S1b-37 Bulgaria | S1b-112 Indonesia | S1b-187 Poland | |
| S1b-38 Burkina Faso | S1b-113 Iran | S1b-188 Portugal | |
| S1b-39 Burma | S1b-114 Iraq | S1b-189 Puerto Rico | |
| S1b-40 Burundi | S1b-115 Ireland | S1b-190 Qatar | |
| S1b-41 Cambodia | S1b-116 Isle of Man | S1b-191 Reunion | |
| S1b-42 Cameroon | S1b-117 Israel | S1b-192 Romania | |
| S1b-43 Canada | S1b-118 Italy | S1b-193 Russia | |
| S1b-44 Cape Verde | S1b-119 Jamaica | S1b-194 Rwanda | |
| S1b-45 Cayman Islands | S1b-120 Jan Mayen | S1b-195 Saint Helena | |
| S1b-46 Central African Republic | S1b-121 Japan | S1b-196 Saint Kitts and Nevis | |
| S1b-47 Chad | S1b-122 Jersey | S1b-197 Saint Lucia | |
| S1b-48 Chile | S1b-123 Jordan | S1b-198 Saint Pierre and Miquelon | |
| S1b-49 China | S1b-124 Juan de Nova Island | S1b-199 Saint Vincent and the Grenadines | |

(*Continued*)

**TABLE 5.6    (Continued)**

**S1b: List of Countries**

S1b-50 Christmas Island

S1b-51 Clipperton Island

S1b-52 Cocos (Keeling) Islands

S1b-53 Colombia

S1b-54 Comoros

S1b-55 Congo, Democratic
Republic of the

S1b-56 Congo, Republic of the

S1b-57 Cook Islands

S1b-58 Coral Sea Islands

S1b-59 Costa Rica

S1b-60 Cote d'Ivoire

S1b-61 Croatia

S1b-62 Cuba

S1b-63 Cyprus

S1b-64 Czech Republic

S1b-65 Denmark

S1b-66 Dhekelia

S1b-67 Djibouti

S1b-68 Dominica

S1b-69 Dominican Republic

S1b-70 Ecuador

S1b-71 Egypt

S1b-72 El Salvador

S1b-73 Equatorial Guinea

S1b-74 Eritrea

S1b-75 Estonia

S1b-125 Kazakhstan

S1b-126 Kenya

S1b-127 Kiribati

S1b-128 Korea, North

S1b-129 Korea, South

S1b-130 Kuwait

S1b-131 Kyrgyzstan

S1b-132 Laos

S1b-133 Latvia

S1b-134 Lebanon

S1b-135 Lesotho

S1b-136 Liberia

S1b-137 Libya

S1b-138 Liechtenstein

S1b-139 Lithuania

S1b-140 Luxembourg

S1b-141 Macau

S1b-142 Macedonia

S1b-143 Madagascar

S1b-144 Malawi

S1b-145 Malaysia

S1b-146 Maldives

S1b-147 Mali

S1b-148 Malta

S1b-149 Marshall Islands

S1b-150 Martinique

S1b-200 Samoa

S1b-201 San Marino

S1b-202 Sao Tome and Principe

S1b-203 Saudi Arabia

S1b-204 Senegal

S1b-205 Serbia and Montenegro

S1b-206 Seychelles

S1b-207 Sierra Leone

S1b-208 Singapore

S1b-209 Slovakia

S1b-210 Slovenia

S1b-211 Solomon Islands

S1b-212 Somalia

S1b-213 South Africa

S1b-214 South Georgia and the
South Sandwich Islands

S1b-215 Spain

S1b-216 Spratly Islands

S1b-217 Sri Lanka

S1b-218 Sudan

S1b-219 Suriname

S1b-220 Svalbard

S1b-221 Swaziland

S1b-222 Sweden

S1b-223 Switzerland

S1b-224 Syria

S1b-225 Taiwan

**TABLE 5.7**

**Normal Weights of Internal Organs, Standard Deviation and Range for Males**

(Age)

(Organ)

(Standard Deviation)

(Range)

| | 11–20 | 21–30 | 31–40 | 41–50 | 51–60 |
|---|---|---|---|---|---|
| Brain | 1315 | 1340 | 1337 | 1334 | 1309 |
| | 133.14 | 113 | 110 | 120 | 118 |
| | 870–1500 | 1040–160 | 1080–1640 | 1030–1550 | 1000–1590 |
| R. Lung | 445 | 579 | 609 | 621 | 607 |
| | 99 | 151 | 163 | 162 | 171 |
| | 195–530 | 210–580 | 210–835 | 260–755 | 230–760 |
| L. Lung | 411 | 532 | 548 | 555 | 540 |
| | 104 | 146 | 156 | 160 | 183 |
| | 172–510 | 180–545 | 205–810 | 235–730 | 210–745 |
| Heart | 248 | 289 | 301 | 315 | 319 |
| | 62 | 55 | 58 | 68 | 81 |
| | 90–420 | 140–440 | 180–465 | 120–480 | 130–490 |
| R. Kidney | 114 | 129 | 137 | 133 | 131 |
| | 24 | 22 | 32 | 30 | 32 |
| | 50–145 | 56–180 | 78–265 | 60–260 | 80–290 |

**TABLE 5.7   (Continued)**
**Normal Weights of Internal Organs, Standard Deviation and Range for Males**

(Age)
(Organ)
(Standard Deviation)
(Range)

| | 11–20 | 21–30 | 31–40 | 41–50 | 51–60 |
|---|---|---|---|---|---|
| L. Kidney | 124 | 139 | 146 | 141 | 142 |
| | 25 | 23 | 31 | 35 | 30 |
| | 55–160 | 65–190 | 75–295 | 70–280 | 100–260 |
| Liver | 1420 | 1494 | 1545 | 1591 | 1486 |
| | 175 | 169 | 361 | 269 | 109 |
| | 909–1645 | 835–1816 | 903–1890 | 1120–2032 | 830–1588 |
| Spleen | 130 | 162 | 164 | 169 | 146 |
| | 30 | 43 | 63 | 70 | 28 |
| | 70–180 | 76–270 | 89–316 | 110–330 | 102–310 |
| Pancreas | 106 | 131 | 132 | 133 | 130 |
| | 14 | 33 | 19 | 22 | 10 |
| | 80–127 | 80–144 | 71–165 | 112–190 | 115–145 |

*Source:*   Koehler, SA, *Forensic Epidemiology*, CRC Press, Boca Raton, FL, 2010.
*Note:*   The weight of female organs are 10% less than males.

## CONSTRUCT RISK FACTOR IDENTIFICATIONS

The first step and last check is to select one category W1–W7. Step 2: Identify which mechanistic risk factor(s) for death via SUDEP appears to be appropriate for a given patient or victim. Read left to right and select 1 for brain, 2 for cardiac, and/or 3 for respiratory & hypoxia pathophysiologic mechanisms pertinent to a given case; some victims have more than one mechanism. Note that scoring interaction terms will increase data needs approximately exponentially. Select category 4 if unknown. For each case dead or alive (W1 to W7), select all relevant categorical subsets of risk factor identifiers A through W in SUDEP Cluster Chart.

## RISK CLUSTERS FOR SUDEP

Classification methods, such as recursive partitioning, will be used for exploratory data analysis and initial rule generation for predictive modeling of SUDEP from the Cluster Risk Factors. These preliminary results can be used to create subsets for more advanced modeling. Given the large number of variables defined in our risk factor method, 100% match of identical groups is expected to be very rare. The purpose of modeling using partitioning, logistic regression, or whatever tool, is to sort out the probabilities in one group vs. another. Not even the best diagnostic screening methods or assays have 100% sensitivity and specificity. Evaluation will be done for overlap of Cluster IDs among groups. Cases illustrate SUDEP Cluster IDs in Chapter 8. Retrospective Preliminary Data epilepsy cases or SUDEP victims total 115–174 cases with Cluster ID risk factor data found in

Chapters 6 through 10. Cluster IDs for animal models to study SUDEP are found in Chapters 11 and 12.

Table 5.1 presents SUDEP Syndrome Cluster Risk Identifiers, Risk Factor Classification Method developed by Lathers et al. (2015).

We developed 7 categories for persons who died and for those alive. The first 5 categories include: W. SUDEP definite (W1), SUDEP probable (W2), possible SUDEP (W3), or non-SUDEP (W5): All people who died. For living people with epilepsy, there are three categories for classification: SUDEP prevented (W4) or a person who is alive and diagnosed with epilepsy and must be medically evaluated to determine what preventive actions should be taken in the day-to-day events to protect the person from becoming a victim of SUDEP at some time in the future; this person is classified in the sixth category of W6. W7 is a survivor, non epileptic.

W1: Definite SUDEP with postmortem
W2: Probable SUDEP with or without postmortem
W3: Possible SUDEP
W4: SUDEP prevented: For living people with epilepsy
W5: Non-SUDEP victims who were thought to have epilepsy but did not or were diagnosed with epilepsy but died of another cause such as a glial brain tumor
W6: Diagnosed with epilepsy and must be medically evaluated to determine what preventive actions should be taken in the day-to-day events to protect the person from becoming a victim of SUDEP at some time in the future
W7: Survivor, non epilepsy

## REFERENCES

Alkadhi KA, Alzoubi KH. Synaptic plasticity of autonomic ganglia: Role of chronic stress and implication in cardiovascular disease and sudden death. Chapter 26 In: Lathers CM, Schraeder PL, Bungo MW, Leestma JE, editors. *Sudden Death in Epilepsy: Forensic and Clinical Issues*. Boca Raton, FL: CRC Press/Taylor & Francis; 2011, pp. 395–426.

Aridon P, Marini C, Di Resta C, Brilli E, De Fusco M, Politi F, Parrini E, Manfredi I, Pisano T, Pruna D, Curia G, Cianchetti C, Pasqualetti M, Becchetti A, Guerrini R, Casari G. Increased sensitivity of the neuronal nicotinic receptor alpha 2 subunit causes familial epilepsy with nocturnal wandering and ictal fear. *Am J Hum Genet* 2006 Aug;79(2):342–50.

Aurlien D, Taubøll E, Gjerstad L. Lamotrigine in idiopathic epilepsy-increased risk of cardiac death? *Acta Neurol Scand* 2007;115(3):199–203.

Baulac S, Huberfeld G, Gourfinkel-An I, Mitropoulou G, Beranger A, Prud'homme JF, Baulac M, Brice A, Bruzzone R, LeGuern E. First genetic evidence of GABA(A) receptor dysfunction in epilepsy: A mutation in the gamma2-subunit gene. *Nat Genet* 2001;28(1):46–8.

Bealer SL, Metcalf CS, Little JG, Vatta M, Brewster A, Anderson AE. Sympathetic nervous system dysregulation of cardiac function and myocyte potassium channel remodeling in rodent seizure models: Candidate mechanism for SUDEP. Chapter 38 In: Lathers CM, Schraeder PL, Bungo MW, Leestma JE, eds. *Sudden Death in Epilepsy: Forensic and Clinical Issues*. Boca Raton, FL: CRC Press/Taylor & Francis; 2011, pp. 333–46.

Calderazzo L, Arida RM, Cysneiros RM, Cavalheiro EA, Scorza FA. From sardines to salmon: Influence of climate fluctuations on sudden unexpected death in epilepsy. *Epilepsy Behav* 2009;14(3):567–8.

Carnel SB, Schaeder PL, Lathers CM. Effect of phenobarbital pretreatment on cardiac neural discharge and pentylenetetrazol-induced epileptogenic activity in the cat. *Pharmacology* 1985;30(4):225–40.

Charlier C, Singh NA, Ryan SG, Lewis TB, Reus BE, Leach RJ, Leppert M. A pore mutation in a novel KQT-like potassium channel gene in an idiopathic epilepsy family. *Nat Genet* 1998;18(1):53–5.

Chen L, Marquardt ML, Tester DJ, Sampson KJ, Ackerman MJ, and Kass RS. Mutation of an A-kinase-anchoring protein causes long-QT syndrome. *Proc Natl Acad Sci U S A* 2007;104(52):20990–5.

Claes L, Del-Favero J, Ceulemans B, Lagae L, Van Broeckhoven C, De Jonghe P. De novo mutations in the sodium-channel gene SCN1A cause severe myoclonic epilepsy of infancy. *Am J Hum Genet* 2001;68(6):1327–32. Epub 2001 May 15.

Claycamp HG. Decision analysis and risk management. Chapter 55 In: Lathers CM, Schraeder PL, Bungo MW, Leestma JE, eds. *Sudden Death in Epilepsy: Forensic and Clinical Issues*. Boca Raton, FL: CRC Press/Taylor & Francis; 2011, pp. 887–904.

Cossette P, Liu L, Brisebois K, Dong H, Lortie A, Vanasse M, Saint-Hilaire JM, Carmant L, Verner A, Lu WY, Wang YT, Rouleau GA. Mutation of GABRA1 in an autosomal dominant form of juvenile myoclonic epilepsy. *Nat Genet* 2002;31(2):184–9.

De Fusco M, Becchetti A, Patrignani A, Annesi G, Gambardella A, Quattrone A, Ballabio A, Wanke E, Casari G. The nicotinic receptor beta 2 subunit is mutant in nocturnal frontal lobe epilepsy. *Nat Genet* 2000;26(3):275–6.

Dhillon PS, Behr ER. Sudden Arrhythmogenic, respiratory, and psychological risk factors for sudden unexpected death and epilepsy: Case histories. Chapter 45, In: Lathers CM, Schraeder PL, Bungo MW, Leestma JE, eds. *Sudden Death in Epilepsy: Forensic and Clinical Issues*. Boca Raton, FL: CRC Press/Taylor & Francis; 2011, pp. 721–742.

Dodd-O JM, Lathers CM. Characterization of lock step phenomenon. Chapter 29 In: Lathers CM, Schraeder PL, Bungo MW, Leestma JE, eds. *Sudden Death in Epilepsy: Forensic and Clinical Issues*. Boca Raton, FL: CRC Press/Taylor & Francis; 2011, pp. 465–80.

Escayg A, MacDonald BT, Meisler MH, Baulac S, Huberfeld G, An-Gourfinkel I, Brice A, LeGuern E, Moulard B, Chaigne D, Buresi C, Malafosse A. Mutations of SCN1A, encoding a neuronal sodium channel, in two families with GEFS+2. *Nat Genet* 2000 Apr;24(4):343–5.

Finsterer J, Stollesburg C. Cardiac and pulmonary risk factors and pathomechanisms of sudden unexplained death in epilepsy patients. Chapter 42 In: Lathers CM, Schraeder PL, Bungo MW, Leestma JE, eds. *Sudden Death in Epilepsy: Forensic and Clinical Issues*. Boca Raton, FL: CRC Press/Taylor & Francis; 2011, pp. 679–92.

Ghali N, Nashef L. Genetics of sudden death in epilepsy. Chapter 18 In: Lathers CM, Schraeder PL, Bungo MW, Leestma JE, eds. *Sudden Death in Epilepsy: Forensic and Clinical Issues*. Boca Raton, FL: CRC Press/Taylor & Francis; 2011, pp. 267–283.

Hanna J, Panelli R. Challenges in overcoming ethical, legal, and communication barriers. Chapter 58 In: Lathers CM, Schraeder PL, Bungo MW, Leestma JE, eds. *Sudden Death in Epilepsy: Forensic and Clinical Issues*. Boca Raton, FL: CRC Press/Taylor & Francis Group; 2011, pp. 915–36.

Harkin LA, Bowser DN, Dibbens LM, Singh R, Phillips F, Wallace RH, Richards MC, Williams DA, Mulley JC, Berkovic SF, Scheffer IE, Petrou S. Truncation of the GABA(A)-receptor gamma2 subunit in a family with generalized epilepsy with febrile seizures plus. *Am J Hum Genet* 2002;70(2):530–6.

Haug K, Warnstedt M, Alekov AK, Sander T, Ramírez A, Poser B, Maljevic S, Hebeisen S, Kubisch C, Rebstock J, Horvath S, Hallmann K, Dullinger JS, Rau B, Haverkamp F, Beyenburg S, Schulz H, Janz D, Giese B, Müller-Newen G, Propping P, Elger CE, Fahlke C, Lerche H, Heils A. Mutations in CLCN2 encoding a voltage-gated chloride channel are associated with idiopathic generalized epilepsies. *Nat Genet* 2003;33(4):527–32.

Hedley PL, Jorgensen P, Schlamowitz S, Moolman-Smook J, Kanters JK, Corfield VA, and Christiansen M. The genetic basis of Brugada syndrome: A mutation update. *Hum Mutat* 2009;30(9):1256–66.

Heron SE, Crossland KM, Andermann E, Phillips HA, Hall AJ, Bleasel A, Shevell M, Mercho S, Seni MH, Guiot MC, Mulley JC, Berkovic SF, Scheffer IE. Sodium-channel defects in benign familial neonatal-infantile seizures. *Lancet* 2002;360(9336):851–2.

Herreros B. Cardiac channelopathies and sudden death. Chapter 19 In: Lathers CM, Schraeder PL, Bungo MW, Leestma JE, eds. *Sudden Death in Epilepsy: Forensic and Clinical Issues*. Boca Raton, FL: CRC Press/Taylor & Francis; 2011, pp. 285–302.

Hofman N, Wilde AA, and Tan HL. Diagnostic criteria for congenital long QT syndrome in the era of molecular genetics: Do we need a scoring system? *Eur Heart J* 2007;28(11):1399.

Hughes JD, Sato S. Sudden death in epilepsy: Relationship to sleep-wake circadian cycle and fractal physiology. Chapter 23 In: Lathers CM, Schraeder PL, Bungo MW, Leestma JE, eds.

*Sudden Death in Epilepsy: Forensic and Clinical Issues*. Boca Raton, FL: CRC Press/Taylor & Francis; 2011, pp. 333–46.

Jay GW, Leestma JE. Sudden death in epilepsy: A comprehensive review of the literature and proposed mechanisms. *Acta Neurol Scand* 1981;63(Suppl 82):S1–66.

Johnston SC, Horn JK, Valente J, Simon RP. The role of hypoventilation in a sheep model of epileptic sudden death. *Ann Neurol* 1995;37:531–7.

Johnston SC, Siedenberg R, Min JK, Jerome EH, Laxer KD. Central apnea and acute cardiac ischemia in a sheep model of epileptic sudden death. *Ann Neurol* 1997;42:588–94.

Kalachikov S, Evgrafov O, Ross B, Winawer M, Barker-Cummings C, Martinelli Boneschi F, Choi C, Morozov P, Das K, Teplitskaya E, Yu A, Cayanis E, Penchaszadeh G, Kottmann AH, Pedley TA, Hauser WA, Ottman R, Gilliam TC. Mutations in LGI1 cause autosomal-dominant partial epilepsy with auditory features. *Nat Genet* 2002;30(3):335–41.

Koehler SA. Normal weights of the internal organs, standard deviation and range for males. *Forensic Epidemiology*. Boca Raton, FL: CRC Press; 2010.

Koehler SA, Schraeder PL, Lathers CM Wecht CH. One-year postmortem forensic analysis of deaths in persons with epilepsy. Chapter 9 In: Lathers CM, Schraeder PL, Bungo MW, Leestma JE, eds. *Sudden Death in Epilepsy: Forensic and Clinical Issues*. Boca Raton, FL: CRC Press/Taylor & Francis; 2011, pp. 145–59.

Lathers CM. Arrhythmogenic, respiratory and psychological risk factors for sudden unexpected death in epilepsy: Case histories. Chapter 44 In: Lathers CM, Schraeder PL, Bungo MW, Leestma JE, eds. *Sudden Death in Epilepsy: Forensic and Clinical Issues*. Boca Raton, FL: CRC Press/Taylor & Francis; 2011, pp. 713–14.

Lathers CM, Koehler SA, Wecht CH, Schraeder PL. Forensic antiepileptic drug levels in autopsy cases of epilepsy. *Epilepsy Behav* 2011;22(4):778–85.

Lathers CM, Leestma JE, Schachter SC, Verrier R, Koehler SA, Claycamp HG, Wannamaker BB, Schraeder PL. SUDEP syndrome related cluster risk identification. Journal to be determined. 2015 1–149, A1.

Lathers CM, Schraeder PL. Animal model for sudden unexpected death in persons with epilepsy. Chapter 27 In: Lathers CM, Schraeder PL, Bungo MW, Leestma JE, eds. *Sudden Death in Epilepsy: Forensic and Clinical Issues*. Boca Raton, FL: CRC Press/Taylor & Francis; 2011, pp. 437–64.

Lathers CM, Schraeder PL. Antiepileptic drugs benefit/risk clinical pharmacology: Possible role in cause and/or prevention of SUDEP. Chapter 47 In: Lathers CM, Schraeder PL, Bungo MW, Leestma JE, eds. *Sudden Death in Epilepsy: Forensic and Clinical Issues*. Boca Raton, FL: CRC Press/Taylor & Francis; 2011, pp. 755–89.

Lathers CM, Schraeder PL. Autonomic dysfunction in epilepsy: Characterization of autonomic cardiac neural discharge associated with pentylenetetrazol-induced epileptogenic activity. *Epilepsia* 1982;23(6):633–47.

Lathers CM, Schraeder PL. Review of autonomic dysfunction, cardiac arrhythmias, and epileptogenic activity. *J Clin Pharmacol* 1987 May–Jun;27(5):346–56.

Lathers CM, Schraeder PL. Clinical Pharmacology: Drugs as a benefit and/or risk in sudden unexpected death in epilepsy? *J Clin Pharmacol* 2002;42:123–36.

Lathers CM, Schraeder PL. Stress and sudden death. *Epilepsy Behav* 2006;9(2):236–42.

Lathers CM, Schraeder PL, Bungo MW. The mystery of sudden death: Mechanisms for risks. *Epilepsy Behav* 2008;12(1):3–24.

Lathers CM, Schraeder PL, Bungo MW. Neurocardiologic mechanistic risk factors in sudden unexpected death in epilepsy. Chapter 1 In: Lathers CM, Schraeder PL, Bungo MW, Leestma JE, eds. *Sudden Death in Epilepsy: Forensic and Clinical Issues*. Boca Raton, FL: CRC Press/Taylor & Francis; 2011, pp. 3–36.

Lathers CM, Schraeder PL, Bungo MW. Unanswered questions: SUDEP clinical studies needed. Chapter 4 In: Lathers CM, Schraeder PL, Bungo MW, Leestma JE, eds. *Sudden Death in Epilepsy: Forensic and Clinical Issues*. Boca Raton, FL: CRC Press/Taylor & Francis; 2011, pp. 67–76.

Lathers CM, Schraeder PL, Bungo MW. Syncope, seizures and SUDEP: Case histories. Chapter 22 In: Lathers CM, Schraeder PL, Bungo MW, Leestma JE, eds. *Sudden Death in Epilepsy: Forensic and Clinical Issues*. Boca Raton, FL: CRC Press/Taylor & Francis; 2011, pp. 325–32.

Lathers CM, Schraeder PL, Claycamp HG. Clinical pharmacology of topiramate versus lamotrigine versus phenobarbital and side effects using odds ratios. *J Clin Pharmacol* 2003;43(5):491.

Lathers CM, Schraeder PL, Claycamp HG. Odds ratios study of antiepileptic drugs: A possible approach to SUDEP prevention? Chapter 46 In: Lathers CM, Schraeder PL, Bungo MW, Leestma JE, eds. *Sudden Death in Epilepsy: Forensic and Clinical Issues*. Boca Raton, FL: CRC Press/Taylor & Francis; 2011, pp. 743–54.

Lathers CM, Schraeder PL, Weiner FL. Synchronization of cardiac autonomic neural discharge with epileptogenic activity: The lock step phenomenon. *Electroencephalogr Clin Neurophysiol* 1987;67(3):247–59.

Leestma JE, Walczak T, Hughes JR, Kalelkar MB, Teas SS. A prospective study on sudden unexpected death in epilepsy. *Ann Neurol* 1989;26(2):195–203.

Mameli O, Alessandro CM. Sudden epileptic death in experimental animal models. In: Lathers CM, Schraeder PL, Bungo MW, Leestma JE, eds. *Sudden Death in Epilepsy: Forensic and Clinical Issues*. Boca Raton, FL: CRC Press/Taylor & Francis; 2011, pp. 591–614.

Neville KA, Blake MJ, Reed MD, Kearns GL. Pediatric pharmacology. Chapter 17 In: Waldman SA, Terzik A, eds. *Pharmacology and Therapeutics: Principles to Practice*. Philadelphia, PA: Saunders, Elsevier; 2009, p. 240.

O'Rourke D, Lathers CM. Interspike interval histogram characterization of synchronized cardiac sympathetic neural discharge and epileptogenic activity in electrocorticogram of cat. Chapter 31 In: Lathers CM, Schraeder PL, Bungo MW, Leestma JE, eds. *Sudden Death in Epilepsy: Forensic and Clinical Issues*. Boca Raton, FL: CRC Press/Taylor & Francis; 2011, pp. 495–512.

Ryvlin P, Tomson T, Montavont A. Excess mortality and sudden unexpected death in epilepsy. *Presse Med* 2009;38(6):905–10.

Schraeder PL, Lathers CM. Cardiac neural discharge and epileptogenic activity in the cat: An animal model for unexplained death. *Life Sci* 1983;32(12):1371–82.

Schraeder PL, Lathers CM. Paroxysmal autonomic dysfunction, epileptogenic activity and sudden death. *Epilepsy Res* 1989 Jan–Feb;3(1):55–62.

Scorza FA, Albuquerque M, Arida RM, Cavalheiro EA. Sudden unexpected death in epilepsy: Are winter temperatures a new potential risk factor? *Epilepsy Behav* 2007;10(3):509–10.

Scorza FA, Cysneiros RM, Arida RM, Terra-Bustamante VC, Albuquerque M, Cavalheiro EA. The other side of the coin: beneficiary effect of omega-3 fatty acids in sudden unexpected death in epilepsy. *Epilepsy Behav* 2008;13(2):279–83.

Scorza FA, Cavalheiro EA, Arida RM, Terra-Bustamente VC, Sonoda EYF, Cysneiros, RM. Omega 3 fatty acids ins sudden unexpected death in epilepsy. Chapter 3 In: Lathers CM, Schraeder PL, Bungo MW, Leestma JE, eds. *Sudden Death in Epilepsy: Forensic and Clinical Issues.* Boca Raton, FL: CRC Press/Taylor & Francis; 2011, pp. 57–66.

Sedý J, Zicha J, Kunes J, Jendelová P, Syková E. Mechanisms of neurogenic pulmonary edema development. *Physiol Res* 2008;57(4):499–506.

Simon RP, Bayne LL, Tranbaugh RF, Lewis FR. Elevated pulmonary lymph flow and protein content during status epilepticus in sheep. *J Appl Physiol Respir Environ Exerc Physiol* 1982;52(1):91–5.

Singh NA, Charlier C, Stauffer D, DuPont BR, Leach RJ, Melis R, Ronen GM, Bjerre I, Quattlebaum T, Murphy JV, McHarg ML, Gagnon D, Rosales TO, Peiffer A, Anderson VE, Leppert M. A novel potassium channel gene, KCNQ2, is mutated in an inherited epilepsy of newborns. *Nat Genet* 1998;18(1):25–9.

So EL, Sam MC, Lagerlund TL. Postictal central apnea as a cause of SUDEP: Evidence from near-SUDEP incident. *Epilepsia* 2000;41(11):1494–7.

Splawski I, Shen J, Timothy KW, Lehmann MH, Priori S, Robinson JL, Moss AJ et al. Spectrum of mutations in long-QT syndrome genes. KVLQT1, HERG, SCN5A, KCNE1, and KCNE2. *Circulation* 2000;102(10):1178–85.

Stauffer AZ, Dodd-O JM, Lathers CM. Relationship of the lock step phenomenon and precipitous changes in mean arterial blood pressure. *Electroencephalogr Clin Neurophysiol* 1989;72(4):340–5.

Stauffer AZ, Dodd-O JM, Lathers CM. Relationship of lock step phenomenon and precipitous changes in blood pressure. Chapter 30 In: Lathers CM, Schraeder PL, Bungo MW, Leestma JE, eds. *Sudden Death in Epilepsy: Forensic and Clinical Issues.* Boca Raton, FL: CRC Press/Taylor & Francis; 2011, pp. 481–94.

Steinlein OK, Mulley JC, Propping P, Wallace RH, Phillips HA, Sutherland GR, Scheffer IE, Berkovic SF. A missense mutation in the neuronal nicotinic acetylcholine receptor alpha 4 subunit is associated with autosomal dominant nocturnal frontal lobe epilepsy. *Nat Genet* 1995;11(2):201–3.

Stewart M. The urethane/kainate seizure model as a tool to explore physiology and death associates with seizures. Chapter 39 In: Lathers CM, Schraeder PL, Bungo MW, Leestma JE, eds. *Sudden Death in Epilepsy: Forensic and Clinical Issues.* Boca Raton, FL: CRC Press/Taylor & Francis; 2011, pp. 625–45.

Striano P, Bordo L, Lispi ML, Specchio N, Minetti C, Vigevano F, Zara F. A novel SCN2A mutation in family with benign familial infantile seizures. *Epilepsia* 2006 Jan;47(1):218–20.

Terra-Bustamante VC, Scorza CA, de Albuquerque M, Sakamoto AC, Machado HR, Arida RM, Cavalheiro EA, Scorza FA. Does the lunar phase have an effect on sudden unexpected death in epilepsy? *Epilepsy Behav* 2009;14(2):404–6.

Terrence CE, Rao GR, Perper JA. Neurogenic pulmonary edema in unexpected, unexplained death in epileptic patients. *Neurol* 1981;25:594–5.

Tester DJ and Ackerman MJ. The role of molecular autopsy in unexplained sudden cardiac death. *Curr Opin Cardiol* 2006;21(3):166–72.

Tester DJ, Ackerman MJ. Postmortem long QT syndrome genetic testing for sudden unexplained death in the young. *J Am Coll Cardiol* 2007;49(2):240–46.

Tester DJ, Will ML, Haglund CM, and Ackerman MJ. Compendium of cardiac channel mutations in 541 consecutive unrelated patients referred for long QT syndrome genetic testing. *Heart Rhythm* 2005;2(5):507–17.

Tomson T. Compliance with antiepileptic drug treatment and the risk of sudden unexpected death in epilepsy. Chapter 51 In: Lathers CM, Schraeder PL, Bungo MW, Leestma JE, eds. *Sudden Death in Epilepsy: Forensic and Clinical Issues.* Boca Raton, FL: CRC Press/Taylor & Francis; 2011, pp. 845–52.

Ueda K, Valdivia, Medeiros-Domingo A, Tester DJ, Vatta M, Farrugia G, Ackerman MJ, and Makielski JC. Syntrophin mutation associated with long QT syndrome through activation of the nNOS-SCN5A macromolecular complex. *Proc Natl Acad Sci U S A* 2008;105(27):9355–60.

Verrier RL, Schachter SC. Neurocardiac interactions in sudden unexpected death in epilepsy: Can ambulatory electrocardiogram-based assessment of autonomic function and T-wave alternans help to predict risk? Chapter 43 In: Lathers CM, Schraeder PL, Bungo MW, Leestma JE, eds. *Sudden Death in Epilepsy: Forensic and Clinical Issues.* Boca Raton, FL: CRC Press/Taylor & Francis; 2011, pp. 693–710.

Walczak TS. Risk factors for sudden death in epilepsy. Chapter 12 In: Lathers CM, Schraeder PL, Bungo MW, Leestma JE, eds. *Sudden Death in Epilepsy: Forensic and Clinical Issues.* Boca Raton, FL: CRC Press/Taylor & Francis; 2011, pp. 187–200.

Wallace RH, Wang DW, Singh R, Scheffer IE, George AL Jr, Phillips HA, Saar K, Reis A, Johnson EW, Sutherland GR, Berkovic SF, Mulley JC. Febrile seizures and generalized epilepsy associated with a mutation in the Na+-channel beta1 subunit gene SCN1B. *Nat Genet* 1998;19(4):366–70.

Wannamaker BB. SUDEP: Medicolegal and clinical experiences. Chapter 24 In: Lathers CM, Schraeder PL, Bungo MW, Leestma JE, eds. *Sudden Death in Epilepsy: Forensic and Clinical Issues.* Boca Raton, FL: CRC Press/Taylor & Francis; 2011, pp. 347–62.

# 6 Forensic Cases Classified as SUDEP Cluster Risk Factor Identifiers

*Claire M. Lathers, Paul L. Schraeder, and Steven A. Koehler*

## CONTENTS

The purpose of the current chapter is to use our published data in the literature with our new methodological tool to construct Cluster Risk Factors IDs for our Allegheny SUDEP study (Koehler et al. 2011; Lathers et al. 2011). We used the Risk Factors in Table 5.1 in Chapter 5, and the data from our Allegheny Study of 2001 (Lathers et al. 2011) to develop a Cluster ID scored summary of the 12 deaths in this study. Please note that although our published 2011 SUDEP studies reported on antiepileptic drug (AED) levels found postmortem, in this chapter we are not focused on the forensic AED levels. A brief discussion of the AED findings is included here. The AED data are published in 2011 by Lathers et al. and Koehler et al. In Chapter 32 of this book, Tomson discusses compliance, AEDs and SUDEP. The role of AEDs and SUDEP is also discussed in Chapters 1 through 10, 12, 15, 16, 17, and 34. Part of the published method and results of our Allegheny SUDEP paper published in 2011 follows.

## METHOD TO CONSTRUCT SUDEP CLUSTER RISK FACTOR, IDENTIFIERS USING 2001 ALLEGHENY COUNTY, PA, OF THE CORONER'S OFFICE

Lathers et al. (2011) published "Retrospective SUDEP Study: Forensic Antiepileptic Drug Levels in Autopsy Cases of Epilepsy" in *Epilepsy and Behavior*. A one-year retrospective coroner-based forensic examination of causes of death among persons with a history of epilepsy were examined at the Allegheny County Coroner's Office to evaluate for the phenomenon of sudden unexpected death in epilepsy (SUDEP), a diagnosis of exclusion. All cases were examined at the Coroner's Office from January 1, 2001 through December 31, 2001. The Allegheny County Coroner's Office has forensic jurisdiction to investigate all deaths within Allegheny County, located in Western Pennsylvania, which encompasses a population of ~1.2 million. The office investigates over 6000 cases and conducts over 1200 autopsies

annually. All deaths investigated by the office from January 1, 2001 to December 31, 2001 were reviewed. Allegheny County Coroner's Office protocol defined how this study was conducted. All cases with a history of seizure disorders indicated in the past medical history or the word "seizure" or phrase "seizure disorder" listed in Part I or Part II of the death certificate were identified by conducting a computer analysis and a hand search of the case files by the forensic epidemiologist. The information available for review included the data contained within the Death Investigation Report, the death certificate, and the available medical records. Inclusion criteria included all cases where seizure was listed in either Part 1: Immediate Cause of Death or in Part 2: Conditions Contributing to the Death on the death certificate. This study began with identifying all death certificates with "seizure" listed on it and worked backward. One hundred percent of the cases were listed as having a diagnosis of seizures. None of the cases listed epilepsy on the death certificates with differentiation of type of seizure. The final conclusion was "yes" or "no" for SUDEP based on the postmortem data. All seizure types would be grouped together in the category of seizures on the death certificates and reinforces one of the most important issues in determining SUDEP as a cause of death, namely, the incomplete nature of the history of type and frequency of seizures in the victims, including those subjected to autopsy. Although the presence of intractable epilepsy and the history of grand mal seizures have been described as two of the most important factors for SUDEP, this type of information relative to this differentiation was not available in the death certificates. The following epidemiological information was collected: Age, sex, race, and time/date last seen alive, and the time/date of death. Seizure-related information collected included past medical history, a list of prescribed medications including all AED medications, and who witnessed the event. Pathological information collected was obtained from the forensic autopsy report.

Toxicological analysis was conducted on the blood, bile, urine, and eye fluid recovered during autopsy. The blood used for the toxicological analysis was collected from the heart during autopsy. The number and level of drugs detected in the body fluids were obtained from the Toxicological Report. The toxicological analysis included the number of detected drugs, blood concentration, and determination if the levels were therapeutic, subtherapeutic, above the therapeutic range, or absent. The data were entered and analysis by Statistical Package for the Social Services® software (11.0) (Chicago, IL). The toxicological data for all deaths with a diagnosis of epilepsy were summarized. On the basis of the data, the cases that met the criteria for SUDEP were identified.

## CLUSTER RISK FACTOR METHOD USING RETROSPECTIVE SUDEP AUTOPSY STUDY

To construct Cluster Risk Factor IDs for the above study (Koehler et al. 2011; Lathers et al. 2011), we used the Risk Factor in Table 6.1 and data from Tables 6.2 through 6.5 in the Allegheny Study of 2001 (Lathers et al. 2011), filled in blank Table 6.6 to create data in Tables 6.1 and 6.7 of this chapter and developed a scored summary of the 12 deaths in this study using the Cluster Risk Factors in Table 5.1. For example, our SUDEP Cluster Risk Factor ID methodology in Table 5.1 demonstrates the use of Cluster ID for AEDs prescribed prescriptions as K1a1 for yes, given AED benzodiazepines were prescribed. K1a2 for no and K1a3 for unknown. Cluster ID K2b1 indicates postmortem toxicology found therapeutic levels, K2a2 subtherapeutic, K2a3 undetected, K2a4 no sample available. Cluster ID K3 is the number of AEDs prescribed by the physician, K4 is the number of AEDs detected postmortem. Cluster ID K5d is for compliant, K5d1 for noncompliant, K5e too high levels, K5e1 no changes in Rx, and K5e2 change in Rx, with K5e3 no documentation. K5f is toxic, K5g tampering and process changing AED, K6 AEDs withdrawn, K7 AEDs unknown, and K8 no postmortem. Use the SUDEP Cluster Chart in Table 5.1 to find appropriate Cluster IDs for all SUDEP risk factors.

Thus, Table 6.1 is an example of SUDEP Cluster ID methodology using actual data from Tables 6.2 through 6.5 Allegheny Study of 2001 (Lathers et al 2011; Koehler et al. 2011). Full discussion of data is found in the published studies of Lathers et al. (2011) and Koehler et al. in 2011 SUDEP book (editors Lathers, Schraeder, Bungo, and Leestma). Note that the attending neurologist, emergency medical physician, and/or personnel from the medical examiner's or coroner's offices may use data such as those found in Tables 6.2 through 6.5 to fill in the blank form in Table 6.6 to identify known risk factors and categories for a given patient with epilepsy: Alive or dead and to build the Cluster IDs in Tables 6.1 and 6.7.

## RESULTS RETROSPECTIVE SUDEP STUDY 2001 ALLEGHENY COUNTY, PA

A total of 1200 autopsied deaths revealed 12 cases with a past medical history of seizure disorder on death certificates that listed seizure disorder as the immediate cause of death or contributory cause of the death. Of the seven males with seizure disorders, five were categorized as definite SUDEP and two as possible SUDEP. Of the five females with seizure disorders, two were listed as definite SUDEP, two as possible SUDEP, and one as not SUDEP as the convulsive seizures developed from a Grade II Glial tumor. Postmortem findings were evaluated for 11 cases; 1 body was decomposed.

### DATA SUMMARY

- 1-year forensic retrospective study of death certificates/coroner autopsies for SUDEP
- 12 of 1200: Persons with epilepsy history and/or seizures
- Deaths: 11 SUDEP, 1 grade II glial tumor
- 7 M: 5 definite SUDEP, 2 possible; 5 F: 2 definite, 2 possible, 1 not
- AED levels blood, bile, urine, eye fluids in all 12, with 7 detectable, 5 no AEDs
- AED levels detected in 7: 4 subtherapeutic, 2 therapeutic, 1 above therapeutic
- 1 decomposed body, no postmortem.

### INCIDENCE OF SUDEP: 0.917%

Incidence of SUDEP: 0.917%. 11 of 1200 autopsied cases. 12 identified with a medical history of seizure disorder on death certificates. Seizure was listed as immediate or contributory to death. 11 of 12 deemed definite or probable SUSWP, 1 non-SUDEP.

Table 6.7 summarizes all 12 death categories (W1-7) for the 2001 Allegheny County SUDEP study. The 99 stands for unknown information. Risk Factor Cluster Identifiers are from Table 5.1 nclude A and C Brain unknown Epilepsy Localization Categories. B99 stands for Refractory unknown. D99 means that the age of onset of epilepsy is unknown. E99 refers to the fact that the frequency of seizures before and near to the time of death is unknown. F99 means that cardiac arrhythomogenic risks are unknown. G99 cardiac unknown, I99 syncope unknown, J99 genetic structural channelopathies unknown, N99 refers to unknown status of psychological risk factors such as stress, anxiety, depression, biopolar disorder, etc. O99 refers to the fact that unusual, others, environment/circumstances at time of death were not known. In particular, O4 is the month of death and O5 is the day of the week, and both are unknown.

Note that H99 for respiratory and hypoxia pathology unknown is not in Table 6.2 as lung autopsies were done; these data appear in Table 6.1. Likewise, AEDS, K, and non AEDs, L, were analyzed for postmortem and are in Table 6.1. Risk factor M was addressed by the coroners' office and appears in Table 6.1. The numerous unknown risk factor parameters in Table 6.7 reveal the lack of data even with a coroners' office conducting the examination of

**TABEL 6.1**

**SUDEP Allegheny Study (Lathers et al. 2011; Koehler et al. 2011). Variables A–E, F–J, K, L, M, Mnp, N, Q, T, U, and V**

| W1-7 W1 Definite SUDEP | Brain Path 1 | Cardiac Path 2 | Respiratory Hypoxia Path 3 | A-E, F-J | K AED | L Postmortem non AED | Mnp Normal Postmortem | M Concomitant diseases Mp Mc | N | Q Age T, U | V post-mortem |
|---|---|---|---|---|---|---|---|---|---|---|---|
| Males P1 Case # 1 | 1 Sz disorder Mp7, Mp7c (SAH) | 2, Mp3, Mp3b | 3, Mp4, Mp4e | A | K1L1, K2L3, K3b, K4a, | L2a4 | | M, Mp7, Mp7c, Mp3, Mp3b, Mp4, Mp4e | N99 | 46 Q5 | V3a |
| # 2 | 1 Sz disorder | 2, Mp3, Mp3b | | A | K1a1, K1c1, K2c2, K2j2. K3b, K4c | L1a3 L1a2 L1a6, L1a7 | Mnp4a, Mnp5 | Mp3, Mp3b | N99 | 49 Q5 | V1a |
| # 3 | 1 Sz disorder | 2, Mp3, Mp3b | 3, Mp4, Mp4e | A | K1L1, K2L1 K3b, K4B, | L1 L2a2 | Mnp5 | M, M6d liver cirrhosis | N99 | 49 Q5 | V1a |
| # 4 | 1 Sz disorder | 2, Mp3, Mp3b | 3, Mp4, Mp4e | A | K1L1, K2L3 K3b, K4b | L1a4 | Mnp5 | M, Mp6b, Mp6d | N99 | 50 Q5 | V1a |
| # 5 | 1 Sz disorder | 2, Mp3, Mp3b | Mp4b | A | K1f1, K1L1, K2f3, K2L2 K3b, K3c, K4b, K5a | L1a1 L1a2 L1a4 L2a4 | Mnp4 w nl wt | M | N99 | 43 Q5 | V3a |
| Females P2 Case # 1 | 1 Sz disorder | 2, Mp3, Mp3b | | A | K1g1, K1L1 K2g1, L2L2, K3c | L2a8a | Mnp4, Mnp5 | M, Non contrib. M10 | N99 | 41 Q5 | V1a |
| # 2 | 1 Sz disorder only with death | 2, Mp3, Mp3b | | A, C4a, E1g | k1B1, KIF1, K1L1, K2c5f, K3d, | | Mnp4, Mnp5 | | N99 | 42 Q5 | V1a |
| W2 Prob SUDEP Males P1 Case # 6 | 1 Sz disorder Mp5g | 2, Mp3, Mp3b | 3, Mp4b: Chronic obstruct pulmonary disease | A | K3f Unknown What AEDs prescribed | L1a2 | Mc2c, Mp5g | M, M2c, Mp3e (putrified, no postmortem data) M4 M10 | N, N4 | 43 Q5 | V3a |
| # 7 | 1 Sz disorder | 2, Dilated cardiomyopathy arteriosclerotic Mp3 | 3, acute pneumonia, emphyse ma Mp4, Mp4e, Mp4f | A | K2L2, K2p2, K3f | L1a3 L2a4 | Mnp5 | M | N, N3 | 38 Q4 | V1a |
| Females P2 Case # 3 | 1 Sz disorder | 2, Mp3, Mp3b | 3, Mp4, Mp 4e | A | K3a | L2a2 | Mnp5 | M, Amyotrophic lateral sclerosis | N, N3, N5b | 39 Q4 | V3a |
| # 4 | 1 Sz disorder | 2, Mp3, Mp3b | 3, Mp4, Mp4e | A | K3f, K4a Trazodone Venlfaxine (antidepressant) | L1a2 | Mnp5 | Mp3e M, M2b, M12, M13, M2c, Asthma | N, N5b | 48 Q5 | V1a |
| W4 Non-SUDEP Females P2 Case # 5 | 1. Convulsive Sz due glial tumor | 2, Mp3, Mp3b | 3, Mp4, Mp4e | A | K1b3, K1L3 K2b1, K2L1, K3b | L1a3 | Mnp5, Mp5c | M, M12, TMJ, Osteocervical fusion | N, N5c, N7 | 54 Q6 | V1a |

**TABLE 6.2**

**Immediate and Contributory Cause of Death for Males**

| Case No.<br>Death Certificate | 1<br>Definite<br>SUDEP | 2<br>Definite<br>SUDEP | 3<br>Definite<br>SUDEP | 4<br>Definite<br>SUDEP | 5<br>Definite<br>SUDEP | 6<br>Possible<br>SUDEP | 7<br>Possible<br>SUDEP |
|---|---|---|---|---|---|---|---|
| Part I<br>Immediate cause<br>of death | Seizure<br>disorder | Seizure<br>disorder<br>(clinical) | Seizure<br>disorder | Seizure<br>disorder | Seizure<br>disorder | Seizure<br>disorder | Dilated cardiomyopathy +<br>arteriosclerotic cardiovascular<br>disease, acute pneumonia,<br>emphysema |
| Part II<br>Contributory cause<br>of death | | | Liver<br>cirrhosis<br>disease | Liver<br>cirrhosis | Chronic obstructive<br>pulmonary<br>disease | Chronic obstructive<br>pulmonary<br>disease | Seizure disorder |

**TABLE 6.3**

**Immediate and Contributory Cause of Death for Females**

| Case No.<br>Death Certificate | 1<br>Definite SUDEP | 2<br>Definite SUDEP | 3<br>Possible SUDEP | 4<br>Possible SUDEP | 5<br>Non-SUDEP |
|---|---|---|---|---|---|
| Part I<br>Immediate cause<br>of death | Seizure disorder | Seizure disorder<br>(clinical) | Seizure disorder (clinical)<br>with arteriosclerotic<br>cardiovascular disease | Seizure disorder w<br>hypertensive + arterioscleortic<br>cardiovascular disease | Convulsive seizure<br>developed from<br>Grade II glial tumor |
| Part II<br>Contributory<br>cause of death | – | – | – | – | – |

**TABLE 6.4**

**Past Medical History, Prescribed Medication, Toxicology Screen, and Pathological Features among Males**

| Males Past Medical<br>History | Prescribed<br>Medications | Drugs Identified and Level in Toxicology<br>Screen (AED drugs) | Level of Postmortem<br>Compounds | Pathological Features |
|---|---|---|---|---|
| 1. Seizures | Dilantin | Acetone (6 mg%)<br>Acetone (5 mg%) | —<br>— | Alive: 1/7/01.<br>Found dead: 1/11/01<br>12:30 PM. Body<br>moderately decomposed |
| 2. Seizures | Prinvil Clonazepam<br>K-Dur Oramorph<br>Depo Medrol<br>Provential inhaler | Doxylamine (0.014 mg%)<br>Benzodiazepines:<br>  Nordiazepam (0.01 mg%)<br>  Chlordiazepoxide (0.013 mg%)<br>  Demoxepam (0.023 mg%)<br>  Oxazepam (0.010 mg%)<br>  Clonazepam (Too low to quantitative)<br>  Morphine (0.087 ug/mL)<br>Dextromethorphan-positive, ibuprofen-<br>positive, diphenhydramine-positive | Above therapeutic<br><br><br>Therapeutic<br>Subtherapeutic<br>—<br>Subtherapeutic<br>—<br>Subtherapeutic<br>— | Alive: 1/17/01 4:30 PM<br>Dead: 1/18/01 12:30 PM |
| 3. Seizures | Dilantin | Phenytoin (8.31 ug/mL) | Subtherapeutic | Alive: 1/18/01 7:30 AM |
| 4. DVT, seizures<br>alcoholism | Dilantin Keflex | None detected | — | Alive: 2/11/01 1:00 AM<br>Found dead: 8:00 PM<br>Decomposed |
| 5. Seizures alcoholism | Celexa<br>Neurontin<br>Phenytoin<br>Indomethacin | Ethanol (0.04%)<br>Phenytoin (1.05 ug/mL) | —<br>Subtherapeutic l | |
| 6. HIV, seizures chronic<br>lung disease<br>bipolar depression | Unknown | Citalopram-positive<br>  Desmethylcitalopram-positive | —<br>— | Putrification |
| 7. Epilepsy depression | Unknown | Ethanol (0.02%)<br>Phenytoin (2.45 ug/mL)<br>Olanzapine (0.041 mg%)<br>Sertraline (0.021 mg%)<br>Valproic Acid (TDX) (8.99 ug/mL) | —<br>Subtherapeutic<br>Above therapeutic<br>Therapeutic<br>Subtherapeutic | Alive: 10/16/01 11:00 PM<br>Found dead: 10/16/01<br>12:00 PM |

## TABLE 6.5
## Past Medical History, Prescribed Medication, Toxicology Screen and Pathological Features among Females

| Females Past Medical History | Prescribed Medications | Drugs Identified in Toxicology Screen (AED drug) | Level of Postmortem Compounds | Pathological Features |
|---|---|---|---|---|
| 1. Hysterectomy seizures | Dilantin Lamotrigine | Phenytoin (5.36 ug/mL) Lamotrigine (0.79 mg%) Ibuprofen (0.81 mg%) | Subtherapeutic Therapeutic Subtherapeutic | Alive: 6/7/01 evening Found dead: 6/8/01 3:30 PM |
| 2. Seizures | Neurontin Tegretol Dilantin | Clonazepram (8.37 ug/mL) | Above therapeutic | Alive: 7/6/01 12:20 AM Dead: 7/6/01 12:21 AM Witnesses seizure |
| 3. Amyotrophic lateral sclerosis depression seizures | Bupropion Ditropanxl Zanaflex Baclofen Rilutek | Bupropion (0.006 mg%) Threoaminobupropion- Positive | Therapeutic — | Alive: Unknown Found dead: 8/7/01 5:37 PM moderate putrification |
| 4. Diabetes seizures Hypertension asthma | Unknown | Trazodone (0.296 mg%) Venlfaxine (0.175 mg%) O-Desmethylvenlafaxine (0.025 mg%) | Therapeutic Therapeutic | Alive: 9/28/01 11:30 PM. Found dead: 9/29/01 9:31 AM |
| 5. Hypertension Seizures TMJ Osteoporosis Cervical Psych Hx | Prempro Gybutynin Butslbital-apac- caff-tap | Carbamazepine (4.56 ug/mL) Phenytoin (14.68 ug/mL) Butalbital (0.246 mg%) Acetaminophen (14.05 g%) | Therapeutic Therapeutic Subtherapeutic Nearly toxic | Alive: 9/4/01 2:30 PM Found dead: 9/5/01 11:32 PM |

## TABLE 6.6
## SUDEP Cases, Definite, Probable, Possible, Non-SUDEP, Prevented, or Alive Patients

| 7 Categories Dead or Alive Patient Table 1A | Brain 1 | Cardiac 2 | Respiratory Hypoxia 3 4 = Unknown' | A–E | F–G | H | I | J | K AED | L | M1 Contributory cause death M2 non-SUDEP | N | O | Q Age | R S T U | V Post-mortem V1A autopsy,+ V4 genetics |
|---|---|---|---|---|---|---|---|---|---|---|---|---|---|---|---|---|
| Definite SUDEP W1 | | | | | | | | | | | | | | | | |
| Males P1 | | | | | | | | | | | | | | | | |
| Case# | | | | | | | | | | | | | | | | |
| 1 | | | | | | | | | | | | | | | | |
| 2 | | | | | | | | | | | | | | | | |
| 3 | | | | | | | | | | | | | | | | |
| 4 | | | | | | | | | | | | | | | | |
| 5 | | | | | | | | | | | | | | | | |
| Females P2 Case # | | | | | | | | | | | | | | | | |
| 1 | | | | | | | | | | | | | | | | |
| 2 | | | | | | | | | | | | | | | | |
| Probable SUDEP W2 | | | | | | | | | | | | | | | | |
| Males P1 Case # | | | | | | | | | | | | | | | | |
| 6 | | | | | | | | | | | | | | | | |
| 7 | | | | | | | | | | | | | | | | |
| Females P2 Case # | | | | | | | | | | | | | | | | |
| 3 | | | | | | | | | | | | | | | | |
| 4 | | | | | | | | | | | | | | | | |
| Possible SUDEP W3 | | | | | | | | | | | | | | | | |

(Continued)

**TABLE 6.6**   (*Continued*)

**SUDEP Cases, Definite, Probable, Possible, Non-SUDEP, Prevented, or Alive Patients**

| 7 Categories Dead or Alive Patient Table 1A | Brain 1 | Cardiac 2 | Respiratory Hypoxia 3 4 = Unknown' | A–E | F–G | H | I | J | K AED | L | M1 Contributory cause death M2 non-SUDEP | N | O | Q Age | R S T U | V Post-mortem V1A autopsy,+ V4 genetics |
|---|---|---|---|---|---|---|---|---|---|---|---|---|---|---|---|---|
| Males P1 Case # | | | | | | | | | | | | | | | | |
| 8 | | | | | | | | | | | | | | | | |
| 9 | | | | | | | | | | | | | | | | |
| Females P2 | | | | | | | | | | | | | | | | |
| Case # | | | | | | | | | | | | | | | | |
| 5 | | | | | | | | | | | | | | | | |
| 6 | | | | | | | | | | | | | | | | |
| Non-SUDEP W5 | | | | | | | | | | | | | | | | |
| Males | | | | | | | | | | | | | | | | |
| P1 Case # | | | | | | | | | | | | | | | | |
| 10 | | | | | | | | | | | | | | | | |
| Females P2 Case # | | | | | | | | | | | | | | | | |
| 7 | | | | | | | | | | | | | | | | |
| SUDEP | | | | | | | | | | | | | | | | |
| Pre-vented W4 | | | | | | | | | | | | | | | | |
| Males | | | | | | | | | | | | | | | | |
| P1 Case # | | | | | | | | | | | | | | | | |
| 11 | | | | | | | | | | | | | | | | |
| Females P2 Case # | | | | | | | | | | | | | | | | |
| 8 | | | | | | | | | | | | | | | | |
| Alive Patient W6 | | | | | | | | | | | | | | | | |
| Males P1 Case # | | | | | | | | | | | | | | | | |
| 12 | | | | | | | | | | | | | | | | |
| Females P2 Case # | | | | | | | | | | | | | | | | |
| 9 etc. | | | | | | | | | | | | | | | | |
| Survivor, not epilepsy W7 | | | | | | | | | | | | | | | | |

**TABLE 6.7**

**SUDEP Allegheny Unknown Factors (Lathers et al. 2011; Koehler et al. 2011)**

| W1-7 | A | B | C | D | E | F | G | I | J | N | O4 | O5 |
|---|---|---|---|---|---|---|---|---|---|---|---|---|
| W1 Definite SUDEP Males P1 Case # 1 | A11 c5 | B99 | | D99 | E1x | F99 | G99 | I99 | J99 | N99 | O4a99 | O5a99 |
| # 2 | A11 | B99 | | D99 | E1x | F99 | G99 | I99 | J99 | N99 | O4a99 | O5a99 |
| # 3 | A11c | B99 | | D99 | E1x | F99 | G99 | I99 | J99 | N99 | O4a99 | O5a99 |
| # 4 | A11 | B99 | | D99 | E1x | F99 | G99 | I99 | J99 | N99 | O4a99 | O5a99 |
| # 5 | A11c | B99 | | D99 | E1x | F99 | G99 | I99 | J99 | N99 | O4a99 | O5a99 |
| Females P2 Case # 1 | A11 c5 | B99 | | D99 | E1x | | G99 | I99 | J99 | N99 | O4a99 | O5a99 |
| # 2 | A11 | B99 | | D99 | E1g | F99 | G99 | I99 | J99 | N99 | O4a99 | O5a99 |
| W2 Prob SUDEP Males P1 Case # 6 | A11 c5 | B99 | | D99 | E1x | F99 | G99 | I99 | J99 | N, N4 | O4a99 | O5a99 |
| # 7 | A11 | B99 | | D99 | E1x | F99 | G99 | I99 | J99 | N, N3 | O4a99 | O5a99 |
| Females P2 Case # 3 | A11 c5 | B99 | | D99 | E1x | F99 | G99 | I99 | J99 | N, N3, N5b | O4a99 | O5a99 |
| # 4 | A11 | B99 | | D99 | E1x | F99 | G99 | I99 | J99 | N, N5b | O4a99 | O5a99 |
| W4 Non-SUDEP Females P2 Case # 5 | A11 c5 | B99 | | D99 | E1x | F99 | G99 | I99 | J99 | N, N5c, N7 | O4a99 | O5a99 |

the death of the person. It is noteworthy that only forensic deaths fall within this category. See Chapter 11 for Dr. Koehler's full discussion of forensic investigations.

## THE RISK FACTOR CLUSTER IDS FOR ALL 12 DEATHS IN THE 2001 ALLEGHENY COUNTY STUDY FOLLOW

### HUMAN DEFINITE SUDEP CASES-SUDEP SYNDROME CLUSTER IDENTIFIERS

Males all on AEDs

1. 1, 2, 3, A11c5, B99, D99, E1x, G99, I99, J99, K1L1, K2L3, K3b, K4a, L2a4, M, Mp3, Mp3b,Mp4, Mp4e, Mp7, Mp7c, N99, O4a99, O5a99, P1, Q5, R3, S2.38, T1, U2, V3a, W1

2. 1, 2, A11c5, B99, D99, E1x, G99, I99, J99, K1a1, K1c1, K2c2, K2j2, K3b, K4c, L1a2, L1a3, L1a6, L1a7, M, Mp3, Mp3b, Mnp4a, Mnp5, N99, O4a99, O5a99, P1, Q5, R3, S2.38, T1, U2, V1a, W1

3. 1, 2, 3, A11c5, B99, D99, E1x, G99, I99, J99, K1L1, K2L1, K3b. K4b, L1, L2A2, M, Mp3, Mp3b, Mp4, Mp4e, M6d, Mnp5, N99, O4a99, O5a99, P1, Q5, R3, S2.38, T1, U2, V1a, W1

4. 1, 2, 3, A11c5, B99, D99, E1x, G99, I99, J99, K1L1, K2L3, K3b, K4b, L1a4, M, Mp3, Mp3b, Mp4, Mp4e, Mp6b, Mp6d, Mnp5, N99, O4a99, O5a99, P1, Q5, R3, S2.38, T1, U2, V1a, W1

5. 1, 2, 3, A11c5, B99, D99, E1x, G99, I99, J99, K1f1, K1L1, K2f3, K2L2, K3b, K3c, K4b, K5a, H, L1a1, L1a2, L1a4, L2a4, M, Mp3, Mp3b, Mp4b w nm wt, Mnp4, N99, O4a99, O5a99, P1, Q5, R3, S2.38, T1, U2, V3a, W1

Females all on AEDs

1. 1, 2, A11c5, B99, D99, E1x, G99, I99, J99, k1g1, k1L1, k2g1, k2L2, K3c, L2a8a, M, Mp3, Mp3b, M10, Mnp4, Mnp5, N99, O4a99, O5a99, P2, Q5, R3, S2.38 T1, U2, V1a, W1

2. 1, 2, A11c5, B99, C4a, D99, E1g, G 99, I 99, J99, K1b1, K1f1, K1L1, K2c5f, K3d, M, Mp3, Mp3b, Mnp4, Mnp5, N99, O4a99, O5a99, P2, Q5, R3, S2.38, T1, U2, V1a, W1,

### HUMAN PROBABLE SUDEP CASES-SUDEP SYNDROME CLUSTER IDENTIFIERS

Males

6. 1, 2, 3, A11c5, B99, D99, E1x, G99, I99, J99, K3f, L1a2, M, Mp5g, Mp3, Mp3B, Mp4B, Mc2c, Mp3e, M2c, M4, M10, N, N4, O4a99, O5a99, P1, Q5, R3, S2.38, T1, U2, V3a, W2 not on AEDs

7. 1, 2, 3, A11c5, B99, D99, E1x, G99, I99, J99, K2L2, K2p2, K3f, L1a3, L2a4, M, Mp3, Mp3b, Mp4, Mp4e, Mp4f, Mnp5, N, N3, O4a99, O5a99, P1, Q4, R3, S2.38, T1, U2, V1a, W2

Females not on AEDs

3. 1, 2, 3, A11c5, B99, D99, E1x, G99, I99, J99, K3a, K2a2, M, Mp3, Mp3b, Mp3e?, Mp4, Mp4e, M5a, Mnp5, M2b, M2c, M3?, N, N3, N5b, O4a99, O5a99, P2, Q4, R3, S2.38, T1, U2, V3a, W2

7. 1, 2, 3, A11c5, B99, D99, E1x, G99, I99, J99, K3f, K4a, L1a2, M, Mp5c, Mp3, Mp3b, Mp4, Mp4e, Mnp5, M5c, M12, M13?, N, N5, N5b, O4a99, O5a99, P2, Q5, R3, S2.38, T1, U2, V1a, W2

### HUMAN NON-SUDEP CASE-SUDEP SYNDROME CLUSTER IDENTIFIER

Males: None

Female

5. 1, 2, 3, A11c5, B99, D99, G99, I99, J99, K1b3, K1L3, K2b1, K2L1, K3b, L1a3, M, Mp3, Mp3b, Mp4, Mp4e, Mp5c,M12, Mnp5, Mp5c, N, N5c, N7, O4a99, O5a99, P2, Q6, R3, S2.38, T1, U2, V1a, W5 AEDs found after death.

## DISCUSSION

In our 2011 Allegheny study, toxicological screens were carried out on the blood, bile, urine, and eye fluids for all 12. Data in Tables 6.4 and 6.5 were used. AED levels detected in postmortem toxicological analysis were examined. AED levels were detected in seven cases. Four of seven had subtherapeutic AED levels, two had therapeutic levels, and only one SUDEP victim had levels above the therapeutic range. Five cases had no detectable AED levels. AED levels at autopsy were either absent or subtherapeutic in 9 of 10 SUDEP cases, findings consistent with the likelihood of poor AED compliance. Subtherapeutic levels of AED's may be a Risk Factor for SUDEP that could contribute to increased interictal and/or ictal epileptiform activity with associated autonomic dysfunction leading to disturbance of heart rate, rhythm, and/or blood pressure.

One of our research goals is to build a database with enough SUDEP cases to allow us to group like or similar SUDEP Cluster Risk Factor IDs and cases together. To date, we have a total of 115 – 173 + human cases summarized in this chapter and in Chapters 7 through 10.

### PRELIMINARY DATA: 115 – 173 + CASES. HUMAN DATA SUDEP SYNDROME CLUSTER IDENTIFIERS

1. Multiple cases of SUDEP
   a. 12 cases. (Lathers et al. 2011) 2001 Allegheny County, PA, Retrospective SUDEP 1: Forensic AEDs Autopsy Cases of Epilepsy. Lathers et al. 2011.

b.  8 cases. 1978–79 Allegheny County, PA, Retrospective SUDEP Study: Forensic Neurogenic Pulmonary Edema in Unexpected, Unexplained Death of Epileptic Patients. Terrence et al. 1981. 111413 Presented below and also discussed in Chapter 7.

2.  Single cases of SUDEP
    a.  21 cases from *Sudden Death Epilepsy Forensic: Clinical Issues,* eds., Lathers, Schraeder, Bungo, Leestma. Presented in Chapter 8.
    b.  40 cases. Table 2X-Z Case Reports of Schachter and Verrier in Chapter 9.
    c.  14 cases. 2011 SUDEP Book ibid Schraeder.
    d.  15 cases identified in the literature. Not analyzed yet.
    e.  39 cases. 1974–2013 South Carolina SUDEP CASES Neurology Practice Collected ~40-year Non-forensic Data (Wannamaker). Chapter 10.

Another of our research goals is to determine the incidence of SUDEP, particularly for a given area to ascertain whether "modern medicine" has caused the incidence to decrease. We, therefore, analyzed the data of Terrence et al. 1981 for Allegheny County, PA, for the years 1978–1979 to compare it with our 2001 SUDEP Cluster ID and incidence data for the same County.

3.  1978–79 Allegheny County, PA, Retrospective SUDEP Study: Forensic Neurogenic Pulmonary Edema in Unexpected, Unexplained Death of Epileptic Patients. Cluster ID Analysis of 8 Cases from Terrence et. al. 1981

**Case 1**. 1, A11c5, B99, C99, D5, E1x, F99, G99, H3, I99, K1k1, K1l1, K2k3, K2l3, K3c, K4a, K5d1, K7b, L1b, L2c, M3, Mnp3, Mnp4, Mnp5, Mc2a, N99, O4a99, O5a99, O7a, O8a, P2, Q3, R3, S2.38, T1, U2, V1a, W1

**Case 2**. 1, 2, A11c5, B99, C99, D4, E1x, F99, G99, H3, I99, K1k1, K1l1, K2r1, K2k3, K2l3, K2r3, K3d, K4a, K5d1, K7b, L1b, L2c, M3, Mnp3, Mnp4, Mnp5, Mnp7, Mp3b, Mp5b, Mc2a, N99, O4a99, O5a99, O7a, O8a, P2, Q3, R3, S2.38, T1, U3, V1a, W1

**Case 3**. 1, A11c5, B99, C99, D5, E1x, F99, G99, H3, I99, K1k1, K1l1, K1r1, K2k1, K2l3, K2s3, K3d, K4b, K5d1, K7a, L1b, L2b, M3, Mnp3, Mnp4, Mnp5, Mnp7, Mp7a, Mc2a, N99, O4a99, O5a99, O7a, O8a, P2, Q3, R3, S2.38, T1, U2, V1a, W1

**Case 4**. 1, 3, A11c5, B99, C99, D2, E1x, F99, G99, H3, I99, K1k1, K1L1, K1s1, K2r1, K2l1, K3d, K4c, K5d1, L1b, L2b, M3, Mnp3, Mnp4, Mnp5, Mnp6, Mp4e, Mc2a, N99, O4a99, O5a99, O7a, O8a, P2, Q3, R3, S2.38, T1, U3, V1a, W1

**Case 5**. 1, A11c5, B99, C99, D4, E1x, F99, G99, H3, I99, K1k1, K1L1, K1r1, K2k1, K2l1, K2s3, K3d, K4c, K5d1, K7a, L1b, L2b, M3, Mnp3, Mnp4, Mnp5, Mnp7, Mp5fe, Mc2a, N99, O4a99, O5a99, O7a, O8a, P2, Q3, R3, S2.38, T1, U2, V1a, W1

**Case 6**. 1, 2, 3, A11c5, B99, C99, D5, E1x, F99, G99, H3, I99, K1k1, K1l1, K2k3, K2l3, K3c, K4a, K5d1, K7a, L1b, L2b, M3, Mnp3, Mnp4, Mnp5, Mnp7, Mp3b, Mp4e, Mc2a, N99, O4a99, O5a99, O7a, O8a, P2, Q3, R3, S2.38, T1, U3, V1a, W1

**Case 7**. 1, 2, 3, A12a, D4, E1x, F2A, H1b, K1, K1k1, K1kL1, K2k2, K2L2, K3c, K4c, K5b, K5d1, L1a4, M3, Mnp3, Mp3b, Mnp4, Mp4e, O4a99, O5a99, O7a, O8c, O9, P1, Q2, R3, T1, U2, V1a, W1; ? Add B99, C99, G99, H3, I99, Mnp5, Mnp7, Mc2a, N99?

**Case 7**. Revised 1, 2, 3, A12a, D4, E1x, F2A, H1b, K1, K1k1, K1kL1, K2k2, K2L2, K3c, K4c, K5b, K5d1, L1a4, M3, Mnp3, Mp3b, Mnp4, Mp4e, O4a99, O5a99, O7a, O8c, O9, P1, Q2, R3, T1, U2, V1a, W1; and add B99, C99, G99, H3, I99, Mnp5, Mnp7, Mc2a, N99

**Case 8**. Revised 1, 3, A11c3, B, D3, E1e, O7d, O8c, K4e, K1b1, K1k1, K1L1, K1p1, K1m1, K2b3, K2k2, K2L3, Kep3, K2m3, K5a, K5d1, Mp4e, Mp5b, O4a99, O5a99, O8c, O9c, P2, Q1, R2, S2.38, T1, U3, V1a, W1; and add C99, F99, G99, H3, I99, K1s1, K2k1, K2s3, K3e, K7a, L1b, L2b, Mnp3, Mnp4, Mnp5, Mnp7, Mp5b, Mc2a, N99

For the 2001 forensic study of Lathers et al. 2011, the incidence of SUDEP was 0.917%. Eleven of 1200 autopsied cases were identified with past medical history seizure disorder on death certificates. Seizure was listed as immediate or contributory to death. Eleven of 12 were deemed definite or probable SUDEP; 1 non-SUDEP. The incidence of SUDEP was 0.267% for Allegheny County for 1978–79 reported by Terrence et al. in 1981. Additional SUDEP incidence data are reported in Chapter 13.

As we reviewed our own published data and cases of others in the literature, several observations were made. A major dilemma associated with trying to analyze published SUDEP case reports is that of insufficiently detailed information in the case narratives and in any data tables provided. The insufficiencies often included absence of EEG data, description of the seizure phenomenology, quantification of seizure frequency, onset date of epilepsy, AED prescription history, compliance history, and AED levels over time as a profile of compliance, and imaging data. Relative to cases lacking EEG data, the analysis of mechanism of generalized tonic-clonic seizure mechanism in a given patient, that is, whether it is primarily generalized or secondarily generalized vs. complex partial vs.

simple partial, depends solely on the clinical judgment of the reviewers of the available data in any particular case. An example of this dilemma is in case 7 of the Terrence et al. (1981). Without the EEG data, the choices are that of primarily generalized vs. secondarily generalized seizures vs. unknown. The onset at age 5 with a history of infrequent generalized seizures despite at time poor compliance, could be interpreted as being consistent with primarily generalized epilepsy, as there is no description of any auras or other focal onset phenomena nor of postictal events such as brief weakness. Thus, although age of onset and infrequent seizures despite history of poor medication compliance may be somewhat consistent with primarily generalized epilepsy, it is not possible to make a definitive diagnosis within a degree of reasonable certainty and therefore presents an analytical dilemma. Case evaluation from published cases in Terrence et al. (1981) and for data in Lathers et al. (2011) and Koehler et al. (2011) emphasizes the need for accurate, detailed clinical history even in cases with complete postmortem examination data. Comparison of data in published tables with the narrative case description may reveal that each contains important separate data. Both detailed clinical data as well as postmortem examination data are equally important and needed to obtain the fullest possible picture for SUDEP Cluster Risk Factor analysis. Analysis of clinical medical records is ideal but is obviously not possible except for cases submitted by clinicians who cared for the patient. An additional in-depth discussion of two cases in the study of Terrence et al. (1981) is found in Chapter 7 by Schraeder and Lathers.

## CONCLUSIONS

Chapters 8, 9, and 10 contain additional Cluster IDs for SUDEP victims. All these data are needed for our new Cluster Risk Factor Method. We developed a very new, different physiological and pharmacological mechanistic perspective of SUDEP; this innovative method is a new forensic risk factor classification. The ultimate goal is to improve individual patient management via better understanding of the relative risk of death in SUDEP and knowledge of its risk factors. Individual risk IDs define risk factors, including central and peripheral autonomic nervous system changes, for SUDEP. Related or similar clusters will identify the types of risk factors for persons with similar risk Cluster IDs and ultimately will allow better medical management before, during, and after seizures.

## REFERENCES

Koehler SA, Schraeder PL, Lathers CM, Wecht CH. One-year postmortem forensic analysis of deaths in persons with epilepsy. In: Lathers CM, Schraeder PL, Bungo MW, Leestma JE, eds. *Sudden Death in Epilepsy: Forensic and Clinical Issues.* Boca Raton, FL: CRC Press/Taylor & Francis Group; 2011, pp. 145–59.

Lathers CM, Leestma JE, Schachter SC, Koehler SA, Claycamp HG, Wannamaker BB, Schraeder PL. SUDEP syndrome related cluster risk identification. *Epilepsy and Behavior* 2014;1–149.

Lathers CM, Koehler SA, Wecht CH, Schraeder PL. Forensic antiepileptic drug levels in autopsy cases of epilepsy. *Epi Behav* 2011;22(4):778–85.

Terrence CE, Rao GR, Perper JA. Neurogenic pulmonary edema in unexpected, unexplained death in epileptic patients. *Neurol* 1981;25:594–5.

# 7 How to and How Not to Use Cluster ID Method

*Paul L. Schraeder and Claire M. Lathers*

## CONTENTS

While using the sudden unexpected death in epilepsy (SUDEP) Cluster Identification (Cluster ID) method, we have learned that the determination of clinical risk factors and possible commonality of mechanisms for SUDEP is an effort fraught with many gaps in data and limitations in analysis. For such an analysis to be relevant there is a need for large numbers of patients. While prospective studies are the "gold standard" for accumulating such data, they require many years. The reality is that most currently available clinical SUDEP databases come from published case summaries that are retrospective and therefore, by their very nature, incomplete. While many, if not most, published SUDEP cases have summarized clinical and pathological data, potentially useful specific descriptors are often omitted, such as the specific description of the patient's individual seizure phenomenology, seizure frequency, electroencephalogram (EEG) data, the details of age of onset and possible etiology of the seizures, imaging data, the type and dosage of antiepileptic drugs (AEDs) at the time of death, the history of AEDs prescribed, the patient's compliance history, as would be documented by sequential AED blood level data, family history of epilepsy, and family history of any sudden deaths. The circumstances of death are, however, usually described. Relative to the postmortem data, there are usually just summary data that often consist of a statement that no cause of death was found. However, even when more details are available, explanations for observed putatively minor pathological findings are not included. The latter point is at times emphasized when tables summarizing the postmortem findings provide more data than was mentioned in the case narrative.

Our proposed cluster grouping analysis of the available published retrospective clinical data attempts to maximize the ability to correlate and compare what is available in the literature. While specific clinical details vary across case reports, they nonetheless are sufficient for cross comparison using our proposed cluster grouping analysis. That is, despite inconsistencies among case reports, with sufficient numbers of cases there is the potential to recognize data clusters and patterns that may provide useful insights.

This chapter demonstrates the complexity of analysis and subsequent details that were obtained from the cases published by Terrence et al. (1981). These cases are used as a prototypical example of how to conduct such analyses.

## EXEMPLARY CASES

A key detail often left out of SUDEP case reports is the EEG findings. This impacs the ability of the reader to assess the patient's potential seizure type(s); for example, whether the patient may have had primary or secondarily generalized tonic–clonic seizures. An example of this dilemma is in case 7 of the Terrence et al. 1981. Without the EEG data, the choices are that of primarily generalized versus secondarily generalized seizures versus unknown. The onset at age 5 with a history of infrequent generalized seizures despite poor compliance at times could be interpreted as being consistent with primarily generalized epilepsy, as there is no description of any auras or other focal onset phenomena nor of lateralizing postictal events such as one-sided weakness. Thus, although age of onset and infrequent seizures despite history of poor medication compliance may be somewhat consistent with primarily generalized epilepsy, it is not possible to make such a definitive diagnosis within a degree of reasonable certainty, and this presents an analytical dilemma. In such ambiguous instances on option, suggested by Barbara Schraeder, would be to have a small panel of neurologists who would try to reach a consensus relative to the seizure category. Otherwise, "unknown" would be assigned as the category.

Relative to the issue of patient compliance with prescribed AEDs, there is thought to be an association with poor compliance and an infrequent occurrence of seizures. One must ask whether or not the occurrence of infrequent seizures in some individuals provides the patient with an excuse or an inappropriate personal incentive to be lax in taking medications as prescribed—"I'm not having any seizures, so maybe I do not need the drugs, so why take them?" This behavior or attitude leading to poor compliance with AED(s) may leave the patient at risk for seizures and/or SUDEP.

Two cases of deaths, containing more detail than just the summary tabular data of all deaths, were published by Terrence et al. (1981). We have added Cluster IDs for these two cases below.

### Terrence et al. 1981 Case 7 Detailed Analysis with Comment as per Cluster ID Classification

1, 2, 3 Brain, cardiac, and pulmonary (history of seizures with cardiopulmonary arrest and agonal pulmonary edema on postmortem).

A12A-Idiopathic: generally genetic or perhaps A11C5 (undetermined epilepsy localization category)

D4-Onset age 5

E1x-Seizure frequency unknown

F2A-Asystolic (cardiopulmonary arrest)

G99 by selecting Cluster ID F2A then it is also assumed that G99 means any cardiac-based predisposition is unknown

H1b-Lung edema was only postmortem finding

K1-AEDs were prescribed

K1k1-AED prescribed phenobarbital

K1L1-AED prescribed phenytoin

K2k2-Subtherapeutic phenobarb level postmortem

K2L2-Sub therapeutic phenytoin level postmortem

K3c-Number of AEDs prescribed 2

K4c-Number of AEDs found postmortem 2

K5b-Penobarbital and phenytoin were subtherapeutic postmortem

K5D1-Noncompliant

L1a4-Alcohol use

M3-Brain, heart, lungs examined on postmortem

MnP3-Increased heart weight

Mp3b-Brain normal

MnP4-Lung edema present postmortem

Mp4E-Increased lung weight/congestion

O4a99-Month of death unknown

O5a99-Day of week of death unknown

O7a-Fatal event occurred at home

O8c-Pronounced dead in hospital (Presumably ER)

O9-Posture of body unknown on discovery

P1-Male

Q2-Age 19 years

R3-Smoker unknown

S2.38 PA

T1-Human

U2 Caucasian

V1a-Complete postmortem

W1-Definite SUDEP

In addition to reading the case history, also add the following Cluster IDs from Table 5.1, Chapter 5.

B99 Refractory unknown

C99 Unknown epileptogenic activity EEG source

I99 Unknown if syncope history

Mnp5 Normal postmortem pathology of brain

Mnp7 Normal postmortem pathology of brain vascular

Mc2a History of epilepsy

N99 Unknown if psychological medical history

### Terrence et al. 1981 Case 8 Data from Narrative and from Table

Terrence case 8

1, 3

Cluster 1 and 3 (Epilepsy and hemorrhagic pulmonary edema on autopsy)

A11c EEG origin undetermined

A11c3 Generalized tonic–clonic and absence seizures

B Refractory epilepsy

D3 Onset 4 months of age

E1e One generalized tonic–clonic seizure per week. Frequency of absence unknown

K1b1 Carbamazepine

K1k1 Phenobarbital

K1L1 Phenytoin

K1p1 Valproic acid

K1m1 Mephenytoin. Mephenytoin is a prodrug that is metabolized to Nirvinol, which provides over 90% of the antiepileptic effect. The half-life of Nirvinol is over 96 hours. A major idiosyncratic effect is that of aplastic anemia. Mephenytoin was removed from the market and is not currently available for use.

K2b3 CBZ undetected postmortem

K2k2 Phenobarb level 14.6, barely therapeutic compared to the above level of 41. The implication of this degree of decrease in level is that the patient stopped taking the phenobarb approximately 1 week earlier (half-life of ~ 96 hours) or that the drug was not taken consistently after the levels 6 months earlier were obtained

K2L3 PHT undetected postmortem

Kep3 VPA undetected postmortem

K2m3 Mephenytoin undetected, but need to consider that the Nirvinol metabolite was not tested

K4e number of AEDs detected postmortem >3 = 4 AEDs prescribed

K5a Therapeutic phenobarb (41 ug/mL), valproate (89 ug/mL), and carbamazepine (11.6 ug/mL) levels 6 months prior to death. These levels were in the high range of therapeutic. Mephenytoin level was not measurable, but it is not clear if the active AED metabolite Nirvinol level was performed or was even available in the laboratory. The other question is why no phenytoin level was performed at that time. This latter question would imply that it had not been prescribed at that time, perhaps later. Since 6 months prior to death, phenobarbital, valproate, and carbamazepine levels were therapeutic, the authors should have addressed the mephenytoin metabolite Nirvinol and why it was not measured.

K5d1 Apparently noncompliant prior to death

Mp4e Lung hemorrhage and edema. Lung weight of 350 g (do not know normal weight) range for 9 years old. Presumption of increased weight based on observed edema but normal data are not available. Note that as per Koehler 2011, ch. 9, normal combined lung weight for a female is 650–950 g

Mp5b Brain edema

O4a99 Month of death unknown

O5a99 Day of week unknown

O7d Event occurred in automobile as passenger

O8c Pronounced death in hospital

O9c Sitting at time of death in passenger seat

P2 Female

Q1 Nine years old

R2 Nonsmoker (age 9 years)

S2.38 PA

T1 Human

U3 Black of African American

V1a Complete postmortem and toxicology screen, nondecomposed

W1 Definite SUDEP

Cluster ID data above are obtained from first reading of the case description. Additional Cluster IDs to be added include:

C99 Unknown epileptogenic activity EEG Source

F99 Unknown if cardiac arrhythomogenic history (and subcategories)

G99 Cardiac unknown

H3? Not positive

I99 Syncope unknown

J99 Genetic structural channelopathies unknown

K1s1 Tiagabine prescribed

K2k1 Postmortem therapeutic phenobarbital

K2s3 Postmortem undetected tiagabine

K3e Number of AEDs prescribed by physician >3

K7a AEDs unknown

L1b Not certain

L2b Not certain

Mnp3 Normal postmortem pathology of heart

Mnp4 Normal postmortem pathology of lung

Mnp5 Normal postmortem pathology of brain

Mnp7 Normal postmortem pathology of brain vascular

Mp5b Postmortem pathology edema

Mc2a History of epilepsy

N99 Unknown if psychological history

Please note that these two forensic SUDEP patient cases and their SUDEP Cluster IDs are summarized in Chapter 6, which contains the Cluster IDs for all eight victims of SUDEP in the 1978–79 time period for Allegheny County, Pennsylvania, included in the study of Terrence et al. (1981). Terrence et al. (1981) conclude that postmortem examination of heart and lungs in these eight deaths revealed that lung weights uniformly exceeded the expected value, with gross evidence of hemorrhagic pulmonary edema with moderate-to-severe pulmonary edema with protein-rich fluid as well as alveolar hemorrhage found. They comment that although death due to a seizure is usually considered almost instantaneous, the finding of neurogenic pulmonary edema in these cases suggests that time is required for this state to occur and thus death may be preventable. Evidence of current or past myocardial disease was not evident in these eight deaths. Absent or nontherapeutic AED levels at the time of death may play a role in a possible centrally mediated adrenergic cause of the neurogenic pulmonary edema and ventricular arrhythmia.

## CONCLUSION

These case evaluations and addition of Cluster IDs of two deaths from the published study of Terrence et al. (1981) indicate that an accurate, detailed clinical history is very important, even in cases with complete postmortem examination data. Comparison of data in the published tables with the narrative case description clearly indicates that each contained important separate data. Detailed clinical data as well as postmortem examination data are equally important and are needed to get the fullest possible picture for analysis. Clearly, analysis of clinical medical records is the ideal but is obviously not possible except in cases that are submitted by clinicians who cared for the patient.

## REFERENCES

Koehler SA, Schraeder PL, Lathers CM, Wecht CH. One-year postmortem forensic analysis of deaths in persons with epilepsy. In: Lathers CM, Schraeder PL, Bungo, MW, Leestma JE, eds. *Sudden Death in Epilepsy: Forensic and Clinical Factors.* Boca Raton, FL: CRC Press/Taylor & Francis Group. 2011, p145–158.

Terrence CE, Rao GR, Perper JA. Neurogenic pulmonary edema in unexpected, unexplained death in epileptic patients. *Neurology* 1981;25:594–5.

# 8 Clinical Cases Classified as SUDEP Cluster Risk Factor Identifiers

*Claire M. Lathers, Paul L. Schraeder, Steven C. Schachter,*
*Richard L. Verrier, and Braxton B. Wannamaker*

## CONTENTS

## RISK FACTOR CLUSTER IDENTIFICATIONS FOR SUDEP CASES: DEFINITE, PROBABLE, PREVENTED, AND NON-SUDEP CASES

The cases in this chapter, from the literature or practicing neurologists, illustrate the use of our sudden unexpected death in epilepsy (SUDEP) cluster identifier (ID) for definite, probable, prevented, and non-SUDEP cardiac cases, both prevented and cardiac sudden death. Single cases of epilepsy and SUDEP with cluster IDs and SUDEP classifications follow.

Cluster IDs for the aforementioned cases follow and will be added to the total human database for analysis.

## SUDEP PROBABLE CASE

Common ion channel dysfunction may underlie both seizures and cardiac arrhythmias. Genetic screen SUDEP syndrome cluster identifier: 1, 2, A8, B, C4a, C91, C92, C98, D5, J2a3, k1g1, G1, k5g, k5b, O7a, O8a, O9a, P2, Q3, R3, T1, U1, V4, W2.

SUDEP classification: SUDEP probable. Authors deemed the case definite SUDEP, which is W1, but our classification requires autopsy for a definite SUDEP.

### CASE SUMMARY

Aurlien et al. (2009). A female teenage patient, at age of 17 years, described symptoms of déjà vu, feeling of fear, sensation of electric current in chest, palpitations, and flushing; last few seconds with some impairment of awareness. Subsequently experienced generalized seizure, and some myoclonic events were identified. At age 24, she was diagnosed with epilepsy, EEG bilateral spike and waves. No EKG was recorded.

AED carbamazepine monotherapy, changes to valproic acid and lamotrigine. Taper valproic acid due to side effects tremor and tiredness. Only 100 mg once a day lamotrigine. At the age of 25 she was found dead in bed, and the cause of death was determined to be SUDEP.

## AUTHOR COMMENTS

Mechanisms of death via SUDEP.

a. Postmortem molecular genetic analysis found heterozygous for DNA sequencing of LQTS-associated new missense mutation of *SCN5A* gene, the gene that codes for cardiac sodium channel, voltage-gated, type V, α subunit.

b. Note that ion channel mutations involving *SCN5A* gene are associated with Brugada syndrome and LQTS. Idiopathic epilepsy is also thought to be associated with ion channelopathies. The cardiac *SCN5A* mutation detected may well have been a factor in explaining death of the patient, possibly in combination with a terminal seizure.

c. AED confounding is use of lamotrigine, a drug that blocks sodium channel function with widening of QRS complex and right-axis deviation.

d. Mechanism of death may have been multifactorial (seizures, predisposition to cardiac channelopathy related arrhythmia, and effects of medication)

e. Question with unknown answer: whether certain people with epilepsy have a predisposition to cardiac arrhythmias that is the result of an ion channel gene mutation that affects both the heart and the brain.

## COMMENTS BY LATHERS, SCHRAEDER, AND BUNGO (2011, PP. 327–8)

a. The mechanism of death may have been multifactorial (seizures; predisposition to cardiac channelopathy related arrhythmia; and effects of medication, including a subtherapeutic lamotrigine dose once the valproic acid was tapered and discontinued).

b. The issue of a common ion channel dysfunction that may underlie both predisposition to seizures and cardiac arrhythmias is an important potential area for investigation. However, the potential role for inherited ion channel dysfunction as a factor in the occurrence of seizures may be operative in primary generalized epilepsy (Mulley et al. 2003). The patient in this case had both complex partial and generalized seizures, with the latter being those overwhelmingly associated with the risk of SUDEP. While the patient had temporal lobe symptoms, i.e., déjà vu; feelings of fear; and self-described "electric," i.e., most probably tingling sensations, the fact that she also had myoclonic events in combination with generalized tonic-clonic seizures raises the possibility that she may have had two types of epilepsy, namely, localization-related temporal lobe seizures with or without secondary generalization and juvenile myoclonic epilepsy. The phenotype of the latter may be determined by a number of genes on chromosome 6p including a locus in the human leukocyte antigen region and in some instances on 1p (Berkokovic 1998). The potential for interactions between genetic

defects that affect ion channel function in the heart and the brain needs to be the subject of future research, especially when combined with the potential for AED-related effects at the ion channel level.

Another possibility should be considered about this case. Her sensation of an electric current in her chest, palpitations, and flushing, lasting a few seconds with some impairment of awareness, suggests a need for ECG evaluation. Further, rather than diagnose two types of epilepsy in the same patient, she may have had bifrontal epilepsy. EEG/video monitoring would have been a good idea for diagnostic purposes.

## SUDEP DEFINITE CASE STRESS (BETTS 1997)

SUDEP syndrome cluster identifier: 1, A11a1, B, C1, C4a, K1bi, K5b, N1, P2, Q4, R3, S2.3, T1, U2, V1b, W1. SUDEP classification: SUDEP definite. Case of SUDEP with a premorbid diagnosis of nonepileptic seizures and stress (PLS).

### CASE SUMMARY

A 35-year-old Caucasian woman was found dead in bed by her parents. She had a long-standing psychiatric history with the occurrence of seizure-like events. The patient was stressed, being a very anxious person. On one occasion, she had a nonepileptic seizure in her neurologist's office consisting of sliding to the floor with bizarre asynchronous bilateral motor activity without loss of consciousness. This event occurred consequent to an emotionally tense situation at her home. Complicating the history was the past observation of another type of event that consisted of some automatisms and post-ictal confusion. Multiple routine EEGs over the years were unremarkable save for one that showed unequivocal isolated left temporal interictal discharges. The patient was placed on carbamazepine and found to have consistently therapeutic levels. The patient recognized that the complex partial events were no longer occurring, but the others continued. After the retirement of her neurologist, the patient was seen at another center and subjected to several days of inpatient EEG monitoring. During the inpatient monitoring there were multiple clinical events but there was no epileptiform activity documented on any of the EEG recordings. As a result, the patient was informed that her seizures were nonepileptic and was advised to taper her antiepileptic medications. Several weeks later, her parents notified her former neurologist (PLS) of her tragic demise. There was no postmortem examination.

### COMMENTS BY LATHERS, SCHRAEDER, AND BUNGO

People with only nonepileptic seizures would, by definition, not be at risk for SUDEP. However, the unfortunate reality is that 10%–30% of patients who appear to have long-established nonepileptic seizures also have epilepsy (Betts 1998). Thus, although the majority of people with nonepileptic seizures do not have concurrent epilepsy, in those who also have a bona fide seizure disorder, as demonstrated in this case, there is a risk of SUDEP associated with withdrawal of antiepileptic drugs based on the observation of only nonepileptic events. The physician must consider all aspects of the history and all prior EEG data before having confidence that the antiepileptic medication can be safely withdrawn. One should also keep in mind that rapid discontinuation of medication that was at a therapeutic serum level could induce a withdrawal seizure even in a person without epilepsy, further clouding the issue of diagnosis. Stress is a risk factor for SUDEP (Lathers and Schraeder 2006, 2008b). A verbal autopsy (Lathers and Schraeder, 2009) may be obtained from family and friends and provides one method of ascertaining if "stress" was a risk factor in a given SUDEP victim. A verbal autopsy is one option if, as for this patient, there was no postmortem examination.

## SUDEP CASES (LANGAN ET AL. 2000; LATHERS 2011)

A series of witnessed SUDEP deaths.

### CASE SUMMARY

Fifteen witnessed deaths were included in a total group of 125 cases of SUDEP identified by coroners, neurologists, and families of victims (Langan et al. 2000). Twelve of the deaths occurred in association with convulsive seizures. One victim exhibited a generalized seizure and then collapsed about 5 minutes later. Of the last two witnessed deaths, one victim died during what was thought to be a "probable postictal state" and one died after experiencing an aura. The witnesses reported that 12 of the 15 cases experienced respiratory difficulty.

### COMMENTS BY LANGAN ET AL. (2000)

The majority of sudden deaths in people with epilepsy were not witnessed, i.e., only 15 of 125 SUDEP cases were witnessed. Most of the deaths that were witnessed occurred in conjunction with a seizure. Respiratory difficulty/compromise was reported to be the prominent problem observed. The authors suggest that repositioning of the patient and/or stimulation of respiration may be important in helping to prevent sudden deaths in people with epilepsy.

### COMMENTS BY LATHERS

The possible mechanisms of SUDEP are several and include central and obstructive apnea and cardiovascular changes, including cardiac arrhythmias. Caution must be exerted when concluding that respiratory changes alone are the primary mechanism of death. At the first onset of the clinical problem, cardiac arrhythmias may be felt by the patient but may not be visually detected by a witness. "Invisible" cardiac arrhythmias may be initiated and then followed by "visible" respiratory distress. Therefore, in addition to repositioning the patient to ensure ease of respiration and/or stimulation of respiration, it is important, if possible, to simultaneously monitor and medically support cardiac rate and rhythm. The answer to the question of "which is the cart and which is the horse?" or "which is the egg and which is the chicken?" will vary from patient to patient depending on the type of the initiating clinical event. However, if an event is witnessed it is of upmost importance to support all vital systems, i.e., respiratory, cardiac, and circulatory. If intravenous access is difficult to obtain in an adult, and even more so in a pediatric patient during a witnessed event, it is possible that the intraosseous route of drug administration would allow rapid access to the circulation to provide anticonvulsant drugs and/or drugs used to treat cardiac arrest (Jim et al. 1988, 1989; Lathers et al. 1989a, b, c; Schoffstall et al. 1989; Spivey et al. 1987a, b).

## SUDEP PROBABLE CASE STRESS RELEVANCE (LATHERS AND SCHRAEDER 2011A)

SUDEP syndrome cluster identifier: 1, A11c3, C4a, D5, E1f, K1b1, K5d, N1, P2, Q2, R2, S2.38, T1.
U3, V1b, W2. SUDEP classification: SUDEP probable.

### CASE SUMMARY

A case of SUDEP associated with a positive life event (PLS).

An 18-year-old black female high school student had a history of infrequent (less than once yearly) generalized tonic-clonic seizures that were controlled with moderate doses of carbamazepine with therapeutic blood levels. She was an outstanding student, and during her senior year she was offered admission to an Ivy League school with a full scholarship. Her social circumstances were modest in that her father worked as a municipal trash collector and she was the first family member to go to college.

Shortly thereafter, her distraught parents notified her neurologist (PLS) that their daughter was found dead in bed. As no postmortem examination was performed, and no other cause of death was evident, the diagnosis of probable SUDEP was applied. This case may demonstrate that intensely positive surprise life events can produce as much stress as negative events.

### DISCUSSION BY LATHERS AND SCHRAEDER

Heart–brain interactions function during normal daily routine actions and during times of stress. The occurrence of stress itself is a powerful change initiator and may trigger transient ischemia and acute coronary syndrome in some people (Pickworth et al. 1990; Lathers and Schraeder 2006; Lathers et al. 2008b; Soufer and Burg 2007). These individuals are at increased risk for recurrent cardiac events and early death. Psychosocial stress can become an acute trigger of myocardial infarction in patients with preexisting coronary artery disease. Stress, via actions on the central and autonomic nervous systems, may produce a cascade of physiologic responses in individuals at risk that may lead to myocardial ischemia, ventricular fibrillation, plaque rupture, or coronary thrombosis (Krantz et al. 1996). Use of simultaneous single-photon emission computed tomography imaging with technetium-99m tetrofosmin myocardial perfusion imaging and transthoracic echocardiography was done at rest and during mental stress induced in patients with stable coronary artery disease (Shah et al. 2006). Nevertheless, today we still do not understand the pathophysiology of mental stress–induced ischemia, what diagnostic tests are needed to identify susceptible people, nor how to develop risk stratification algorithms to be applied in the clinical workplace. Research is needed to define the brain–heart relationship during the occurrence of mental stress that underlies the cognitive and emotional aspects of mental stress as the distinct patterns of brain activity occurring during mental stress may trigger silent myocardial ischemia (Soufer 2006; Soufer and Burg 2007; Rozanski et al. 1988).

## PROBABLE SUDEP CASES

SUDEP syndrome cluster identifier: 1, 3, A11e, B, C3, D4, E1g, H1, P2, Q2, S2.46?, T1, U1, V1c, W2. SUDEP classification: SUDEP probable.

Sudden death of Patsy Custis: George Washington on SUDEP.

### CASE SUMMARY

Patsy Custis, the stepdaughter of George Washington, suffered from what, by description, was convulsive epilepsy that began at age 6. The seizures were uncontrolled by treatment of the time, which included bleeding, purging, mercury, and cinchona along with other decoctions. She was taken to the healing baths in what is now Berkeley Springs, West Virginia, and was made to wear an iron ring, since such a ring was thought to protect against seizures. All of these interventions, unsurprisingly, were of no avail. Despite being described by George Washington as being in "better health and spirits" than in the past, on June 19, 1773, at age 17, she died in the afternoon within 2 minutes of "one of her usual fits," "with scarcely a sigh."

### COMMENTS BY DOHERTY (2004)

Patsy's demise met the criteria for probable SUDEP as established by Leestma and Koenig (1968) and Jay and Leestma (1981). In summary, she had epilepsy, was in a reasonably good state of health, the fatal event was sudden with or without a concurrent seizure but was not status epilepticus as it occurred during normal activity, and no other obvious explanation for the sudden death was extant. Her death is one of the first documented cases of SUDEP, as described by her stepfather, George Washington.

### COMMENTS BY LATHERS ET AL. (2011, CH. 22, PP. 329–330)

George Washington clearly was a witness to the fatal event as he described her as having "one of her usual fits," also noting that she manifested "scarcely a sigh" at the time of her demise, a description that implies apnea. From the distance of almost a quarter of a millennium, Patsy seemed to have met the published criteria for probable SUDEP. Although presently we are not much further along in our understanding of the mechanism of death in SUDEP than we were in

the eighteenth century, the witnessed description is consistent with seizure-related apnea as the probable mechanism in this case in that George Washington observed his stepdaughter as having manifested "scarcely a sigh" at the time of her demise.

Although having had uncontrolled convulsive seizures since childhood puts her into a higher risk category, the possibility of the risk factor of an underlying nonprogressive brain disease is unknown. While being female had a slight mitigating effect on risk of SUDEP, she was a young adult and, as mentioned earlier, had uncontrolled seizures.

SUDEP is not a function of the victims' social or socioeconomic status.

Note: DeToledo et al. (1999) notes from George Washington's diaries on the illness and death of Martha Parke-Custis.

## PREVENTED SUDEP CASE AND SYNCOPE AND A SURVIVOR, NONEPILEPTIC CASE WITH SYNCOPE (STRZELEZYK ET AL. 2008)

SUDEP syndrome cluster identifier: 2, B, C3, C4a, D99, E1X, F2a, F2a1, F2b, I, P1, Q5, R3, S2, T1, U1, W4.

SUDEP syndrome cluster identifier: 2, C4a, F2a, F2a1, F2b, G, N1, P1, Q3, R3, S2, T1, U1, W7.

SUDEP classification: SUDEP prevented case 1 and survivor, not epilepsy case 2.

Ictal asystole in temporal lobe epilepsy before and after pacemaker implantation.

### CASE SUMMARY

A 41-year-old male presented with refractory partial seizures resulting in syncope leading to severe head trauma. Presurgical video-EEG monitoring demonstrated two episodes of ictal bradycardia followed by asystole and syncope. Implantation of a cardiac pacemaker provided a seizure-free, syncope-free 9-month follow-up period.

### COMMENTS BY STRZELCZYK, BAUER, KNAKE, OERTEL, HAMER, AND ROSENOW

Ictal bradycardia or asystole in patients with epilepsy presenting with ictal falls may be a factor in some cases of SUDEP. This case documents that cardiac pacemaker implantation in addition to continuation of AEDs may optimize seizure control while preventing ictal syncope and/or trauma associated with a fall.

### COMMENTS BY LATHERS ET AL. (2011, CH. 22, PP. 328–9)

When treating patients with epilepsy and a known previous history of ictal falls and/or ictal bradycardia or asystole, one must also consider the psychological stress related to fear of falling and injury consequent to having a seizure. One case study in a nonepileptic individual (Schraeder et al. 1983) described how a young athletic male who was listening to his minister's sermon describing gory details of how martyrs were tortured for their beliefs passed out and exhibited what appeared to be a generalized tonic-clonic seizure. Subsequent repetition of the offending verbal passages with EEG monitoring confirmed that the clinical seizures were the consequence of psychologically induced asystole lasting over 30 seconds with resultant electrocerebral silence. No epileptiform activity occurred on the EEG. This patient became seizure free after implantation of a cardiac pacemaker. This nonepileptic case emphasizes the strong contribution of cerebral output to cardiac function. Stress itself may be a risk factor for SUDEP (Lathers and Schraeder 2006). SUDEP cluster identifier is given above. The W7 category indicates that this person was a survivor who did not have epilepsy. Stress factors will not show up on autopsy.

Carinci et al. (2007) note that the clinical distinction between cardiovascular and epileptic causes of loss of consciousness may be difficult to discern. This becomes a diagnostic challenge when a primary epileptic seizure secondarily causes asystole. The ictal bradycardia syndrome refers to correlation of epilepsy with severe bradycardia or asystole, both of which may be a mechanism of SUDEP. Nonetheless, Carinci et al. (2007) conclude that asystole induced by partial seizures is rarely a cause of syncope.

Patients with potentially fatal mechanisms of syncope may be diagnosed inaccurately to have seizures and people with epilepsy may be at risk for ictal arrhythmias as a cause for sudden death (Al Aloul et al. 2007). It is clinically important to diagnose accurately patients in both categories. Al Aloul et al. (2007) cited the fact that the emergence of Brugada pattern on the electrocardiogram in response to administration of class IA or IC antiarrhythmic agents has been routinely recognized as a means of inducing concealed Brugada syndrome, which is a risk factor for sudden cardiac death. They reported a case in which the patient demonstrated induced Brugada pattern after phenytoin, a class IB antiarrhythmic agent, was administered. Phenytoin levels were supratherapeutic. The authors recommended that all patients with supratherapeutic phenytoin levels should be evaluated for emergence of the Brugada pattern in the electrocardiogram. Britton and Benarroch (2006) also emphasized that, although pathophysiologically distinct, syncope and seizures often exhibit the same clinical phenomena, making it difficult to diagnosis clinically the cause of a patient's seizure-like activity. Furthermore, in some patients both seizure and syncope may coexist. Syncope may be associated with seizure-like motor manifestations, and seizure may be complicated by cardiac arrhythmia and syncope. Combined EEG/ECG telemetry is necessary to establish the accurate diagnosis and allow evaluation of neuroanatomic circuitry involved in the production of cardiovascular manifestations of seizures.

## PREVENTED SUDEP CASE (LATHERS 2011)

SUDEP syndrome cluster identifier: 3, A7, A11c3, B, C3, C4c, D4, E1e, H1a, H2, O7f, O8h, P1, Q5, R3, S2.35, T1, U1, W4. SUDEP classifications: SUDEP prevented.

Postictal laryngospasm as one potential mechanism for SUDEP.

## CASE SUMMARY

A 1-minute generalized tonic-clonic seizure occurred as a 42-year-old male patient diagnosed with refractory epilepsy was being monitored in an epilepsy-monitoring unit (EMU) (Tavee and Morris 2008). This episode was followed by persistent inspiratory stridor and cyanosis. Cardiac parameters remained stable during the event. However, the respiratory status declined rapidly, despite the administration of oxygen via bag-valve-mask. As the emergency code team proceeded with intubation, they noted severe laryngospasm as the endotracheal tube was being inserted. Resuscitation was successful. This case demonstrated that postictal laryngospasm may be one potential cause of sudden unexpected death in people with epilepsy (Lathers 2011, ch. 44).

## COMMENTS BY LATHERS (2011, CH. 44)

As discussed by Abu-Shaweesh (2007), activation of laryngeal mucosa results in apnea mediated through, and elicited via, electrical stimulation of the superior laryngeal nerve. The inhibitory reflex is thought to be involved in the pathogenesis of apnea of prematurity and sudden infant death syndrome. Theophylline and block of γ-aminobutyric acid (GABA) (A) receptors attenuate the inhibitory reflex. Phrenic nerve response to increasing levels of superior laryngeal nerve stimulation was examined in ventilated, vagotomized, decerebrate, and paralyzed newborn piglets. Phrenic activity decreased with increased stimulation of the superior laryngeal nerve and resulted in apnea and hypotension with higher levels of stimulation. It was concluded that activation of adenosine A (2A) receptors enhances superior laryngeal nerve stimulation-induced apnea. This may occur via a GABAergic pathway. The authors hypothesize that superior laryngeal nerve stimulation may cause endogenous release of adenosine to activate A (2A) receptors on GABAergic neurons, resulting in the release of GABA at inspiratory neurons and subsequent respiratory inhibition.

## PREVENTED SUDEP CASE (SO ET AL. 2000; LATHERS 2011)

SUDEP syndrome cluster identifier: 2, 3, A11c3, C3, C4c, D4, F2a1, F2b, H1, H2, P2, Q2, T1, U1, W4. SUDEP classifications: SUDEP prevented.

Postictal central apnea as one potential Mechanism for SUDEP.

## CASE SUMMARY

A 55-second convulsive seizure occurred in a 20-year-old female as she underwent video-EEG monitoring (So et al. 2000). Persistent apnea then developed. Electrocardiogram-monitored rhythm was not altered for the first 10 seconds; then it gradually and progressively slowed and stopped 57 seconds later. Cardiorespiratory resuscitation was successful. No evidence of airway obstruction or pulmonary edema was noted.

## Comments by So et al. (2000)

One previous cardiorespiratory arrest after a complex partial seizure without secondary generalization had been reported for this patient. So et al. (2000) note that although epileptic seizures may be associated with arrhythmogenic actions at the heart, in this patient the mechanism of marked central suppression of respiratory activity after seizures was clearly involved and almost resulted in sudden death.

## Comments by Lathers (2011, ch. 44)

Psychological factors, including stress (Lathers and Schraeder 2006; Lathers et al. 2008a, b; Schraeder et al. 1983), are risk factors for SUDEP (Lear-Kaul et al. 2005; Fenwick 1994; Wannamaker 1985; Stopper et al. 2007; Owada et al. 1999; Scorza et al. 2008). Some people with epilepsy may experience stress during video-EEG monitoring, especially since monitoring protocols often include reduction or withdrawal of antiepileptic drugs to increase the likelihood of triggering seizures and the unwanted respiratory and/or cardiac events. Fortunately, in this patient and in the patient of Tavee and Morris successful resuscitation occurred and SUDEP appears to have been prevented. Unlike the finding by Tavee and Morris (2008) discussed earlier, So et al. (2000) do not mention any observation of severe laryngospasm as the endotracheal tube was being inserted. We do not know if severe laryngospasm did occur in this 20-year-old female with epilepsy, and the emergency code team did not detect it if it did actually occur. In the future, it will be important for emergency teams to note if a given person with known epilepsy exhibits severe laryngospasm. In any event, these case histories highlight the fact that both respiratory and cardiac changes occur in people with epilepsy. The timing of events such as seizures, respiratory and/or laryngospasm, and cardiac EKG changes varies among patients. The physician must consider risk factors for a given individual patient and prescribe procedures to protect the person from future unwanted events that may result in SUDEP. The question must be asked as to whether a person first experienced seizures and respiratory events and then cardiac events or if the person experienced seizures and arrhythmia and then respiratory events. Published case reports support both cardiac and respiratory events as initiating mechanisms of sudden death. Obviously, rapid reversal of these changes is essential and the "availability of resuscitation methods on the spot where the victim is located" certainly increases the likelihood that SUDEP will be prevented. It is also important to note that interictal discharges, just like ictal discharges, have been reported in association with cardiac arrhythmias and/or respiratory changes and/or sudden death (Lathers and Schraeder 1982; Schraeder and Lathers 1983). The people administering the EEG/EKG video monitoring must watch for both interictal and ictal discharges as warning signs of unwanted events that may be triggered.

## Prevented Sudep Case (Novakova et al. 2013; Lathers and Schraeder 2011c)

SUDEP syndrome cluster identifier: 1, A11, A11a1, C3, C4a, C9, C91, C95, C96, D4, K1, K1p1, K1b1, L1a1, N, N1, N2, N3, N4, N5a, P1, Q4, R3, S2, T1, U1, W6. SUDEP classification: SUDEP prevented.

Case report of postictal aggressive behavior.

### Case Summary

A 37-year-old man had complex partial seizures, consisting of an olfactory aura followed by alteration of consciousness, since age 5, with occasional tonic-clonic seizures. He also had a history of depression and bipolar affective disorder. During the postictal period, at times he would feel threatened and harmed and would focus his aggressive response by attacking any individual in his immediate environment, often resulting in physical injury to that person. The patient's postictal confusion would remit usually after 1 hour; but the fear of harm and sense of being threatened would last for 24 hours, after which he felt great remorse. He had been charged with aggravated assault several times. His magnetic resonance imaging image was unremarkable, but sleep-deprived EEG manifested left anterior temporal spikes and sharp waves. The aggressive postictal episodes ended with control of his seizures resulting from addition of carbamazepine to his original regimen of valproic acid and sertraline.

### Discussion by Mendez

The author describes aggressive acts as a direct consequence of seizures, occurring directly during seizures or postictally (Mendez 1998). He also emphasizes that postictal violence is most commonly resistive behavior during the postictal delirium and is associated with attempts at restraint. He also discussed the observation that seemingly violent automatisms such as flailing or spitting can occur during complex partial seizures and that secondary violent automatisms can be behavioral responses to ictal fear, hallucinations, or other disagreeable seizure-related experiences.

### Discussion by Lathers and Schraeder (2011, ch. 17)

Another issue to consider in relationship to the occurrence of putative ictal or postictal violent behavior is that of the possible induction of an excited delirium syndrome when attempts are made to restrain the behavior of an individual who is manifesting actual or seemingly violent behavior. As discussed by DiMaio and DiMaio (2006), excited delirium syndrome "involves the sudden death of an individual, during or following an episode of excited delirium, in which an autopsy fails to reveal evidence of sufficient trauma or natural disease to explain the death. In virtually all cases, the episode of excited delirium is terminated by a struggle with police of medical personnel, and the use of physical restraint. Typically, within a few to several minutes following cessation of the struggle, the individual is noted to be in cardiopulmonary arrest. Attempts at resuscitation are usually unsuccessful." During state of delirium, there are varying transient disturbances of consciousness and cognition with disorientation; disorganized and inconsistent thought processes; inability to distinguish reality from hallucinations; speech disturbance; and disorientation to time, place, and person. The deaths occur most commonly in individuals who have abused stimulants such as cocaine and methamphetamine, and also in people with endogenous mental disease who have not used these drugs. The majority of deaths occur between the ages of 17 and 35 years. Although the mechanism of death in these individuals is not defined, it was concluded that stimulation of the sympathetic nervous system causes release of norepinephrine at the synapses and in combination with epinephrine it is released into the bloodstream from the adrenal glands. This response then results in a subsequent increase in myocyte activity and oxygen demand in combination with decreased myocardial blood flow secondary to coronary artery constriction.

We need to be aware of the potential for induction of this potentially fatal state of agitation when attempts are made to restrain people with epilepsy who manifest ictal or postictal agitation or seemingly violent behavior. This is a highly stressful state and in combination with the history of epilepsy could be contributory to the occurrence of SUDEP in these individuals. Since both ictal and postictal states are self-limited, it is imperative for family members, police, and emergency care personnel to understand that watchful observation to keep the affected individual out of harm's way, rather than the high risk intervention of physical restraint, is the most appropriate intervention.

## PREVENTED SUDEP CASE (FAUCHIER ET AL. 2000)

SUDEP syndrome cluster identifier: 1, 2, A11 e, C4a, D4, F1b, I, J2a12, K1d1, K1L1, L2, P1, Q3, R3, S2, T1, U1, W6. SUDEP classifications: SUDEP prevented.

Epilepsy and Brugada syndrome in a man with a history of generalized tonic-clonic seizures. Case summary. A 24-year-old man had an EEG-confirmed diagnosis of generalized tonic-clonic epilepsy since age 7, at times associated with tongue biting and urinary incontinence. He was treated with phenobarbital and diazepam. Since age 17, he also had some seizures that seemed to be related to alcohol abuse. At age 24, he was observed by his wife to have a syncopal episode without generalized clinical seizure activity. An ECG found right bundle branch block and ST segment elevation in V2 and V3, findings consistent with Brugada syndrome. All other cardiac studies, Doppler echocardiography, radionuclide tomography, coronary angiography, contrast ventriculography, cardiac MRI, 24-hour ambulatory ECG, and electrophysiological studies, were normal. After implantation of a cardioverter-defibrillator, no syncope, no seizure, nor any appropriate therapy by the defibrillator occurred.

## DISCUSSION BY AUTHORS (FAUCHIER ET AL. 2000)

Fauchier et al. (2000) make the point that epilepsy may occur concurrently with the Brugada syndrome, which is attributable to defects of the cardiac sodium channel gene *SCN5* and is associated with a high risk of cardiac sudden death from ventricular arrhythmias. They noted that, as in SUDEP, there is young male predominance. In patients with the Brugada syndrome, an implantable defibrillator is indicated. Patients treated only with amiodarone and/or β-blockers were not protected against sudden death, as there was a death rate of 26% during follow-up. An emphasis was placed on the fact that people with cardiac syncope usually do not experience tongue biting unless a hypoperfusion-related secondary seizure occurs. Finally, they commented that the previous ECGs of SUDEP victims should be reviewed, when available, to help in determining whether Brugada syndrome was a factor contributing to the death.

## DISCUSSION BY LATHERS, SCHRAEDER, AND BUNGO (2011, CH. 20)

This is one of the first case reports to document the concurrence of epilepsy and Brugada syndrome. However, the authors did not discuss the physiological connection in the form of sodium channel dysfunction that is extant in both entities. One of the most important clinical points that Fauchier et al. (2000) made was the need to review the previous ECGs of victims of SUDEP to look for evidence of subtle cardiac abnormalities that either could have been the primary disorder that was mimicking seizures or were concurrent with a bona fide seizure disorder. However, the next obvious step, namely, considering screening ECGs in all people with a diagnosis of seizure disorder, should be addressed. A primary diagnosis of Brugada syndrome indicates implantation of a cardioverter-defibrillator, whereas the finding of coexisting Brugada syndrome and epilepsy would suggest that the patient should also be continued on antiepileptic medication. The authors did not clarify whether or not the patient in their case report was continued on antiepileptic medication.

Lathers et al. (2011, ch. 20). Constructed from Fauchier et al. (2000).

## PREVENTED SUDEP CASE SODIUM CHANNEL DYSFUNCTION (SANDORIFI ET AL. 2013)

SUDEP syndrome cluster identifier: 1, 2, A11b?, A11c3, C4c, J2a12, K1g1, K11h1, K1L1, k1N1, K1f, P2, R3 Q4, S2, T1, U1, W4. SUDEP classifications: SUDEP prevented.

### CASE SUMMARY (GIRARD ET AL. 2008)

A woman with Brugada syndrome and epilepsy. A 40-year-old woman had recurrent episodes of dizziness followed by remitting episodes of hearing loss. It was suspected that the episodes of dizziness might be seizures and that the transient hearing loss might be a postictal phenomenon. An ECG on admission found ST elevation in V1 through V3 consistent with a diagnosis of Brugada syndrome. She was placed on long-term EEG and ECG monitoring. Several episodes of jerking movements and confusion followed by hearing loss were observed on video. As there were no apparent EEG or telemetry abnormalities, a diagnosis of pseudoseizures was entertained. It was determined that the patient should be weaned off of her antiepileptic medications of phenytoin, lamotrigine, levetiracetam, and topiramate. During the process of being weaned off of lamotrigine, she experienced a tonic-clonic seizure accompanied by generalized polyspike and wave activity. The EEG discharges persisted for 24 hours but resolved after the lamotrigine dosage was increased. No cardiac arrhythmia was observed on telemetry, and in fact the ECG changes consistent with Brugada syndrome improved but did not resolve as the phenytoin dose was reduced. The patient suffered no further attacks and she was maintained on lamotrigine and low-dose phenytoin. At no time during her hospital stay were any arrhythmias observed.

## Discussion by Authors (Girard et al. 2008)

The authors hypothesize that their patient may have a presumably genetic underlying systemic sodium channel dysfunction. They acknowledge that both Brugada syndrome and epilepsy are associated with the risk of sudden death. They also note that even though seizures may occur in patients with Brugada syndrome, they are secondary to arrhythmia-related cerebral hypoperfusion.

## Discussion by Lathers, Schraeder, and Bungo (SUDEP Book 2014)

This case is another example of a group of patients with sodium channelopathies that have a potential for both Brugada syndrome and epilepsy. However, in this case, the Brugada component appeared to be clinically silent, whereas the epilepsy was clinically manifest. An important question to consider is whether or not the presence of ECG markers of Brugada syndrome without related ventricular arrhythmias increases the risk of a seizure-related fatal cardiac event. As discussed in the case described by Fauchier et al. (2000), the question can be raised about the possible need for implantation of a defibrillator in a patient with a heretofore clinically silent set of ECG findings consistent with Brugada syndrome. Another question raised by the observation that the ECG changes in the V1 through V3 leads lessened with a decrease in the dose of phenytoin is whether certain antiepileptic drugs increase risk for cardiogenic ventricular arrhythmias. The aforementioned two cases illustrate that some patients will exhibit both Brugada syndrome and some types of epilepsy produced by sodium channel dysfunction. Brugada syndrome is produced by a mutation in gene *SCN5A*, which encodes the α subunit of cardiac sodium channel (Antzelevitch et al. 2005). Herreros

et al. note that some epileptic syndromes (Graves 2006) are due to different mutations in genes encoding α subunits of neuronal sodium channels (*SCN1A* and *SCN2A*) or in the β subunit (*SCN1B*), common for both cardiac and neuronal isoforms (Lehmann-Horn and Jurkat-Rott 1999). Additional clinical, electrocardiographic, and genetic studies are needed to improve risk stratification for a given patient and to determine whether or not there is a relationship among sodium channel dysfunction, Brugada ECG, and idiopathic epilepsy. The response of the two patients presented in the aforementioned cases appears to support the possibility that a common pathophysiologic mechanism is associated with sodium channel dysfunction and may be common to ECG abnormalities of Brugada syndrome and some types of epilepsy. Many more patients must be screened to confirm this possibility. Prospective electrocardiographic and genetic studies must be performed to determine which individuals with epilepsy are at risk for SUDEP compared with patients with cardiac disease at risk for sudden cardiac death. The risks factors for SUDEP must be defined and linked with mechanisms for death (Lathers et al. 2008a, b; Herroes 2011, ch. 19). Parameters must be developed regarding what drugs should be avoided. One patient has been reported with two ion channel disorders in heart and brain.

## PREVENTED SUDEP (GILMAN ET AL. 1993; LATHERS AND SCHRAEDER 2011B)

SUDEP syndrome cluster identifier: 1, K1, K1b1, K5e, P?, Q1, R2, S2, T1, U1, W4. SUDEP classifications: SUDEP prevented. Statistically: use cluster ID two times.

Case history of generic carbamazepine.

### Case Summary

Two 6-year old children exhibited carbamazepine toxicity resulting from generic substitution (Gilman et al. 1993). Increases in the maximum serum carbamazepine concentrations, one of 22% and one of 41%, occurred. When serum concentrations were decreased in both patients, the two patients became asymptomatic and residual effects did not occur. Summarized from Gilman et al. (1993). Lathers and Schraeder (2011b, ch. 47).

### Questions Raised by Lathers and Schraeder

That reduced serum concentrations and seizure exacerbation followed generic substitution of Tegretol is a well-established phenomenon. Increased carbamazepine levels could possibly be a risk factor for SUDEP. As cited later, carbamazepine has been shown on Holter monitoring to produce intermittent complete atrioventricular block. At higher blood levels, carbamazepine can interfere with cardiac electrical conduction and increase the risk of conduction block. Devinsky et al. (1994) found that variations in blood pressure and heart rate during orthostasis and cold face test were higher in epilepsy patients than in controls with or without carbamazepine. People with epilepsy exhibited higher initial increase in blood pressure and greater subsequent decreases in blood pressure than nonmedicated controls during the cold face test.

Controls treated with carbamazepine demonstrated higher heart rates during orthostasis and cold face test with apnea than those without the drug. The carbamazepine levels correlated with baseline, orthostatic blood pressure, and heart rate during deep breathing in sinus arrhythmia. The authors conclude that people with epilepsy have greater blood pressure and heart rate variability and reactivity than controls and that these characteristics are attributable in part to carbamazepine levels. If carbamazepine levels decrease, there is a possibility of increased uncontrolled interictal discharges and/or seizures developing and these events may increase the chance of SUDEP via impaired autonomic cardiac sympathetic discharges/nonuniformity (Lathers and Schraeder 1982; Schraeder and Lathers 1983). See chapter 28 in our 2011 SUDEP book (Lathers and Schraeder 2011c, ch. 28) for a full discussion on this animal model. Aside from the generic question, there is also a formulation difference. Ficker et al. (2005) found that switching patients to an extended-release formulation from an immediate-release formulation of carbamazepine diminished the risk of adverse events, improved quality of life measures, and was associated with improved seizure control.

Could carbamazepine-induced hyponatremia contribute to the occurrence of SUDEP in some patients by lowering the threshold for arrhythmia? Hyponatremia lowers seizure threshold and increases frequency of seizures. Thus, carbamazepine-induced hyponatremia may contribute to the occurrence of SUDEP in some patients.

## PREVENTED SUDEP INDUCED QRS PROLONGATION (HEROLD 2006; LATHERS AND SCHRAEDER 2011B)

SUDEP syndrome cluster identifier: 1, 2, A11c3?, C4a, G1, K1, K1e1, K1g1, K5e, P2, Q3, R3, S2, T1, U1, W4. SUDEP classifications: SUDEP prevented.

Paradoxical seizures due to toxic AED levels.

Case history: lamotrigine-induced QRS prolongation.

### CASE SUMMARY

A 22-year-old female had two seizure-like episodes consisting of tonic-clonic activity of the upper extremities with no sphincter incontinence and presented to the emergency room. On examination, she was found to have horizontal nystagmus on lateral gaze and ataxia, with widening of the QRS complex and right-axis deviation on the ECG. There was no history of her taking more than her prescribed dose of lamotrigine (200 mg t.i.d.). A lamotrigine level of 57.8 μmol/L was detected (therapeutic range is 3.9–15.6 μmol/L).

### SUMMARIZED FROM HEROLD (2006)

As lamotrigine blocks sodium channels, sodium bicarbonate administered intravenously resulted in improvement of the QRS narrowing. The patient was also taking felbamate 600 mg t.i.d. and had no laboratory evidence of any other medication that could have produced QRS prolongation. The author suggested that a drug interaction may have been responsible for the toxic lamotrigine level. She left the emergency room against medical advice.

### COMMENTS BY LATHERS AND SCHRAEDER (2011B, CH. 47)

QRS prolongation may be a possible contributory risk factor for sudden death (Lathers et al. 2008a). Lamotrigine toxicity secondary to acute intentional or unintentional overdose may be, as Herold (2006) notes, a possible cause of QRS prolongation in a patient with a seizure disorder. If a drug inhibits the human cardiac delayed rectifier potassium current, prolongation of the cardiac QT interval may occur. This change is associated with a potentially fatal, polymorphic ventricular tachycardia called torsades de pointes. Lamotrigine inhibits the human cardiac delayed rectifier potassium current in vitro, and it has been hypothesized that QT prolongation may contribute to the risk of SUDEP. Dixon et al. (2008) studied QT/QTc and found the QTc interval was not prolonged by therapeutic doses of lamotrigine (50–200 mg b.d.) in healthy subjects. The patient described by Herold (2006) had been taking a therapeutic dose of lamotrigine (200 mg t.i.d.) and was found to have a toxic level, which in all likelihood was the cause of the EKG changes.

## PREVENTED SUDEP (LATHERS AND SCHRAEDER 2011A)

SUDEP syndrome cluster identifier: 1, 2, C4a, G, G1, K1b1 (K5g), K1p1 (substituted), P2, Q7, R3, S2, T1, U1, W4. SUDEP classifications: SUDEP prevented.

### CASE: CARBAMAZEPINE INTERMITTENT COMPLETE AV BLOCK

A 66-year-old female with epilepsy and no history of heart disease went to the hospital complaining of frequent episodes of sudden dizziness (summarized by Ide and Kamijo [2007]). She had taken a low dose of carbamazepine, 200 mg daily, for 1 year. The carbamazepine level on admission was subtherapeutic at 4 μg/mL (therapeutic range is 6–12 μg/mL). Holter monitoring showed intermittent complete atrioventricular block of up to 10 seconds duration with ventricular escape. The patient reverted to a normal sinus rhythm after the carbamazepine was discontinued with substitution of valproic acid 600 mg daily. The authors note that this case demonstrates that although complete atrioventricular block may occur in association with a high carbamazepine level, it may also occur long after the initiation of carbamazepine therapy in an "older" woman even if the serum concentration of carbamazepine is subtherapeutic.

## COMMENTS BY LATHERS AND SCHRAEDER (2011B, CH. 47)

This case report raises the possibility that some people without any history of heart disease may have a genetic predisposition to atrioventricular block when exposed to carbamazepine and emphasizes the potential role for an as yet undeveloped genetic methodology to screen for patients who might be at risk for antiepileptic drugs–related cardiac conduction disturbances or arrhythmias.

In another study, both carbamazepine and oxycarbamazepine used as monotherapy were associated with reduced serum thyroid hormone concentrations in 78 girls diagnosed with epilepsy (Vainionpää et al. 2004). An earlier study found similar changes for carbamazepine. Phenytoin was also shown to decrease serum thyroid hormone levels and similar to carbamazepine was theorized to accelerate hepatic plasma clearance of these hormones due to induction of hepatic microsomal enzyme systems by these antiepileptic drugs (Isojärvi et al. 1992). Nonetheless, since the subjects were clinically euthyroid, the implication of the decreased thyroid hormone levels is unknown. Increased QT interval dispersion (QTd) is an EKG parameter associated with malignant ventricular arrhythmias and sudden death (Backiner et al. 2008). QT dispersion corrected for heart rate is thought to be one predictor of cardiac death. Thyroid-stimulating hormone level in overt hypothyroidism is associated with increased QTd. Backiner et al. (2008) investigated QTc in subclinical hypothyroidism and monitored changes when TSH levels were normalized with L-thyroxine. The prolonged QTc found in the females was corrected when TSH levels reach 10 mIU/I or more. Thus, even though there is, as yet, no known clinical implications for the female patients with epilepsy taking carbamazepine, oxycarbamazepine, or phenytoin, it is likely that they should be observed for changes in QTd/QTc as prolonged QTc may place these patients at a greater risk for SUDEP.

## PREVENTED SUDEP SYNCOPE SECONDARY TO HYPONATREMIA: ELECTROLYTE CHANGES (RUIZ ET AL. 2007; LATHERS AND SCHRAEDER 2011A)

SUDEP syndrome cluster identifier: 1, B, I, K11b1, K1g1, L, N, N3, N5b1, P2, Q4, R3, S2, T, U1, W4. SUDEP classifications: SUDEP prevented.

Symptomatic secondary hyponatremia due to combined treatment with carbamazepine, lamotrigine, and venlafaxine: risk of sudden death in epilepsy?

### CASE SUMMARY

A 37-year-old female presented with an episode of syncope secondary to symptomatic hyponatremia. She had refractory epilepsy associated with exogenous depressive syndrome and was receiving combined treatment with carbamazepine; lamotrigine; and venlafaxine, an antidepressant.

## COMMENT BY RUIZ ET AL. (2007)

The hyponatremia was generated by inappropriate secretion of antidiuretic hormone. The electrolytic anomaly can result in secondary neurological and cardiovascular effects and may contribute to sudden death secondary to the risk of cardiac arrhythmia in patients with epilepsy. The authors recommend "strict ionic control" in patients requiring a combined antiepileptic drugs and antidepressant treatment to avoid "paroxysmal vascular episodes" and to minimize the risk of SUDEP.

## COMMENT BY LATHERS AND SCHRAEDER

Readers are referred to a paper by Kloster et al. (1998) that reported sudden death in two patients with epilepsy and the syndrome of inappropriate antidiuretic hormone. The two patients, one with complex partial and the other with secondarily generalized seizures, were both taking oxcarbazepine and vigabatrin. One of the two patients was also taking lamotrigine. The authors note that both oxcarbazepine and carbamazepine may cause inappropriate secretion of antidiuretic hormone and recommend review of SUDEP cases and the antiepileptic drugs prescribed to determine if an inappropriate secretion of antidiuretic hormone may have been involved in the mechanism of death.

## NON-SUDEP CASES (LATHERS, SCHRAEDER, AND BUNGO 2011)

SUDEP syndrome cluster identifier: 2, G, G1, I, J2a1, P2, Q2, R3, S2, T1, U1, W7. A 10-year-old girl presented with recurrent episodes of syncope while swimming. She was diagnosed with type 1 LQTS.

SUDEP syndrome cluster identifier: 2, G, G1, I (family history), J2a2, P1, Q4, R3, S2, T1, U1, W7. A 36-year-old asymptomatic male was unexpectedly diagnosed with type 2 LQTS. Familial history revealed audio-triggered syncope and sudden death at a young age.

SUDEP syndrome cluster identifier: 2, G, G1, J2a3, P1, Q2, R3, S2, T1, U1, V, V1b, V2, W5. A 16-year-old male died in his sleep. Postmortem testing revealed type 3 LQTS.

SUDEP classifications: non-SUDEP

Congenital long QT-syndrome, recurrent syncope, and sudden death at young age

### COMMENTS BY AKKERHUIS ET AL. (2007)

A leading cause of sudden death at a young age is congenital LQTS. Gene mutation for encoding myocardial ion channel proteins leads to prolonged QT-interval and abnormal ST-T segments demonstrated in 12-lead ECG.

Syncope or sudden cardiac death due to ventricular tachyarrhythmias may occur. Genotype-specific differences in ECG abnormalities and triggers for cardiac events may differentiate the type of LQTS and trigger initiation of genotype-specific treatment before the results of genetic testing are known. Genetic testing to determine the genetic substrate, genotype-specific treatment, and possibility of treatment with an implantable cardioverter-defibrillator all contribute to improved prognosis of patients with LQTS. The authors recommend that young patients with unexplained recurrent syncope after specific stimuli and those with atypical forms of epilepsy undergo a cardiological evaluation.

## COMMENTS BY LATHERS ET AL. (2011, CH. 22, PP. 326–7)

Readers are also referred to another case of the video monitoring of long QT syndrome–related aborted sudden death by Rossenbacker et al. (2007). The congenital long QT syndrome is an alteration in cardiac polarization that results in an increased risk of cardiac arrhythmias in young people. As a result of hypoperfusion, syncope, often with convulsive activity, occurs, so that up to 10% of cases may have an erroneous diagnosis of epilepsy. Typically, the clinical events are associated with preceding physical exertion with initiation of ventricular tachycardia, including torsades de pointes. The high mortality of long QT syndrome and the potential for prevention with an implanted defibrillator emphasize the importance of accurate diagnosis from the clinical history of exercise-related loss of consciousness and ECG recording (Medina-Villanueva et al. 2002). The overlapping diagnoses of long QT syndrome and epilepsy occur when the patient presents with what appears to be a convulsive seizure. The risk of death resulting from an incorrect diagnosis is obvious. However, the observation that up to 10% of these patients, who are at risk for premature demise, are diagnosed as having epilepsy raises two questions. The first is whether some people with epilepsy whose deaths are attributed to SUDEP in fact had long QT syndrome. The second is whether some people with epilepsy may also have long QT syndrome, predisposing them for neurogenically induced arrhythmias. It is well known that the long QT interval syndrome is familial and that family members of an index case should be screened with ECG and genetic testing. Research needs to be undertaken to address the potential need for screening family members of victims of SUDEP for long QT and other genetically determined ion channel disorders.

Recommendation: congenital LQTS. Gene mutation for encoding myocardial ion channel proteins leads to prolonged QT interval and abnormal ST-T segments in 12-lead EKG. Syncope or sudden cardiac death due to VT may occur. Genotype-specific differences in ECG abnormalities and triggers for cardiac events may differentiate the subtypes of LQTS and trigger initiation of genotype-specific treatment before results of genetic testing are known. Genetic testing to determine genetic substrate, genotype-specific treatment, and possible implantable cardioverter-defibrillator all contribute to improved therapy. Young patients with unexplained recurrent syncope after specific stimuli and those with atypical forms of epilepsy should undergo a cardiological evaluation.

## NON-SUDEP CASE

SUDEP syndrome cluster identifier: 2, L, G?, G1, M, N2, N3, P2, Q6, R3, S2, T, U1, W7.

SUDEP classifications: non-SUDEP.

Heart–brain interplay: a 53-year-old woman recovering from mitral valve repair.

## CASE SUMMARY (CALLAHAN ET AL. 2008)

A 53-year-old woman had an uncomplicated mitral valve repair, after which she refused to use the incentive spirometer, ambulate, or even sit in a chair. She experienced unexplained episodes of shortness of breath and tachycardia. At 4 weeks postoperatively, the ejection fraction, which was 50% preoperatively, remained at 40%. She was complaining of more postoperative pain and fatigue than was usual for this type of successful surgery. The patient experienced tearful episodes and, reluctantly, was interviewed by a psychiatrist. Although the initial diagnosis was adjustment disorder with anxious features, subsequent evaluation established a diagnosis of depression. Ultimately, the patient agreed to take an SSRI, citalopram. After several weeks of treatment, she had a profound improvement in her mental and physical states, with the patient and her family concurring that she had returned to her "old self."

## DISCUSSION BY LATHERS AND SCHRAEDER (2011A, CH. 17, P. 253)

This case illustrates how postoperative cardiac rehabilitation can be significantly affected by an adverse psychological state. Anxiety, panic, fatigue, and depression can have a profound adverse effect on physical well-being. This case illustrated how these adverse psychological symptoms interfered with recovery from mitral valve surgery. Psychiatric issues are risk factors for both SUDEP and cardiac sudden death. While the pathophysiological mechanism of SUDEP is not established, acute cardiac dysfunction is thought to be a major factor. Cardiologists have long known of the physical risks of adverse mental states in cardiac patients including unexpected sudden cardiac death. Stress and other psychological disturbances require consideration as possible risk factors associated with SUDEP. However, in contrast to the interest cardiologists have manifested in psychogenic risks associated with cardiac sudden death, little research has been undertaken on the subject of psychological issues relative to the risk of SUDEP.

A lesson from cardiology for those taking care of people with epilepsy is that there is a need for more data on psychogenic risks in persons with epilepsy as these risk factors include stress, and a better understanding of this risk should help to manage persons at risk for SUDEP by minimizing the consequence of this risk factor category, i.e., psychogenic risks, including stress.

## SUMMARY OF SINGLE CASES OF SUDDEN UNEXPECTED DEATH IN EPILEPSY

Of the preceding SUDEP Epilepsy cases in this chapter, from *Sudden Death in Epilepsy: Forensic and Clinical Issues:*

W1: Definite SUDEP with postmortem.
Female

1, A11a1, B, C1, C4a, K1bi, K5b, N1, P2, Q4, R3, S2.3, T1, U2, V1b, W1

W2: Probable SUDEP with or without postmortem.

Female

1, 2, A8, B, C4, C91, C92, C98, D5, J2a3, k1g1, G1, k5g, k5b, O7a, O8a, P2, Q3, R3, S2, T1, U1, V4, W2 (W1 per author but no autopsy as in our classification)

1, A11c3, C4a, D5, E1f, K1b1, K5d, N1, P2, Q2, R2, S2.38, T1, U3, V1b, W2

1, 3, A11e, B, C3, D4, E1g, H1, P2, Q2, S2.46?, T1, U1, V1c, W2

W3: Possible SUDEP 0

W4: SUDEP prevented: for people with epilepsy who are alive.

Male

3, A7, A11c3, B, C3, C4c, D4, H1a, H2, P1, Q5, R3, S2, T1, U1, W4

2, B, C3, C4a, D99, E1X, F2a, F2a1, F2b, I, P1, Q5, R3, S2, T1, U1, W4

Female

2, 3, A11a1, C3, C4c, F2a, F2b, H1, H2, P2, Q2, S2, T1, U1, W4 So et al.

1, 2, A11b?, A11c3, C4c, J2a12, K1g1, K11h1, K1L1, k1N1, K1f, P2, R3 Q4, S2, T1, U1, W4

1, 2, A11c3?, C4a, G1, K1, K1e1, K1g1, K5e, P2, Q3, R3, S2, T1, U1, W4

1, 2, C4a, G, G1, K1b1 (K5g), K1p1 (substituted), P2, Q7, R3, S2, T1, U1, W4

1, B, I, K11b1, K1g1, L, N, N3, N5b1, P2, Q4, R3, S2, T, U1, W4

Sex not known

1, K1, K1b1, K5e, P?, Q1, R2, S2, T1, U1, W4. Statistically: use cluster ID two times (Gilman et al. 1993; Lathers and Schraeder 2011b, ch. 47, p. 773).

1, K1, K1b1, K5e, P?, Q1, R2, S2, T1, U1, W4. Statistically: use cluster ID two times (Gilman et al. 1993; Lathers and Schraeder 2011b, ch. 47, p. 773).

W5: Non-SUDEP victims who were thought to have epilepsy but did not have epilepsy or were diagnosed with epilepsy but died of another cause such as a glial brain tumor.

Male

2, G, G1, J2a3, P1, Q2, R3, S2, T1, U1, V, V1b, V2, W5

W6: Diagnosed with epilepsy and must be medically evaluated to determine what preventive actions should be taken in the day-to-day events to protect a person from becoming a future victim of SUDEP.

Male

1, A11, A11a1, C3, C4a, C9, C91, C95, C96, D4, K1, K1p1, K1b1, L1a1, N, N1, N2, N3, N4, N5a, P1, Q4, R3, S2, T1, U1, W6

1, 2, A11 e, C4a, D4, F1b, I, J2a12, K1d1, K1L1, L2, P1, Q3, R3, S2, T1, U1, W6

W7: Survivor, nonepilepsy.

Male

2, C4a, F2a, F2a1, F2b, G, N1, P1, Q3, R3, S2, T1, U1, W7

2, G, G1, I (family history), J2a2, P1, Q4, R3, S2, T1, U1, W7

Female

2, G, G1, I, J2a1, P2, Q2, R3, S2, T1, U1, W7

2, L, G?, G1, M, N2, N3, P2, Q6, R3, S2, T, U1, W7

In the aforementioned cases, brief comments from the authors are found and are accompanied by discussion points from chapter authors. SUDEP risk factor cluster IDs have now been added to each case and then have been summarized on the previous page in a format usable for statistical analysis. The following 40 cases are from the published medical literature and illustrate a third method to present cluster IDs for each patient.

**Cases from Aurlien et al., 2007:**

*Patient 1:*
C4a: Clinical EEG
D5: Seizure onset age 17
E1c: Seizure frequency 1.5/month.
H1b: Lung edema
O7a: Died at home
O8a: Pronounced dead at residence.
O9a: Prone
P2: Female
Q3: Age at death 25 years
V1b: Postmortem exam performed.
W1: Definite SUDEP

*Patient 2:*
C4a: Clinical EEG
D5: Seizure onset at age 13.
E1a: Seizure free for 6 months.
E1g: Seizure just prior to death.
H1b: Lung edema
O7a: Died at home
O8a: Pronounced dead at residence.
O9a: Pone
P2: Female
Q2: Died at age 16
V1b: Postmortem exam performed.
W1: Definite SUDEP

*Patient 3:*
C4a: Clinical EEG
D6: Seizure onset at age 23.
E1a: Seizure free for 7 months.
E1g: Seizure just prior to death

E2a: Average frequency of seizures less than one/year.
O7a: Died at home
O8a: Pronounced dead at residence.
P2: Female
Q4: Died at age 37
V1b: Postmortem exam performed.
W1: Definite SUDEP

*Patient 4:*
  D5: Seizure onset at age 17
  E1: Two seizures in 1 week, otherwise seizure free for
  3 months.
  H1b: Lung edema
  O7a: Died at home
  O8a: Pronounced dead at residence.
  P2: Female
  Q3: Age at SUDEP 24 years
  V1b: Postmortem exam performed.
  W1: Definite SUDEP

**Case from Aurlien et al., 2009:**

Case A
1: Brain A8 juvenile myoclonic
2: Cardiac G1 function long QT
A8: Juvenile myoclonic epilepsy
B: Refractory
C4a: Clinical EEG
D5: First seizure at age 17 years
J2a3 LQT3, SCN5a
K1g1: Prescribed lamotrigine
K5b: Subtherapeutic
K5g: Tapering, process change
G1: Cardiac function long QT
O7a: Died at home
O8a: Pronounced dead at residence.
O9a: Prone position
P2: Female
Q3: Died at age 25 years
R3: Smoking unknown
T1: Human
U1: Race unknown
V4: Genetic screen
W2: Lack autopsy
W1: Definite SUDEP

**Cases from Bateman et al., 2010:**

*Patient 1:*
  A11c3: Generalized seizure.
  C4c: EMU
  D7: Seizure onset at age 35 years.
  E1g: Seizure preceded death.
  F2a: Asystole
  O7f: Site of fatal event = hospital.
  O8c: Pronounced dead in hospital.
  O8h: Asleep
  O9a: Prone.
  P2: Female

Q5: Age 42 years at death
S, W1: Definite SUDEP

*Patient 2:*
  A11c3: Generalized seizure.
  C4c: EMU setting
  C97: Snxiety
  D4: Seizure onset at age 6
  O7f: Site of fatal event = hospital.
  O8c: Pronounced dead in hospital.
  O8h: Asleep
  O9a: Prone.
  P1: Male
  Q6: Age 62 years at death
  S, W1: Definite SUDEP

**Case from Breningstall, 2001:**

*Patients 1–6: Not SUDEP cases*
*Patient 7:*
  D4: 9 years old at seizure onset.
  E1b: Less than or equal to one seizure/month before death
  E2d: One seizure in 2 years prior to event.
  O7a: Died at home
  O8a: Pronounced dead at home.
  O8h: Found dead in bed
  P2: Male
  Q2: Age 11
  S, W1: Definite SUDEP

**Case from Dasheiff and Dickinson, 1986:**

C4a: Clinical EEG
D6: Age 27 years at seizure onset.
E1g: Seizure just prior to death
E2d: Six seizures per month.
F1a: Ventricular fibrillation.
G: Cardiomegaly
G3b1: Myocardial infarction.
H1b: Pulmonary edema.
O7a: Died at home
O8a: Pronounced dead at residence.
O8h: Awake, daytime
Q5: Age 48 years at death
S, W1: Definite SUDEP.
S2.49: Wisconsin
V1b: Autopsy

**Case from Doherty and Sloan, 2010:**

A11b: Seizure had right frontal origin.
C4a: Clinical EEG
D5: Seizure onset at age 17 years.
E2a: No seizures in 6 months.
G: Cardiomyopathy
Q3: Age 23 years
O7a: Died at home
O8a: Pronounced dead at residence.
P1: Male

V1b: Autopsy performed.
S, W1: Definite SUDEP

### Case from Espinosa et al., 2009:

A11b1: Seizure activity in right temporal region.
C4c: Recordings in EMU during video monitoring
D4: Seizures began at age 3
E2d: Two to three seizures per week.
F1a: Ventricular fibrillation
F1b: Cardiac defibrillator implanted.
H2: Defibrillated
O7f: Event in hospital.
O8h: Event in sleep.
P2: Female
Q6: Age 51 years at case report.
W4: SUDEP prevented

### Case from Ferlisi et al., 2013:

A11b1: Right temporal lobe.
A11c3: Generalized seizure.
D6: 27 years old
E2d: Three to four seizures per year.
F1a: Ventricular fibrillation
F1b: Cardiac defibrillator implanted.
H2: Defibrillation successful
P1: Male
Q5: Age 44 years at case report.
W4: SUDEP prevented

### Case from Hindocha et al., 2008:

*Patient 1 ("V.8"):*
  A11c3: Generalized seizures
  D5: Seizure onset during teens.
  P2: Female
  O7a: Found dead at home
  O8a: Pronounced dead at residence.
  V1c: No postmortem exam
  W2: Probable SUDEP

*Patient 2 ("VI.4")*
  D4: Seizure onset at 14 months.
  E1g: Seizure just prior to death.
  O7a: Found dead at home
  O8a: Pronounced dead at residence.
  P2: Female
  V1b: Postmortem exam performed.
  W1: Definite SUDEP

### Case from Howell and Blumhardt Aurlien et al., 1989:

C4a: Clinical EEG
D9: Age at onset 55 years.
F2a: Ictal asystole
F2a1: Cardiac pacemaker implanted but no change in seizure frequency.
P1: Male
Q7: Age at death 69 years.

V1c: No postmortem exam.
W1: Definite SUDEP

### Case from Hunt and Tang, 2005:

D8: Age at onset 50 years.
E2d: Seizure frequency three or more per year
F2a1: Pacemaker implanted, seizure free.
G1: Long QT, torsades de pointes, AV block.
P2: Female
W5: Non-SUDEP; sudden cardiac death (SCD) prevented

### Case from Johnson et al., 2010:

C4a: Clinical EEG
D4: Age at epilepsy diagnosis = 4 years.
E1g: Seizure shortly before death
E2d: Three or more seizures per year.
O7c: Died outside
O8b: Pronounced dead outside.
P2: Female
Q1: Age at death = 8 years.
R2: Nonsmoker
V2: Genetic screen positive for RYR2-encoded ryanodine receptor.
W1: Definite SUDEP

### Cases from Kloster et al., 1998:

*Patient 1:*
D2: Age 14 years at seizure onset.
E1e: 2 Seizures in 5 days
E2d: One complex partial seizure per day + one generalized tonic-clonic seizure per 3 months.
H1b: Pulmonary edema
O7f: Died in hospital
O8c: Pronounced dead in hospital
P1: Male
Q5: Age 45 years at death.
V1b: Autopsy
W3: SUDEP or inappropriate antidiuretic hormone secretion (SIADH)

*Patient 2:*
D5: Age 20 at seizure onset
E1b: Less than or equal to one seizure per month near time of death.
E2b, E2c: One to two seizures per year
H1b: Pulmonary edema.
O7a: Died at home
O8a: Pronounced dead at residence.
O9a: Prone
P1: Male.
V1b: Autopsy
W5: Potential non-SUDEP; could be inappropriate antidiuretic hormone secretion (SIADH)

### Case from Kuroiwa et al., 1994:

A11c3: Generalized seizures.

C4b: Intensive care unit.
D4: 6 to 7 years old at onset
E1g: Seizure just prior to lethal arrhythmia.
E2d: Three seizures in 1 year
G1: Long QT, torsades de pointes.
H1c: Respiratory arrest/apnea.
H2: Successful resuscitation
P2: Female
W5: Non-SUDEP; SCD prevented

## Case from Le Gal et al., 2010:

C4a: Clinical EEG
D3: Age at onset = 5 months.
Q2: Age at death = 11 years.
O9b: Supine position
P1: Male
V2: Genetic testing
W1: Definite SUDEP

## Case from McLean and Wimalaratna, 2007:

C4a: Clinical EEG recording.
D4: Age 4 years for first seizure.
H1b: Pulmonary edema
Q6: Age 50–59 years
O7a: Died at home
O8a: Pronounced dead at residence.
O8h: Died at night
O9a: Prone.
P2: Female
S, W1: Definite SUDEP.
V1b: Autopsy

## Cases from Nelson and Ray, 1968:

*Patient 1: Did not die, report is on respiratory arrest not SUDEP*

*Patient 2:*
C4b or C4c: EEG in intensive care unit or EMU.
D5: Age at onset = 18 years
E2a: Less than one average yearly seizure.
H1c: Obstructive apnea
H2: Successful resuscitation.
P1: Male
W4: SUDEP prevented

## Cases from Pacia et al., 1994:

*Patient 1:*
C4a: Clinical EEG
D5: Seizure onset at age 13 years.
G1: Long QT syndrome.
G3b: SCD.
O7a: Found dead at home
O8a: Pronounced dead at residence.
P2: Female
Q2: Death at age 19 years
W5: Non-SUDEP

*Patient 2:*
C4a: Clinical EEG
D4: Seizure onset at age 4 years
E2d: Seizures monthly during past year.
F1b: ICD implanted
G1: Long QT syndrome.
P1: Male
W5: Non-SUDEP; SCD prevented

## Case from Pezzella et al., 2009:

A11c3: Generalized seizure.
D5: Age 14 at seizure onset
E2a: Average yearly frequency of seizures less than or equal to one (first event).
G: Cardiomegaly
H1b: Pulmonary edema.
P1: Male
W4: SUDEP prevented

## Case from Pinto et al., 2011:

A11c3: Generalized seizure
C4c: EEG in EMU
D4: Age at epilepsy onset = 5 years.
E1e: Less than 3 seizures per month
E2d: Three or more seizures per year.
P1: Male
Q2: Age at death = 16 years
V1: Postmortem examination negative for cardiac causes.
W1: Definite SUDEP

## Case from Rauscher et al., 2011:

A11a2, A11b2: Right and left temporal lobes.
C4a: Clinical EEG source
D6: Age 17 years at first seizure
E2d: Three or more seizures in a year.
Q4: Age 33 years at death
O7a: Died at home
O8a: Pronounced dead at residence.
O9a: Prone
P1: Male
S, W1: Definite SUDEP.
V1b: Autopsy

## Case from Rossenbacker et al., 2007:

C4c: EEG recording in EMU.
D5: Age at onset = 11 years. F1b: ICD implanted
G1: Long QT syndrome, torsades de pointes.
P2: Female
W5: Non-SUDEP; SCD prevented

## Case from Schuele et al., 2011:

A11a1, A11b1: Right and left temporal lobe involvement.
E1e: Four seizures in 2 weeks
H1: Central apnea.
O7a: Died at home

O8a: Pronounced dead at residence.
O8h: Died in sleep
O9a: Prone.
P2: Female
Q3: Age 30 years at death
S, W1: Definite SUDEP.
V1b: Autopsy

**Case from So et al., 2000:**

Case 2H
A11c3: Generalized seizures
C3: Ictal
C4c: EMU
D4: Age 1 year at seizure onset
F2a1: Cardiac pacemaker implanted (not ICD)
F2b: Ictal bradycardia
H1: Respiratory arrest
H2: Successful resuscitation
P2: Female
Q2: Age 20 years
T1
U1: Race unknown
W4: SUDEP prevented

**Case from Swallow et al., 2002:**

A11c3: Generalized seizure activity.
D4: Age 9 years at seizure onset.
E1g: Seizure prior to death.
E2c: Two seizures in a year.
F1a: Ventricular fibrillation.
H1: Apnea
H1b: Pulmonary edema.
O7f: Died in hospital
O8c: Pronounced dead in hospital.
P1: Male
Q2: Age 18 years at death
8S, W1: Definite SUDEP.
V1b: Autopsy

**Cases from Swinghamer et al., 2012:**

*Patient 1:*
    A11c3: Generalized seizure activity
    C4b: Intensive care unit.
    D4: Age 4 years at seizure onset
    E1g: Complex partial seizure prior to death.
    E2b, E2c: One to two generalized seizures per year.
    F2b: Bradycardia
    H1b: Pulmonary edema.
    H1d: Hypoxia
    O7f: Died in hospital
    O8c: Pronounced dead in hospital.
    Q3: Age 27 years at death
    P1: Male
    S, W1: Definite SUDEP.
    V1b: Autopsy

*Patient 2:*
    A11c3: Generalized seizure activity.
    C9: Aura
    D5: Age 14 years at seizure onset.
    E1g: Seizure prior to death.
    H1: Apnea
    O7c: Died outdoors, walking to car.
    O8c: Pronounced dead in hospital.
    P2: Female
    Q4: Age 36 years at death
    S, W1: Definite SUDEP.
    V1b: Autopsy

**Case from Tao et al., 2010:**

A11b1: Right temporal lobe seizure activity.
A11c3: Generalized seizure activity
C4c: Video EEG recording in EMU.
D5: Age 19 years at seizure onset
E1g: Seizure just prior to death.
E2c, E2d: Two to three seizures per month.
F, H: Cardiorespiratory arrest
H1d: Ictal hypoxemia, hypercapnia.
O7f: Died in hospital
O8c: Pronounced dead in hospital.
O8h: Died in sleep
O9a: Prone.
P2: Female
Q4: Age 35 years at death
S, W1: Definite SUDEP

**Case from Tavee and Morris, 2008:**

A11c3: Generalized seizure activity
A7: Idiopathic generalized epilepsy (IGE)
B: Refractory
C3: Ictal
C4c: EEG in EMU
D4: Age 6 years at first seizure.
E1e: Four seizures per month
H1a: Laryngospasm
H2: Successful resuscitation.
O7f: Event in hospital
O8h: Event during sleep
P1: Male
Q5: Age 42 years at event
R3: Smoking unknown
S2.35: Ohio
T1: Human
U1: Race unknown
W4: SUDEP prevented

**Case from Tigaran et al., 2002:**

C4c: EEG recording in EMU.
D5: Epilepsy onset at age 17 years.
E2d: Three or more seizures per year
F2a1: Pacemaker implant but not seizure free.
G1: Atrioventricular block

P1: Male
W4: SUDEP prevented

**Case from Wilder-Smith, 1992:**

C4a: Clinical EEG
D9: Age at onset = 56 years.
E2d: Five recent seizure episodes.
G1: Atrioventricular block.
P2: Female
W4: SUDEP prevented.
X2: Caucasian

**Case from Wittekind et al., 2012:**

C4c: EEG in EMU
D7: Epilepsy onset at age 32 years.
E2c: Seizures averaged two per year.

F2a: Ictal asystole
F2a1: Pacemaker implanted; seizure-free period not known.
P1: Male
W4: SUDEP prevented

**Case from Zarraga and Ware, 2007:**

D8: Seizure onset age 49 years.
F2a1: Pacemaker implanted.
G1: Atrioventricular block
P2: Female
W4: SUDEP prevented

The following 37 SUDEP (definite, probable, and possible) cases are from the cohort data for 3000 de-identified patients in Dr. Wannamaker's practice in South Carolina and illustrates a fourth method to present cluster IDs for each case (Tables 8.1 through 8.3).

---

**TABLE 8.1**

**Risk Factors Derived from Medical Records of 35 Patients with SUDEP, Probable SUDEP and Possible SUDEP. Part I**

| ID | A Epilepsy | B Refractory | C Epi Activity C1–C4 | D Age at Onset | E Frequency | Brain |
|---|---|---|---|---|---|---|
| 001 | A8(JME), A11e, A12d | B | C1, C3, C4a, C4c | D4 | F1d | 1 |
| 002 | A11a, A12e | B | C1, C1a | D5 | E1c | 1 |
| 003 | A11a, A12f | B | C1, C4a | D4 | E1b | 1 |
| 004 | A11b, A12e | B | C1, C4a | D5 | | 1 |
| 005 | A11c, A12F | | C1, C4a | D4 | E1a | 1 |
| 006 | A11a, A12f (MTS) | B | C1, C4a | D5 | E1f (2/yr) | 1 |
| 007 | A11a, A12f | B | C1, C4a | D6 | E1f (1/6 mo) | 1 |
| 008 | A11a, A12f | B | C1, C3, C4a, C4c | D3 | E1f (4/yr), E1g | 1 |
| 009 | A11a, A12e | B | C1, C4a | D5 | E1d | 1 |
| 010 | A11c, A12e | B | C4a(NL) | D3 | E1b | 1 |
| 011 | A11a, A12f | B | | D5 | | 1 |
| 012 | A11b, A12e | B | C1, C4a, C4c | D4 | E1e, E1g | 1 |
| 013 | A11c, A12e | | C(NL), C1, C4a | D9 | E1f | 1 |
| 014 | A11c, A12f | | C1, C4a | D4 | | 1 |
| 015 | A11c(NL), A12f | | C1(NL), C4a | D7 | | 1 |
| 016 | A8(JME), A11e, A12d | B | C1, C3, C4a, C4b, C4c | D3 | E1f | 1 |
| 017 | A11b, A12f | | C1, C4a | D6 | | 1 |
| 018 | A8(JME), A11e, A12d | | C, C4 | D4 | E1b | 1 |
| 019 | A11b, A12e | | C1, C4a | UTD | E1d | 1 |
| 020 | A11c, A12f | | C1, C4a | D6 | | 1 |
| 021 | A11c, A12f | | C1, C4a | D5 | | 1 |
| 022 | A11a, A12e | | C1, C4a | D4 | | 1 |
| 023 | A11a, A12f | | C1, C4a | D3 | | 1 |
| 024 | A11b, A12e | | C1, C4a | D6 | | 1 |
| 025 | A11d, A11e, A12f | B | C1, C4 | D5 | E1e | 1 |
| 026 | A11e, A12e | B | C1, C4a | D7 | | 1 |
| 027 | A11b, A12f | B | | D5 | E1e | 1 |
| 028 | A11c, A11d, A12f | B | C1 | D2 | E1e, E1g | 1 |
| 029 | A11a, A11e, A12f | B | C1, C4, C4a | D4 | E1b | 1 |
| 030 | A11c, A12e | B | | D7 | E1f | 1 |
| 031 | A8(JME), A11e, A12d | B | | D5 | E1c | 1 |
| 032 | A8(JME), A11e, A12d | | | D4 | | 1 |
| 033 | A11b, A12e | B | C1, C4a | D5 | E1f | 1 |
| 034 | A11b, A12f | B | C1, C3, C4a, C4c | D5 | E1b | 1 |
| 035 | A11f, A12e | B | C1, C3, C4a, C4c | D4 | E1e* | 1 |

*Note:* K1 - therapy at last visit before death. Where there is a blank, the answer is unknown (B) or no information (C,E).

* *Refers to patient who had no contact 2 or more years before death.*

**TABLE 8.2**

**Risk Factors Derived from Medical Records of 35 Patients with SUDEP, Probable SUDEP and Possible SUDEP. Part II**

| ID | Cardiac | H Resp | I Syncope | K Therapy | L Non-AED | M Contributory Causes* | N Psych |
|---|---|---|---|---|---|---|---|
| 001 | | | | K1aPHT, VPA, K1d, K2 | | | N3 |
| 002 | | | | K1aCBZ, GPN, K1d, K2, K1f | | | N3 |
| 003 | | | | K1aPHT, PB, VPA, K1d, K2 | caffeine | | N3 |
| 004 | | | | K1aCBZ, VPA, K2 | | | |
| 005 | | | | K1CBZ, K1c, K1d | | | |
| 006 | | | | K1a PRM, VPA, K1d, K2 | | | N3 |
| 007 | | | | K1aPB, PHT, K1d, K2 | | | |
| 008 | | | | K1aVPA, LMT, CBZ, K1d, K2 | | M1(ID) | |
| 009 | | | | K1aCBZ, PHT, PB, K1d, K2 | | | |
| 010 | | | | K1aVPA, CBZ, PB, K1d, K2, K3, K1f | | | N2 |
| 011 | | | | K1 PHT, K1c | | M1(TBI) | N3 |
| 012 | | | | K1aCBZ, K2 | | | N2 |
| 013 | | | | K1B PHT, K2 | L1 | | |
| 014 | | | | K1a PB, K1d, K2 | | M1(ID) | |
| 015 | | | | K None | L1 | | |
| 016 | | | | K1aVPA, K1d, K2 | | M1(Sleep Apnea) | |
| 017 | | | | K1bPB, PHT, K2 | L1 | M1(TBI) | |
| 018 | | | | K1a CBZ, VPA, K1d, K2 | | | N2 |
| 019 | | | | K1a CBZ, VPA, K2 | | | N2 |
| 020 | | | | K1b PHT, K3 | L1 | M1(Pychosis) | |
| 021 | | | | K1aVPA, PRM, Kd, K2 | | M1(ID) | |
| 022 | | | | K1a PHT, K2 | | | |
| 023 | | | | K1b PB, PHT, CBZ, K2 | | M1(ID) | |
| 024 | | | | K1PHT, PB | | | |
| 025 | | | | K1aVPA, LMT, K1a, K1d, K2 | | M1(ID) | N3 |
| 026 | | | | K1a, VPA, PRM, Kd, K2 | | | |
| 027 | | | | K1aPHT, K1d, K2 | | | |
| 028 | | | | K1a VPA, CBZ, K1d, K2 | | M1(ID) | |
| 029 | | | | K1aPHT, PRM, K1d, K2 | | M1(Thought Disorder) | N3 |
| 030 | | | | K1aPHT, K2 | | | N3 |
| 031 | | | | K1aPHT, CBZ, K2 | | | |
| 032 | | | | K1aVPA, K2 | L1 | | |
| 033 | | H1b | | K1aPHT, K1d, K2 | | | |
| 034 | | | | K1aLMT, PHT, K1d, K2 | | | N3 |
| 035 | | | | K1aPHT, CLZ, K1d, K2 | | | N1 |

* ID = intellectual disability, TBI = traumatic brain injury.

**TABLE 8.3**

**Risk Factors Derived from Medical Records of 35 Patients with SUDEP, Probable SUDEP and Possible SUDEP. Part III**

| ID | O Other | P Gender | Q Age at Death | R Smoker | S Incidence | V Autopsy[a] | SUDEP Class W1–W7 | Clusters for SUDEP |
|---|---|---|---|---|---|---|---|---|
| 001 | 8 | P1 | Q4 | R2 | SUDEP | no | W2 | |
| 002 | 8 | P1 | Q5 | R2 | SUDEP | no | W2 | |
| 003 | 8 | P1 | Q3 | R1 | SUDEP | no | W2 | |
| 004 | | P1 | Q4 | R3 | Prob SUDEP | Vu | W2 | |
| 005 | 8 | P1 | Q6 | R2 | Poss SUDEP | no | W2 | |
| 006 | 8 | P2 | Q6 | R2 | Prob SUDEP | no | W2 | |
| 007 | 8 | P1 | Q6 | R2 | Poss SUDEP | no | W3 | |
| 008 | 8 | P1 | Q3 | R2 | SUDEP | no | W3 | |
| 009 | 8 | P1 | Q5 | R1 | Prob SUDEP | Vu | W2 | |
| 010 | 8 | P2 | Q5 | R2 | SUDEP | V1a | W1 | |
| 011 | 12(ED) | P1 | Q5 | R3 | Prob SUDEP | Vu | W2 | |
| 012 | 8 | P1 | Q4 | R2 | SUDEP | no | W3 | |
| 013 | 8 | P2 | Q7 | R3 | Prob SUDEP | no | W3 | |
| 014 | 8 | P2 | Q3 | R2 | Prob SUDEP | Vu | W3 | |
| 015 | 12(ED) | P1 | Q5 | R3 | Prob SUDEP | no | W3 | |
| 016 | 8 | P1 | Q6 | R2 | SUDEP | no | W2 | |
| 017 | 8 | P1 | Q4 | R3 | SUDEP | Vu | W3 | |
| 018 | 8 | P2 | Q5 | R2 | Prob SUDEP | no | W2 | |
| 019 | 8 | P1 | Q4 | R3 | Prob SUDEP | Vu | W2 | |
| 020 | 8 | P1 | Q5 | R3 | SUDEP | Vu | W3 | |
| 021 | 12(ED) | P1 | Q4 | R2 | SUDEP | Vu | W3 | |
| 022 | 8 | P1 | Q4 | R3 | Prob SUDEP | Vu | W3 | |
| 023 | 8 | P1 | Q4 | R2 | SUDEP | no | W3 | |
| 024 | 8 | P2 | Q5 | R2 | Poss SUDEP | no | W3 | |
| 025 | 8 | P1 | Q3 | R2 | SUDEP | no | W2 | |
| 026 | 8 | P2 | Q6 | R1 | Prob SUDEP | no | W2 | |
| 027 | 8 | P1 | Q6 | R3 | SUDEP | no | W3 | |
| 028 | 12(ED) | P1 | Q1 | R2 | SUDEP | no | W2 | |
| 029 | 8 | P1 | Q5 | R1 | SUDEP | no | W2 | |
| 030 | 8 | P2 | Q4 | R2 | SUDEP | no | W2 | |
| 031 | 12(Dorm) | P1 | Q3 | R3 | SUDEP | no | W2 | |
| 032 | 12(ED) | P1 | Q5 | R1 | Poss SUDEP | no | W2 | |
| 033 | 8 | P1 | Q3 | R2 | SUDEP | V1a | W1 | |
| 034 | 8 | P2 | Q3 | R1 | SUDEP | Vu | W2 | |
| 035 | 8 | P2 | Q3 | R2 | SUDEP | V2b | W2 | |

*Abbreviations:* ED = emergency department; Dorm = dormitory.

[a] *Vu = Autopsy, results unknown.*

## CONCLUSION

In this chapter, we have presented four ways to illustrate SUDEP risk factor cluster IDs. As illustrated in the sections at the beginning of this chapter, the first way is to publish the complete case history with author comments and reviewer discussions and cluster IDs. The second method is to publish the cluster IDs only, allowing at a quick glance a summary of the pertinent medical facts relevant to a case. This method is shown for 40 cases from the medical literature. The third method to report cluster IDs is a summary format using only the numerical and alphabetical designations. This latter method is used for our statistical analysis. The fourth method of Dr. Wannamaker uses a spreadsheet format. The first page begins with category A Epilepsy and continues with B Refractory through E Frequency of seizures of our SUDEP Risk Factor Cluster Method found in Table 5.1. Subsequent pages contain the rest of the risk factors found in Table 5.1. Data for all SUDEP cases are included on each page. The spreadsheet format allows the reader, at a quick glance, to determine how many SUDEP victims fell into the given risk factor category. This method provides a very nice visual summary of risk factors for these particular SUDEP cases. The S or Incidence column represents a clinical diagnosis based on particular circumstances, death certificate information, and/or verbal autopsy. This classification is discrepant with the "W" classification, which adheres to the requirement for autopsy for definite SUDEP.

## REFERENCES

Abu-Shaweesh JM. Activation of central adenosine A (2A) receptors enhances superior laryngeal nerve stimulation-induced apnea in piglets via a GABAergic pathway. *J Appl Physiol* (1985) 2007;103(4):1205–11.

Akkerhuis JM, Baars HF, Marcelis CL, Akkerhuis KM, Wilde AA. Congenital long QT-syndrome: The cause of recurrent syncope and sudden death at a young age. *Ned Tijdschr Geneeskd* 2007; 151(43):2357–64.

Al Aloul B, Adabag AS, Houghland MA, Tholakanahalli V. Brugada pattern electrocardiogram associated with supratherapeutic phenytoin levels and the risk of sudden death. *Pacing Clin Electrophysiol* 2007;30(5):713–5.

Antzelevitch C, Brugada P, Borggrefe M, Brugada J, Brugada R, Corrado D, Gussak I, LeMarec H, Nademanee K, Perez Riera AR, Shimizu W, Schulze-Bahr E, Tan H, Wilde A. Brugada syndrome: Report of the second consensus conference. *Heart Rhythm* 2005;2(4):429–40.

Aurlien D, Leren TP, Tauboll E, Gjerstand L. New SCN5A mutation in a SUDEP victim with idiopathic epilepsy. *Seizure* 2009;18:158–60.

Aurlien D, Taubøll E, Gjerstad L. Lamotrigine in idiopathic epilepsy—increased risk of cardiac death? *Acta Neurol Scand* 2007;115(3):199–203.

Backiner O, Ertorer ME, Haydardedeogiu FE, Bozkirli E, Tutuncu NB, Demirag NG. Subclinical hypothyroidism is characterized by increase QT interval dispersion among women. *Med Princ Pract* 2008;17:390–4.

Bateman LM, Spitz M, Seyal M. Ictal hypoventilation contributes to cardiac arrhythmia and SUDEP: Report on two deaths in video-EEG-monitored patients. *Epilepsia* 2010;51(5):916–20.

Berkokovic SF, Scheffer IE. Febrile seizures: Genetics and relationship to other epilepsy syndromes. *Curr Opin Neurol* 1998;11(2):129–34.

Betts T. Psychiatric aspects of nonepileptic seizures. In: Engel J, TA Pedley, eds. *Epilepsy: A Comprehensive Textbook.* Philadelphia: Lippincott-Raven; 1997.

Betts T, Betts H. John Hall and his epileptic patients—epilepsy management in early 17th century England. *Seizure* 1998;7(5):411–4.

Breningstall GN. Mortality in pediatric epilepsy. *Pediatr Neurol* 2001;25(1):9–16.

Britton JW, Benarroch E. Seizures and syncope: Anatomic basis and diagnostic considerations. *Clin Auton Res* 2006;16(1):18–28.

Callahan TD, Khokhar U, Pozuelo L, Young JB. Case study in heart-brain interplay: A 53-year-old woman recovering from mitral valve repair. *Cleve Clin J Med* 2008;75 Suppl 2:S10–4.

Carinci V, Barbato G, Baldrati A, Di Pasquale G. Asystole induced by partial seizures: A rare cause of syncope. *Pacing Clin Electrophysiol* 2007;30(11):1416–9.

Dasheiff RM Dickinson LJ. Sudden unexpected death of epileptic patient due to cardiac arrhythmia after seizure. *Arch Neurol* 1986;43(2):194–6.

DeToledo J C, DeToledo MB, Lowe MR. Epilepsy and sudden death: Notes from George Washington's diaries on the illness and death of Martha Parke-Custis (1756–1773). *Epilepsia* 1999;40:1835–6.

Devinsky O, Kelley K, Yacubian EM, Sato S, Kufta CV, Theodore WH, Porter RJ. Postictal behavior. A clinical and subdural electroencephalographic study. *Arch Neurol* 1994; 51(3):254–9.

DiMaio TG, DiMaio VJM. *Excited Delirium Syndrome.* Boca Raton: CRC Press/Taylor & Francis Group; 2006.

Dixon R, Job S, Oliver R, Thompson D, Wright JG, Maltby K, Lorch U, Taubel J. Lamotrigine does not prolong QTc in a thorough QT/QTc study in healthy subjects. *Br J Clin Pharmacol* 2008;66(3)396–404.

Doherty MJ. The sudden death of Patsy Custis, or George Washington on sudden unexplained death in epilepsy. *Epilepsy Behav* 2004;4:598–600.

Doherty MJ, Sloan D. Tourette syndrome and epilepsy: A strange case of possible sudden unexpected death. *Epilepsy Behav* 2010;17(2):285–6.

Espinosa PS, Lee JW, Tedrow UB, Bromfield EB, Dworetzky BA. Sudden unexpected near death in epilepsy: Malignant arrhythmia from a partial seizure. *Neurology* 200912;72(19):1702–3.

Fauchier L, Babuty D, Cosnay P. Epilepsy, Brugada syndrome, and the risk of SUDEP. *J Neurol* 2000;247:643–4.

Fenwick P. The behavioral treatment of epilepsy generation and inhibition of seizures. *Neurol Clin* 1994;12(1):175–202.

Ferlisi M, Tomei R, Carletti M, Moretto G, Zanoni T. Seizure induced ventricular fibrillation: A case of near-SUDEP. *Seizure* 2013;22(3):249–51.

Ficker DM, Privitera M, Krauss G, Kanner A, Moore JL, Glauser T. Improved tolerability and efficacy in epilepsy patients with extended-release carbamazepine. *Neurology* 2005;23;65(4):593–5.

Gilman JT, Alvarez LA, Duchowny M. Carbamazepine toxicity resulting from generic substitution. *Neurol* 1993;43:2696–7.

Girard S, Cadnea A, Acharya Y. Women with Brugada syndrome and epilepsy: A unifying diagnosis? *South Med J* 2008;101:1150–3.

Graves TD. Ion channels and epilepsy. *QJM* 2006;99(4):201–17.

Herold TJ. Lamotrigine as a possible cause of QRS prolongation in a patient with known seizure disorder. *CJEM* 2006;8:361–4.

Herreros B. Cardiac channelopathies and sudden death. Chapter 19 In: Lathers CM, Schraeder PL, Bungo MW, Leestma JE, eds. *Sudden Death in Epilepsy: Forensic and Clinical Issues.* Boca Raton: CRC Press/Taylor & Francis Group; 2011, pp. 285–302.

Hindocha N, Nashef L, Elmslie F, Birch R, Zuberi S, Al-Chalabi A, Crotti L, Schwartz PJ, Makoff A. Two cases of sudden unexpected death in epilepsy in a GEFS+ family with an SCN1A mutation. *Epilepsia* 2008; 49(2):360–65.

Howell SJ, Blumhardt LD. Cardiac asystole associated with epileptic seizures: A case report with simultaneous EEG and ECG. *J Neurol Neurosurg Psychiatry* 1989; 52:795–8.

Hunt DP, Tang K. Long QT syndrome presenting as epileptic seizures in an adult. *Emerg Med J* 2005;22:600–1.

Ide A, Kamijo Y. Intermittent complete atrioventricular block after long term low-dose carbamazepine therapy with a serum concentration less than the therapeutic level. *Intern Med* 2007;46(9):627–9.

Isojärvi JI, Pakarinen AJ, Myllylä VV. Thyroid function with antiepileptic drugs. *Epilepsia* 1992;33(1):142–8.

Jay GW, Leestma JE. Sudden death in epilepsy: A comprehensive review of the literature and proposed mechanisms. *Acta Neurol Scand* 1981;63Suppl 82:S1–66.

Jim KF, Lathers CM, Farris VL, Pratt LF, Spivey WH. Suppression of pentylenetetrazol elicited seizure activity by intraosseous lorazepam in pigs. *Epilepsia* 1989;30:480–6.

Jim KF, Lathers CM, Spivey WH, Matthews WD, Kahn C, Dolce K. Suppression of pentylenetetrazol-elicited seizure activity by intraosseous propranolol in pigs. *J Clin Pharmacol* 1988;28(12):1106–11.

Johnson JN, Tester DJ, Bass NE, Ackerman MJ. Cardiac channel molecular autopsy for sudden unexpected death in epilepsy. *J Child Neurol* 2010;25(7):916–21.

Kloster R, Børresen HC, Hoff-Olsen P. Sudden death in two patients with epilepsy and the syndrome of inappropriate antidiuretic hormone secretion (SIADH). *Seizure* 1998; 7(5):419–20.

Krantz DS, Kop WJ, Santiago HT, Gottdiener JS. Mental stress as a trigger of myocardial ischemia and infarction. *Cardiol Clin* 1996;14(2):271–87.

Kuroiwa T, Morita H, Tanabe H, Ohta T. Life threatening epilepsy in a child [letter]. *J Neurol Neurosurg Psychiatry* 1994;57(11):1440–1.

Langan Y, Nashef L, Sander JW. Sudden unexpected death in epilepsy: A series of witnessed deaths. *J Neurol Neurosurg Psychiatry* 2000;68(2):211–3.

Lathers CM. Arrhythmogenic, respiratory and psychological risk factors for sudden unexplained death and epilepsy: Case histories. Chapter 44 In: Lathers CM, Schraeder PL, Bungo MW, Leestma JE, eds. *Sudden Death in Epilepsy: Forensic and Clinical Issues*. Boca Raton: CRC Press/Taylor & Francis Group; 2011, pp. 713–4.

Lathers CM, Bungo MW, Schraeder PL. Sodium channel dysfunction. common pathophysiologic mechanism associated with sudden death ECG abnormalities in Brugada syndrome and some types of epilepsy: Case histories. Chapter 20 In: Lathers CM, Schraeder PL, Bungo MW, Leestma JE, eds. *Sudden Death in Epilepsy: Forensic and Clinical Issues*. Boca Raton: CRC Press/Taylor & Francis Group; 2011, pp. 303–10.

Lathers CM, Jim KF, High WB, Spivey WH, Matthews WD, Ho T. An investigation of the pathological and physiological effects of intraosseous sodium bicarbonate in pigs. *J Clin Pharmacol* 1989a;29(4):354–9.

Lathers CM, Jim KF, Spivey WH. A comparison of intraosseous and intravenous routes of administration for antiseizure agents. *Epilepsia* 1989b;30(4):472–9.

Lathers CM, Schraeder PL. Autonomic dysfunction in epilepsy: Characterization of autonomic cardiac neural discharge associated with pentylenetetrazol-induced epileptogenic activity. *Epilepsia* 1982;23(6):633–47.

Lathers CM, Schraeder PL. Stress and sudden death. *Epilepsy Behav* 2006;9(2):236–42.

Lathers CM, Schraeder PL. Verbal autopsies and SUDEP. *Epilepsy Behav* 2009;14:573–6.

Lathers CM, Schraeder PL. Stress and SUDEP. Chapter 17 In: Lathers CM, Schraeder PL, Bungo MW, Leestma JE, eds. *Sudden Death in Epilepsy: Forensic and Clinical Issues*. Boca Raton: CRC Press/Taylor & York: CRC Press/Taylor & Francis Group, 2011a, pp. 253–67.

Lathers CM, Schraeder PL. Antiepileptic drugs benefit/risk clinical pharmacology: Possible role in cause and/or prevention of SUDEP. Chapter 47 In: Lathers CM, Schraeder PL, Bungo MW, Leestma JE, eds. *Sudden Death in Epilepsy: Forensic and Clinical Issues*. Boca Raton: CRC Press/Taylor & Francis Group; 2011b, pp. 755–88.

Lathers CM, Schraeder PL. Animal model for sudden unexpected death in persons with epilepsy. Chapter 28 In: Lathers CM, Schraeder PL, Bungo MW, Leestma JE, eds. *Sudden Death in Epilepsy: Forensic and Clinical Issues*. Boca Raton: CRC Press/Taylor & Francis Group; 2011c, pp. 437–64.

Lathers CM, Schraeder PL, Bungo MW. Reply. *Epilepsy Behav* 2008a;13:265–9.

Lathers CM, Schraeder PL, Bungo, MW. Sudden death: Neurocardiologic mystery. Chapter 13 In: Sher L, ed. *Psychological Factors and Cardiovascular Disorders: Role of Stress and Psychosocial Influences*. New York: Nova Biomedical Books; 2008b, pp. 263–311.

Lathers CM, Schraeder PL, Bungo MW. Syncope, seizures and SUDEP: Case histories. Chapter 22 In: Lathers CM, Schraeder PL, Bungo MW, Leestma JE, eds. *Sudden Death in Epilepsy: Forensic and Clinical Issues*. Boca Raton: CRC Press/Taylor & Francis Group; 2011, pp. 325–32.

Lathers CM, Tumer N, Schoffstall JM. Plasma catecholamines, pH, and blood pressure during cardiac arrest in pigs. *Resuscitation* 1989c;18(1):59–74.

Lear-Kaul KC, Coughlin L, Dobersen MJ. Sudden unexpected death in epilepsy: A retrospective study. *Am J Forensic Med Pathol* 2005;26:11–7.

Leestma JE, Koenig KL. Sudden death and phenothiazines: A current controversy. *Arch Gen Psychiat* 1968;18:137–48.

Le Gal F, Korff CM, Monso-Hinard C, Mund MT, Morris M, Malafosse A, Schmitt-Mechelke T. A case of SUDEP in a patient with Dravet syndrome with SCN1A mutation. *Epilepsia* 2010;51(9):1915–8.

Lehmann-Horn F, Jurkat-Rott K. Voltage-gated ion channels and hereditary disease. *Physiol Rev* 1999;79(4):1317–72.

McLean BN, Wimalaratna S. Sudden death in epilepsy recorded in ambulatory EEG. *J Neurol Neurosurg Psychiatry* 2007;78(12):1395–7.

Medina-Villanueva A, Rey-Galán C, Concha-Torre A, Gutiérrez-Martínez JR. Long QT syndrome presented as epilepsy. *Rev Neurol* 2002;35(4):346–8.

Mendez MF. Postictal violence and epilepsy. *Psychosomatics* 1998;39(5):478–80.

Mulley JC, Scheffer IE, Petrou S, Berkovic SF. Channelopathies as a genetic cause of epilepsy. *Curr Opin Neurol* 2003; 16(2):171–6.

Nelson DA, Ray CD. Respiratory arrest from seizure discharges in limbic system. *Arch Neurol* 1968;19:199–207.

Novakova B, Harris PR, Ponnusamy A, Reuber M. The role of stress as a trigger for epileptic seizures: A narrative review of evidence from human and animal studies. *Epilepsia* 2013;54(11):1866–76.

Owada M, Aizawa Y, Kurihara K, Tanabe N, Aizaki T, Izumi T. Risk factors and triggers of sudden death in the working generation: An autopsy proven case-control study. *Tohoku J Exp Med* 1999;189:245–58.

Pacia SV, Devinsky O, Luciano DJ, Vasquez B. The prolonged QT syndrome presenting as epilepsy: A report of two cases and literature review. *Neurology* 1994;44:1408–10.

Pezzella M, Striano P, Ciampa C, Errichiello L, Penza P, Striano S. Severe pulmonary congestion in a near miss at the first seizure: Further evidence for respiratory dysfunction in sudden unexpected death in epilepsy. *Epilepsy Behav* 2009; 14(4):701–2.

Pickworth WB, Gerard-Ciminara J, Lathers CM. Stress, arrhythmias, and seizures. In: Lathers CM, Schraeder PL, eds. *Epilepsy and Sudden Ddeath*. New York: Marcel Dekker; 1990, pp. 261–92.

Pinto KG, Scorza FA, Arida RM, Cavalheiro EA, Martins LD, Machado HR, Sakamoto AC, Terra VC. Sudden unexpected death in an adolescent with epilepsy: All roads lead to the heart? *Cardiol J* 2011;18(2):194–6.

Rauscher G, DeGiorgio AC, Miller PR, DeGiorgio CM. Sudden unexpected death in epilepsy associated with progressive deterioration in heart rate variability. *Epilepsy Behav* 2011;21(1):103–5.

Rossenbacker T, Nuyens D, Van Paesschen W, Heidbüchel H. Epilepsy? Video monitoring of long QT syndrome-related aborted sudden death. *Heart Rhythm* 2007;4(10):1366–7.

Rozanski A, Bairey CN, Krantz DS, Friedman J, Resser KJ, Morell M, Hilton-Chalfen S, Hestrin L, J. Bietendorf, D. S. Berman. Mental stress and the induction of silent myocardial ischemia in patients with coronary artery disease. *N Engl J Med* 1988;318(16):1005–12.

Ruiz GMA, García GS, Ruiz GJA, Tze KE, Fernández RE. Symptomatic secondary hyponatraemia due to combined treatment anticonvulsant and antidepressant: Risk of sudden death in epilepsy? *An Med Interna* 2007;24(7):335–8.

Sandorfi G, Clemens B, Csanadi Z. Electrical storm in the brain and in the heart: Epilepsy and Brugada syndrome. *Mayo Clin Proc* 2013;88(10):1167–73.

Schoffstall JM, Spivey WH, Davidheiser S, Lathers CM. Intraosseous crystalloid and blood infusion in a swine model. *J Trauma* 1989;29(3):384–7.

Schraeder PL, Lathers CM. Cardiac neural discharge and epileptogenic activity in the cat: An animal model for unexplained death. *Life Sci* 1983;32:1371–82.

Schraeder PL, Pontzer R, Engel TR. A case of being scared to death. *Arch Intern Med* 1983;143(9):1793–4.

Schuele SU, Afshari M, Afshari ZS, Macken MP, Asconape J, Wolfe L, Gerard EE. Ictal central apnea as a predictor for sudden unexpected death in epilepsy. *Epilepsy Behav* 2011;22(2):401–3.

Scorza FA, Arida RM, Cavalheiro EA. Preventive measures for sudden cardiac death in epilepsy beyond therapies. *Epilepsy Behav* 2008; 13(1):263–4; author reply 265–9.

Shah R, Burg MM, Vashist A, Collins D, Liu J, Jadbabaie F, Graeber B, Earley C, Lampert R, Soufer R. C-reactive protein and vulnerability to mental stress-induced myocardial ischemia. *Mol Med* 2006 Nov-Dec;12(11–12):269–74.

So EL, Sam MC, Lagerlund TL. Postictal central apnea as a cause of SUDEP: Evidence from near-SUDEP incident. *Epilepsia* 2000;41(11):1494–7.

Soufer R. C-reactive protein and vulnerability to mental stress- induced myocardial ischemia. *Mol Med* 2006;12(11–12): 269–74.

Soufer R, Burg MM. The heart brain interaction during emotionally provoked myocardial ischemia: Implications of cortical activation in CAD and gender interactions. *Cleve Clinic J Med* 2007;74:Suppl 1:S59–S62.

Spivey WH, Unger HD, Lathers CM, McNamara RM. Intraosseous diazepam suppression of pentylenetetrazol-induced epileptogenic activity in pigs. *Ann Emerg Med* 1987a;16(2):156–9.

Spivey WH, Unger HD, McNamara RM, LaManna MM, Ho T, Lathers CM. The effect of intraosseous sodium bicarbonate on bone in swine. *Ann Emerg Med* 1987b;16(7):773–6.

Stopper M, Joska T, Burg MM, Batsford WP, McPherson CA, Jain D, Lampert R. Electrophysiologic characteristics of anger-triggered arrhythmias. *Heart Rhythm* 2007;4(3):268–73.

Strzelczyk A, Bauer S, Knake S, Oertel WH, Hamer HM, Rosenow F. Ictal asystole in temporal lobe epilepsy before and after pacemaker implantation. *Epileptic Disord* 2008;10:39–44.

Swallow RA, Hillier CE, Smith PE. Sudden unexplained death in epilepsy (SUDEP) following previous seizure-related pulmonary oedema: Case report and review of possible preventative treatment. *Seizure* 2002;11(7):446–8.

Swinghamer J, Devinsky O, Friedman D. Can post-ictal intervention prevent sudden unexpected death in epilepsy? A report of two cases. *Epilepsy Behav* 2012;24(3):377–9.

Tao JX, Qian S, Baldwin M, Chen XJ, Rose S, Ebersole SH, Ebersole JS. SUDEP, suspected positional airway obstruction, and hypoventilation in postictal coma. *Epilepsia* 2010;51(11):2344–7.

Tavee J, Morris H 3rd. Severe postictal laryngospasm as a potential mechanism for sudden unexpected death in epilepsy: A near-miss in an EMU. *Epilepsia* 2008;49(12):2113–7.

Tigaran S, Molgaard H, Dam M. Atrio-ventricular block: A possible explanation of sudden unexpected death in epilepsy. *Acta Neurol Scand* 2002;106(4):229–33.

Vainionpää LK, Mikkonen K, Rättyä J, Knip M, Pakarinen AJ, Myllylä VV, Isojärvi JI. Thyroid function in girls with epilepsy with carbamazepine, oxcarbazepine, or valproate monotherapy and after withdrawal of medication. *Epilepsia* 2004;45(3):197–203.

Wannamaker B. B. Autonomic nervous system and epilepsy. *Epilepsia* 1985;(S1)26:31–9.

Wilder-Smith E. Complete atrio-ventricular conduction block during complex partial seizure. *J Neurol Neurosurg Psychiatry* 1992;55(8):734–6.

Wittekind SG, Lie O, Hubbard S, Viswanathan MN. Ictal asystole: An indication for pacemaker implantation and emerging cause of sudden death. *Pacing Clin Electrophysiol* 2012; 35(7):e193–6.

Zarraga IGE, Ware DL. Syncope, seizure, or both? An unusual case of complete heart block. *J Electrocardiol* 2007;40:493–5.

# 9 SUDEP
## Continued Forensic Challenges

*Jan E. Leestma and Claire M. Lathers*

## CONTENTS

At one time, the concept of sudden unexpected (unexplained) deaths in people suffering from epilepsy (SUDEP) was not accepted by many physicians and certainly not by the forensic pathology community, but this outlook has changed. Judging by the number and scope of publications relating to some aspect of SUDEP, acceptance of the phenomenon is much wider than it once was. The problem of SUDEP, whether it is called this or something else, confronts forensic pathologists in any number of ways, and like forensic sciences in general, SUDEP is ever-changing. This chapter provides an overview of the forensic issues associated with the evaluation of sudden death and provides an example of the complexities that can be encountered.

At the outset, there is the problem of recognition and identification of a given case as probably being classified as SUDEP distinct from other conditions that could explain or contribute to the death (Schraeder et al. 2006). This differentiation begins before the autopsy is done and takes into consideration the circumstances of the death of an apparently healthy adult individual who has usually died at home in the course of normal activities. Such individuals are often found in bed or the bedroom, in the bath or bathroom, or in other rooms of the home, and show evidence of rapid collapse without any suspicious activity (Leestma et al. 1989). Medications for epilepsy are often found, and this evidence should alert investigators to the possibility of SUDEP. Of course, family members or scene witnesses can provide a history of epilepsy in the victim as well. Next there are the results of the autopsy and toxicology studies, which are either noncontributory, negative, or unsatisfactory in explaining the death or its mechanism (Leestma 1990).

There is a tendency for forensic pathologists or contract pathologists performing coroner's work to list such deaths with ambiguous, imprecise, or incorrect labels such as "heart failure," "heart attack," "cardiac arrhythmia," "undetermined," or "unknown," rather than linking the death to epilepsy (Schraeder et al. 2006, 2009). Some pathologists will use the term SUDEP or some other label that connotes the same condition. Quite often the history and relationship to epilepsy is never mentioned in the official documents; thus, it can escape public health notice or statistics.

More pressing are the situations with confounding variables in the presence of known or newly discovered disease conditions such as underlying heart disease, pneumonia or other infections, the use of illicit drugs, or polypharmacy. Within this group also fall the pediatric population and individuals with advanced age whose death might be ascribed as being due to the pathologies of old age. The presence of these confounders does not mean that SUDEP does not occur in the very young or the very old, but only that differentiation from other disease mechanisms may be difficult.

Perhaps the most vexing forensic challenges are the deaths in patients with epilepsy who have become violent, delusional, delirious, intoxicated, and agitated. In these circumstances, the individual may be physically involved with police, emergency medical personnel, firemen, family members, or passersby. The contribution of restraint struggles, hog-tying, overlaying, and the use by law enforcement of "rubber" bullets or electronic darts to subdue the victim makes the analysis of such cases very complex. In these cases, there is always the specter of civil litigation and the glare of publicity with accusations of police brutality hovering over the forensic determinations. The following case illustrates many of these issues.

A man in his middle 30s was driving on a freeway during the day in an suburban utility vehicle (SUV), swerved and sideswiped two other vehicles, crashing into a median concrete barrier and coming to rest on the barrier. A police officer in a cruiser witnessed the crash and immediately stopped to investigate. The driver of the SUV was apparently uninjured and still wearing his seat belt, but the vehicle was still running and drive train engaged. The officer was unable to get the driver to respond although he appeared conscious, and he had to break the driver's side window to turn off the ignition. The driver began to struggle with the officer, who attempted to get him out of the vehicle. The struggle continued on the roadway, with the driver attempting to crawl under his vehicle or into the roadway. The police officer, despite repeated efforts to gain control of the driver, deployed his electronic control device (ECD), commonly called a "stun gun" and shocked the driver multiple times without apparent effect. Handcuffs were eventually placed on the driver and he was placed in a prone position. A passing motorist with medical training stopped to render assistance. With no one physically upon the driver, it was noted that the driver had ceased struggling and was quiet. The physician noted that the driver was cyanotic and in cardiac arrest and began cardiopulmonary resuscitation (CPR) until emergency medical personnel arrived. The driver was unresponsive and was transported to a hospital, where about 30 minutes after the crash event, he was pronounced dead.

The deceased driver was a resident physician and he had apparently had epilepsy for many years and had taken a number of anticonvulsant medications, possibly self-prescribed. He had had at least two prior traffic accidents in which it was supposed that he had experienced a seizure while driving, yet he continued to drive his car. The driver at the time of one of these events had indicated that he had had an aura while driving, and it was concluded that he had suffered a generalized convulsion. Electrocardiography (EKG) at the time of one of these incidents showed sinus tachycardia with possible anterior fascicular block.

An autopsy revealed that the driver was 33 years old, weighed 220 lbs, and was 74 in. tall. There were abrasions on the wrists and punctuate wounds on the left upper and lower chest where the electronic darts had entered. The heart weighed 470 g and had arteriosclerotic narrowing of 10%–20% in left anterior descending coronary artery. The lungs together weighed 2140 g. The brain weighed 1550 g and showed possible ectopic gray matter in the temporal horn of the lateral ventricle. Toxicological testing showed a blood level of gabapentin of 31 ug/mL.

It is not immediately clear what form of seizure disorder this victim had. He apparently had never told his family that he had epilepsy. It is possible that as a child he had nonconvulsive seizures that nobody, perhaps even the victim himself, realized were actually seizures. Sometime in his early adult years the victim realized that he had seizures and apparently consulted a neurologist, who was never found. He had been taking several anticonvulsant medications, which he may have prescribed for himself, with varying degrees of success, but apparently recently his seizures interfered with his education and employment. Given his apparent postictal behavior, it seems reasonable to suppose that he suffered from some form of complex/partial seizure disorder with secondarily generalized seizures. There was no electroencephalogram (EEG) ever found for the victim. Given the incomplete information, no one will know precisely what kind of epilepsy he had. One possible clue is his behavior. Individuals with complex partial seizures may display agitation and bizarre behavior, often with aggression in the postictal state. This behavior is usually disordered, disorganized, and obviously erratic. When individuals approach such victims, their approach or proximity appears to be threatening to the victim and may prompt some physical response or attempt to

flee, even though the victim is not capable of organizing this activity or perhaps even being aware of it.

It is difficult to assess whether a given level of anticonvulsant is therapeutic for a given individual in the absence of more history. Thus, this man's gabapentin level may or may not have controlled his seizures. In a lawsuit involving this case there was discussion about what a normal therapeutic level for gabapentin is. It is also worth considering whether this drug in any way contributed to the victim's delirium or death (Kruszewski et al. 2009; Peterson 2009; Walczak 2003). The role of the physical struggle with the police officer and the subsequent use of an ECD device is of course the central issue in the case.

In many deaths in which some form of excited delirium is present (absent known epilepsy background), the stress of the encounter may have resulted in excessive catecholamine release with pathological consequences (Rona 1985; Pedal et al. 1999; Ho et al. 2010). The same issue arises during an epileptic seizure with the same potential risks and complications (Shimizu et al. 2008; Kerling et al. 2009). When excited delirium exists in a person with epilepsy who is postictal and who may be subjected to an ECD device, it is conceivable that stress-related sympathetic nervous system activity may be exaggerated, with possible fatal consequences.

The increasing prevalence of ECD devices in the hands of security and law enforcement personnel has inevitably given rise to deaths with the inevitable civil lawsuits (Strote and Range Hutson 2006). The scientific issues that surround the effect of ECD devices on the heart are many with the expected pro and con positions regarding the safety of ECD devices (Swerdlow et al. 2009; Vilke et al. 2009). It appears that most accounts of death associated with ECD deployment are rarely subjected to robust analysis and are similarly unevenly reported in the medical literature. Zipes (2012) reported eight cases of fatality with ECD devices and reviewed the experimental and case literature relating to these devices. He concluded that in some circumstances the ECD shocks can cause "electrical capture of the heart," leading to cardiac arrest. When EKG recordings were taken in ECD victims, ventricular tachycardia and in some cases fibrillation were noted. It should be noted that Zipes participated in litigation of these cases; nevertheless, the data reported appear compelling (Myerburg et al. 2012). Swerdlow et al. (2009) analyzed 200 cases in which victims collapsed within 15 minutes of ECD shocks. In 56 subjects on whom EKG records were collected, 4 subjects had ventricular fibrillation and 52 subjects had bradycardia–asystole. It is interesting to note that the large majority of the 56 subjects studied (91%) collapsed more than a minute after the ECD. Swerdlow et al. concluded that ventricular fibrillation is not a common mechanism of sudden death with ECD devices.

A number of animal studies of the effects of ECDs (Lakkireddy et al. 2007, 2008; Jenkins et al. 2013) have shown that in the porcine model, ventricular fibrillation is uncommon and if it occurs it may be related to certain shock parameters (frequency, voltage, duration, and cycling–repetition rate) as well as proximity to the heart of the ECD discharges.

The problem in the forensic analysis of ECD-related fatalities is that the processes involved are physiological and thus not discoverable postmortem. If, however, EKG records exist, this evidence may be used in the analysis, which also must incorporate any cardiac pathology as well as toxicological evidence. A proper question to ask in any given case, with and without the ECD use, is whether the outcome is different in any respect from other epilepsy-related sudden deaths.

The proper assignment of medical cause of death which is part of the responsibility of the forensic pathologist in medical examiner's or Coroner's cases may be difficult if not impossible in SUDEP and SUDEP-like cases, with or without ECD use. The likely mechanisms for SUDEP deaths have been discussed many times and include cardiac arrhythmia and sudden right heart failure with pulmonary failure and edema. Behind these mechanisms may lurk inherited genetic abnormalities such as a membrane "channelopathy," (Langlois 2009) which might be discoverable. It may be appropriate to be imprecise here, using terms such as probable heart failure associated with a seizure disorder.

As for the manner of death, which in common forensic practice is categorized as homicide (death at the hands of another), suicide, accident, natural, or undetermined, one may encounter similar difficulty. In the above case, the death could be labeled as a homicide, an accident, natural, or, of course, undetermined.

Other case histories, recounted elsewhere, have in common the apparent postictal state of someone, most likely with some form of complex partial epilepsy (temporal lobe seizures), who was delusional, agitated, and struggling with someone else (DiMaio and DiMaio 2006). In many of these histories, it was perceived by witnesses and police that the individual was a danger to himself and to others, and this observation prompted restraint procedures and may have involved "piling on" of personnel over the victim. In some of the cases, anticonvulsant drugs were present and in others not. Sometimes victims were drug abusers using a variety of illicit drugs such as cocaine, phencyclidine, and related drugs. Common to virtually all of these cases was the issue of catecholamine stress.

This and other similar cases raise the obvious questions: what type of seizure disorder did this man have? Did his behavior have some relationship to being in a postictal state? Was his medication at therapeutic levels or have any influence on the outcome? What role did the physical struggle with the police officer and/or the ECD discharges have in the death? What is the medical cause of death? What is the proper manner of death classification for this case?

The next section of this chapter illustrates how to read this case and evaluate all data to assign the appropriate Cluster Identifications (Cluster IDs) using Table 5.1. Each relevant word in the case text is underlined and the appropriate Cluster ID number and definition is shown in the comment box of Figure 9.1. The Cluster IDs are then constructed in list form as follows.

## CLUSTER IDENTIFICATION FOR SUDEP VICTIM

A11e Generalized convulsions concluded after prior traffic accidents

Or A11a1 and A11 b1 (left and right temporal lobes, respectively)

B99 Refractory epilepsy: unknown

C3 Ictal

C4a Clinical EEG changes

C9 Auras reported after previous driving accidents

C91 Fear, postictal agitation

C95 Disconnected feelings; police officer unable to get person to respond although he appeared conscious

C97 Anxiety

D5 Estimate for 11–20 years since died age 33. Noted he "had epilepsy for many years."

F Cardiac arrhythmogenic, EKG at the time of one of the several previous driving accident incidents showed sinus tachycardia with possible anterior fascicular block

F Autonomic

F1 Sympathetic

F2a Asystolic cardiac arrest

G Cardiac. Arteriosclerotic narrowing of 10–20% in left anterior descending coronary artery. Congestive heart failure (CHF) occurs when your heart muscle does not pump blood as well as it should. Conditions such as narrowed arteries in your heart (coronary artery disease) or high blood pressure gradually leave your heart too weak or stiff to fill and pump efficiently.

G1 Function atrioventricular (AV) block

H Respiratory and hypoxia pathology

H1b Lung edema

H1d Ictal hypoxemia, hypercapnia

H1e: Began CPR until emergency medical personnel arrived. The driver was unresponsive; in respiratory arrest

K1f3 Unknown as a physician, self-prescribed antiepileptic drugs (AEDs).

K2f1 Gabapentin detected. Uncertain if therapeutic level for this patient

Mp Postmortem pathology

Mp3 Postmortem cardiac pathology

MP3b Cardiomegaly. Heart of a different male SUDEP victim weighed 455 g and he weighed 240 lbs; should have had a normal heart weight of 406 g. Victim in this case weighed 220 lbs and had a heart weight of 470 g (so he weighed less but had a heavier heart) so weight of the SUDEP victim heart was above that of the expected heart weight (values from Koehler et al. 2011, ch. 9).

Mp4 Lung pathology.

Mp4e Congestion/increased weight both lungs 2140 g so heavy; normal male 720–1140 g (Koehler et al. 2011).

| Actual Clinical History of SUDEP Victim | Risk Factor Cluster Identifiers |
|---|---|
| A man in his middle 30s was *driving* on a freeway during the day in an SUV, swerved and sideswiped two other vehicles, crashing into a median concrete barrier and coming to rest on the barrier. A police officer in a cruiser witnessed the crash and immediately stopped to investigate. The driver of the SUV was apparently uninjured and still wearing his seat belt, but the vehicle was still running and drive train engaged. The officer was *unable* to get the driver to respond, although he appeared conscious and had to break the driver's side window to turn off the ignition. The driver began to *struggle* with the officer who attempted to get him out of the vehicle. The struggle continued on the roadway with the driver attempting to crawl under his vehicle or into the *roadway*. The police officer despite repeated efforts to gain control of the driver, *deployed* his ECD, commonly called "stun gun" and shocked the driver multiple times without apparent effect. *Handcuffs* were eventually placed on the driver and he was placed in a *prone position*. A passing motorist with medical training stopped to render assistance. With no one on the driver, it was noted that the driver had ceased struggling and was quiet. The physician noted that the driver was *cyanotic* and in cardiac *arrest* and began *CPR* until emergency medical personnel arrived. The driver was unresponsive and was transported to a hospital where about 30 minutes after the crash event, he was pronounced *dead*. | O7 site of fatal event, O7d driving<br><br>C95 Police officer unable to get person to respond though he appeared conscious<br><br>C3 ictal, C4a clinical, C91 fear, Postictal agitation, C95 disconnected feelings, C97 anxiety<br>As above O7<br>N1 stress Deployed stun gun, shocked driver multiple times, without apparent effect. Nevertheless, this is a type of stress and we do not know what driver did or did not perceive<br>O8g Restraint with handcuffs<br>O9a prone position<br><br>H1d Ictal hypoxemia, hypercapnia<br>F2a Asystolic cardiac arrest<br>H1e: began CPR until emergency medical personnel arrived. The driver was unresponsive. Respiratory arrest<br>O8c pronounced dead at hospital |
| The history of the deceased driver, who was a resident physician, was that he *apparently had epilepsy for many years* and had taken a number of anticonvulsant medications, possibly self-prescribed. He had had at least two prior traffic accidents in which it was supposed that he had experienced a seizure while driving, yet he continued to drive his car. The driver at the time of one of these events had indicated that he had had an aura while driving, and it was concluded that he had suffered a *generalized convulsion. EKG at the time of one of these incidents showed sinus tachycardia with possible anterior fascicular block.* | D5 estimate for 11–20 years since died age 33. Noted he "had epilepsy for many years."<br><br>C9 auras<br>A11e generalized convulsions and/or complex/partial seizure disorder with secondarily generalized seizures.<br>F. cardiac arrhythmogenic, F. Autonomic, F1 Sympathetic, EKG at the time of the previous driving accident incidents |
| An autopsy revealed that the male driver was *33 years* old, weighed 220 lbs, and was 74 in. tall. There were abrasions on the wrists and punctuate wounds on the left upper and lower chest, where the electronic darts had entered. *The heart weighed 470 g* and had *arteriosclerotic narrowing of 10–20% in left anterior descending coronary artery.* The lungs together weighed 2140 g. *The brain weighed 1550 g* and *showed possible ectopic gray matter in the temporal horn of the lateral ventricle.* Toxicological testing showed *a blood level of gabapentin of 31 ug/mL.* | V. Postmortem Examination, V1a Non-Decomposed body: complete<br>P1 Male victim<br>Q4 Age at death 33 years<br>Mp Post mortem pathology. Mp3b Cardiomegaly. Heart of a different male<br>G. Cardiac, Function. arteriosclerotic narrowing of 10–20% in left anterior<br>Mp4 lung pathology. Mp4e congestion/increased wt Both lungs 2140gm so<br>Mnp5 Normal Brain weight 1550 gm brain weight normal since range normal<br>Mp5 possible. No expert agreement. Brain may have showed possible ectopic gray matter in the temporal horn of lateral ventricle.<br>V1a toxicological testing and Non-Decomposed body: complete external and<br>K1f3 Unknown Self prescribed AED. K2f1 gabapentin detected. No expert agreement if therapeutic level<br>W1 Definite SUDEP |
| This and other similar cases raise the obvious questions: what type of seizure disorder did this man have? Did his behavior have some relationship to being in a postictal state? Was his medication at therapeutic levels or have any influence on the outcome? What role did the physical struggle with the police officer and/or the ECD discharges have in the death? What is the medical cause of death? What is the proper manner of death classification for this case? | |

FIGURE 9.1 Clinical findings and derivation of sudden unexpected death in epilepsy (SUDEP) risk factor Cluster Identifications IDs.

Mnp5 Normal brain weight 1550 g brain weight normal since range normal male brain weight is 1100–1700 g

Mp5 Brain showed possible ectopic gray matter in the temporal horn of the lateral ventricle. It should be noted that there were differences of expert opinion since not everyone, including Dr. Leestma (JEL), agreed that the victim had this

N1 Stress police officer deployed stun gun, shocked driver multiple times, without apparent effect. Nevertheless, this is a type of stress and we do not know what the driver did or did not perceive in his agitated state

O7 Site of fatal event

O7d Driving

O8c Pronounced dead at hospital

O8g Restraint with handcuffs

O9a Prone position

P1 Male victim

Q4 Age at death 33 years

R3 Smoking history unknown

S2.28 Nevada

T1 Human

U2 Caucasian

V Postmortem examination

V1a Nondecomposed body: complete external and internal postmortem autopsy with toxicological analysis

## SUDEP CLASSIFICATION: W1 DEFINITE SUDEP WITH POSTMORTEM EXAMINATION

To determine Cluster IDs for postmortem examination of heart, lung, and brain weights, Table 9.1 was constructed. Normal organ weight values for males and females are found in Koehler et al. 2011, ch. 9, p. 150. The appropriate Cluster ID was then added to the table and to the list.

To determine the mechanisms that most likely contributed to death in this patient, Table 9.2 was constructed and the appropriate Cluster IDs were added.

The final Cluster ID for this victim is 1, 2, 3, A11e, Or A11a1 and A11 b1 (left and right temporal lobes, respectively), B99, C3, C4a, C9, C91, C95, C97, D5, F, F, F1, F2a, G, G1, H, H1b, H1d, H1e, K1f3, K2f1, Mp, Mp3, MP3b, Mp4, Mp4e, Mnp5, Mp5?, N1, O7, O7d, O8c, O8g, O9a, P1, Q4, R3, S2.28, T1, U2, V, and V1a

The data in Table 9.1 suggest that several medical issues may have been present in this patient—cardiac and the stress of the postictal state combined with the confrontation with the police officer.

Cardiomegaly is a general term used to describe any condition that results in an enlarged heart. There are two types of cardiomegaly: (1) Dilative: The heart can become enlarged due to dilation of the myocardium. An example is dilated cardiomyopathy (DCM), which is the most common form of nonischemic cardiomyopathy. In DCM, the heart becomes weakened and enlarged, and CHF quickly follows. Signs and symptoms are those of left and/or right heart failure, and signs on autopsy would include central hemorrhagic necrosis in the liver. In this patient, a liver autopsy was not done. (2) Hypertrophic: In response to increased demand, cardiac muscle undergoes hypertrophy when placed under a high workload for a prolonged period of time. Some cardiac hypertrophy is normal and reversible, such as that seen in athletes and pregnant women. Pathologic hypertrophy is the result of diseases that place increased demand on the heart, such as chronic hypertension, myocardial infarction, and valvular damage. Left ventricular hypertrophy (LVH) is the most common type of hypertrophic heart disease. A common cause of LVH is chronic hypertension, which increases the afterload on the left ventricle. This means the left ventricle has to increase contractility and/or preload to maintain the same stroke volume. Over time the added stress on the left ventricular myocardium results in muscle hypertrophy and remodeling of the left ventricle to a less efficient size and shape. This leads to a diminishing ejection fraction, meaning the heart must work even harder to maintain cardiac output.

## TABLE 9.1
## Postmortem Examination of Heart, Lung, and Brain Weights

| Sex | Weight (lbs) | Weight Heart (g) | Normal Heart Weight (g)[a] | Weight Both Lungs (g) | Normal Weight Both Lungs (g)[b] | Weight of Brain (g) | Normal Weight Brain (g) Male[c] |
|---|---|---|---|---|---|---|---|
| Male | | 470 | | 2140 | | 1550 | |
| This case | 220 | Heavy | ~406 for 240 lb male | Heavy | 720–1140 | Normal | 1100–1700 |
| | | Mp3b | | H1b | | Mnp5 | |
| Male | | 455 | | | | | |
| Koehler et al. 2011 | 240 | Heavy | 406 | | | | |
| | | Mp3b | | | | | |

[a] Normal heart range (mean expected heart weight based on body weight and sex).

[b] Normal combined weights of lungs: males, 720–1140 g; females, 650–960 g.

[c] Normal brain weights: males, 1100–1700 g; females, 1050–1550 g.

**TABLE 9.2**

**Risk Factors and Suspected Underlying Mechanism of Death**

| 1 Brain Clinical Diagnosis | 1 Brain Postmortem Autopsy Weight (g) | 2 Cardiac Clinical Diagnosis | 2 Cardiac Postmortem Autopsy Weight (g) | 3 Respiratory Hypoxia Clinical Diagnosis | 3 Respiratory Hypoxia Postmortem Autopsy Weight (g) |
|---|---|---|---|---|---|
| A11e generalized convulsions Epilepsy Seizures Postictal seizures, flatline | Mp5 possible. No expert agreement. Brain may have showed possible ectopic gray matter in the temporal horn of lateral ventricle. Weight: normal | F Cardiac arrhythmogenic, EKG at the time of one of the several previous driving accident incidents showed sinus tachycardia with possible anterior fascicular block F Autonomic F1 Sympathetic G1 Function AV block | F2a Asystolic cardiac arrest G Cardiac. Mpb3 arteriosclerotic narrowing of 10%–20% in left anterior descending coronary artery. Heart failure (CHF) occurs when your heart muscle does not pump blood as well as it should. Conditions such as narrowed arteries in your heart (coronary artery disease) or high blood pressure gradually leave your heart too weak or stiff to fill and pump efficiently Weight: heavy | H1b lung edema H1d ictal hypoxemia, hypercapnia H1e: Began CPR until emergency medical personnel arrived. The driver was unresponsive; in respiratory arrest | Mp4 lung pathology Mp4e congestion/ increased weight both lungs 2140 g so heavy Weight: heavy |
| 1 A11e Or A11a1 A11b1 | 1 Mnp5 wt, Mp5 | 2 F, F1, G, G1 | 2 F2a, G Mp, Mp3b | 3 H1b, H1d, H1e | 3 Mp4 lung pathology Mp4e |

*Note:* 1. Brain: A11e, Mnp5 wt, Mp5, Or A11a1, A11b1; 2. Cardiac: F, F1, F2a, G, G1, Mp, Mp3b; 3. Respiratory/hypoxia: H1b, H1d, H1e, Mp4, Mp4e.

In some patients with cardiomegaly, some degree of CHF develops. However, even though this patient did have both a heavy heart and heavy lungs as identified on autopsy, he did not have CHF. Coronary artery disease, which was identified on autopsy, or high blood pressure, could contribute to organ weight increase. Heart failure, sometimes known as CHF, occurs when the heart muscle does not pump blood as well as it should. Conditions such as narrowed arteries in the heart (coronary artery disease) or high blood pressure gradually leave the heart too weak or stiff to fill and pump efficiently. Not all conditions that lead to heart failure can be reversed, but treatments can improve the signs and symptoms of heart failure and help one to live longer. Lifestyle changes, such as exercising, reducing salt in the diet, managing stress and especially losing weight, can improve the quality of life. The best way to prevent heart failure is to control conditions that cause heart failure, such as coronary artery disease, high blood pressure, diabetes, or obesity.

Mendez (1998) describes aggressive acts as direct consequence of seizures, occurring directly during seizures or postictally. He emphasizes that postictal violence is most commonly resistive behavior during the postictal delirium and is associated with attempts at restraint. The observation that seemingly violent automatisms such as flailing or spitting can occur during complex partial seizures and that secondary violent automatisms can be behavioral responses to ictal fear, hallucinations, or other disagreeable seizure-related experiences is discussed.

As discussed by Lathers and Schraeder 2014, ch. 8:

Another issue to consider in relationship to the occurrence of putative ictal or postictal violent behavior is that of the possible induction of an excited delirium syndrome when attempts are made to restrain the behavior of an individual who is manifesting actual or seemingly violent behavior. As defined by DiMaio and DiMaio (DiMaio and DiMaio 2006) excited delirium syndrome "involves the sudden death of an individual, during or following an episode of excited delirium, in which an autopsy fails to reveal evidence of sufficient trauma or natural disease to explain the death. In virtually all cases, the episode of excited delirium is terminated by a struggle with police of medical personnel, and the use of physical restraint. Typically, within a few to several minutes following cessation of the struggle, the individual is noted to be in cardiopulmonary arrest. Attempts at resuscitation are usually unsuccessful." During state of delirium, there are varying transient disturbances of consciousness and cognition with disorientation, disorganized and inconsistent thought processes, inability to distinguish reality from hallucinations, speech disturbance, and disorientation to time, place and person.

Please see "SUDEP Probable Case" and related discussion in Chapter 8 for a prevented SUDEP who exhibited postictal agitation similar to that observed by the attending traffic police officer for the SUDEP victim described in the current chapter. We need to be aware of the potential for induction of this potentially fatal state of agitation when attempts are made to restrain persons with epilepsy who manifest ictal or postictal agitation or seemingly violent behavior. This is a highly stressful state and in combination with the history of epilepsy could be contributory to the occurrence of SUDEP in these individuals. Since both ictal and postictal states are self-limited, it is imperative for family members, police, and emergency care personnel to understand that watchful observation to keep the affected individual out of harm's way, rather than the high-risk intervention of physical restraint, is the most appropriate intervention (Novakova et al. 2013; Lathers and Schraeder 2011, ch. 17).

## CONCLUSION

This chapter presents a definite SUDEP case illustrating one problem for those confronted by patients with epilepsy who have become violent, delusional, delirious, intoxicated, and agitated. The individual may be physically involved with police, emergency medical personnel, firemen, family members, or passersby. The contribution of restraint struggles and use by law enforcement of electronic darts to subdue the victim makes the forensic analysis of these cases difficult, especially since there is always the concern of civil litigation and glare of publicity with accusations of police brutality.

We have also used this case to teach the readers how to read a SUDEP case and evaluate all data to assign the appropriate cluster IDs using.

## REFERENCES

DiMaio TG, DiMaio VJM. *Excited Delirium Syndrome.* Boca Raton, FL: CRC Press/Taylor & Francis Group; 2006.

Ho JD, Dawes DM, Nelson RS, Lundin EJ, Ryan FJ, Overton KG, Zeiders AJ, Miner JR. Acidosis and catecholamine evaluation following simulated law enforcement "use of force" encounters. *Acad Emerg Med* 2010;17(7):e60–8.

Jenkins DM Jr., Murray WB, Kennett MJ, Hughes EL, Werner JR. The effects of continuous application of the TASER X26 waveform on Susscrofa. *J Forensic Sci* 2013;58(3):684–92.

Kerling F, Dutsch M, Linke R, Kuwert T, Stefan H, Hilz MJ. Relation between ictal asystole and cardiac sympathetic dysfunction shown by MIBG-SPECT. *Acta Neurol Scand* 2009;120(2):123–9.

Koehler SA, Schraeder PL, Lathers CM, Wecht CH. One-year postmortem forensic analysis of deaths in persons with epilepsy. Chapter 9 In: Lathers CM, Schraeder PL, Bungo MW, Leestma JE, eds. *Sudden Death in Epilepsy: Forensic and Clinical Issues.* Boca Raton, FL: CRC Press/Taylor & Francis Group; 2011, pp. 145–59.

Kruszewski SP, Paczynski RP, Kahn DA. Gabapentin-induced delirium and dependence. *J Psychiatr Pract* 2009;15(4):314–9.

Lathers CM, Schraeder PL. Stress and SUDEP. Chapter 17 In: Lathers CM, Schraeder PL, Bungo MW, Leestma JE, eds. *Sudden Death in Epilepsy: Forensic and Clinical Issues.* Boca Raton, FL: CRC Press/Taylor & Francis Group; 2011, pp. 253–67.

Lathers CM, Schraeder PL. Clinical cases classified as SUDEP Cluster Risk Factor Identifiers. Chapter 8 In: Lathers CM, Schraeder PL, Leestma JE, Wannamaker BB, Verrier RL, Schachter SC, eds. *Sudden Death in Epilepsy: Risk Analyses.* Boca Raton, FL: CRC Press/Taylor & Francis Group; 2014.

Leestma J. Sudden unexpected death associated with seizures: A pathological review. Chapter 5 In: Lathers CM, Schraeder P, eds. *Epilepsy and Sudden Death.* New York, NY: Marcel Dekker; 1990, pp. 61–88.

Leestma JE, Walczak T, Hughes JR, Kalelkar MB, Teas SS. A prospective study on sudden unexpected death in epilepsy. *Ann Neurol* 1989;26(2):195–203.

Mendez MF. Postictal violence and epilepsy. *Psychosomatics* 1998;39(5):478–80.

Myerburg RJ, Goodman KW, Ringe TB 3rd. Electronic control devices: Science, law, and social responsibility. *Circulation* 2012;125(20):2406–8.

Novakova B, Harris PR, Ponnusamy A, Reuber M. The role of stress as a trigger for epileptic seizures: A narrative review of evidence from human and animal studies. *Epilepsia* 2013;54(11):1866–76.

Pedal I, Zimmer G, Mattern R, Mittmeyer HJ, Oehmichen M. [Fatal incidences during arrest of highly agitated persons]. *Arch Kriminol* 1999;203(1–2):1–9.

Peterson BL. Prevalence of gabapentin in impaired driving cases in Washington State in 2003–2007. *J Anal Toxicol* 2009;33(8):545–9.

Rona G. Catecholamine cardiotoxicity. *J Mol Cell Cardiol* 1985;17(4):291–306.

Schraeder PL, Delin K, McClelland RL, So EL. Coroner and medical examiner documentation of sudden unexplained deaths in epilepsy. *Epilepsy Res* 2006;68(2):137–43.

Schraeder PL, Delin K, McClelland RL, So EL. A nationwide survey of the extent of autopsy in sudden unexplained death in epilepsy. *Am J Forensic Med Pathol* 2009;30(2):123–6.

Shimizu M, Kagawa A, Takano T, Masai H, Miwa Y. Neurogenic stunned myocardium associated with status epileptics and postictal catecholamine surge. *Intern Med* 2008;47(4):269–73.

Strote J, Range Hutson H. Taser use in restraint-related deaths. *Prehosp Emerg Care* 2006;10(4):447–50.

Swerdlow CD, Fishbein MC, Chaman L, Lakkireddy DR, Tchou P. Presenting rhythm in sudden deaths temporally proximate to discharge of TASER conducted electrical weapons. *Acad Emerg Med* 2009;16(8):726–39.

Vilke GM, Sloane CM, Suffecool A, Kolkhorst FW, Neuman TS, Castillo EM, Chan TC. Physiologic effects of the TASER after exercise. *Acad Emerg Med* 2009;16(8):704–1.

Walczak T. Do antiepileptic drugs play a role in sudden unexpected death in epilepsy? *Drug Saf* 2003;26(10):673–83.

Zipes DP. Sudden cardiac arrest and death following application of shocks from a TASER electronic control device. *Circulation* 2012;125(20):2417–2.

# 10 A South Carolina Cohort of Epilepsy Patients

*Angela M. Malek and Braxton B. Wannamaker*

## CONTENTS

Several of the key methods for understanding sudden unexpected death in epilepsy (SUDEP) are the creation of large registries, development of cohorts, and the use of retrospective studies. A cohort of epilepsy patients in South Carolina was established over a 30-year period. This dataset is unique in that it includes over 3000 cases, both alive and deceased, some of whom have died from SUDEP. The inclusion of living patients as a comparison group is highly desirable and will be used in the forthcoming SUDEP cluster risk identification study.

Efforts to identify the mechanisms of SUDEP have not been successful yet much useful information has been ascertained. Risk factors appear to be relevant for some patients such as noncompliance to medications, duration of epilepsy, frequent seizures, generalized tonic–clonic seizures (GTCS), refractoriness to medication, and nocturnal seizures. Table 10.1 presents a list of the risk factors identified by a number of studies. The prevalence of these risk factors in any one series is variable and not seen in all SUDEP victims. In the decade ahead, we will move toward better clinical analyses, recognizing risk factors and understanding the integrative pathophysiological interactions of brain, epileptic foci, heart, and pulmonary mechanisms. All these components are influenced by genetics, medications, and basal and pathological health status. SUDEP results when some or all of these underlying conditions coalesce. This chapter presents the mortality studies from SUDEP among children and adults, an overview of prospective and retrospective SUDEP studies, risk factors associated with SUDEP, and a summary of the South Carolina Epilepsy Cohort study.

## MORTALITY

### MORTALITY IN CHILDREN

Approximately 120,000 new cases of childhood epilepsy are diagnosed in the United States each year (Hauser and Hesdorffer 1990). Although most achieve remission, epilepsy remains active for 20,000–45,000 children (Hauser and Hesdorffer 1990; Berg 1995; Shinnar and Pellock 2002). The prevalence of epilepsy in children under the age of 17 is 0.5%–1% (Hauser and Hesdorffer 1990; Hauser et al. 1993; Berg 1995; Camfield et al. 1996; Sillanpaa et al. 1998). Mortality rates among children with epilepsy have been found to range from 2.7 to 6.9 deaths per 1000 person-years (Sillanpaa et al. 1998; Callenbach et al. 2001; Berg et al. 2004; Camfield and Camfield 2005). This is due to SUDEP, status epilepticus (SE), accidents due to seizures, aspiration during seizures, progression of underlying disease, suicide (Ficker 2000), frequency of tonic–clonic seizures in the past year (Walczak et al. 2001), mental retardation/neurological deficit (Walczak et al. 2001; Camfield et al. 2002), number of anticonvulsant medications (Walczak et al. 2001), abnormal neurologic examination (Nickels et al. 2012), structural/metabolic causes of epilepsy (Nickels et al. 2012), and poor control of seizures (Berg et al. 2004).

In 2013, Sillanpaa and Shinnar investigated risk factors for SUDEP among a cohort of 245 children with incident and prevalent epilepsy who were followed for 40 years. Using the Nashef criteria, 38% ($n = 23$) of deaths were classified as SUDEP. An increased risk of SUDEP was found for individuals without localization-related epilepsy (hazard ratio [HR] = 3.0, 95% confidence interval [CI]: 1.2–7.6) and for failure to attain remission within 5 years (HR = 5.1, 95% CI: 1.5–17.3) (Sillanpaa and Shinnar 2013).

When persons with symptomatic childhood epilepsy were studied, significantly more deaths were observed (standard mortality ratio [SMR] = 4.9, 95% CI: 1.8–19.4) compared with non-epileptic cohort members (Chin et al. 2011). Mortality among individuals with idiopathic epilepsy was similarly increased (SMR = 1.2, 95% CI: 1.0–4.3) (Chin et al. 2011). Several causes of death were observed and none

**TABLE 10.1**
**Risk Factors for SUDEP**

| Author (Year, Location) | Design | Study Population | SUDEP-Related Findings |
|---|---|---|---|
| Hirsch (1970, United States) (Hirsch and Martin 1971) | Descriptive | 55 Deaths due to epilepsy, 19 SUDEP cases, aged 6–30 years | + Epilepsy duration >6 years although seizures occurred infrequently<br>+ Mild-to-moderate intellectual disability in 6 cases |
| Terrence (1975, United States) (Terrence et al. 1975) | Descriptive | 37 SUDEP cases, aged 2–73 years | + Epilepsy duration >1 year<br>+ Most had <1 seizure per month<br>+ Generalized seizure diagnosis |
| Leestma (1989, United States) (Leestma et al. 1989) | Descriptive | 60 SUDEP cases | + The majority of cases were African American adult males, had frequent generalized seizures, structural brain lesions, poor AED compliance, and alcohol abuse |
| Earnest (1992, United States) (Earnest et al. 1992) | Descriptive | 44 SUDEP cases, 39 were adults | + Monotherapy for most adults although noncompliance was common<br>+ Adults experienced seizures less often |
| Timmings (1993, New Zealand) (Timmings 1993) | Retrospective case–control | 14 SUDEP cases and 18 controls | + 2:1 ratio of males to females<br>+ >6 years duration of epilepsy for 25% of patients |
| Tennis (1995, Canada) (Tennis et al. 1995) | Descriptive | 3688 Patients with epilepsy (163 deaths) 39 cases of SUDEP among | + Male<br>+ History of hospitalization for intellectual disability<br>+ Psychotropic drugs<br>+ Use of ≥2 concurrent AEDs<br>+ In maximum SUDEP cases: hospitalization for alcohol abuse and older age (35–49 vs. 15–34 years) |
| Derby (1996, United Kingdom) (Derby et al. 1996) | Nested case–control | 63 Deaths among 4150 refractory epilepsy patients, aged ≤50; 15 possible/probable SUDEP cases, 4 matched controls per case | − Three AEDs concurrently within 30 days vs. two AEDs not associated with SUD<br>− Intellectual disability not associated with SUD |
| Nilsson (1999, Sweden) (Nilsson et al. 1999) | Nested case–control | 57 Cases, 171 matched controls, aged 15–70 years | + Dementia and injuries (non-CNS)<br>+ Early epilepsy onset (all and men)<br>+ Frequency of seizures in last year (vs. ≤2) (all and men)<br>+ Polytherapy with AEDs (vs. 1) (all, men, and women)<br>+ 3–5 changes in dose of AEDs per year (all and women)<br>+ Antipsychotics (women)<br>+ Anxiolytics (all and men)<br>+ After adjustment for covariables: frequency of seizures, polytherapy with AEDs, and 3–5 AED dose changes per year<br>− Cerebrovascular disease<br>− Localization-related symptomatic epilepsy (vs. generalized symptomatic epilepsy) |
| Walczak (2001, United States) (Walczak et al. 2001) | Nested case–control | 4578 Patients (111 deaths) 20 SUDEP cases and 80 controls with epilepsy | + Higher incidence in women<br>+ ≥50 seizures per month<br>+ 1–3 tonic–clonic seizures in past year<br>+ ≥30 years duration of epilepsy<br>+ IQ <70 or too impaired to test<br>+ Use of >2 AEDs at last clinic visit<br>+ After adjustment for covariables: 1–3 tonic–clonic seizures in past year, IQ <70, number of AEDs |
| Chin (2011, United Kingdom) (Chin et al. 2011) | Prospective | 101 Adults with childhood epilepsy and >12,000 cohort members without childhood epilepsy | + More deaths occurred among persons with symptomatic and idiopathic epilepsy compared to children without epilepsy; however, no SUDEP deaths were observed |
| Hesdorffer (2011, United States, England, Scotland, Sweden) (Hesdorffer et al. 2011) | Combined case–control | 289 Cases and 958 controls with epilepsy | + Men<br>+ <16 Years at age on onset<br>+ >15 Years duration of epilepsy (overall and <16 years)<br>+ Polytherapy (overall and <16 years)<br>+ Lamotrigine (United States, England, and Scotland analysis) (Overall and <16 years) |

**TABLE 10.1    (Continued)**
**Risk Factors for SUDEP**

| Author (Year, Location) | Design | Study Population | SUDEP-Related Findings |
|---|---|---|---|
| | | | + ≥1 (or unknown frequency) GTCS per year (overall and <16 years) |
| | | | + Various GTCS frequency and therapy combinations (overall and <16 years) |
| | | | + Learning difficulty (aged <16 years) |
| | | | − Idiopathic generalized epilepsy (Overall and women in cohort and in those <16 years) |
| | | | − Not taking lamotrigine therapy (England and Scotland) |
| Hesdorffer (2012, United States, England, Sweden) (Hesdorffer et al. 2012) | Combined case–control | 216 Cases and 831 controls (carbamazepine, phenytoin, valproic acid, other AEDs, and GTCS frequency analysis); 160 cases and 674 controls (lamotrigine and GTCS frequency analysis) | + GTCS frequency (not use of AEDs) <br> − After adjustment for covariables: Individual AEDs (carbamazepine, phenytoin, valproic acid, and other AEDs) or number of AEDs used <br> − After adjustment for covariables: Number of AEDs (none, monotherapy, polytherapy) |
| Holst (2013, Denmark) (Holst et al. 2013) | Historical cohort | 33,022 Patients with epilepsy, aged 1–35 years (685 deaths) 50 definite/probable SUDEP cases; 37 possible SUDEP | + Higher proportion of comorbidities among possible SUDEP cases than definite/probable SUDEP cases <br> + Deaths more likely to be witnessed for definite/probable SUDEP cases |
| Sillanpaa and Shinnar (2013, Finland) (Sillanpaa and Shinnar 2013) | Prospective | 245 children followed (60 deaths) 23 SUDEP | + Individuals without localization-related epilepsy <br> + Failure to attain remission within 5 years |

*Note:* + = Positive association, − = Negative association

were found to be SUDEP related. Of the deaths, five were not due to epilepsy and those that were related to epilepsy varied and included an infection of the central nervous system ($n = 1$), carbon monoxide poisoning ($n = 1$), metastatic lung cancer ($n = 1$), inhaled foreign body ($n = 1$), aspiration pneumonia ($n = 1$), bronchopneumonia ($n = 1$), and convulsive SE ($n = 4$). Cerebral palsy was present among one of the convulsive SE deaths.

Various studies in children have demonstrated an increase in mortality but not all studies have found a high incidence of SUDEP. The outcome and course of pediatric SE was investigated prospectively over a period of 5 years by the Dutch Study of Epilepsy in Children (Stroink et al. 2007). Incident epilepsy cases ($n = 494$) involved children aged 1 month through 15 years. Of the 494 cases, 47 were diagnosed with SE. Mortality among children with SE (4.3%) did not differ significantly from children without SE (1.6%) (Stroink et al. 2007). The underlying etiology of epilepsy was responsible for two deaths occurring during the study, both of which initially presented with SE. However, the two children had different experiences. The first child died from aspiration pneumonia after 1.5 follow-up years and had experienced only one SE. The second child, who was diagnosed with Ohtahara syndrome, had seven prior SE episodes, some of which occurred with fever, and had generally poor compliance. This child succumbed to pneumonia after 4.8 follow-up years.

A prospective study investigating outcomes for secondarily generalized epilepsies with an onset in childhood was conducted in Nova Scotia and involved 80 children, aged 1 month to 15 years (Camfield and Camfield 2007). Most participants were male (54%) and the onset age ranged from 1 to 144 months with a mean of 22 months. During the first year of life, the majority (59%) of children experienced their first seizure. Deaths occurred among nearly 1/4 of patients ($n = 19$) and were due to underlying neurologic disorders. Deceased patients ranged in age from 17 to 243 months, with a mean age of $139 \pm 75$ months (Camfield and Camfield 2007). Epilepsy was diagnosed during the first year of life for most who had died (79%). Cognitive dysfunction or intellectual disability was a comorbid condition among all the deaths; 2 were diagnosed with mental retardation and 17 with a neurological handicap that was severe. At the time of death, intractable seizures were present in 11 of the 19 children. The other eight children had either stopped taking antiepileptic drugs (AEDs) about 97 months into remission or had seizures that were persistent yet nonintractable.

## MORTALITY IN ADULTS

The elderly are known to have the greatest excess mortality in SUDEP (Hauser and Tomson 2005); however, the majority of studies report a mean age of 25–39 years (Tomson et al. 2005). In 1989, Leestma et al. described characteristics of SUDEP cases in 60 adults. The greatest proportion of SUDEP cases involved African American males (mean age of 35 years) with frequent generalized seizures and structural brain lesions (Leestma et al. 1989). This group was also described as having poor AED compliance and abuse of alcohol.

A study by Hirsch and Martin in 1971 identified 19 SUDEP cases among 55 deaths due to epilepsy in Cleveland, Ohio. The cases ranged in age from 6 to 30 years, and there were 12 adults. Seizures occurred infrequently and duration of epilepsy was >6 years for most of the SUDEP cases. Therapy varied by case, and mild-to-moderate intellectual disability was present in six cases.

A total of 37 SUDEP cases ranging in age from 2 to 73 years were described for Allegheny County, Pennsylvania, by Terrence et al. in 1975. The mean age was 32 years, and all cases were diagnosed with epilepsy for >1 year. Several different therapies were reported, nearly all cases experienced <1 seizure per month, and a diagnosis of generalized seizures was made for 59%.

In 1986, Schwender and Troncoso reviewed natural death records in epilepsy ($n = 29$) in Maryland over a 2-year period and found that most were male and African American, <50% had neuropathological lesions, and the median age was 26 years.

Earnest et al. in 1992 examined SUDEP among 44 patients in Colorado, 39 of whom were adults. Most commonly, the adults were on monotherapy, although noncompliant, and their seizures occurred less often.

In 1993, Timmings investigated 14 SUDEP cases and found a 2:1 ratio for males to females. The majority were aged 20–40 years with a mean age of 35 years, and >6 years duration of epilepsy duration was reported by 25% of all SUDEP patients (Timmings 1993). The authors also compared demographics and clinical factors among SUDEP cases with 1806 patients with epilepsy; the two groups did not differ with regard to seizure frequency, epilepsy duration, age, or number of medications.

A descriptive study evaluating risk factors for SUDEP was carried out in Canada by Tennis et al. in 1995 and involved 3688 patients with epilepsy. Sixty-one percent of the cohort was aged ≥25 years, and a total of 163 deaths were observed. Of the 39 SUDEP cases, 21 were classified as possible SUDEP and 18 as definite or probable SUDEP. Six additional deaths, of the nine in which SUDEP status was undocumented or unknown (and based on the proportion of SUDEP among deaths outside of the hospital), were presumed to be possible SUDEP cases and were added to the total thus increasing the number of possible, probable, or definite SUDEP cases to 45. In the 39 SUDEP cases (minimum) and 45 maximum cases (including the 6 presumed cases), the incidence of SUDEP was elevated in the presence of the following characteristics for those with definite, possible, or probable SUDEP: male, history of hospitalization for intellectual disability, psychotropic drugs, and use of ≥2 concurrent AEDs (Tennis et al. 1995). History of

hospitalization for alcohol abuse and older age (35–49 years compared to 15–34) increased incidence in the 45 maximum cases with SUDEP (Tennis et al. 1995).

Derby et al. (1996) examined sudden unexplained death (SUD) cases among refractory epilepsy patients ($n = 4150$) aged ≤50 years. Of the 63 deaths, 23 were initially classified as potential SUD. However, after reviewing available autopsy reports and clinical and death records, only 15 cases were determined to be possible or probable sudden unexplained death (Derby et al. 1996). Six of the 15 cases were between 40 and 49 years of age, four were 30–39 years, three were 20–29 years, and two were younger than 20 years. In addition, potential SUD risk factors (intellectual disability and count of concurrent AEDs in a 30-day period) were compared in a nested case–control study conducted by Derby et al. that involved a 1:4 ratio of patients with SUD (cases) to patients without SUD (controls), matched by age and sex. Epilepsy severity was approximated by number of AEDs in a 30-day period. Neither three AEDs concurrently within 30 days (vs. two AEDs) (relative risk [RR] = 0.04, 95% CI: 0.1–3.5) nor intellectual disability (RR = 1.04, 95% CI: 0.3–8.0) was found to be associated with SUD among cases compared to non-SUD controls (Derby et al. 1996).

In 1998, Ficker et al. reported a total of nine definite or probable SUDEP cases and one possible SUDEP case among 535 deaths in a cohort of 1535 patients. In addition, there was nearly a 24-fold risk of mortality from SUDEP in persons aged 20–40 years in Rochester, Minnesota, compared with sudden death in persons without epilepsy in the general population (SMR = 23.7, 95% CI: 7.7–55) (Ficker et al. 1998).

## COHORT AND CASE–CONTROL STUDIES

A cohort study involves following a group of individuals without the disease of interest, either prospectively or retrospectively, over time (usually for a period of years) to observe incident cases of specific health outcomes. Due to the temporal relationship between exposure and disease in prospective cohort studies, causality may be assessed. Qualities of a good prospective cohort study include: (1) accurate case identification; (2) a comparison group (unexposed or less exposed), which differs from the exposed group only with regard to the exposure(s) of interest (i.e., potential confounding factors are similar); (3) thorough design of data collection materials measuring exposure of interest and potential confounders prior to disease onset; (4) standardized data collection procedures in both groups (exposed and unexposed/less exposed); (5) complete follow-up of participants including if and when they develop the outcome, die, or are lost to follow-up, with 80%–90% follow-up ideal as bias can result from loss to follow-up; and (6) documentation of any changes in an individual's exposure. A prospective study is pivotal in determining the true incidence of disease as well as establishing the relationship between potential exposures or risk factors and the outcome of interest.

Case–control studies begin by identifying persons with an outcome of interest (cases) and persons without the outcome of interest (controls) to retrospectively investigate exposures. Frequency of the exposure(s) in cases is then compared to frequency of the exposure(s) in controls. This study design is ideal for rare diseases/outcomes and for outbreaks. In general, case–control studies are less expensive and quicker to conduct than cohort studies. When designing a case–control study, the case and control groups must be chosen carefully. In addition, overmatching should be avoided, bias minimized, and confounding taken into account.

## PREVIOUS RESEARCH ON RISK FACTOR IDENTIFICATION

Over the past years, several risk factors for SUDEP have been identified. A nested case–control study was carried out by Nilsson et al. in 1999 in Sweden to investigate potential risk factors for SUDEP among cases ($n = 57$) and age- and sex-matched epilepsy patient controls ($n = 171$) aged 15–70 years. Cases were identified by chart review and epilepsy as a cause of death on the death certificate and included definite and probable SUDEP. Those not taking a major AED (sodium valproate, phenytoin, carbamazepine) or taking AEDs <1 year before death were excluded. The presence of dementia and injuries (noncentral nervous system) were associated with SUDEP in cases compared to controls, while the risk was lower for cerebrovascular disease (Nilsson et al. 1999). In addition, a relationship was found for the following clinical factors and SUDEP: early epilepsy onset (vs. late) (RR = 7.72, 95% CI: 2.13–27.96), frequency of seizures in last year (vs. ≤2) with >50 seizures having the greatest risk (RR = 10.16, 95% CI: 2.94–35.18), polytherapy with AEDs (3 vs. 1) (RR = 9.89, 95% CI: 3.20–30.60), and AED dose changes per year (vs. none) (RR = 6.08, 95% CI: 1.99–18.56) (Nilsson et al. 1999). Compared to generalized idiopathic epilepsy, the risk of SUDEP was significantly decreased for localization-related symptomatic epilepsy. The risk of SUDEP was nearly 16-fold for those with >2 seizures and taking >1 AED; the risk was fivefold higher in those with >2 seizures with monotherapy (Nilsson et al. 1999). Following adjustment for all covariates in a multivariate model, the findings remained significant for seizure frequency (3–12 and >12) in last year (vs. 0–2 seizures), 3 AEDs (vs. 1), and 3–5 changes in doses of AEDs per year.

Further examination of clinical characteristics by sex found a higher risk of SUDEP for men with increased seizure frequency in the past year (vs. ≤2), earlier epilepsy onset, and therapy with two or three AEDs, whereas risk was highest for women who were taking three AEDs and had more AED dose changes per year (Nilsson et al. 1999). Overall and in men, use of anxiolytic medications was associated with SUDEP (RR = 3.00, 95% CI: 1.16–7.76) (Nilsson et al. 1999). SUDEP risk was significantly elevated in women taking antipsychotic medication, but the risk was not increased for men or overall.

A prospective study and a nested case–control study were carried out by Walczak et al. in the United States in 2001 to describe the incidence of SUDEP and to investigate risk factors among 20 SUDEP cases and 80 epilepsy controls from 3 epilepsy centers. The proportion of deaths due to SUDEP was 18%. The incidence of SUDEP in women was 1.45 per 1000 patient-years and slightly lower overall at 1.21 per 1000 patient-years (Walczak et al. 2001). Relationships were found between the risk of SUDEP and the occurrence of >50 seizures per month (odds ratio [OR] = 11.5, 95% CI: 1.3–99.3), 1–3 tonic–clonic seizures in the past year (OR = 2.4, 95% CI: 1.8–30.5), >3 tonic-clonic seizures per year (OR = 8.1, 95% CI: 2.2–30.0), ≥30 years duration of epilepsy (OR = 13.9, 95% CI: 3.4–57.1), intelligence quotient (IQ) <70 or too impaired to test (OR = 5.0, 95% CI: 1.3–19.3), and use of >2 AEDs at last clinic visit (OR = 4.0, 95% CI: 1.4–11.7) (Walczak et al. 2001). Further adjustment was performed and found similar results for the number of tonic–clonic seizures, intellectual disability based on IQ <70, and number of AEDs.

In 2011, Hesdorffer et al. combined four case–control studies to investigate risk factors for SUDEP among cases ($n = 289$) compared to epilepsy controls ($n = 958$). A relationship was found for male sex (OR = 1.42, 95% CI: 1.07–1.88), <16 years at age of onset (OR = 1.72, 95% CI: 1.23–2.40), >15 years duration of epilepsy (OR = 1.95, 95% CI: 1.45–2.63), polytherapy (OR = 1.95, 95% CI: 1.08–3.47), lamotrigine (England, United States, and Scotland analysis) (OR = 1.86, 95% CI: 1.22–2.84), and for 1–2 GTCS per year (OR = 5.07, 95% CI: 2.94–8.76) with the risk higher for ≥3 seizures and unknown seizure frequency and risk of SUDEP after adjustment for age, gender, study type, and epilepsy duration (Hesdorffer et al. 2011). Risk of SUDEP was also significantly elevated for various combinations of number of GTCS per year and AED therapies. Decreased associations were observed for idiopathic generalized epilepsy overall (OR = 0.69, 95% CI: 0.49–0.98) and for females (OR = 0.39, 95% CI: 0.23–0.67), and for those without lamotrigine therapy in England and Scotland (OR = 0.50, 95% CI: 0.33–0.74) (Hesdorffer et al. 2011).

Potential risk factors were also assessed by age of epilepsy onset (<16 vs. ≥16 years) with adjustment for data source. In those less than 16 years of age, a relationship was found for >15 years duration of epilepsy (OR = 3.20, 95% CI: 2.07–4.97), polytherapy (OR = 7.90, 95% CI: 2.37–26.37), lamotrigine (OR = 2.32, 95% CI: 1.33–4.03), learning difficulty (OR = 2.44, 95% CI: 1.52–3.90), GTCS frequency per year (≥1 and unknown) (ORs range from 3.91 to 18.92), and various combinations of GTCS frequency per year (≥1 or unknown) and AED therapy (none, monotherapy, or polytherapy) (ORs range from 3.12 to 37), and risk of SUDEP (Hesdorffer et al. 2011). In those aged <16 years, the risk of SUDEP was decreased overall and for females with idiopathic generalized epilepsy. Among those aged ≥16 years, a relationship was reported for male sex (OR = 1.88, 95% CI: 1.20–2.94), GTCS frequency per year (≥1 and unknown)

(ORs range from 3.46 to 10.18), various combinations of GTCS frequency per year and AED therapy (none, monotherapy, or polytherapy) (ORs ranged from 3.07–12.57), and alcohol abuse (OR = 2.71, 95% CI: 1.50–4.88) and SUDEP (Hesdorffer et al. 2011). Alcohol was no longer associated with SUDEP following adjustment for age at death and GTCS frequency per year. Duration of epilepsy >15 years, idiopathic etiology, monotherapy, and idiopathic generalized epilepsy (overall and females) were associated with a lower risk of SUDEP among those aged ≥16 years. In addition, the authors commented that the pooled results confirmed some findings from the original studies as well as reported on newly identified risk factors.

Hesdorffer et al. also examined AED use and risk of SUDEP in a 2012 pooled analysis of four studies. No association was found for individual AEDs (carbamazepine, phenytoin, valproic acid, and other AEDs) or number of AEDs categorized as none, monotherapy, polytherapy, or other, and risk of SUDEP after adjustment for data source, gender, age at death, and GTCS frequency (Hesdorffer et al. 2012). The authors concluded that SUDEP risk was influenced by GTCS frequency rather than use of AEDs.

A Danish historical cohort study carried out by Holst et al. in 2013 investigated the risk of SUDEP among subjects aged 1–35 years with epilepsy and SUD among patients without epilepsy from 2000 to 2006 with a median follow-up of 3.7 and 7 years, respectively. In subjects with epilepsy ($n$ = 33,022), 50 cases of definite or probable SUDEP and 37 cases of probable SUDEP occurred among a total of 685 deaths (Holst et al 2013). The incidence rate for definite and probable SUDEP was 41.1 (95% CI: 31.6–54.9) per 100,000 person-years; the rate increased with age to 73.8 (95% CI: 52.5–103.8) for those aged 24 to <35 (Holst et al. 2013). Compared to definite and probable cases, the proportions of comorbidities were higher for cases with possible SUDEP. Deaths were more often witnessed among definite and probable SUDEP cases (12%) than those with possible SUDEP (5%) ($p$ < 0.001) (Holst et al. 2013).

In summary, previous studies investigating risk factors for SUDEP have consistently reported relationships with frequency of seizures in the past year, AED polytherapy, generalized seizures, early onset of epilepsy, and AED dose changes per year, although one study did not find an association with AED use. Other associations have been reported by a small number of studies such as IQ <70, lamotrigine therapy, >1 seizure type, dementia, noncentral nervous system injuries, various seizure frequencies in combination with number of AEDs, and certain medications (antipsychotics in women and anxiolytics in men) and are in need of replication. Lamotrigine therapy was associated with an increased risk of SUDEP by one study and a decreased risk by another. Good seizure control, effectiveness of the AED (s), and use of the fewest number of AEDs as necessary may perhaps be important risk reduction strategies in the prevention of SUDEP.

## A SOUTH CAROLINA COHORT OF EPILEPSY PATIENTS

In 1996 it was appreciated that there were a number of patients in private practice who had died of sudden death. Records on patients who had died were returned to a file for later review. Through written agreement and with approval of the South Carolina Department of Health and Environmental Control, death certificates of the SUDEP victims were obtained from the Bureau of Vital Statistics. It was also apparent that to obtain information about all patients who had died, and especially those with SUDEP, it would be necessary to have comparative data with those patients who had not died. In collaboration with two epidemiologists, Dr. Alan Gross and Dr. Donna Daniel, we asked how questions could be best addressed in the setting of private practice. It was thought best to compare SUDEP patients with matched controls of patients living and all in the same practice. Dr. Daniel developed a data abstraction tool (see Appendix) along with a data dictionary. The goal was to abstract pertinent demographic, diagnostic, testing, and treatment information from each record of the SUDEP patients and from the records of living epilepsy cohorts.

The patient records were from a private practice in a university epilepsy clinic from 1974 to 1984 and another private practice from 1984 to 2004, all in South Carolina. The private practices were unique in that the patients were predominantly those with epilepsy. During those periods, various epileptologists worked with this cohort of patients, yet the manner of practice was that of maintaining a single physician in charge of individual patients. Ninety-five percent of the patient records constituting a cohort of slightly over 3090 patients were under the care of a single epileptologist. The records of 3090 patients with epilepsy from a private clinical practice were gathered and their personal identifiers were collated. Essentially all were South Carolina residents.

In 2006, a digitized list was screened by the Bureau of Vital Statistics to determine death (Lineberry et al. 2006). There were 407 deaths (263 male and 144 female) of epilepsy patients of all causes. Over a period of approximately 8 years, data had been abstracted from 881 records of living patients and 407 deceased patients.

In the group of 881 living epilepsy controls, there were 53.2% women ($n$ = 469) and 46.8% males ($n$ = 412) (see Table 10.2). The median age at onset of epilepsy was 14 years (birth to 82 years), and the median duration of epilepsy was 15 years (birth to 82 years). Patients were followed for an average of 5 years. We were able to determine the category of epilepsy as partial for 61.2% and generalized in 27.6%. The category could not be determined in 10.1%. The database also revealed that reports of electroencephalograms were available in 537 patients with 37.3% abnormal and 22.6% normal. Much more information from the database and the original records is also available and being analyzed.

**TABLE 10.2**

**Characteristics of Patients with Epilepsy from the Living Cohort (*n* = 881), 1974–2004**

| Characteristic | *n* (%) |
|---|---|
| Male | 412 (46.8) |
| Epilepsy category | |
|    Partial | 539 (61.2) |
|    Generalized | 243 (27.6) |
|    Undetermined | 89 (10.1) |
|    Unknown/missing | 10 (1.1) |
| Age at onset, median (range) | 14 (Birth–82) |
| Neonatal (birth–1 month) | 11 (1.2) |
| Infantile (2–18 months) | 69 (7.8) |
| Childhood (19 months–10 years) | 254 (28.8) |
| Adolescence (11–17 years) | 166 (18.8) |
| Adult | 341 (38.7) |
| Unknown | 40 (4.5) |
| Duration of epilepsy (years), median (range) | 15 (Birth–82) |
| EEGs[a] | |
|    Normal | 199 (22.6) |
|    Abnormal | 329 (37.3) |
|    Normal/abnormal | 7 (0.8) |
|    Unknown | 344 (39.0) |

[a] One EEG was borderline and one was unsatisfactory.

## PLAN

The South Carolina Cohort of Epilepsy Patients has been assimilated over a 40-year period. The patients are representative of epilepsy and its treatment in this area. Many patients have required subspecialty evaluation and care and thus were followed on average about 5 years. The abstracted data and other charted features from the records of the patients and of SUDEP victims in this cohort will be de-identified. The information pertaining to the SUDEP victims will be submitted for SUDEP Risk Factor Identification. We also will submit de-identified patient data from those living patients with epilepsy matched for specific SUDEP victims from our cohort and from those of other centers for SUDEP Risk Factor Identification. This method will be useful in determining the prevalence of potential demographic, behavioral, and clinical risk factors that may be associated with SUDEP and which are described in more detail in Chapters 4 and 5.

Mortality is higher among persons with epilepsy than that of the general population. Among known epilepsy deaths, the most common cause of death is due to SUDEP (England et al. 2012), for which the mechanisms are largely unknown and few risk factors have been consistently identified. Previous studies attempting to explain this phenomenon have mostly involved a small number of cases ranging from possible to definite SUDEP. Larger studies are needed to identify risk factors for SUDEP and to prevent the occurrence of future SUDEP deaths. Through provision of a large number of SUDEP cases, living epilepsy controls, and use of the SUDEP Risk Factor Cluster Identifiers classification, the proposed South Carolina Cohort of Epilepsy Patients study will be instrumental in filling an important gap in the literature regarding mechanisms of and risk factors for SUDEP. To better understand and ultimately prevent SUDEP, coroners and medical examiners must work together to improve the accuracy of reporting of SUDEP on death certificates, which will in turn increase the amount of information available thereby allowing for more accurate findings.

## REFERENCES

Berg A. The epidemiology of seizures and epilepsy in children. In: Shinnar S, Amir N, Branski D, eds. *Childhood Seizures.* Basel, Switzerland: Karger; 1995.

Berg AT, Shinnar S, Testa FM, Levy SR, Smith SN, Beckerman B. Mortality in childhood-onset epilepsy. *Arch Pediatr Adolesc Med* 2004;158(12):1147–52.

Callenbach PM, Westendorp RG, Geerts AT, Arts WF, Peeters EA, van Donselaar CA, Peters AC, Stroink H, Brouwer OF. Mortality risk in children with epilepsy: The Dutch study of epilepsy in childhood. *Pediatrics* 2001;107(6):1259–63.

Camfield CS, Camfield PR, Gordon K, Wirrell E, Dooley JM. Incidence of epilepsy in childhood and adolescence: A population-based study in Nova Scotia from 1977 to 1985. *Epilepsia* 1996;37(1):19–23.

Camfield CS, Camfield PR, Veugelers PJ. Death in children with epilepsy: A population-based study. *Lancet* 2002;359 (9321):1891–5.

Camfield P, Camfield C. Sudden unexpected death in people with epilepsy: A pediatric perspective. *Semin Pediatr Neurol* 2005;12(1):10–4.

Camfield P, Camfield C. Long-term prognosis for symptomatic (secondarily) generalized epilepsies: A population-based study. *Epilepsia* 2007;48(6):1128–32.

Chin RF, Cumberland PM, Pujar SS, Peckham C, Ross EM, Scott RC. Outcomes of childhood epilepsy at age 33 years: A population-based birth-cohort study. *Epilepsia* 2011;52(8):1513–21.

Derby LE, Tennis P, Jick H. Sudden unexplained death among subjects with refractory epilepsy. *Epilepsia* 1996;37(10):931–5.

Earnest MP, Thomas GE, Eden RA, Hossack KF. The sudden unexplained death syndrome in epilepsy: Demographic, clinical, and postmortem features. *Epilepsia* 1992;33(2):310–6.

England MJ, Liverman CT, Schultz AM, Strawbridge LM, Committee on the Public Health Dimensions of the Epilepsies; Board on Health Sciences Policy. *Summary. Epilepsy across the Spectrum: Promoting Health and Understanding.* Washington, DC: Institute of Medicine, National Academy of Sciences; 2012.

Ficker DM. Sudden unexplained death and injury in epilepsy. *Epilepsia* 2000;41(Suppl 2):S7–12.

Ficker DM, So EL, Shen WK, Annegers JF, O'Brien PC, Cascino GD, Belau PG. Population-based study of the incidence of sudden unexplained death in epilepsy. *Neurology* 1998;51(5):1270–4.

Hauser WA, Annegers JF, Kurland LT. Incidence of epilepsy and unprovoked seizures in Rochester, Minnesota: 1935–1984. *Epilepsia* 1993;34(3):453–68.

Hauser WA, Hesdorffer DC. *Epilepsy: Frequency, Causes and Consequences.* New York, NY: Demos; 1990.

Hauser WA, Tomson T. Conclusions and recommendations summary of workshop proceedings. *Epilepsia* 2005;46(Suppl 11):62–3.

Hesdorffer DC, Tomson T, Benn E, Sander JW, Nilsson L, Langan Y, Walczak TS, et al. Combined analysis of risk factors for SUDEP. *Epilepsia* 2011;52(6):1150–9.

Hesdorffer DC, Tomson T, Benn E, Sander JW, Nilsson L, Langan Y, Walczak TS, et al. Do antiepileptic drugs or generalized tonic-clonic seizure frequency increase SUDEP risk? A combined analysis. *Epilepsia* 2012;53(2):249–52.

Hirsch CS, Martin DL. Unexpected death in young epileptics. *Neurology* 1971;21(7):682–90.

Holst AG, Winkel BG, Risgaard B, Nielsen JB, Rasmussen PV, Haunso S, Sabers A, Uldall P, Tfelt-Hansen J. Epilepsy and risk of death and sudden unexpected death in the young: A nationwide study. *Epilepsia* 2013;54(9):1613–20.

Leestma JE, Walczak T, Hughes JR, Kalelkar MB, Teas SS. A prospective study on sudden unexpected death in epilepsy. *Ann Neurol* 1989;26(2):195–203.

Lineberry LA, Wannamaker BB, Ferguson, PL, Selassie AW, Smith GM. *Sudden Unexplained Deaths (SUDEP) and Cohort Study from a 30 Year Epilepsy Practice Population. Epilepsia* 2006;47(S4):280.

Nickels KC, Grossardt BR, Wirrell EC. Epilepsy-related mortality is low in children: A 30-year population-based study in Olmsted County, MN. *Epilepsia* 2012;53(12):2164–71.

Nilsson L, Farahmand BY, Persson PG, Thiblin I, Tomson T. Risk factors for sudden unexpected death in epilepsy: A case-control study. *Lancet* 1999;353(9156):888–93.

Schwender LA, Troncoso JC. Evaluation of sudden death in epilepsy. *Am J Forensic Med Pathol* 1986;7(4):283–7.

Shinnar S, Pellock JM. Update on the epidemiology and prognosis of pediatric epilepsy. *J Child Neurol* 2002;17(Suppl 1):S4–17.

Sillanpaa M, Jalava M, Kaleva O, Shinnar S. Long-term prognosis of seizures with onset in childhood. *N Engl J Med* 1998;338(24):1715–22.

Sillanpaa M, Shinnar S. SUDEP and other causes of mortality in childhood-onset epilepsy. *Epilepsy Behav* 2013;28(2):249–55.

Stroink H, Geerts AT, van Donselaar CA, Peters AC, Brouwer OF, Peeters EA, Arts WF. Status epilepticus in children with epilepsy: Dutch study of epilepsy in childhood. *Epilepsia* 2007;48(9):1708–15.

Tennis P, Cole TB, Annegers JF, Leestma JE, McNutt M, Rajput A. Cohort study of incidence of sudden unexplained death in persons with seizure disorder treated with antiepileptic drugs in Saskatchewan, Canada. *Epilepsia* 1995;36(1):29–36.

Terrence CF Jr., Wisotzkey HM, Perper JA. Unexpected, unexplained death in epileptic patients. *Neurology* 1975;25(6):594–8.

Timmings PL. Sudden unexpected death in epilepsy: A local audit. *Seizure* 1993;2(4):287–90.

Tomson T, Walczak T, Sillanpaa M, Sander JW. Sudden unexpected death in epilepsy: A review of incidence and risk factors. *Epilepsia* 2005;46(Suppl 11):54–61.

Walczak TS, Leppik IE, D'Amelio M, Rarick J, So E, Ahman P, Ruggles K, Cascino GD, Annegers JF, Hauser WA. Incidence and risk factors in sudden unexpected death in epilepsy: A prospective cohort study. *Neurology* 2001;56(4):519–25.

# 11 Measuring the Incidence of SUDEP Using Forensic and National Data

*Steven A. Koehler, Claire M. Lathers, and Paul L. Schraeder*

## CONTENTS

In the fields of medicine, epidemiology, research, and public health, it is critically important to be able to ascertain the number of individuals at risk for a specific disease or condition as well as the number of individuals who die from that disease or condition. These numbers are used to monitor the general state of health for a specific area and the country at large. Public health researchers use these data to measure the impact of prevention programs, identify emerging diseases, locate hot spots. If we cannot identify cases of sudden unexpected death in epilepsy (SUDEP), we will be unable to determine the number of deaths from SUDEP, if the rates are increasing or decreasing, or if current treatment programs are beneficial or increasing the risk of death.

There are several methods to measure the number of individuals at risk for a disease and the number of deaths for a specific condition/disease. Common methods of reporting these numbers are incidence, mortality, and prevalence. Incidence is a measure of the risk of developing some new condition within a specified period of time. Typically expressed simply as the number of new cases during some period, it is better expressed as a proportion or a rate with a denominator. The incidence of any disease is vital for the understanding of a disease, identifying populations at risk, and identifying risk factors. Incidence is a measure of morbidity or mortality, whereas prevalence is only a measure of morbidity (Woodward 2005). Mortality is the number of deaths from a specific disease divided by the total population. Prevalence is the number of existing cases of a disease at a particular point in time.

In the case of SUDEP, relative risk can be examined on a number of levels. Seizure risk can be examined by age, etiology, location, type, and antiepileptic drugs (AEDs). The role of AEDs has received much attention focusing on determining if there is an increased risk of SUDEP associated with compliance, increased number of AEDs, and the interaction between AEDs and other drugs. The main question is as follows: "Is the risk of SUDEP a function of the actual medications taken by patients with epilepsy?" or "Is SUDEP risk correlated better with a measure of the severity of seizure disorder?" Because of the importance of this issue, the SUDEP Syndrome Cluster Identification matrix included the incidence of SUDEP, the number of AEDs, and risk factors based on the pathological mechanisms involved in SUDEP.

SUDEP is by definition a diagnosis after death; therefore, mortality data are the focus of this chapter and, in particular, two main sources of mortality data relating to deaths from SUDEP: epilepsy and other seizure-related disorders. These data are obtained directly from the medical examiner/coroners (ME/C) offices and the Centers for Disease Control and Prevention (CDC) National Mortality Database. This chapter describes how such data can be utilized to ascertain the number of deaths from SUDEP and the mortality rates from SUDEP and presents the total number and mortality rates (1,000,000) for SUDEP, status epilepticus, and episodic and paroxysmal disorders from forensic data and the CDC database for Allegheny County, Pennsylvania; the state of Pennsylvania; and the United States. Finally, it discusses the strengths and weakness of both ascertainment methods and suggestions to improve the identification of SUDEP deaths.

## FORENSIC DATA FROM MEDICAL EXAMINER/CORONERS OFFICES

ME/C offices are charged by state and/or county laws to conduct investigations into deaths that are unexpected, sudden, or suspicious, or that lack significant past medical history to determine the cause and manner of death. ME/C investigation is composed of three parts: Death Scene Investigation, Autopsy, and Toxicology Analysis. The Death Scene Investigation Report contains basic epidemiological information of the victim, a summary of the circumstances surrounding the death, and other relative information. The Autopsy Report contains the weight and description of the internal organs, and anatomical and pathological findings. The Toxicology Report contains a list and concentration of all compounds detected in the body fluids. Each ME/C office serves a well-defined population demographic, typically a county or state. Not all deaths undergo a forensic investigation; only about 20% of all deaths are investigated by the ME/C office. For example, most persons who die from natural causes such as heart disease, cancers, or pneumonia are transported from the place of death directly to the funeral home for burial/cremation. Natural deaths that are investigated by the ME/C include deaths where the physician refused to sign the death certificate, the victim has no physician, or there is a lack of significant past medical history to determine the cause. In the case of death attributed to SUDEP, by definition the death was sudden and unexpected and therefore should undergo a forensic death investigation.

## NATIONAL MORTALITY DATABASE: CENTERS FOR DISEASE CONTROL AND PREVENTION

A certificate of death is completed on every individual whose death occurs in the United States. The death certificate contains epidemiological information, the place of birth, the place of death, the cause of death, the manner of death, and other information. For a complete list of information contained in the death certificate, see the work by Koehler (2011). Information contained on the death certificate is coded by a nosologist and entered into the CDC's mortality database. The information is coded using the International Classification of Diseases (ICD). The ninth revision of the International Classification of Diseases and Clinical Modification (ICD-9-CM) was used to code cases until 1999. The tenth revision of the International Classification of Diseases and Clinical Modification (ICD-10-CM) are

used to code cases after 1999. ICD-9 and ICD-10 are the official system for assigning codes to diagnoses and procedures associated with hospital utilization in the United States. The ICD-9 coding system was used to code and classify mortality data from death certificates until 1999. The ICD-10 coding classification system was initiated in 2000. The CDC mortality database allows researchers to search for the number of deaths by specific codes and contains the totals numbers and rates of deaths by state, county, year, sex, and other variables.

## ICD CODING OF DISORDERS OF THE CENTRAL NERVOUS SYSTEM AND EPILEPSY, EPISODIC AND PAROXYSMAL DISORDERS, AND SUDEP

Under the ICD-9 coding system, deaths relating to epilepsy are classified under the heading Other Disorders of the Central Nervous System and are identified by codes 340–349. Appendix A presents a complete listing of codes 340–349. Under the ICD-10 coding system, deaths associated with Epilepsy and Episodic and Paroxysmal Disorders are identified by codes G40–G47. Appendix B presents a complete listing of codes G40–G47.

Sudden unexplained death (SUD) in individuals with epilepsy, referred to as SUDEP, has been recognized in the medical community for decades; however, there is no specific code for SUDEP in either ICD-9 or ICD-10. Therefore, when using the CDC National Mortality Database identifying deaths that could represent deaths from SUDEP, one must use deaths coded as either 340 under ICD-9 or G40 under ICD-10.

## METHODS OF MEASURING DISEASE/DEATH IN SUDEP

As discussed earlier, methods to measure a disease include incidence, prevalence, morbidity, and mortality (Woodward 2005).

### INCIDENCE

Incidence is a measure of disease that allows one to determine a person's probability of being diagnosed with a disease during a given period. Incidence rate is the number of new cases of a disease divided by the number of persons at risk for the disease. If, over the course of 1 year, 5 women are diagnosed with breast cancer out of a total female study population of 200 (who do not have breast cancer at the beginning of the study period), then we would say that the incidence of breast cancer in this population was 0.025 (2,500 per 100,000).

Determining the incidence of SUDEP requires the number of deaths from SUDEP and ascertaining the number at risk for SUDEP. There are many challenges in determining the accurate number of deaths from SUDEP. The use of forensic information, which is the most reliable, allows for independent review of a death but is time consuming and labor intensive. The data from the CDC National Mortality Database provide access to millions of deaths but cannot undergo an independent reevaluation.

Ascertaining an estimate of the number of individuals at risk for SUDEP is easier. Data from physicians, hospitals, insurance claims, and large university studies provide a reliable number of individuals with epilepsy. Current research such as the SUDEP Syndrome Cluster Risk Identification Method (discussed elsewhere in the book) is refining methods to identify those individuals with epilepsy at risk for SUDEP. Previous studies have reported that SUDEP is not uncommon, with the estimated incidence varying from 1/1100 to 1/5000 (Jay et al.1981; Leestma et al. 1984).

## PREVALENCE

Prevalence allows one to determine a person's likelihood of having a disease. Prevalence rate is the total number of cases of a disease existing in a population divided by the total population. If a measurement of cancer is taken in a population of 40,000 people and 1,200 were recently diagnosed with cancer and 3,500 are living with cancer, then the prevalence of cancer is 0.118 (1,200 + 3,500/40,000) or 11,750 per 100,000. The prevalence rate of SUDEP cannot be determined because it is a diagnosis after death. However, the prevalence of individuals with epilepsy can be calculated and serves as the number of individuals at risk for SUDEP.

## MORBIDITY

Morbidity is another term for illness. A person can have several comorbidities simultaneously. So, morbidities can range from Alzheimer's disease to cancer to traumatic brain injury. Morbidities are not deaths. Prevalence is a measure often used to determine the level of morbidity in a population.

## MORTALITY

Mortality is another term for death. Mortality rate is the number of deaths due to a disease divided by the total population. If there are 25 lung cancer deaths in 1 year in a population of 30,000, then the mortality rate for that population is 83 per 100,000.

The mortality rates for SUDEP can be calculated by two different methods. The first is by using forensic data from ME/C offices. Ideally, all sudden and unexpected deaths, such as SUDEP, should be examined by the local or state ME/C office. ME/C offices serve a specific population, therefore allowing for the calculation of local and state mortality rates. The second method involves the use of the CDC National Mortality Database. This database allows one to search different causes of death using the ICD codes, by variables such as location, age, sex, and other parameters. In addition, the database provides the total number of deaths and mortality rates.

## FORENSIC INVESTIGATION OF SUDEP: ALLEGHENY COUNTY

ME/C offices are the only sources of detailed information on deaths from SUDEP. As noted earlier, ME/C offices collect information during Death Scene Investigation, Autopsy, and Toxicology Analysis, including epidemiological data, anatomical abnormalities, organ descriptions/weights, toxicological analysis of body fluids, information relating to the circumstances surrounding the death, past medical history, and medical treatment including a list of prescribed medication.

Two retrospective forensic studies were conducted in Allegheny County. The first was conducted by the Allegheny County Coroners' Office, which has forensic jurisdiction within Allegheny County, located in Western Pennsylvania and encompassing a population of approximately 1.2 million. The office investigates over 6000 cases and conducts over 1200 autopsies annually. The first study investigated deaths from SUDEP occurring from 1978 to 1979 (Terrance et al. 1981). The details of the investigation methodology are presented elsewhere in the literature (Koehler 2011, ch. 9). In brief, all deaths that were included in the forensic autopsy were those that were unexplained and unexpected, and where there was a history of epilepsy. The results are summarized in Table 11.1. During this 2-year period, approximately 3000 deaths were investigated and 8 were classified as SUDEP (0.267%).

The second forensic investigation was conducted in Allegheny County in 2001 (Lathers et al. 2011) as a retrospective review of all deaths examined by the medical examiners from January 1, 2001 to December 31, 2001. This study began by first identifying all death certificates with the word "seizure" listed. These cases then underwent a reevaluation to identify deaths that met the definition of a SUDEP. Inclusion criteria further included a history of seizure disorders indicated in the past medical history, as indicated by the word seizure or phrase "seizure disorder" appearing in Part I (Immediate Cause of Death) or Part II (Conditions Contributing to the Death) of the death certificate. In addition, cases were identified by conducting a computer analysis and a hand search of the case files by the forensic epidemiologist. The information available for review included the Death Investigation Report, Toxicology Report, death certificates, and available medical records. The following epidemiological information was collected: age, sex, race, time/date last seen alive, and the time/date of death. The seizure-related information collected included past medical history, a list of prescribed medications including all AEDs, and all who witnessed the event. Pathological information was obtained from the forensic autopsy report. Toxicological analysis was conducted on the blood, bile, urine, and eye fluid recovered during the autopsy. The blood used for the toxicological analysis was collected from the heart during the autopsy. The number and level of drugs detected in the body fluids were obtained from the Toxicological Report. The toxicological analysis included the number of detected drugs; blood concentrations; and determination if the levels were therapeutic,

**TABLE 11.1**

**Total Number and Mortality Rates for SUDEP, Seizures, and Epilepsy-Type Deaths in Allegheny County, 1978–1979 and 2001**

| Year<br>Population<br>Source | Total Number of Deaths in the<br>Study Population<br>Total Number of Deaths by Type<br>(SUDEP, Seizure, or Epilepsy Type) | Incidence of SUDEP, Seizure,<br>and Epilepsy-Type Deaths in<br>Study Population (%) | Total Population<br>Total Number of Deaths |
|---|---|---|---|
| 1978–1979<br>Allegheny County<br>Coroners' Office (Forensic)[a] | 3000[b]<br>8-SUDEP[b] | 0.267% SUDEP | 2,911,382[c]<br>31,218[c] |
| 2001<br>Allegheny County<br>Medical Examiners' Office (Forensic)[d] | 1200<br>12-Seizures<br>11-SUDEP[e] | 1.0% Seizures<br>0.917% SUDEP[e] | 1,272,576<br>15,235 |

[a]  Terrance et al. (1981).
[b]  Estimation based on 1500 cases per year.
[c]  Estimations.
[d]  Lathers et al. (2011) (modified from Koehler et al. [2011]).
[e]  These are the only SUDEP data cited. The rest of the numbers in Tables 6, 6B, and 7 of the Allegheny study refer to seizure deaths but have not been evaluated to identify victims of SUDEP.

subtherapeutic, above the therapeutic range, or absent. The data were entered and analyzed using the Statistical Package for the Social Services® software (SPSS 11.0, Chicago, Illinois).

Among the 1200 forensic investigations conducted by the medical examiner's office in 2001, 12 (1%) deaths had a death certificate listing seizure as either the immediate cause of death or the contributory cause of death. The results of the 2001 study are summarized in Table 11.1. All 12 cases had an established diagnosis of seizures. For a detailed examination of the 12 deaths, see Chapter 6, "Forensic Antiepileptic Drug Levels in Autopsy Cases of Epilepsy" (Lathers et al. 2011). None of the cases listed "epilepsy" on the death certificates or provided the victim's seizure types. All seizure types would be grouped together in the category of seizure on the death certificates, and this reinforces one of the most important issues in determining SUDEP as a cause of death, namely, the incomplete nature of the history of type and frequency of seizures in the victims, including those subjected to autopsy. Although the presence of intractable epilepsy and the history of generalized tonic-clonic seizures have been described as one of the most important factors for SUDEP, this information was not available in the death certificates.

Based on a reevaluation of the available forensic data, 11 of these deaths met the definition of SUDEP. In summary, 1% of the deaths investigated by the medical examiner's office were signed out as seizure. Of these deaths, 11 met the current definition of SUDEP, representing less than 1% (0.917%) of the deaths investigated by the medical examiners' office. Based on these results and the county's population, less than 0.072% of all deaths would be classified as SUDEP in Allegheny County.

Both studies highlight two important features of deaths investigated by ME/C offices. First, deaths caused by

epilepsy, seizures, and other related conditions are rarely encountered in the forensic community. Second, deaths that meet the criteria of a SUDEP are signed out on the death certificates as "Seizures" or "Seizure Disorders."

## FORENSIC INVESTIGATION OF SUDEP: ROLES OF THE MEDICAL EXAMINERS/ CORONERS AND MEDICAL COMMUNITY

ME/C offices have a legal duty to investigate all sudden and unexpected deaths and determine the cause and manner of death in these cases. Part of the death scene investigation involves obtaining medical records and interviewing the victim's family and physician. However, this protocol is not always followed by the ME/C office. The main reason given is to spare the victim's family the emotional stress of an autopsy. This practice, while more common in the past, does a disservice to the victim's family, limits our understanding of SUDEP, and limits the collection of key information about the condition.

Four cases from Chapter 8 illustrate failures in the forensic investigation system of SUDEP and highlights the importance of the role played by all those involved in the care, treatment, and investigation of victims with SUDEP to ensure that a proper and thorough forensic investigation is conducted and that all available information is provided and considered. Physicians must advocate for a forensic autopsy and death investigation and explain to the family the importance of such an investigation. Medical examiners or coroners must begin to investigate all cases of sudden and unexpected deaths and understand and search for the features of SUDEP, especially the roles of subtherapeutic levels of AEDs, changes in AED medications, and the roles of stress and life events as they relate to sudden death.

# NATIONAL DATABASES INVESTIGATION OF SUDEP: CDC MORTALITY DATABASE

As mentioned previously, all information contained in the death certificates issued in the United States is coded and entered into the CDC National Mortality Database. Nosologists first code the information and then enter the data into the database. The cause of death is coded using the ICD-9 or ICD-10 codes, depending on the year.

## CENTERS FOR DISEASE CONTROL AND PREVENTION MORTALITY DATABASE

Using the CDC National Mortality Database, a search was conducted using ICD-9 and ICD-10 codes for the number of deaths from epilepsy, status epilepticus, and episodic and paroxysmal disorders within Allegheny County, the state of Pennsylvania, and the United States between 1979 and 2010 (Centers for Disease Control and Prevention, National Center for Health Statistics; CDC WONDER On-line Database, compiled from Compressed Mortality File 1979–1998 and Centers for Disease Control and Prevention, National Center

for Health Statistics; CDC WONDER On-line Database, compiled from Compressed Mortality File 1999–2010).

## ALLEGHENY COUNTY

During the years 1979–1998, ICD-9 code 345 was used for deaths from epilepsy. Table 11.2 shows the total number of deaths and deaths rates for Allegheny County from 1979 to 1998. Allegheny County had a population of 1.2 million and 15,000 deaths per year. An average of 15 (range 2–22) deaths per year from epilepsy occurred. No deaths from epilepsy were recorded for the years 1991–1995. The rate (per 1,000,000) ranged from a low of 1.4 in 1981 to a high of 16.2 in 1987. In 1999, the ICD-9 codes were replaced by the ICD-10 codes, allowing for tabulation of death from epilepsy (G-40), status epilepticus (including grand mal status epileptics, petit mal status epilepticus, complex partial, other, status epilepticus) (G41), and episodic and paroxysmal disorders (G40–G47). Between the years 1999 and 2010, there were no recorded deaths from epilepsy and there were a total of 65 deaths from status epilepticus. A breakdown by year was not available. A breakdown by year for deaths coded episodic and paroxysmal disorders

---

**TABLE 11.2**

**Total Number of Deaths and Rates (per 1,000,000) Using ICD-9 Code 345.0 and ICD-10 Codes G40–G47 for Allegheny County, and the State of Pennsylvania, 1979–1998, 1999-2007, and 2008–2010**

| Location Years | Total Number of Deaths and Rates Code 345.0 | Total Number of Deaths and Rates Code G40 | Total Number of Deaths and Rates Code G41 | Total Number of Deaths and Rates Codes G40–G47 |
|---|---|---|---|---|
| **Allegheny County** | | | | |
| 1979 | 15 (10.3) | | | |
| 1980 | 17 (11.7) | | | |
| 1981 | 2 (1.4) | | | |
| 1982 | 14 (9.8) | | | |
| 1983 | 7 (4.9) | | | |
| 1984 | 17 (12.1) | | | |
| 1985 | 19 (13.8) | | | |
| 1986 | 22 (16.1) | | | |
| 1987 | 22 (16.2) | | | |
| 1988 | 20 (14.8) | | | |
| 1989 | 16 (11.9) | | | |
| 1990 | 16 (12.0) | | | |
| 1991 | None | | | |
| 1992 | None | | | |
| 1993 | None | | | |
| 1994 | None | | | |
| 1995 | None | | | |
| 1996 | 12 (9.1) | | | |
| 1997 | None | | | |
| 1998 | None | | | |
| **Allegheny County** | | | 1999–2000 = 47 | Number Rate () |
| 1999 | | | | 11 (8.5) |
| 2000 | | | | 12 (9.4) |

*(Continued)*

**TABLE 11.2**    (*Continued*)

**Total Number of Deaths and Rates (per 1,000,000) Using ICD-9 Code 345.0 and ICD-10 Codes G40–G47 for Allegheny County, and the State of Pennsylvania, 1979–1998, 1999-2007, and 2008–2010**

| Location Years | Total Number of Deaths and Rates Code 345.0 | Total Number of Deaths and Rates Code G40 | Total Number of Deaths and Rates Code G41 | Total Number of Deaths and Rates Codes G40–G47 |
|---|---|---|---|---|
| 2001 | | | | 13 (10.0) |
| 2002 | | | | 12 (9.4) |
| 2003 | | | | 13 (10.0) |
| 2004 | | | | 14 (11.0) |
| 2005 | | | | 18 (15.00) |
| 2006 | | | | 10 (8.2) |
| 2007 | | | | 14 (17.0) |
| Allegheny County | | | 2008–2010 = 18 | Number Rate () |
| 2008 | | | | 20 (16.0) |
| 2009 | | | | 13 (11.0) |
| 2010 | | | | 10 (8.2) |
| Pennsylvania | | | | |
| 1979 | 89 (7.5) | | | |
| 1980 | 80 (6.7) | | | |
| 1981 | 67 (5.6) | | | |
| 1982 | 81 (6.8) | | | |
| 1983 | 82 (6.9) | | | |
| 1984 | 92 (7.8) | | | |
| 1985 | 101 (8.6) | | | |
| 1986 | 95 (8.1) | | | |
| 1987 | 98 (8.3) | | | |
| 1988 | 100 (8.4) | | | |
| 1989 | 92 (7.7) | | | |
| 1990 | 84 (7.1) | | | |
| 1991 | 81 (6.8) | | | |
| 1992 | 69 (5.7) | | | |
| 1993 | 55 (4.5) | | | |
| 1994 | 66 (5.4) | | | |
| 1995 | 80 (6.6) | | | |
| 1996 | 54 (4.4) | | | |
| 1997 | 46 (3.8) | | | |
| 1998 | 49 (4.0) | | | |
| Pennsylvania | | | | |
| 1999 | | 28 (2.3) | 27 (2.2) | 94 (7.7) |
| 2000 | | 23 (2.0) | 34 (2.8) | 89 (7.2) |
| 2001 | | 19 (1.5) | 40 (3.2) | 91 (7.4) |
| 2002 | | 22 (1.8) | 31 (2.5) | 93 (7.5) |
| 2003 | | 18 (1.4) | 34 (2.7) | 101 (8.2) |
| 2004 | | 26 (2.1) | 12 (0.9) | 80 (6.5) |
| 2005 | | 24 (1.9) | 39 (3.1) | 125 (10) |
| 2006 | | 30 (2.4) | 24 (1.9) | 103 (8.2) |
| 2007 | | 20 (1.6) | 42 (3.3) | 99 (7.9) |
| 2008 | | 19 (1.5) | 32 (2.5) | 102 (8.1) |
| 2009 | | 25 (2.0) | 39 (3.1) | 108 (8.5) |
| 2010 | | 25 (2.0) | 33 (2.6) | 107 (8.4) |

*Notes:* ICD-9 coding for epilepsy: 345.0.

   ICD-10 code G40.0: epilepsy.

   ICD-10 code G41.0: status epilepticus: grand mal status epileptics, petit mal status epileptics, complex partial, other, status epilepticus.

   Code G40–G47: episodic and paroxysmal disorders.

(G40–G47) was available and showed that an average of 12 (range 10–20) deaths occurred in Allegheny County annually.

## PENNSYLVANIA

During the years 1979–1998, the ICD-9 code 345 was used for deaths from epilepsy. An average of 78 (range 46–101) deaths from epilepsy occurred in the state of Pennsylvania, which has an average population of 12 million and 123,000 deaths per year. In 1999, the ICD-10 replaced the ICD-9 allowing for the tabulation of death from epilepsy (G-40), status epilepticus (including grand mal status epileptics, petit mal status

epileptics, complex partial, other , status epilepticus) (G41), and episodic and paroxysmal disorders (G40–G47). Between the years 1999 and 2010, there were an average of 23 (range 18–30) deaths from epilepsy, 32 (range 12–42) from status epilepticus, and 99 (range 80–108) from episodic and paroxysmal disorders (G40–G47).

## UNITED STATES

The total number of deaths and death rates (per 1,000,000) using ICD-10 codes G40–G47 for the United States over the period 2000–2010 are shown in Table 11.3. The United

### TABLE 11.3
### Total Number of Deaths and Rates (per 1,000,000) using ICD-10 Code G40-G47 for the United States of America, 2000–2010

| Year | Total Number of Deaths and Rates (per 1,000,000) Coded 345.0 | Total Number of Deaths and Rates (per 1,000,000) Coded G40 | Total Number of Deaths and Rates (per 1,000,000) Coded G41 | Total Number of Deaths and Rates (per 1,000,000) Coded G40–G47 |
|---|---|---|---|---|
| 1979 | 1653 (7.4) | | | |
| 1980 | 1693 (7.5) | | | |
| 1981 | 1731 (7.5) | | | |
| 1982 | 1553 (6.7) | | | |
| 1983 | 1653 (7.1) | | | |
| 1984 | 1619 (6.9) | | | |
| 1985 | 1643 (6.9) | | | |
| 1986 | 1627 (6.8) | | | |
| 1987 | 1595 (6.5) | | | |
| 1988 | 1619 (6.6) | | | |
| 1989 | 1595 (6.5) | | | |
| 1990 | 1627 (6.5) | | | |
| 1991 | 1476 (5.2) | | | |
| 1992 | 1391 (5.4) | | | |
| 1993 | 1337 (5.1) | | | |
| 1994 | 1381 (5.2) | | | |
| 1995 | 1373 (5.2) | | | |
| 1996 | 1331 (4.9) | | | |
| 1997 | 1378 (5.1) | | | |
| 1998 | 1348 (4.9) | | | |
| 1999 | | 841 (3.0) | 497 (1.8) | 2005 (7.2) |
| 2000 | | 812 (2.9) | 511 (1.8) | 2019 (7.2) |
| 2001 | | 799 (2.8) | 493 (1.7) | 2016 (7.1) |
| 2002 | | 887 (3.1) | 492 (1.7) | 2103 (7.3) |
| 2003 | | 925 (3.2) | 491 (1.7) | 2170 (7.5) |
| 2004 | | 847 (2.9) | 500 (1.7) | 2045 (7.0) |
| 2005 | | 949 (3.2) | 521 (1.8) | 2350 (8.0) |
| 2006 | | 919 (3.1) | 510 (1.7) | 2305 (7.7) |
| 2007 | | 919 (3.0) | 522 (1.7) | 2463 (8.2) |
| 2008 | | 847 (2.9) | 524 (1.7) | 2414 (7.9) |
| 2009 | | 945 (3.1) | 606 (2.0) | 2626 (8.6) |
| 2010 | | 994 (3.2) | 612 (2.0) | 2739 (8.9) |

*Notes:* ICD-9 epilepsy = 345.0.
   ICD-10 epilepsy = G40.
   ICD-10 status epilepticus: grand mal status epileptics, petit mal status epileptics, complex partial, other, status epilepticus = G41.
   ICD-10 episodic and paroxysmal disorders = G40–G47.

States has an average population of 238 million and 2 million deaths per year. From 1979–1998, the ICD-9 code 345 was used for epilepsy deaths. An average of 1531 (range 1331–1731) deaths from epilepsy occurred in the United States per year. In 1999, the ICD-10 codes were replaced by ICD-9, allowing for tabulation of deaths from epilepsy (G-40), status epilepticus (including grand mal status epileptics, petit mal status epileptics, complex partial, other, status epilepticus) (G41), and episodic and paroxysmal disorders (G40–G47). Between the years 1999 and 2010, there was an annual average of 890 (range 799–994) deaths from epilepsy, 523 (range 491–612) from status epilepticus, and 2271 (range 2005–2739) from episodic and paroxysmal disorders (G40–G47).

## COMPARING FORENSIC DATA TO THE CDC NATIONAL DATABASE

There are several potential reasons for differences between data from the Allegheny County ME/C offices discussed earlier and the data from the CDC National Mortality Database.

First, it is estimated that only about 20% of all deaths in the United States undergo a forensic investigation. Deaths from homicide, suicide, and a vast majority of deaths from accidents typically receive a forensic investigation. However, the majority of natural deaths do not undergo any form of death investigation. In a large number of these deaths, the cause of death is well documented and expected. Deaths from SUDEP are by definition sudden and unexpected and should receive a forensic investigation. However, family physicians simply issue the death certificate as seizure disorder or some other central nervous system disorders whether to shield the family from an autopsy or because they are unaware of SUDEP. The end result is that the body is transferred to the funeral home, bypassing the ME/C office completely. It is difficult to ascertain the exact number of cases of SUDEP that are mislabeled as simple seizures. A comparison of ME/C records to the CDC data highlights the magnitude of missed cases. Data from the Allegheny County ME/C office from 1978–1979 and 2001 show that deaths from seizures, SUDEP, and related disorders are rarely encountered. Based on CDC data, on average 15 deaths are coded with episodic and paroxysmal disorders. The majority of these deaths never underwent a forensic investigation, an autopsy, or a toxicological analysis. Without a detailed review of each case, ascertaining the number that would meet the definition of SUDEP is difficult.

Second, when the definitions of a disease change, or there is a change in the coding of a specific disease as in the transition from ICD-9 to ICD-10, the number and rate of specific diseases will always be impacted. The magnitude depends on the level of refinement and new definition used to code the disease. At the county level under ICD-9, there were on average 15 deaths per year attributed to epilepsy. However, after

the change to ICD-10, no deaths were signed out as epilepsy between 1999 and 2010 in Allegheny County. Between 1999 and 2010, on average five deaths per year were caused by status epilepticus. During that same period, 160 deaths were coded under the general grouping of deaths called episodic and paroxysmal disorders. At the state level under ICD-9 an annual average of 78 deaths was reported from 1979–1998, whereas after ICD-10 deaths from epilepsy averaged only 23 deaths per year. At the national level, an annual average of 1531 deaths were reported from epilepsy using ICD-9 from 1979–1998, whereas after ICD-10 deaths from epilepsy averaged only 890 deaths per year (1999–2010). Overall, therefore, there was a dramatic impact on the number of deaths and the corresponding death rates attributed to epilepsy after the switch from ICD-9 to ICD-10. This dramatic drop of reported deaths from epilepsy cannot be explained by improved treatment or a reduction in the prevalence of epilepsy.

Third, one would hope that over time as clinicians and the public receive expanded information about SUDEP, the number of epilepsy victims dying from SUDEP would be more consistently reported to the ME/C for investigation. However, the data to date do not support this prediction. At the state level, between 1999 and 2010 the rate of epilepsy remained relatively stable at around 1.9/1,000,000. At the national level also, the rate remained stable at around 3.0/1,000,000. One would have expected that with increased awareness of SUDEP the number of cases signed out as epilepsy would increase.

## STRENGTHS AND WEAKNESSES OF FORENSIC DATA VERSUS CDC NATIONAL DATABASE RELATING TO SUDEP

The great strength of forensic data is the level and detail of information collected and available at the ME/C office. The ME/C office is the only agency that is authorized to investigate sudden and unexpected deaths and has the legal authority to subpoena medical records. Researchers examining SUDEP deaths should always start by obtaining access to ME/C office data. Previous deaths that have been ruled as seizure, seizure disorder, or epilepsy-type deaths should be reexamined to ascertain if they meet the current definition of SUDEP. Both the detailed Death Scene Investigation Report and findings from toxicological analysis of body fluids can provide important information relating to AED compliance, effects of multiple AEDs, and possible interaction of AEDs and non-AED medications.

The main weakness of forensic data is that not every death undergoes a forensic investigation. Therefore, possible cases of SUDEP may never receive a forensic investigation. These cases are signed out by treating physicians as natural deaths under the diagnoses of seizures, seizure disorder, or other central nervous system disorders. A lesser weakness is the time required to search ME/C records for cases of SUDEP.

The clear strength of the CDC National Mortality Database is easy access to millions of death certificates at one time. The total number of deaths and death rates can be obtained for hundreds of diseases broken down by state, county, age, sex, and other variables via the Internet. The main weakness is the inability to reexamine the facts of a death to ascertain if the death meets the criteria for SUDEP. Another major weakness is the lack of detailed information describing the events leading to the death, a list of prescribed medications and dosages, the results of toxicological analysis (if conducted), and detailed past medical history.

## CONCLUSION

All sudden and unexpected deaths among individuals with a past medical history of epilepsy must receive a complete forensic death investigation including an autopsy and a toxicological analysis. Family physicians must explain to the next of kin why an autopsy is required and its importance in our understanding of SUDEP. In addition, the CDC must create a unique code for SUDEP, therefore allowing better ascertainment of the magnitude of SUDEP at local, state, and national levels.

## APPENDIX A: ICD-9 CODES FOR OTHER DISORDERS OF THE CENTRAL NERVOUS SYSTEM (340–349)

- (340) Multiple sclerosis
- (341) Other demyelinating diseases of the central nervous system
  - (341.0) Neuromyelitis optica
  - (341.1) Schilder's disease
  - (341.2) Acute myelitis (transverse myelitis)
- (342) Hemiplegia
  - (342.0) Hemiplegia, flaccid
  - (342.1) Hemiplegia, spastic
- (343) Infantile cerebral palsy
  - (343.0) Cerebral palsy, paraplegic, congenital
  - (343.1) Cerebral palsy, hemiplegic, congenital
  - (343.2) Cerebral palsy, quadriplegic
- (344) Other paralytic syndromes
  - (344.0) Quadraplegia and quadraparesis
  - (344.1) Paraplegia
  - (344.2) Diplegia of upper limbs
  - (344.3) Monoplegia of lower limb
  - (344.4) Monoplegia of upper limb
  - (344.5) Unspecified monoplegia
  - (344.6) Cauda equina syndrome
  - (344.8) Other specified paralytic syndromes
    - (344.81) Locked-in state
  - (344.9) Paralysis unspecified
- (345) Epilepsy
  - (345.0) Epilepsy, absence, w/o intractable epilepsy
  - (345.1) Epilepsy, tonic-clonic, w/o status
  - (345.3) Epilepsy, status

- (345.4) Epilepsy, temporal lobe, w/o status
- (345.9) Epilepsy, unspecified, w/o status
- (346) Migraine
  - (346.0) Migraine, classical, not intractable
  - (346.1) Migraine, common, not intractable
  - (346.2) Headaches, cluster, not intractable
  - (346.9) Migraine, unspecified, not intractable
- (347) Cataplexy and narcolepsy
  - (347.0) Narcolepsy, w/o cataplexy
- (348) Other conditions of brain
  - (348.0) Cerebral cysts
  - (348.1) Anoxic brain damage
  - (348.2) Pseudotumor cerebri
  - (348.3) Encephalopathy, unspecified
    - (348.31) Encephalopathy, metabolic
  - (348.4) Compression of brain
  - (348.5) Cerebral edema
- (349) Other and unspecified disorders of the nervous system
  - (349.0) Headache, postspinal puncture
    - Postdural puncture headache
  - (349.8) Other specified disorders of nervous system
    - (349.81) Cerebrospinal fluid rhinorrhea
    - (349.82) Toxic encephalopathy

## APPENDIX B: ICD-10-CM DIAGNOSIS CODES DISEASES OF THE NERVOUS SYSTEM

### EPILEPSY AND RECURRENT SEIZURES G40–G40.919

#### Clinical Information

- A brain disorder characterized by episodes of abnormally increased neuronal discharge resulting in transient episodes of sensory or motor neurological dysfunction, or psychic dysfunction. These episodes may or may not be associated with loss of consciousness or convulsions.
- A disorder characterized by recurrent episodes of paroxysmal brain dysfunction due to a sudden, disorderly, and excessive neuronal discharge. Epilepsy classification systems are generally based on (1) clinical features of the seizure episodes (e.g., motor seizure), (2) etiology (e.g., posttraumatic), (3) anatomic site of seizure origin (e.g., frontal lobe seizure), (4) tendency to spread to other structures in the brain, and (5) temporal patterns (e.g., nocturnal epilepsy) (from Adams et al. 1998, p.313).
- A disorder characterized by recurrent seizures.
- A group of disorders marked by problems in the normal functioning of the brain. These problems can produce seizures, unusual body movements, loss of consciousness, or changes in consciousness, as well as mental problems or problems with the senses.
- Brain disorder characterized by recurring excessive neuronal discharge, exhibited by transient episodes

of motor, sensory, or psychic dysfunction, with or without unconsciousness or convulsive movements.

- Epilepsy is a brain disorder that causes people to have recurring seizures. The seizures happen when clusters of nerve cells, or neurons, in the brain send out the wrong signals. People may have strange sensations and emotions or behave strangely. They may have violent muscle spasms or lose consciousness. Epilepsy has many possible causes, including illness, brain injury, and abnormal brain development. In many cases, the cause is unknown; doctors use brain scans and other tests to diagnose epilepsy. It is important to start treatment right away. There is no cure for epilepsy, but medicines can control seizures for most people. When medicines are not working well, surgery or implanted devices such as vagus nerve stimulators may help. Special diets can help some children with epilepsy.

## ICD-10 Codes: (G40–G47) Episodic and Paroxysmal Disorders

### Epilepsy

- (G40) Epilepsy
  - (G40.0) Localization-related (focal) (partial) idiopathic epilepsy and epileptic syndromes with seizures of localized onset
    - Benign childhood epilepsy with centrotemporal electroencephalogram (EEG) spikes
    - Childhood epilepsy with occipital EEG paroxysms
      - G40.001 With status epilepticus
      - G40.009 Without status epilepticus
  - (G40.1) Localization-related (focal) (partial) symptomatic epilepsy and epileptic syndromes with simple partial seizures
    - Attacks without alteration of consciousness
    - Seizures
      - G40.101 With status epilepticus
      - G40.109 Without status epilepticus
  - (G40.2) Localization-related (focal) (partial) symptomatic epilepsy and epileptic syndromes with complex partial seizures
    - Attacks with alteration of consciousness, often with automatisms
    - Complex partial seizures developing into secondarily generalized seizures
      - G40.201 With status epilepticus
      - G40.209 Without status epilepticus
  - (G40.3) Generalized idiopathic epilepsy and epileptic syndromes
    - Benign:
      - Myoclonic epilepsy in infancy
      - Neonatal convulsions (familial)
    - Childhood absence epilepsy (pyknolepsy)
    - Epilepsy with grand mal seizures on awakening

- Juvenile:
  - Absence epilepsy
  - Myoclonic epilepsy (impulsive petit mal)
- Nonspecific epileptic seizures:
- Atonic
- Clonic
- Myoclonic
- Tonic
- Tonic clonic
  - G40.301 With status epilepticus
  - G40.309 Without status epilepticus
  - G40.31 Generalized idiopathic epilepsy and epileptic syndromes, intractable
  - G40.311 With status epilepticus
  - G40.319 Without status epilepticus
  - (G40. A) Absence epileptic syndrome
  - G40. A0 Absence epileptic syndrome, not intractable
  - G40. A01 With status epilepticus
  - G40. A09 Without status epilepticus
  - G40. A1 Absence epileptic syndrome, intractable
  - G40. A11 With status epilepticus
  - G40. A19 Without status epilepticus
  - G40. B Juvenile myoclonic epilepsy (impulsive petit mal)
  - (G40. B0) Juvenile myoclonic epilepsy, not intractable
  - G40. B01 With status epilepticus
  - G40. B09 Without status epilepticus
  - G40. B1 Juvenile myoclonic epilepsy, intractable
  - G40. B11 With status epilepticus
  - G40. B19 Without status epilepticus
- (G40.4) Other generalized epilepsy and epileptic syndromes
  - Epilepsy with
    - Myoclonic absences
    - Myoclonic-astatic seizures
  - Infantile spasms
  - Lennox–Gastaut syndrome
  - Salaam attacks
  - Symptomatic early myoclonic encephalopathy
  - West's syndrome
    - G40.401 With status epilepticus
    - G40.409 Without status epilepticus
    - G40.41 Other generalized epilepsy and epileptic syndromes, intractable
    - G40.411 With status epilepticus
    - G40.419 Without status epilepticus
- (G40.5) Special epileptic syndromes
  - Epilepsia partialis continua (Kozhevnikov)
  - Epileptic seizures related to
    - Alcohol
    - Drugs
    - Hormonal changes

- – Sleep deprivation
- – Stress
  - – G40.501 With status epilepticus
  - – G40.509 Without status epilepticus
- (G40.6) Grand mal seizures, unspecified (with or without petit mal)
- (G40.7) Petit mal, unspecified, without grand mal seizures
- (G40.8) Other epilepsy
  - – Epilepsies and epileptic syndromes undetermined as to whether they are focal or generalized
    - – G40.801 Not intractable, with status epilepticus
    - – G40.802 Not intractable, without status epilepticus
    - – G40.803 Intractable, with status epilepticus
    - – G40.804 Intractable, without status epilepticus
    - – G40.81 Lennox–Gastaut syndrome
    - – G40.811 Not intractable, with status epilepticus
    - – G40.812 Not intractable, without status epilepticus
    - – G40.813 Intractable, with status epilepticus
    - – G40.814 Intractable, without status epilepticus
    - – G40.82 Epileptic spasms
    - – G40.821 Not intractable, with status epilepticus
    - – G40.822 Not intractable, without status epilepticus
    - – G40.823 Intractable, with status epilepticus
    - – G40.824 Intractable, without status epilepticus
    - – G40.89 Other seizures
- (G40.9) Epilepsy, unspecified
  - – Epileptic:
  - – Convulsions NOS (not otherwise specified)
  - – Fits NOS
  - – Seizures NOS
    - – G40.90 Epilepsy, unspecified, not intractable
    - – G40.901 With status epilepticus
    - – G40.909 Without status epilepticus
    - – G40.91 Epilepsy, unspecified, intractable
    - – G40.911 With status epilepticus
    - – G40.919 Without status epilepticus
- (G41) Status epilepticus
  - (G41.0) Grand mal status epilepticus
  - (G41.1) Petit mal status epilepticus
  - (G41.2) Complex partial status epilepticus
  - (G41.8) Other status epilepticus
  - (G41.9) Status epilepticus, unspecified

## Migraine G43

### Clinical Information

- A class of disabling primary headache disorders, characterized by recurrent unilateral pulsatile headaches. The two major subtypes are common migraine (without aura) and classical migraine (with aura or neurological symptoms) (Headache Society 2004).
- A common, severe type of vascular headache often associated with increased sympathetic activity, resulting in nausea, vomiting, and light sensitivity.
- If you suffer from migraine headaches, you are not alone. About 12% of the U.S. population gets them. Migraines are recurring attacks of moderate to severe pain. The pain is throbbing or pulsing and is often on one side of the head. During migraines, people are very sensitive to light and sound. They may also become nauseated and vomit. Migraine is three times more common in women than in men. Some people can tell when they are about to have a migraine because they see flashing lights or zigzag lines or they temporarily lose their vision. Many things can trigger a migraine. These include
- Anxiety
- Stress
- Lack of food or sleep
- Exposure to light
- Hormonal changes (in women)

Doctors used to believe that migraines were linked to the opening and narrowing of blood vessels in the head. Now they believe the cause is related to genes that control the activity of some brain cells. Medicines can help prevent migraine attacks or help relieve symptoms of attacks when they happen. For many people, treatments to relieve stress can also help.

- Neural condition characterized by a severe recurrent vascular headache; usually on one side of the head; often accompanied by nausea, vomiting, and photophobia; and sometimes preceded by sensory disturbances. Triggers include allergic reactions, excess carbohydrates or iodine in the diet, alcohol, bright lights, or loud noises.
- (G43) Migraine
  - (G43.0) Migraine without aura (common migraine)
    - – G43.001 With status migrainosus
    - – G43.009 Without status migrainosus
    - – G43.011 With status migrainosus
    - – G43.019 Without status migrainosus
  - (G43.1) Migraine with aura (classical migraine)
    - – G43.10 Migraine with aura, not intractable
      - – G43.101 With status migrainosus
      - – G43.109 Without status migrainosus
    - – G43.11 Migraine with aura, intractable
      - – G43.111 With status migrainosus
      - – G43.119 Without status migrainosus

- (G43.2) Status migrainosus
- (G43.3) Complicated migraine
  - (G43.4) Hemiplegic migraine
    - G43.40 Hemiplegic migraine, not intractable
    - G43.401 With status migrainosus
    - G43.409 Without status migrainosus
    - G43.41 Hemiplegic migraine, intractable
    - G43.411 With status migrainosus
    - G43.419 Without status migrainosus
  - (G43.5) Persistent migraine aura without cerebral infarction
    - G43.50 Persistent migraine aura without cerebral infarction, not intractable
    - G43.501 With status migrainosus
    - G43.509 Without status migrainosus
    - G43.51 Persistent migraine aura without cerebral infarction, intractable
    - G43.511 With status migrainosus
    - G43.519 Without status migrainosus
    - (G43.6) Persistent migraine aura with cerebral infarction
    - G43.60 Persistent migraine aura with cerebral infarction, not intractable
    - G43.601 With status migrainosus
    - G43.609 Without status migrainosus
    - G43.61 Persistent migraine aura with cerebral infarction, intractable
    - G43.611 With status migrainosus
    - G43.619 Without status migrainosus
    - G43.7 Chronic migraine without aura
  - (G43.70) Chronic migraine without aura, not intractable
    - G43.701 With status migrainosus
    - G43.709 Without status migrainosus
  - (G43.71) Chronic migraine without aura, intractable
    - G43.711 With status migrainosus
    - G43.719 Without status migrainosus
  - G43. A Cyclical vomiting
    - G43. A0 Not intractable
    - G43. A1 Intractable
  - G43. B Ophthalmoplegic migraine
    - G43. B0 Not intractable
    - G43. B1 Intractable
  - G43. C Periodic headache syndromes in child or adult
    - G43. C0 Not intractable
    - G43. C1 Intractable
  - G43. D Abdominal migraine
    - G43. D0 Not intractable
    - G43. D1 Intractable
- (G43.8) Other migraine
  - Ophthalmoplegic migraine
  - Retinal migraine
    - G43.801 With status migrainosus
    - G43.809 Without status migrainosus

- G43.81 Other migraine, intractable
  - G43.811 With status migrainosus
  - G43.819 Without status migrainosus
- G43.82 Menstrual migraine, not intractable
  - G43.821 With status migrainosus
  - G43.829 Without status migrainosus
- G43.83 Menstrual migraine, intractable
  - G43.831 With status migrainosus
  - G43.839 Without status migrainosus
- (G43.9) Migraine, unspecified
  - G43.901 With status migrainosus
  - G43.909 Without status migrainosus
  - G43.91 Migraine, unspecified, intractable
    - G43.911 With status migrainosus
    - G43.919 Without status migrainosus
- (G44) Other headache syndromes
  - (G44.0) Cluster headache syndrome
    - Chronic paroxysmal hemicrania
    - Cluster headache:
    - chronic
    - episodic
    - G44.00 Cluster headache syndrome, unspecified
      - G44.001 Intractable
      - G44.009 Not intractable
    - G44.01 Episodic cluster headache
      - G44.011 Intractable
      - G44.019 Not intractable
    - G44.02 Chronic cluster headache
      - G44.021 Intractable
      - G44.029 Not intractable
    - G44.03 Episodic paroxysmal hemicrania
      - G44.031 Intractable
      - G44.039 Not intractable
    - G44.04 Chronic paroxysmal hemicrania
      - G44.041 Intractable
      - G44.049 Not intractable
    - G44.05 Short-lasting unilateral neuralgiform headache with conjunctival injection and tearing
      - G44.051 Intractable
      - G44.059 Not intractable
    - G44.09 Other trigeminal autonomic cephalgias
      - G44.091 Intractable
      - G44.099 Not intractable
  - (G44.1) Vascular headache, not elsewhere classified
  - (G44.2) Tension-type headache
    - Chronic tension-type headache
    - Episodic tension headache
    - Tension headache NOS
    - G44.20 Tension-type headache, unspecified
    - G44.201 Intractable
    - G44.209 Not intractable
    - G44.21 Episodic tension-type headache
      - G44.211 Intractable
      - G44.219 Not intractable

- G44.22 Chronic tension-type headache
  - G44.221 Intractable
  - G44.229 Not intractable
- (G44.3) Chronic posttraumatic headache
- G44.3 Posttraumatic headache
  - G44.30 Posttraumatic headache, unspecified
    - G44.301 Intractable
    - G44.309 Not intractable
  - G44.31 Acute posttraumatic headache
    - G44.311 Intractable
    - G44.319 Not intractable
  - G44.32 Chronic posttraumatic headache
    - G44.321 Intractable
    - G44.329 Not intractable
- (G44.4) Drug-induced headache, not elsewhere classified
  - G44.40 Not intractable
  - G44.41 Intractable
- G44.5 Complicated headache syndromes
  - G44.51 Hemicrania continua
  - G44.52 New daily persistent headache
  - G44.53 Primary thunderclap headache
  - G44.59 Other complicated headache syndrome
- (G44.8) Other specified headache syndromes
  - G44.81 Hypnic headache
  - G44.82 Headache associated with sexual activity
  - G44.83 Primary cough headache
  - G44.84 Primary exertional headache
  - G44.85 Primary stabbing headache

## CEREBROVASCULAR

- (G45) Transient cerebral ischemic attacks and related syndromes
  - (G45.0) Vertebrobasilar artery syndrome
  - (G45.1) Carotid artery syndrome (hemispheric)
  - (G45.2) Multiple and bilateral precerebral artery syndromes
  - (G45.3) Amaurosis fugax
  - (G45.4) Transient global amnesia
  - (G45.8) Other transient cerebral ischemic attacks and related syndromes
  - (G45.9) Transient cerebral ischemic attack, unspecified
    - Spasm of cerebral artery
    - Transient cerebral ischemia NOS
- (G46) Vascular syndromes of brain in cerebrovascular diseases
  - (G46.0) Middle cerebral artery syndrome
  - (G46.1) Anterior cerebral artery syndrome
  - (G46.2) Posterior cerebral artery syndrome
  - (G46.3) Brain stem stroke syndrome
    - Benedikt syndrome
    - Claude syndrome
    - Foville syndrome
    - Millard–Gubler syndrome
    - Wallenberg syndrome
    - Weber syndrome
  - (G46.4) Cerebellar stroke syndrome
  - (G46.5) Pure motor lacunar syndrome
  - (G46.6) Pure sensory lacunar syndrome
  - (G46.7) Other lacunar syndromes
  - (G46.8) Other vascular syndromes of brain in cerebrovascular diseases

## SLEEP DISORDERS G47

### Clinical Information

- A change from the patient's baseline sleeping pattern, either an increase or a decrease in the number of hours slept. This can also refer to alterations in the stages of sleep.
- A disturbance of normal sleep patterns. There are a number of sleep disorders that range from trouble falling asleep to nightmares, sleepwalking, and sleep apnea (problems with breathing that cause loud snoring). Poor sleep may also be caused by diseases such as heart disease, lung disease, or nerve disorders.
- Conditions characterized by disturbances of usual sleep patterns or behaviors. Sleep disorders may be divided into three major categories: dyssomnias (i.e., disorders characterized by insomnia or hypersomnia), parasomnias (abnormal sleep behaviors), and sleep disorders secondary to medical or psychiatric disorders (from Thorpy 1994).
- Conditions characterized by disturbances of usual sleep patterns or behaviors, divided into three major categories: dyssomnias (i.e., disorders characterized by insomnia or hypersomnia), parasomnias (abnormal sleep behaviors), and sleep disorders secondary to medical or psychiatric disorders.
- Is it hard for you to fall asleep or stay asleep through the night? Do you wake up feeling tired or feel very sleepy during the day, even if you have had enough sleep? You might have a sleep disorder. The most common kinds are
  - Insomnia—a hard time falling or staying asleep
  - Sleep apnea—breathing interruptions during sleep
  - Restless legs syndrome—a tingling or prickly sensation in the legs
  - Narcolepsy daytime "sleep attacks"

Nightmares, night terrors, sleepwalking, sleep talking, head banging, wetting the bed, and grinding teeth are kinds of sleep problems called parasomnias. There are treatments for most sleep disorders. Sometimes, just having regular sleep habits can help.

## SLEEP DISORDERS

- (G47) Sleep disorders
  - (G47.0) Disorders of initiating and maintaining sleep (insomnias)
    - G47.00 Unspecified
    - G47.01 Due to medical condition
    - G47.09 Other insomnia
  - (G47.1) Disorders of excessive somnolence (hypersomnias)
    - G47.10 Unspecified
    - G47.11 Idiopathic hypersomnia with long sleep time
    - G47.12 Idiopathic hypersomnia without long sleep time
    - G47.13 Recurrent hypersomnia
    - G47.14 Due to medical condition
    - G47.19 Other hypersomnia
  - (G47.2) Disruptions in circadian rhythm including jet lag
    - Delayed sleep phase syndrome
    - Irregular sleep–wake pattern
      - G47.20 Circadian rhythm sleep disorder, unspecified type
      - G47.21 Circadian rhythm sleep disorder, delayed sleep phase type
      - G47.22 Circadian rhythm sleep disorder, advanced sleep phase type
      - G47.23 Circadian rhythm sleep disorder, irregular sleep–wake type
      - G47.24 Circadian rhythm sleep disorder, free running type
      - G47.25 Circadian rhythm sleep disorder, jet lag type
      - G47.26 Circadian rhythm sleep disorder, shift work type
      - G47.27 Circadian rhythm sleep disorder in conditions classified elsewhere
      - G47.29 Other circadian rhythm sleep disorder
  - (G47.3) Sleep apnea
    - G47.30 Unspecified
    - G47.31 Primary central sleep apnea
    - G47.32 High altitude periodic breathing
    - G47.33 Obstructive sleep apnea (adult) (pediatric)
    - G47.34 Idiopathic sleep–related nonobstructive alveolar hypoventilation
    - G47.35 Congenital central alveolar hypoventilation syndrome
    - G47.36 Sleep-related hypoventilation in conditions classified elsewhere
    - G47.37 Central sleep apnea in conditions classified elsewhere
    - G47.39 Other sleep apnea
  - (G47.4) Narcolepsy and cataplexy
    - G47.41 Narcolepsy
      - G47.411 With cataplexy
      - G47.419 Without cataplexy
    - G47.42 Narcolepsy in conditions classified elsewhere
      - G47.421 With cataplexy
      - G47.429 Without cataplexy
  - G47.5 Parasomnia
    - G47.50 Unspecified
    - G47.51 Confusional arousals
    - G47.52 Rapid eye movement sleep behavior disorder
    - G47.53 Recurrent isolated sleep paralysis
    - G47.54 In conditions classified elsewhere
    - G47.59 Other parasomnia
    - G47.6 Sleep-related movement disorders
    - G47.61 Periodic limb movement disorder
    - G47.62 Sleep-related leg cramps
    - G47.63 Sleep-related bruxism
    - G47.69 Other sleep-related movement disorders
  - (G47.8) Other sleep disorders
    - Kleine–Levin syndrome
  - G47.8 Other sleep disorders
  - G47.9 Sleep disorder, unspecified

## REFERENCES

Adams RD, Victor M, Ropper AH. *Principles of Neurology.* 6th Ed. New York, NY: Mcgraw-Hill; 1998, p. 313.

Centers for Disease Control and Prevention, National Center for Health Statistics. Compresses Mortality File 1979–1998 and 1999–2010. Accessed at http://wonder.cdc.gov/cmf-icd10-archive2006.html, July 27, 2011.

International Headache Society, Headache Classification Subcommittee. The International Classification of Headache Disorders: 2nd edition. *Cephalalgia.* 2004;24 Suppl 1:9–160.

Jay W, Leetman JE. Sudden death in epilepsy. *Acta Neurol Scand* 1981;63(Suppl. 82):1–66.

Koehler SA. *Forensic Epidemiology.* Boca Raton, FL: CRC Press; 2011.

Koehler SA, Schraeder PL, Lathers CM, Wecht CH. One-year postmortem forensic analysis of deaths in persons with epilepsy. Chapter 9 In: Lathers CD, Schraeder PL, Bungo MW, Leestma JE, eds. *Sudden Death in Epilepsy: Forensic and Clinical Issues.* Boca Raton, FL: CRC Press/Taylor & Francis Group; 2011, pp.145–59.

Lathers CM, Koehler SA, Wecht CH, Schraeder PL. Forensic anti-epileptic drug levels in autopsy cases of epilepsy. *Epilepsy Behav* 2011;22(4):778–85.

Leestma JE, Kalelkar MB, Teas, SS, Jay, GW, Hughes JR. Sudden unexpected death associated with seizures: Analysis of 66 cases. *Epilepsia* 1984;25:84–88.

Terrance CD, Rao GR, Perper JA. Neurogenic pulmonary edema in unexpected, unexplained death in epileptic patients. *Neurol* 1981;25:594–5.

Thorpy, MJ. *Practice of Sleep Medicine.* 2nd ed. Philadelphia, PA: WB Saunders;1994.

Woodward M. *Epidemiology: Study Design and Data Analysis.* Chapman & Hall, Boca Raton, FL: CDC Press; 2005.

# 12 Risk Predictor
## *Individual SUDEP Risk Factor Cluster IDs*

*Claire M. Lathers, Steven C. Schachter,*
*Braxton B. Wannamaker, and Jan E. Leestma*

## CONTENTS

Risk factors for and mechanisms of sudden unexpected death in epilepsy (SUDEP) will be established by constructing individual Cluster Identifications (IDs) for SUDEP in drug-refractory patients, which will permit the development of a Classification System by defining risk factors, including central and peripheral autonomic nervous system changes, for SUDEP. Related or similar clusters will identify the types of risk factors for people with similar risk Cluster IDs. This chapter discusses autonomic characteristics that will be studied with several readily available methods and added to the Cluster IDs. Tilt table methods (Lathers et al. 1990, 1991, 1993; Lathers and Charles 1994a,b), the skin conductance response, and heart rate variability measured from electrocardiography (EKG) recordings will help to evaluate patients with greatest risk for sympathetic and parasympathetic activity changes before, during, and after seizures.

## MEASURING AUTONOMIC CHARACTERISTICS

Tilt table methods with the skin conductance response (Scheirer and Picard 1992) is a primary method of measuring autonomic function. Tilt table testing may be used to evaluate autonomic responses in people with cardiac, epilepsy, and other medical problems, such as syncope. Heart rate variability measured by spectral analysis of heart rate may be performed simultaneously with head-up tilt testing to evaluate autonomic function as posture is changed from supine to standing position (Ansakorpi et al. 2011). An inadequate sympathovagal balance in response to orthostasis in patients with unexplained syncope and a positive head-up tilt test was attributed to a major role of the autonomic nervous system in the genesis of vasovagal, neutrally mediated, syncope (Kouakam et al. 1999). Spectral analysis of heart rate variability was used to evaluate changes in autonomic function with and without head-up tilt test in patients exhibiting unexplained syncope. The supine position did not elicit

syncope. In those who demonstrated a positive syncopal response, a head-up tilt test was required. It was concluded that the pathological mechanism triggering vasovagal syncope is related to an abrupt and excessive increase of vagal activity (Wu et al. 2003). A study of power spectral analysis of heart rate and blood pressure and head-up tilt found that anxious people had a higher baseline cardiac sympathetic hyperactivity and low heart rate variability. These changes may explain their susceptibility to sudden cardiac death (Piccirillo et al. 1997). Of diagnostic concern is the fact that syncope, epilepsy, and psychogenic pseudosyncope all present with similar symptoms, including abnormal limb movements. A study in the United Kingdom found that at least 74,000 English patients were misdiagnosed with epilepsy and were prescribed antiepileptic drugs (AEDs) (Petkar et al. 2012). Two other sources that discuss related topics are *Not Seizure but Syncope* by Sharma et al. (2011, ch. 21), and *Syncope, Seizures and SUDEP. Case Histories* by Lathers et al. (2011, ch. 22). "Fatal syncopal events may masquerade as epilepsy but this possibility has yet to be investigated. Syncope results from acute cerebral hypoperfusion and must be differentiated from epileptic seizures in cases where convulsive activity is observed during a syncopal episode" (Lathers et al. 2011, p. 325).

The skin conductance response is measured using bracelets that wirelessly assess skin resistance as a surrogate measure of autonomic function. One such device, the galvactivator, was invented and designed by Scheirer and Picard at the Massachusetts Institute of Technology. The skin conductance response is also known as the electrodermal response and in older terminology as "galvanic skin response." The skin conductance response is the phenomenon occurring when the skin momentarily becomes a better conductor of electricity in response to either external or internal stimuli that are physiologically arousing. Arousal is a broad term referring to overall activation and is widely considered to be one of the two main dimensions of an emotional response. Measuring arousal is, therefore, not the same as measuring emotion but is an important component of it. Arousal has been found to be a strong predictor of attention and memory. Certain groups of individuals have signature patterns of electrodermal baseline activity. Everyone has an individual baseline, but some people tend to have skin conductance signals that vary relatively little when they are at rest and not being stimulated by either external events or internal thoughts. This category of individuals is often referred to as stabiles. Alternatively, some people have high levels of skin conductance responses, even when at rest and when not in the presence of external stimuli; individuals with this pattern are referred to as labiles. Initial attempts to correlate these two physiological predispositions with personality style have been encouraging. The skin conductance response is also known as the electrodermal response. The galvactivator is powered by a 6 V battery and the average value is 0.1–0.4. A custom-built wrist watch sensor device (Poh et al. 2012) is now available for continuous recording of the sympathetically mediated electrodermal activity of patients with refractory epilepsy admitted to epilepsy monitoring units.

Ambulatory EKG-based assessment of autonomic function and T-wave alternans provides tools for quantification of the potential cardioprotective effect of vagus nerve stimulation on cardiac electrical instability (Verrier and Schachter 2011, ch. 43; Chapter 14 of this book). The barocuff device can be used to measure baroreceptor sensitivity, an indicator of vagus nerve activity (Eckberg and Frisch 1991).

The role of AEDs and the Lock Step Phenomenon (LSP) in refractory patients may be examined. The LSP is an animal model discovered in Dr. Lathers' research laboratory at the Medical College of Pennsylvania, which now needs to be studied in humans. (See Hughes and Sato 2011, ch. 23 and Chapters 28 and 29 of this book) All data will be entered in SUDEP autonomic Risk Factor Cluster Classification and IDs.

Noninvasive methods are useful to identify all risk parameters I (Table 5.1), including autonomic factors, environmental characteristics, and others such as site of death, etc., to classify a person with epilepsy in Cluster IDs. The determination can be based on central and peripheral neurological assessments, electroencephalography (EEG), and cardiovascular and pulmonary measurements obtained in supine and seated positions. Risk factors will be used to compare and evaluate risk of a given patient as a candidate for SUDEP.

The autonomic nervous system has functional and neurochemical components that respond differentially to stressors and pathophysiologic events (Goldstein 2013). Seizures produce changes in autonomic nervous system activity. Metcalf et al. (2009) reported that status epilepticus activates the autonomic nervous system to increase control of cardiac function in the short term. Status epilepticus was associated with a chronic shift in sympathovagal balance favoring sympathetic dominance due to decreased parasympathetic activity for 1–2 weeks. The decreased baroreflex response to an increase in

blood pressure was assumed to be due to decreased vagal activation. It was concluded that the status epilepticus produces chronic alterations in cardiac sympathovagal balance that may increase cardiac risk and mortality.

Acute and chronic autonomic changes were also reported following surgical temporal lobectomy. Postoperatively, in patients with intractable temporal lobe epilepsy, the sympathovagal balance was altered in favor of the parasympathetic activity early after surgery but in favor of the sympathetic activity after the first postoperative month (Dericioglu et al. 2013).

Patients respond differently to changes in autonomic function induced by epileptic seizures, nor is the change in a given individual always the same. Eggleston et al. (2014) noted that cardiac signals are potential biomarkers that may serve as an extracerebral indicator of ictal onset in some patients. The parameter of heart rate itself is a biomarker associated with seizures and may be used to detect seizure onset. Increased heart rate, i.e., ictal tachycardia, with ictal events occurs in 82% of patients with epilepsy. Average percent of seizures and significant heart rate changes were similar with generalized (64%) and partial onset seizures (71%) with *intraindividual variability*. The majority of studies reported significant increase in heart rate during seizure in the temporal lobe. The actual magnitude of heart rate changes occurring with seizures exhibited variability among patients. It is appropriate to use multiple modalities simultaneously to assess changes of autonomic activity associated with epileptic seizures.

The autonomic nervous system modulates cardiac electrophysiology and arrhythmogenesis. Mechanisms vary for specific arrhythmias. Shen and Zipes (2014) discuss the potential for modulating autonomic activity for both prevention and treatment of specific arrhythmias using either neural ablation or stimulation.

## CONTROLLED VERSUS INTRACTABLE EPILEPSY AND SUDEP

Mukherjee et al. (2009) address the autonomic imbalance of sympathetic and parasympathetic activity thought to contribute to SUDEP and suggest that people with well-controlled versus intractable epilepsy may present different autonomic responses. They found a higher vasomotor tone, higher sympathetic tone, lower parasympathetic tone, lower parasympathetic reactivity, and more severe dysautonomia in those with intractable epilepsy, suggesting refractoriness may alter cardiovascular autonomic regulation and predispose these individuals to SUDEP. Additional evidence supporting the suggestion that autonomic imbalance of sympathetic and parasympathetic activity may contribute to SUDEP was provided by Poh et al. (2012), who studied autonomic dysfunction, seizures, and postictal EEG suppression in patients with refractory epilepsy. They used custom-built wrist-worn sensors to record sympathetically mediated electrodermal activity of patients with refractory epilepsy. Parasympathetically modulated high-frequency power of heart rate variability was measured simultaneously with EKG recordings. Findings demonstrated that sympathetic activation and parasympathetic suppression increased with the duration of EEG suppression after tonic–clonic seizures. The authors suggested that a critical window of postictal autonomic dysregulation may be pertinent to the pathogenesis of SUDEP.

## THE EFFECT OF YOGA

Treatment regimens for resistant cases of epilepsy and depression include vagal nerve stimulation to reverse the parasympathetic suppression. Streeter et al. (2012) theorized that yoga may correct disorders exacerbated by stress, including the imbalance of the autonomic nervous system, and perhaps decreased activity of the inhibitory gamma aminobutyric acid neurotransmitter, associated with epilepsy and depression.

## CONCLUSIONS

This chapter reviewed autonomic nervous system activity in seizures and described suitable tools that may be used. Autonomic testing to measure end-organ responses to physiological provocation includes assessing parasympathetic and sympathetic nervous system function with heart rate variability. Sympathetic nervous system function may be measured by blood pressure response to physiological stimuli using tilt table testing, with or without pharmacological stimulations, neurological vasovagal syncope, postural tachycardia, and orthostatic hypotension (Freeman and Chapleau 2013). Additional autonomic central and peripheral risk factors and other risk factors for refractory epilepsy patients, using noninvasive methodologies, are presented.

## REFERENCES

Ansakorpi H, Korpelainen JT, Suominen K, Tolonen U, Bloigu R, Myllylä VV, Isojärvi JI. Evaluation of heart rate variation analysis during rest and tilting in patients with temporal lobe epilepsy. *Neurol Res Int* 2011;2011:829365.

Dericioglu N, Demirci M, Cataltepe O, Akalan N, Saygi S. Heart rate variability remains reduced and sympathetic tone elevated after temporal lobe epilepsy surgery. *Seizure* 2013;22:713–8.

Eckberg DL, Frisch J. Human autonomic responses to actual and simulated weightlessness. *J Clin Pharmacol* 1991:31:956–62.

Eggleston KS, Olin BD, Fisher RS. Ictal tachycardia: The head–heart connection. *Seizure* 2014;23:495–505.

Freeman R, Chapleau MW. Testing the autonomic nervous system. *Handb Clin Neurol* 2013;115:115–36.

Goldstein DS. Differential responses of components of the autonomic nervous system. *Handb Clin Neurol* 2013;117:13–22.

Hughes JD, Sato S. Sudden death in epilepsy: Relationship to sleep-wake circadian cycle and fractal physiology. In: Lathers CM, Schraeder PL, Bungo MW, Leestma JE, eds. *Sudden Death in Epilepsy: Forensic and Clinical Issues.* Boca Raton, FL: CRC Press; 2011, pp. 333–46.

Kouakam C, Lacroix D, Zghal N, Logier R, Klug D, Le Franc P, Jarwe M, Kacet S. Inadequate sympathovagal balance in

response to orthostatism in patients with unexplained syncope and a positive head up tilt test. *Heart* 1999;82(3):312–8.

Lathers CM, Charles JB. Orthostatic hypotension in patients, bed rest subjects, astronauts. *J Clin Pharm* 1994a;34:403–17.

Lathers CM, Charles JB. Comparison cardiovascular function during early hours BR and SF. *J Clin Pharm* 1994b;34:489–99.

Lathers CM, Diamandis PH, Riddle JM, Mukai C, Elton KF, Bungo MW, Charles JB. Acute and intermediate cardiovascular response to zero gravity and to fractional gravity levels induced by head-down or head-up tilt. *J Clin Pharm* 1990;30:494–523.

Lathers CM, Diamandis PH, Riddle JM, Mukai C, Elton KF, Bungo MW, Charles JB. Orthostatic function during a stand test before and after head-up or head-down bedrest. *J Clin Pharmacol* 1991:31:893–903.

Lathers CM, Riddle JM, Mulvagh SL, Mukai C, Diamandis PH, Dussack LG, Bungo MW, Charles JB. Echocardiograms during six hours of bedrest at head-down and head-up tilt and during space flight. *J Clin Pharmacol* 1993;33:535–43.

Lathers CM, Schraeder PL, Bungo MW. Syncope, seizures and SUDEP: Case histories. Chapter 22 In: Lathers CM, Schraeder PL, Bungo MW, Leestma JE, eds. *Sudden Death in Epilepsy: Forensic and Clinical Issues.* Boca Raton, FL: CRC Press/Taylor & Francis Group; 2011, pp. 325–32.

Metcalf CS, Radwanski PB, Bealer SL. Status epilepticus produces chronic alterations in cardiac sympathovagal balance. *Epilepsia* 2009;50(4):747–54.

Mukherjee S1, Tripathi M, Chandra PS, Yadav R, Choudhary N, Sagar R, Bhore R, Pandey RM, Deepak KK. Cardiovascular autonomic functions in well-controlled and intractable partial epilepsies. *Epilepsy Res* 2009;85(2–3):261–9.

Petkar S, Hamid T, Iddon P, Clifford A, Rice N, Claire R, McKee D, Curtis N, Cooper PN, Fitzpatrick AP. Prolonged implantable electrocardiographic monitoring indicates a high rate of misdiagnosis of epilepsy—REVISE study. *Europace* 2012;14:1653–60.

Piccirillo G, Elvira S, Bucca C, Viola E, Cacciafesta M, Marigliano V. Abnormal passive head-up tilt test in subjects with symptoms of anxiety power spectral analysis study of heart rate and blood pressure. *Int J Cardiol* 1997 25;60(2):121–31.

Poh MZ, Loddenkemper T, Reinsberger C, Swenson NC, Goyal S, Madsen JR, Picard RW. Autonomic changes with seizures correlate with postictal EEG suppression. *Neurology* 2012;78(23):1868–76.

Scheirer J, Picard R. *The skin conductance response.* Boston, MA: MIT Media Lab; 1992.

Sharma S, Ho T, Kantharia BK. Not seizure but syncope. Chapter 21. In: Lathers CM, Schraeder PL, Bungo MW, Leestma JE, eds. *Sudden Death in Epilepsy: Forensic and Clinical Issues.* Boca Raton, FL: CRC Press/Taylor & Francis Group; 2011, pp. 311–24.

Shen MJ, Zipes DP. Role of the autonomic nervous system in modulating cardiac arrhythmias. *Circ Res* 2014;114(6):1004–21.

Streeter CC, Gerbarg PL, Saper RB, Ciraulo DA, Brown RP. Effects of yoga on the autonomic nervous system, gamma-aminobutyric-acid, and allostasis in epilepsy, depression, and post-traumatic stress disorder. *Med Hypotheses* 2012;78(5): 571–9.

Verrier RL, Schachter SC. Neurocardiac interactions in sudden unexpected death in epilepsy. Chapter 43 In: Lathers CM, Schraeder PL, Bungo MW, Leestma JE, eds. *Sudden Death in Epilepsy: Forensic and Clinical Issues.* Boca Raton, FL: CRC Press Taylor & Francis Group; 2011, pp. 693–709.

Wu XH, Chen SL, Wang XD, Ji XF. Assessment of the changes in autonomic nervous function during head up tilt test in syncopal patients using spectral analysis of heart rate variability. *Zhonghua Nei Ke Za Zhi* 2003;42(12):833–6.

# 13 Intracranial Pressure, Cerebral Edema, and Obstructive Sleep Apnea
## A Risk Factor Cluster for SUDEP?

*Claire M. Lathers, Steven C. Schachter,*
*Braxton B. Wannamaker, and Jan E. Leestma*

## CONTENTS

## SEIZURES AND INTRACRANIAL PRESSURE

Penfield and Erickson (1941) reported that increased intracranial pressure (ICP) did not cause seizures but could be the consequence of seizures. In a pilot study of 17 patients, it was demonstrated that acute increased ICP was not associated with precipitation of subclinical seizures as monitored by 30 minutes of electroencephalogram (EEG) activity following the rise (McNamara et al. 2003). In preparation for this chapter, a PUBMED literature search did not find epilepsy or seizures associated with the syndrome of benign intracranial hypertension (pseudotumor cerebri), except in a few cases with a coexisting condition which in all likelihood was the cause of the seizures.

White et al. (1961) documented that cerebral edema and increased ICP could follow seizures. In 1978, Minns and Brown subsequently recorded ICPs which were coincidental with over 100 seizures in 5 children. Their measurements were obtained by four separate approaches including ventricular cannulation via a burr hole or open fontanelle, existing Pudenz shunts, cerebrospinal fluid reservoir, or lumbar puncture. They found a relatively rapid rise in ICP following seizures that fell and then rose a second time for as long as 20 minutes. Demonstrable changes were even noticed in nonconvulsive atypical absence seizures.

Studies conducted in dogs had shown that ICP increased after electroconvulsive-induced seizures (Hendley et al. 1965) and that these changes were also associated with bradycardia or even cardiac arrest. In other work, generalized tonic–clonic convulsions 7 to 35 seconds after administration of proconvulsant drugs to cats (Goitein and Shohami 1983) were followed by threefold to fivefold increases in ICP, reaching maximal pressures of 20 to 94 mm Hg after 20 seconds to 7 minutes. The ICP remained high for 47 seconds to 10 minutes, then fell gradually and reached preictal levels after 2 to 30 minutes despite the continuation of convulsions.

Observations of ICP and seizures in humans have paralleled the introduction of monitoring activities in neurological/neurosurgical intensive care units and epilepsy monitoring units. Observations of seizures including nonconvulsive seizures followed by increased ICP (Vespa et al. 2007) support proposals for early use of antiepileptic drugs in managing acute traumatic brain injury including swelling. The need for ICP monitoring in children who are undergoing invasive EEG monitoring has been stressed (Shah et al. 2007). Increased ICP in these circumstances can be associated with hemodynamic instability and bradycardia (Agrawal et al. 2008).

Based on these observations, consideration must be given for ICP and its potential implications for relationships with seizures, cardiac dysfunction, peripheral autonomic changes (Poh et al. 2012), and sudden unexpected death in epilepsy (SUDEP). To make this practical, noninvasive monitoring of ICP is a desirable investigational tool. The value of ocular tonometry is controversial. Investigators using handheld tonometry found poor correlation between measures of intraocular pressure with this device and standard lumbar puncture determination of ICP (Golan et al. 2013). Intraocular pressures by tonometry and ICP by invasive pressure transducer were compared in children with traumatic brain injury (Spentzas et al. 2010). There was good sensitivity but limited specificity. A promising noninvasive method recently described by Ragauskas et al. (2012) incorporates a two-depth high-resolution transcranial Doppler isonation of the ophthalmic artery. When compared with ICP by standard lumbar puncture, there was good accuracy and high precision.

It is likely that most seizures are associated with some transient cerebral edema, which may be generalized or localized, depending on the type of seizure. Cerebral edema functionally may equate to increased ICP but is not long-lasting. Neurosurgeons observed swelling/edema of the brain when seizures occur during surgery. With status epilepticus, cerebral edema and increased ICP last as long as the seizures continue.

ICP goes up at night during apneic episodes associated with obstructive sleep apnea (Gücer and Viernstein 1979), which is a common comorbidity in patients with epilepsy (Malow et al. 1997, 2000; Manni and Terzaghi 2010; van Golde et al. 2011). Obstructive sleep apnea acts on the autonomic nervous system during the night, via one or more mechanisms, including brainstem respiratory–cardiac coupling, stimulation of the chemoreflex, baroreflexes, and lung inflation reflexes (Leung 2009). Obstructive sleep apnea modifies the normally dominant parasympathetic control of the heart and greater myocardial electrical stability found at night, resulting in profound vagal activity causing bradyarrhythmias and sympathoexcitation linked to ventricular ectopy. Aytemir et al. (2007) examined patients with obstructive sleep apnea syndrome and found changes in heart rate turbulence, heart rate variability and QT dynamicity, i.e., the QT interval in the electrocardiogram, indications of autonomic imbalance, and increased myocardial vulnerability, which may theoretically predispose an individual to sudden cardiac death. Continuous positive airway pressure does change this imbalance, resulting in decreased nocturnal arrhythmias and autonomic profile.

The evidence, therefore, supports the conclusions that increased ICP may follow clinical generalized tonic–clonic seizures and nonconvulsive electrographic seizures but does not cause epileptic seizures. The relevance of this information to the occurrence of SUDEP may reside in two possibilities. Transient cerebral swelling or edema following seizures could create increased ICP. This, in turn, could subsequently result in bradycardia and apnea (Agrawal et al. 2008), which might potentiate cardiac disturbances already generated by the predominance of sympathetic tone during the postictal state. Furthermore, Hu (2007) characterized interdependency between ICP and heart variability signals, finding a causal spectral measure and a generalized synchronization measure, i.e., between ICP and heart rate variability where the ICP and R-R interval appeared to be coupled with B-waves of the ICP.

## RELATIONSHIP TO BREATHING

As reviewed in other chapters, seizures alone, without obstructive sleep apnea, may alter the function of respiratory control, causing apnea and/or SUDEP in adults or in children. There could conceivably be some interplay between the factors, underlying or associated conditions, which may alter respiratory control in adults, as well as in very young victims of SUDEP and in sudden infant death syndrome (SIDS) victims. Evaluation of SUDEP in infants and young children has inherently been very difficult, owing to the many confounding variables that may be unique to the very young. Examples could include: brain damage related to birth events

(prematurity, placental pathologies, hypoxia, ischemia, intracranial bleeding, and hyperbilirubinemia); congenital malformations of the brain (micropolygyria, schizencephaly, Arnold–Chiari malformation, ectopic neurons); intrauterine and perinatal infections (rubella, herpes simplex, cytomegalovirus, and toxoplasmosis), and many others. The phenomenon of SIDS appears, in part, to involve disorders of respiration (Valdes-Dapena 1986; Prandota 2004; Thach 2008). These can be due to sleeping in the prone position, entrapment by bed clothing or blankets, or abnormality in neural control of respiration. Studies implicate damage to the medullary regions with gliosis and altered neurotransmitter expression in regions in or near the tractus solitarius (Sparks and Hunsaker 1991; Weese-Mayer et al. 2003; Kinney et al. 2005).

Knowledge of the anatomy and neurophysiology of respiratory control has evolved (Petrovicky 1989; Smith et al. 2009; Nattie 2011; Ott et al. 2012). Studies show remarkable concordance between rodent and primate anatomy. The anatomy of respiratory control involves a vertical chain of interconnected nuclei beginning in and near the motor nucleus of the vagus nerve in pontinetegmentum, which connect in a descending course with a group of nuclei and the lateral parabrachial group, which includes the Koelliker–Fuse nucleus. These nuclei connect with the facial nerve nucleus and the superior olivary nucleus at the pontomedullar junction. Below this, the retrotrapezoid group connects with the Boetzinger and pre-Boetzing complex, which in turn descends to connect with the rostral ventral neuronal group, the nucleus ambiguous, and the caudal ventral group in the lower lateral medulla. These nuclei interconnect and project to the hypoglossal nucleus and the phrenic nerve nuclei (not via the pyramidal tract but rather through reticulospinal pathways) and ultimately reach the diaphragm, thoracic, and abdominal musculature, providing the physical–motor aspects of respiration. Control of respiration involves both voluntary and involuntary drive, including sensing changes in blood pH, oxygen tension, and carbon dioxide tension (Darnall 2010; Dean and Putnam 2010; Mulkey and Wenker 2011). The control of inspiration must alternate with expiration to properly function (Alheid and McCrimmon 2008; Fortuna et al. 2008; Hilaire and Dutschman 2009). These "opposite" actions are coordinated by the brainstem nuclei, listed above, with inputs from the cerebellum, higher centers, and sensory inputs from the chest musculature and diaphragm. Structural damage or physiological dysfunctions that impinge on these vital nuclei may result in failure of the respiratory system. Seizures clearly could interfere with this physiology in both adults and young children with epilepsy.

Some hypothesize that damage to these regions may result in dysfunctional breathing, especially during sleep, causing failure of respiratory drive and apnea leading to death. Part of this dysfunction may be impaired chemoreceptor function to pH and oxygen and carbon dioxide tension in the lower pons and medulla (Darnall 2010; Guyenet et al. 2010). Furthermore, if an adult or infant had some underlying damage to the neural respiratory apparatus, a seizure projecting to these areas might trigger or facilitate shut down of respiration and cause death. In such an instance, the result is the same in SUDEP as in SIDS, and probably cannot be differentiated given present technologies and knowledge.

Just one of the pathologies not uncommonly found in autopsies of apparent SUDEP victims is cerebellar atrophy, the cause of which has be variously hypothesized to be on the basis of hypoxia, ischemia, edema, or some effect of anticonvulsant medications (Hagemann et al. 2002; De Marcoset al. 2003). A report of Ebert et al. (1995) describes a series of patients with known cerebellar disease who, in addition to movement disorders, exhibited ataxic breathing patterns. Could patients with epilepsy who have cerebellar atrophy also be vulnerable to expansion or exacerbation of their ataxic breathing into apnea, which may or may not prove to be a fatal event? A recent case report of Scorza et al. (2011) raises this very question, among others, in the death of a child with epilepsy. As reviewed above, seizures can result in raised ICP and cerebral edema. Some element of cerebral edema is commonly found in victims classified as SUDEP. How much of this is due to agonal events or some preagonal event probably cannot be known or determined. If cerebral edema occurred prior to the agonal process, some element of brainstem-elevated pressure could occur. One of the early physiological and clinical signs of this may be some alteration of respiration, associated or followed by some disorder of consciousness. It is reasonable to suppose that if an individual with epilepsy has underlying damage to brainstem structures, they might respond to this challenge in a diminished fashion as compared to a healthy individual.

## SYNTHESIS AND CONCLUSION

Other chapters in this volume have reviewed the relationships of sleep, nonrapid eye movement sleep, nocturnal seizures, the sympathetic nervous system, and potentially fatal cardiac arrhythmias (Chapters 18, 19, 20, 21, 28, 29, and 31 in this book). We have presented evidence that increased ICP occurs during sleep and during seizures (Hendley et al. 1965; Goitein and Shohami 1983), that raised ICP and cerebral edema may occur together and adversely affect brainstem control of respiration, and that obstructive sleep apnea is associated with cardiac instability. One possible terminal sequence of events in patients with epilepsy and obstructive sleep apnea is that nocturnal seizures would cause significantly increased ICP and cerebral edema which, in turn, would produce a sudden pressure-induced decompensation of cardiopulmonary control centers in the brainstem.

Since obstructive sleep apnea is associated with increased nocturnal seizures, ICP, and autonomic dysfunction, we propose that these risk factors, together with time of seizure occurrence, changes in autonomic nervous system function, cardiac arrhythmias, and altered pulmonary function, may represent a risk factor cluster for SUDEP. Definitive experiments are needed so that potentially life-saving interventions can be tested.

## REFERENCES

Agrawal A, Timothy J, Cincu R, Agrawal T, Waghmare LB. Bradycardia in neurosurgery. *Clin Neural Neurosurg* 2008; 110:321–7.

Alheid GF, McCrimmon DR. The chemical neuroanatomy of breathing. *Respir Physiol Neurobiol* 2008;164(1–2):3–11.

Aytemir K, Deniza A, Yavuza B, Demirb AU, Sahinera L, Ciftcia O, Tokgozoglua L, Canc I, Sahinb A, Otoa A. Increased myocardial vulnerability and autonomic nervous system imbalance in obstructive sleep apnea syndrome. *Respir Med* 2007;101:1277–82.

Darnall RA. The role of CO(2) and central chemoreception in the control of breathing in the fetus and the neonate. *Respir Physiol Neurobiol* 2010;173(3):201–12.

Dean JB, Putnam RW. The caudal solitary complex is a site of central CO(2) chemoreception and integration of multiple systems that regulate expired CO(2). *Respir Physiol Neurobiol* 2010;173(3):274–87.

De Marcos FA, Ghizoni E, Kobayashi E, Li LM, Cendes F. Cerebellar volume and long-term use of phenytoin. *Seizure* 2003;12:312–5.

Ebert D, Hefter H, Dohle C, Freund HJ. Ataxic breathing during alternating forearm movements of various frequencies in cerebellar patients. *Neurosci Lett* 1995;193(3):145–8.

Fortuna MG, West GH, Stornetta RL, Guyenet PG. Botzinger expiratory-augmenting neurons and the parafacial respiratory group. *J Neurosci* 2008;28(10):2506–15.

Goitein KJ, Shohami E. Intracranial pressure during prolonged experimental convulsions in cats. *J Neurol* 1983;230:259–66.

Golan S, Kurtz S, Mezad-Koursh D, Waisbourd M, Kesler A, Halpern P. Poor correlation between intracranial pressure and intraocular pressure by hand-held tonometry. *Clin Ophthalmol* 2013;7:1083–7.

Gücer G, Viernstein LJ. Intracranial pressure in the normal monkey while awake and asleep. *J Neurosurg* 1979;51(2):206–10.

Guyenet PG, Stornetta RL, Bayliss DA. Central respiratory chemoreception. *J Comp Neurol* 2010;518(19):3883–906.

Hagemann G, Lemieux L, Free SL, Krakow K, Everitt AD, Kendall BE, Stevens JM, Shorvon SD. Cerebellar volumes in newly diagnosed and chronic epilepsy. *J Neurol* 2002;249:1651–8.

Hendley CD, Spudis EV, Delatorre E. Intracranial pressure during electroshock convulsions in the dog. *Neurology* 1965;15:351–60.

Hilaire G, Dutschmann M. Foreword: Respiratory rhythmogenesis. *Respir Physiol Neurobiol* 2009;168(1–2):1–3.

Hu X, Nenov V, Vespa P, Bergsneider M. Characterization of interdependency between intracranial pressure and heart variability signals: A causal spectral measure and a generalized synchronization measure. *IEEE Trans Biomed Eng* 2007;54:1407–17.

Kinney HC, Myers MM, Belliveau RA, Randall LL, Trachtenberg FL, Fingers ST, et al. Subtle autonomic and respiratory dysfunction in sudden infant death syndrome associated with serotonergic brainstem abnormalities: A case report. *J Neuropathol Exp Neurol* 2005;64(8):689–94.

Leung RST. Sleep-disordered breathing: Autonomic mechanisms and arrhythmias. progress in cardiovascular diseases. *Prog Cardiovasc Dis* 2009;51(4):324–38.

Malow BA, Fromes GA, Aldrich MS. Usefulness of polysomnography in epilepsy patients. *Neurology* 1997;48:1389–94.

Malow BA, Levy K, Maturen K, Bowes R. Obstructive sleep apnea is common in medically refractory epilepsy patients. *Neurology* 2000;55:1002–7.

Manni R, Terzaghi M. Comorbidity between epilepsy and sleep disorders. *Epilepsy Research* 2010;90:171–7.

McNamara B, Ray J, Menon D, Boniface S. Raised intracranial pressure and seizure in the neurological intensive care unit. *Br J Anaesth* 2003;90:39–42.

Minns RA, Brown JK. Intracranial pressure changes associated with childhood seizures. *Dev Med Child Neurol* 1978;20:561–9.

Mulkey DK, Wenker IC. Astrocyte chemoreceptors: Mechanisms of H+ sensing by astrocytes in the retrotrapezoid nucleus and their possible contribution to respiratory drive. *Exp Physiol* 2011;96(4):400–6.

Nattie E. Julius H. Comroe, Jr., distinguished lecture: Central chemoreception: Then and now. *J Appl Physiol* 2011; 110(1):1–8.

Ott MM, Nuding SC, Segers LS, O'Connor R, Morris KF, Lindsey BG. Central chemoreceptor modulation of breathing via multipath tuning in medullary ventrolateral respiratory column circuits. *J Neurophysiol* 2012;107(2):603–17.

Penfield W, Erickson T. *Epilepsy and Cerebral Localization: A Study of the Mechanisms, Treatment and Prevention of Epileptic Seizures*. Springfield, IL: Charles C Thomas; 1941, pp. 344–5.

Petrovicky P. The nucleus Kolliker-Fuse (K-F) and parabrachial-complex (PNBC) in man. Location, cytoarchitectonics and terminology in embryonic and adult periods, and comparison with other animals. *J Hirnforschung* 1989;30(5):551–63.

Poh MZ, Loddenkemper T, Reinsberger C, Swenson NC, Goyal S, Madsen JR, Picard RW. Autonomic changes with seizures correlate with postictal EEG suppression. *Neurology* 2012;78(23):1868–76.

Prandota J. Possible pathomechanisms of sudden infant death syndrome: Key role of chronic hypoxia, infection/inflammation states, cytokine irregularities, and metabolic trauma in genetically predisposed infants. *Am J Ther* 2004;11(6):517–46.

Ragauskas A, Matijosaitis V, Zakelis R, Petrikonis K, Rastenyte D, Piper I, Daubaris G. Clinical assessment of noninvasive intracranial pressure absolute value measurement method. *Neurology* 2012;78(21):1684–91.

Scorza FA, Terra VC, Arida RM, Sakamoto AC, Harper RM. Sudden death in a child with epilepsy: Potential cerebellar mechanisms? *Arq Neuropsiquiatr* 2011; 69:707–17.

Shah AK, Fuerst D, Sood S, Asano E, Ahn-Ewing J, Pawlak C, Chugani HT. Seizures lead to elevation of intracranial pressure in children undergoing invasive EEG monitoring. *Epilepsia* 2007;48:1097–103.

Smith JC, Abdala AP, Rybak IA, Paton JF. Structural and functional architecture of respiratory networks in the mammalian brainstem. *Philos Trans R Soc Lond B Biol Sci* 2009; 364(1529):2577–87.

Sparks DL, Hunsaker JC III. Sudden infant death syndrome: Altered aminergic-cholinergic synaptic markers in hypothalamus. *J Child Neurol* 1991;6(4):335–9.

Spentzas T, Henricksen J, Patters AB, Chaum E. Correlation of intraocular pressure with intracranial pressure in children with severe head injuries. *Pediatr Crit Care Med* 2010;11:593–8.

Thach BT. Some aspects of clinical relevance in the maturation of respiratory control in infants. *J Appl Physiol* 2008;104(6): 1828–34.

Valdes-Dapena M. Sudden infant death syndrome. Morphology update for forensic pathologists—1985. *Forensic Sci Int* 1986;30(2–3):177–86.

vanGolde EGA, Gutter T, de Weerd AW. Sleep disturbances in people with epilepsy; prevalence, impact and treatment. *Sleep Med Rev* 2011;15(6):357–68.

Vespa PM, Miller C, McArthur D, et al. Nonconvulsive electrographic seizures after traumatic brain injury result in a delayed, prolonged increase in intracranial pressure and metabolic crisis. *Crit Care Med* 2007;35:2830–6.

Weese-Mayer DE, Zhou L, Berry-Kravis EM, Maher BS, Silvestri JM, Marazita ML. Association of the serotonin transporter gene with sudden infant death syndrome: A haplotype analysis. *Am J Med Genet A* 2003;122A(3):238–45.

White PT, Grant P, Mosier J, Craig A. Changes in cerebral dynamics associated with seizures. *Neurology* 1961;11(4)(Pt 1):354–61.

# 14 Neurocardiac Interactions in Sudden Unexpected Death in Epilepsy

## Can Ambulatory Electrocardiogram-Based Assessment of Autonomic Function and T-Wave Alternans Help to Evaluate Risk?

*Richard L. Verrier and Steven C. Schachter*

## CONTENTS

## SCOPE OF THE PROBLEM

Sudden unexpected death occurs 20 times more frequently in patients with epilepsy than in the general population (Shorvon and Tomson 2011) and accounts for nearly 17% of premature deaths among individuals with this condition (Lathers et al. 2008). Witnessed cases indicate that death is contemporaneous with seizure activity (Kloster and Engelskjøn 1999; Langan et al. 2005; Tomson et al. 2005; Devinsky 2011). Cardiac dysfunction, primarily in the form of enhanced arrhythmia susceptibility (Leestma et al. 1984; Blumhardt et al. 1986; Opeskin et al. 2000; Opherk et al. 2002; Leutmezer et al. 2003; Ryvlin et al. 2006) with concomitant myocardial ischemia (Tigaran et al. 1997, 2003) has been implicated as a critical factor. Although decreases in heart rate can occur during epileptic seizures, pronounced sinus tachycardia reflecting heightened adrenergic activity is the most common electrocardiographic abnormality associated with seizures. Identification of the influences contributing to enhanced cardiac risk in sudden unexpected death in epilepsy (SUDEP) patients has been elusive, although a number of plausible cardiac pathologic changes have been suggested.

More extensive electrocardiographic monitoring and analysis of paroxysmal clinical events could also ameliorate the reported incidence of misdiagnosis of epilepsy in patients with cardiac pathology. In a series of 74 patients diagnosed with epilepsy, 31 (41.9%) were found to have cardiac disorders rather than epilepsy (Zaidi et al. 2000). Review by consulting physicians confirmed neurogenic syncope, long QT syndrome, and other cardiovascular diagnoses rather than epilepsy in several cases and case series (Table 14.1). Genomic characterization could also help to differentiate cardiac syndromes from epilepsy as a number of genetic characteristics are shared by patients with the cardiac long QT syndrome and individuals with epilepsy (Glasscock et al. 2010; Tu et al. 2011; Glasscock 2013; Partemi et al. 2013). Discussion of this subject is however outside the scope of this chapter.

The goals of this chapter are twofold. The first is to review the basic mechanisms of autonomic control of cardiac electrical function, which could potentially contribute to precipitation of SUDEP. The second is to draw attention to new ambulatory electrocardiogram (ECG)-based tools for assessing autonomic function with heart rate turbulence and cardiac arrhythmia vulnerability with T-wave alternans (TWA).

## IMPORTANCE OF NEUROCARDIAC INTERACTIONS IN TRIGGERING LIFE-THREATENING ARRHYTHMIAS

A major theme in the field of sudden cardiac death research is that although autonomic factors exert potent influences on the stability of heart rhythm, precipitation of life-threatening arrhythmias requires the coexistence of a vulnerable coronary vasculature and myocardial substrate (Figure 14.1). In the general population, enhanced vulnerability of the myocardium to arrhythmic death results from the presence of relatively advanced coronary artery disease due to atherosclerosis, which is an underlying condition in ~80% of cases. The mean age of sudden cardiac death victims is 69 years (Reddy et al. 2009). Patients with epilepsy who die suddenly are generally younger, in the range of 20 to 40 years of age (Tomson et al. 2005) and only 19% of cases have ischemic heart disease (Annegers et al. 1984). Thus, coronary atherosclerosis does not appear to be a major predisposing condition for SUDEP.

Relatively severe cardiac rhythm, conduction, and repolarization abnormalities have been reported in association with seizures, including bradycardia, asystole, bundle-branch block, ST-segment changes indicative of myocardial ischemia, and T-wave inversion (Tigaran et al. 1997, 2003; Opeskin et al. 2000; Opherk et al. 2002; Nei et al. 2000, 2004; Jallon 2004; Surges et al. 2010a, 2010c; Brotherstone et al. 2010).

## TABLE 14.1
## Misdiagnoses of Cardiac Conditions as Epilepsy

| Correct Diagnosis | Investigators |
|---|---|
| Long QT syndrome | Stollberger and Finsterer (2004); Rossenbacker et al. (2007); Johnson et al. (2009) |
| Neurogenic syncope | Linzer et al. (1994); Scheepers et al. (1998); Smith et al. (1999); Zaidi et al. (2000); Josephson et al. (2007); Petkar et al. (2012) |
| Catecholaminergic polymorphic ventricular tachycardia | Johnson et al. (2010) |
| Idiopathic cardiac asystole | Scheepers et al. (1998); Venkataraman et al. (2001) |
| Psychogenic basis | Scheepers et al. (1998); Smith et al. (1999); Zaidi et al. (2000) |
| Migraine | Scheepers et al. (1998); Smith et al. (1999) |
| Bradycardia | Zaidi et al. (2000); Petkar et al. (2012) |
| Transient ischemic episodes | Scheepers et al. (1998) |
| Vertebrobasilar insufficiency | Scheepers et al. (1998) |
| Postural hypotension | Scheepers et al. (1998) |
| Congenital heart disease | Scheepers et al. (1998) |
| Carotid sinus syndrome/sinus node disease | Scheepers et al. (1998); Petkar et al. (2012) |

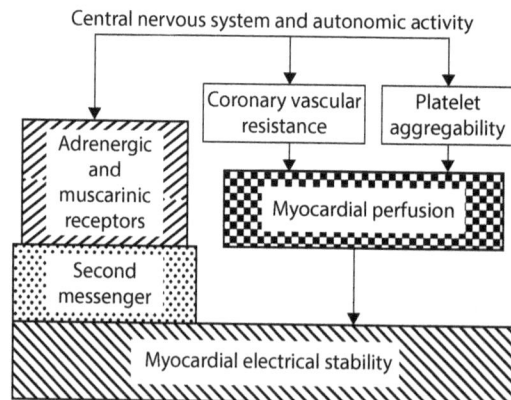

**FIGURE 14.1** The interaction between neural triggers and cardiovascular substrate during autonomic activation. Stimulation of beta$_1$-adrenergic receptors can decrease electrical stability directly as a result of changes in second messenger formation and alterations in ion fluxes. This deleterious influence is opposed by muscarinic receptor stimulation, which inhibits presynaptically the release of norepinephrine and opposes its action at the receptor level. Catecholamines may also alter myocardial perfusion by complex means, including alpha-receptor stimulation of coronary vessels and platelets and by impairing diastolic perfusion time due to adrenergically mediated sinus tachycardia. (From Verrier, RL, Central nervous system modulation of cardiac rhythm, In: Rosen, MR and Palti, Y, editors. *Lethal arrhythmias resulting from myocardial ischemia and infarction*, Boston, MA: Kluwer Academic Publishers, 1988, pp. 149–164. With permission.)

When these abnormalities occur, the length of the seizure is typically prolonged (Zijlmans et al. 2002). The occurrence of bradycardia and asystole in some cases (Rocamora et al. 2003; Rugg-Gunn et al. 2004; Ryvlin et al. 2006) may reflect the indirect influences of seizure-related respiratory disturbances and hypoxia (Lathers et al. 2008), with prone position during sleep a possible factor (Kloster and Engelskjøn 1999). The facts that neural influences play a major role in the stability of heart rhythm and that a number of indicators of autonomic function reveal significant alterations provide a basis for considering the important role of neural triggering of cardiac arrhythmias during epileptic seizures as a factor in SUDEP (Devinsky 2004). Increased cardiac sympathetic nerve activity during a seizure is indicated by surges in heart rates to above 150 beats/min (Blumhardt et al. 1986; Drake et al. 1993; Opherk et al. 2002; Nei et al. 2004; Rugg-Gunn et al. 2004; Moseley et al. 2011, 2013) that persist after the event (Surges et al. 2010b) and by heart rate variability (HRV) analysis (Kenneback et al. 1997; Massetani et al. 1997; Drake et al. 1998; Ansakorpi et al. 2002; Evrengul et al. 2005; Ronkainen et al. 2006; Persson et al. 2005, 2007; Mukherjee et al. 2009; Sevcencu and Struijk 2010; DeGiorgio et al. 2010; Toth et al. 2010; Strzelczyk et al. 2011; Yildiz et al. 2011; Brotherstone and McLellan 2012; Poh et al. 2012; Lotufo et al. 2012; Ponnusamy et al. 2012).

The hyperadrenergic state associated with seizures (Moseley et al. 2013) constitutes a major component of arrhythmia risk, as it is capable not only of directly triggering rhythm disturbances but also of promoting cardiac pathology including myocardial fibrosis (Natelson et al. 1998; Kloster and Engelskjøn 1999; Stollberger and Finsterer 2004; P-Codrea Tigaran et al. 2005) (Figure 14.2) and degeneration in up to 33% of cases as well as left atrial enlargement (Ramadan et al. 2013), which could constitute a vulnerable myocardial substrate for atrial and ventricular arrhythmia. Autopsy investigations have revealed that hearts of SUDEP victims were characteristically dilated and heavier than expected (Falconer and Rajs 1976; Leestma et al. 1989). The changes have been

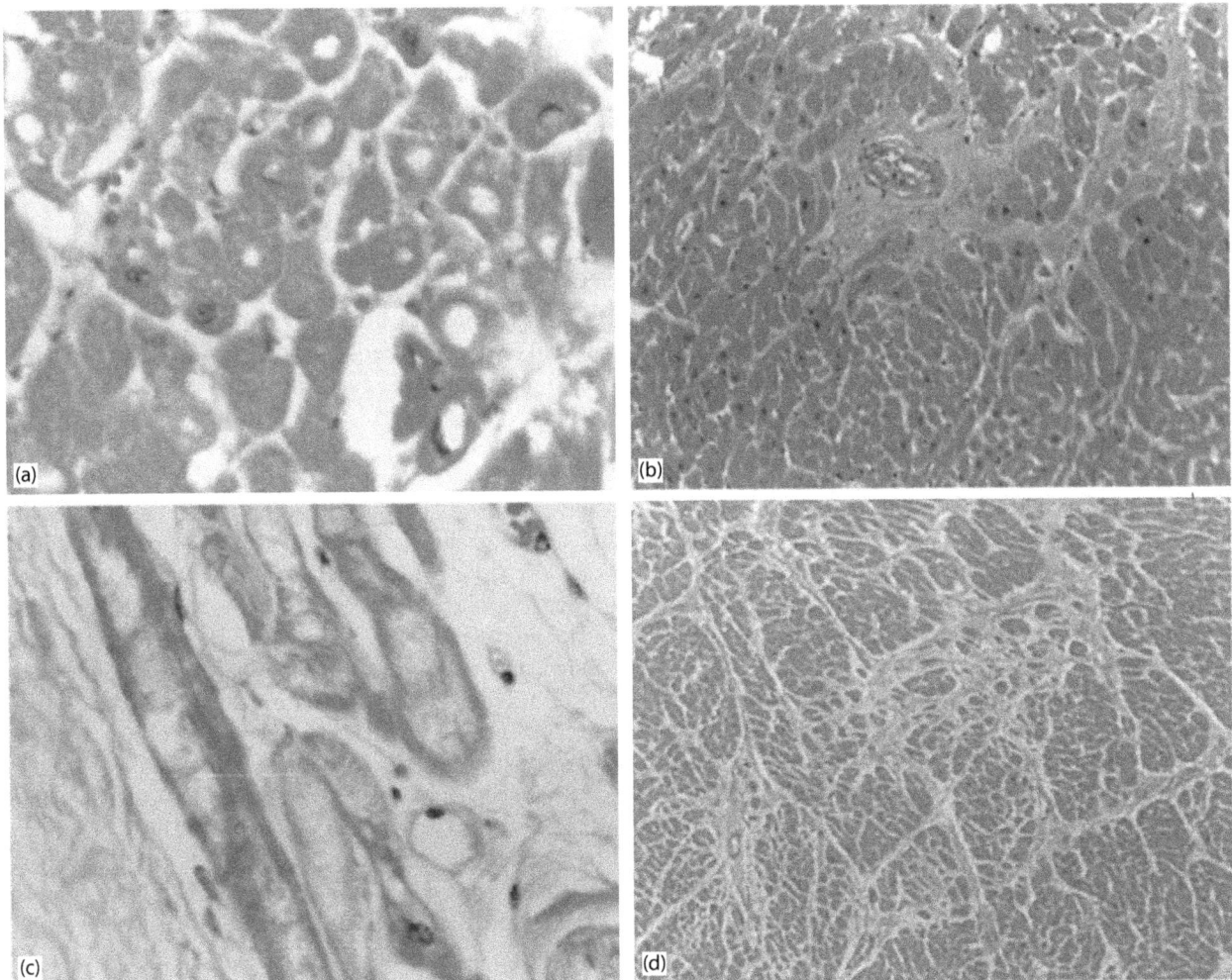

**FIGURE 14.2** Reversible (a, b) and irreversible (c, d) pathologic conditions found at autopsy in patients with epilepsy who died suddenly. (a) Myocytes with vacuolization; note in lower right the nucleus being displaced by vacuole (original magnification × 400). (b) Several longitudinally cut myocytes showing areas of vacuolization (original magnification × 400). (c) Diffuse interstitial fibrosis with multiple areas of myocyte replacement by connective tissue (original magnification × 40). (d) Perivascular fibrosis (original magnification × 100). All specimens were stained with hematoxylin–eosin. (From Natelson, BH et al., *Arch Neurol*, 55, 857–860, 1998. With permission.)

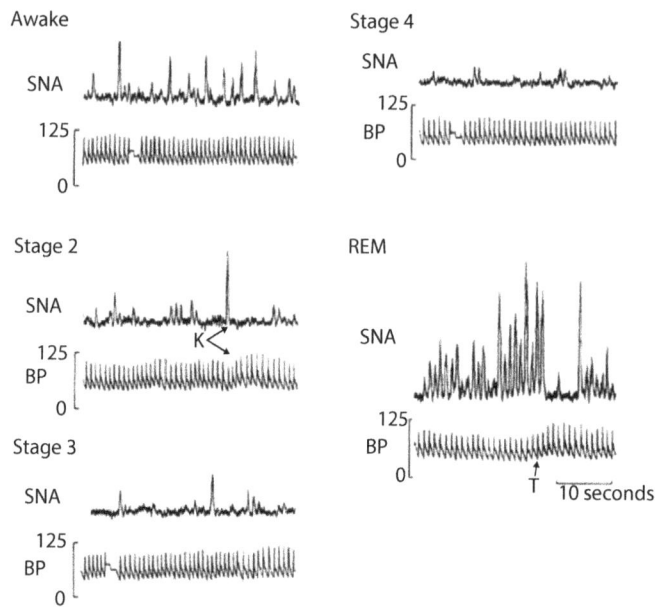

**FIGURE 14.3** Recordings of sympathetic nerve activity (SNA) and mean blood pressure (BP) in a single subject while awake and while in stages 2, 3, 4, and rapid eye movement sleep. As nonrapid eye movement sleep deepened (stages 2 through 4), SNA gradually decreased and BP (measured in millimeters of mercury) and variability in BP were gradually reduced. Arousal stimuli elicited K complexes on the electroencephalogram (not shown), which were accompanied by increases in SNA and BP (indicated by the arrows, stage 2 sleep). In contrast to the changes during nonrapid eye movement sleep, heart rate, BP, and blood pressure variability increased during rapid eye movement sleep, together with a profound increase in both the frequency and the amplitude of SNA. There was a frequent association between rapid eye movement twitches (momentary periods of restoration of muscle tone, denoted by T on the tracing) and abrupt inhibition of sympathetic nerve discharge and increases in BP. (From Somers, VK et al., *N Engl J Med*, 328, 303–307, 1993. With permission.)

attributed to repeated hypoxemia (Blum et al. 2000; Moseley et al. 2013) and/or increased catecholamine levels (Falconer and Rajs 1976; Natelson et al. 1998). Increased serum levels of cardiac troponin I, indicative of myocardial injury, have been documented following uncomplicated epileptic seizures (Hajsadeghi et al. 2009). The incidence of myocardial infarction is greater in patients with epilepsy than in the general population (Annegers et al. 1984; Janszky et al. 2009). Janszky et al. (2009) documented a 4.83-fold increased risk (95% confidence interval [CI], 1.62–14.43) of myocardial infarction in patients with epilepsy after multivariable correction for age, sex, hospital characteristics, education, and established risk factors including diabetes, smoking, hypertension, physical inactivity, obesity, cholesterol, etc.

Ventricular fibrillation has been reported in association with seizures in a number of SUDEP and near-SUDEP cases, despite the evanescence of the arrhythmia and the necessity of active ECG monitoring required for this diagnosis (Bruce and Kluge 1971; Smith and Vieweg 1974; Shaw 1981; Dasheiff and Dickinson 1986; Swallow et al. 2002; Espinosa et al. 2009; Ferlisi et al. 2013; Hocker et al. 2013). Bardai et al. (2012) recently reported the results of the community-based Amsterdam Resuscitation Studies that a diagnosis of epilepsy increased risk for sudden cardiac arrest by threefold (adjusted odds ratio [OR] 2.9 [95% CI 1.1–8.0.], $p = 0.034$) over the general population.

SUDEP often occurs at night (Shorvon and Tomson 2011). Several investigators (Nashef et al. 1996; Walker and Fish 1997; Langan et al. 2000; Eriksson 2011; Devinsky 2011; Li

et al. 2012; Derry and Duncan 2013; Ryvlin et al. 2013) have attributed SUDEP to central or obstructive sleep apnea, which is a risk factor for cardiac mortality (Gami et al. 2005). It is also likely that adrenergic factors play a direct role as higher maximum heart rates and tachycardia associated with seizures are indicative of heightened adrenergic activity and are more frequent during sleep in SUDEP victims by comparison with other patients with epilepsy (Nei et al. 2004; Shorvon and Tomson 2011). This profile suggests a link to sleep-state-related autonomic activity (Verrier and Harper 2010; Verrier and Josephson 2010; Verrier and Mittleman 2010). Although it is generally viewed that sleep is a protected state, bursts in cardiac sympathetic nerve activity have been reported in healthy individuals during rapid eye movement sleep (Somers et al. 1993) (Figure 14.3). These surges are concentrated in short, irregular periods, reach levels higher than during wakefulness, trigger intermittent increases in heart rate and blood pressure, and have been implicated in nocturnal ventricular arrhythmias and myocardial ischemia (Kales and Kales 1970). Investigators have reported variable findings regarding HRV indicators of vagus nerve tone during sleep in patients with epilepsy (Ronkainen et al. 2006; Persson et al. 2007; Surges et al. 2009).

## NEUROCIRCUITRY OF CARDIAC RHYTHM CONTROL

Regulation of cardiac neural activity is highly integrated and is achieved by circuitry at multiple levels (Figure 14.4). Higher brain centers operate through elaborate pathways

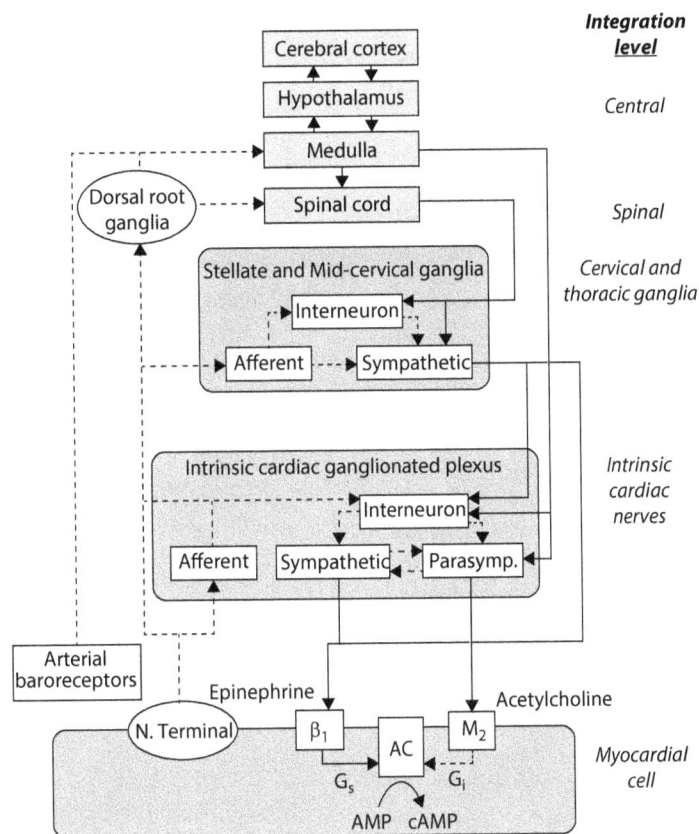

**FIGURE 14.4** Synthesis of new and present views on levels of integration important in neural control of cardiac electrical activity. More traditional concepts focused on afferent tracts (dashed lines) arising from myocardial nerve terminals and reflex receptors (e.g., baroreceptors) that are integrated centrally within hypothalamic and medullary cardiostimulatory and cardioinhibitory brain centers and on central modulation of sympathetic and parasympathetic outflow (solid lines) with little intermediary processing at the level of the spinal cord and within cervical and thoracic ganglia. More recent views incorporate additional levels of intricate processing within the extraspinal cervical and thoracic ganglia and within the cardiac ganglionic plexus, where recently described interneurons are envisioned to provide new levels of noncentral integration. Release of neurotransmitters from postganglionic sympathetic neurons is believed to enhance excitation in the sinoatrial node and myocardial cells through norepinephrine binding to beta1-receptors, which enhances adenyl cyclase (AC) activity through intermediary stimulatory G-proteins (Gs). Increased parasympathetic outflow enhances postganglionic release and binding of acetylcholine to muscarinic (M2) receptors, and through coupled inhibitory G-proteins (Gi), inhibits cyclic AMP production (cAMP). The latter alters electrogenesis and pacemaking activity by affecting the activity of specific membrane Na, K, and Ca channels. New levels of integration are shown superimposed on previous views and are emphasized here to highlight new possibilities for intervention. (From Lathrop, DA and PM Spooner, *J Cardiovasc Electrophysiol*, 12, 841–844, 2001. With permission.)

between and within the hypothalamus and medullary cardiovascular regulatory sites. Baroreceptor mechanisms are integral to autonomic control of the cardiovascular system, as evidenced by HRV and baroreceptor sensitivity testing of both cardiac patients and healthy subjects. The intrinsic cardiac nerves and fat pads provide local neural coordination independent of higher brain centers (Armour 1999). Electrical remodeling of the myocardium by nerve degeneration and regrowth has been documented (Zhou et al. 2004). At the level of the myocardial cell, autonomic receptors influence G proteins to control ionic channels, pumps, and exchangers (Verrier and Antzelevitch 2004). Important aspects of neurocardiac interactions in ventricular arrhythmogenesis have been explored in rat models of epilepsy (Bealer et al., ch. 23; Naggar and Stewart, ch. 25). Clinical markers of arrhythmia vulnerability and autonomic parameters can be monitored

noninvasively during emotional and physical stressors as well as sleep states to identify individuals at heightened risk of lethal cardiac arrhythmias (Kovach et al. 2001; Kop et al. 2004; Lampert et al. 2009).

## AUTONOMIC MECHANISMS IN ARRHYTHMOGENESIS

### ADRENERGIC INFLUENCES

It is well established that adrenergic inputs constitute the primary neural trigger for arrhythmias (Verrier and Antzelevitch 2004). Activation of sympathetic nervous system structures, including the posterior hypothalamus or stellate ganglia, increases susceptibility to ventricular fibrillation. A striking surge in sympathetic nerve activity also occurs within a few minutes of induction of myocardial ischemia by left anterior descending coronary artery occlusion as documented by direct nerve recording in experimental animals (Lombardi et al. 1983). This enhancement in sympathetic nerve activity is associated with a marked increase in susceptibility to ventricular fibrillation, as evidenced by a fall in ventricular fibrillation threshold and by spontaneous occurrence of the arrhythmia. Stellectomy significantly blunts this occlusion-induced surge in vulnerability to ventricular fibrillation (Lombardi et al. 1983; Nearing et al. 1991).

Enhanced sympathetic nerve activity increases cardiac vulnerability in the normal and ischemic heart by complex processes. The major indirect effects include impairment of oxygen supply–demand ratio due to increased cardiac metabolic activity; alpha-adrenergically mediated coronary vasoconstriction, especially in vessels with damaged endothelium; and changes in preload and afterload. The direct arrhythmogenic effects on cardiac electrophysiologic function, which are primarily mediated through beta$_1$-adrenergic receptors, include derangements in impulse formation, conduction, repolarization alternans, and heterogeneity of repolarization (Han and Moe 1964; Janse and Wit 1989; Nearing and Verrier 2003). Increased levels of catecholamines stimulate beta-adrenergic receptors, which in turn alter adenylate cyclase activity and intracellular calcium flux (Opie 2004; Verrier et al. 2009). These effects are probably mediated by the cyclic nucleotide and protein kinase regulatory cascade, which can alter spatial heterogeneity of calcium transients and consequently provoke TWA and dispersion of repolarization. The effects of increased intracellular calcium, with the potential for overload and impaired intracellular calcium cycling by the sarcoplasmic reticulum may be compounded and become especially arrhythmogenic during concurrent myocardial ischemia, which further predisposes to intracellular calcium excess (Verrier et al. 2009).

Cardiac beta$_1$-adrenergic receptor blockade is capable of negating the profibrillatory effect of direct sympathetic nerve stimulation by an action at the neurocardiac effector junction. But cardiac beta$_2$-adrenergic receptors, which control vasodilation in the vasculature and bronchi (Brodde 1991), do not appear to play a significant role in modulating ventricular excitable properties.

## ALPHA-ADRENERGIC RECEPTORS

In the normal heart, alpha-adrenergic receptor stimulation or blockade does not appear to affect ventricular electrical stability, as evidenced by the fact that administration of an alpha-adrenergic agonist such as phenylephrine or methoxamine does not influence excitable properties when the pressor response is controlled to prevent reflex changes in autonomic tone (Kowey et al. 1983). In the setting of myocardial ischemia, alpha-adrenergic blockade may alleviate coronary vasoconstriction and reduce platelet aggregability. Thus, alpha-adrenergic receptor activity exerts direct actions not only on myocardial excitable properties but also on platelet aggregability and coronary hemodynamic function.

## SYMPATHETIC–PARASYMPATHETIC INTERACTIONS

Vagus nerve influences are contingent on the prevailing level of adrenergic tone. When sympathetic tone to the heart is augmented by thoracotomy, sympathetic nerve stimulation, myocardial ischemia, or catecholamine infusion, vagal activation exerts an antiarrhythmic effect. Vagus nerve stimulation is without effect on vulnerability to ventricular arrhythmias when adrenergic input to the heart is ablated by beta-adrenergic blockade, a phenomenon termed "accentuated antagonism" (Verrier and Antzelevitch 2004). The basis for this antagonism of adrenergic effects is presynaptic inhibition of norepinephrine release from nerve endings and a muscarinically mediated action at the second messenger level, which attenuates the response to catecholamines at receptor sites. Also, importantly, vagal influences provide indirect protection against ventricular fibrillation by reducing excess heart rates, which can otherwise increase the ischemic insult by critically compromising diastolic perfusion time during acute myocardial ischemia. However, beneficial effects of vagus nerve activity may be annulled if profound bradycardia and hypotension ensue.

## BAROREFLEXES AND ARRHYTHMIAS

The classic studies by Billman et al. (1982) drew attention to the importance of baroreceptor function in susceptibility to life-threatening arrhythmias associated with myocardial ischemia and infarction. In their initial investigations in canines, they demonstrated that the more brisk was the baroreflex response, the less vulnerable were the animals to ventricular fibrillation during myocardial ischemia superimposed on prior myocardial infarction. The protective effect of the baroreceptor mechanism has been linked primarily to the antifibrillatory influence of vagus nerve activity, which improves diastolic coronary perfusion, minimizing the ischemic insult from coronary artery occlusion. The importance of baroreceptor sensitivity was subsequently documented in human subjects in whom baroreceptor function was evaluated with the pressor agent phenylephrine. La Rovere et al. (1998) demonstrated that following myocardial infarction, patients were less likely to experience sudden cardiac death if their baroreceptor function was preserved.

## BEHAVIORAL STRESS AND ARRHYTHMIAS

Because epilepsy is associated with intense emotions such as anxiety and depression (Earnest et al 1992; Lathers and Schrader 2006), it is relevant to consider experimental evidence of the impact of behavioral state on vulnerability to cardiac arrhythmias. In early studies, we developed aversive behavioral conditioning paradigms and models eliciting natural emotions, notably anger and fear. Aversive conditioning of dogs in a Pavlovian sling with mild chest shock on 3 consecutive days resulted in a >30% reduction in the repetitive extrasystole threshold during subsequent exposure to the environment without shock. The same paradigm elicited a threefold increase in the occurrence of spontaneous ventricular fibrillation when coronary artery occlusion was carried out in the aversive sling compared to the nonaversive cage environment (Lown et al. 1973). In dogs recovering from myocardial infarction, exposure to the aversive environment consistently elicited ventricular tachycardia for several days during the healing process. After this time, the animals continued to exhibit signs of behavioral stress in the aversive environment but no longer experienced ventricular arrhythmias, indicating that the arousal state required an electrically unstable substrate for the induction of rhythm disturbances. The stress-induced increases in arrhythmia vulnerability were largely suppressed by beta-adrenergic receptor blockade with propranolol or metoprolol.

An experimental canine model was developed to emulate anger, which is the emotion most commonly associated with myocardial infarction and sudden death (Mittleman et al. 1995; Verrier and Mittleman 1996). A standardized food-access-denial paradigm provoked intense arousal and pronounced myocardial ischemia in territories of stenosed coronary vessels (Verrier et al. 1987). The anger-like state also elicited severe repolarization abnormalities conducive to life-threatening cardiac arrhythmias (Kovach et al. 2001).

## AMBULATORY ELECTROCARDIOGRAM-BASED TOOLS FOR THE EVALUATION OF AUTONOMIC FUNCTION

As noted above, several studies have indicated that epileptic seizures are associated with reduced HRV, indicative of a hyperadrenergic state. These findings are important because depressed HRV is associated with heightened risk for sudden cardiac death in patients with ischemic heart disease (Tulppo et al. 1996; Lombardi 2002). Lotufo et al. (2012) provided a meta-analysis of HRV studies in patients with epilepsy, which revealed that indicators of vagus nerve activity (high-frequency as well as time-domain measures) were consistently reduced in patients with epilepsy compared to matched healthy controls. Patients with well-controlled seizures who experienced <1 seizure/month also did not exhibit this reduction in high-frequency HRV, suggesting a role for repetitive seizures in HRV levels. In an exploratory study, DeGiorgio et al. (2010) reported that higher SUDEP scores (based on frequency and duration of epilepsy and multiple drug therapy) are associated with reduced vagus nerve activity based on HRV indicators.

Baroreceptor sensitivity is diminished in patients with epilepsy (Dutsch et al. 2006). Depression of this indicator of autonomic activity is associated with heightened risk for arrhythmias and can be noninvasively measured from ambulatory ECG by monitoring heart rate turbulence, which refers to fluctuations of sinus rhythm cycle length after a single ventricular premature beat. These effects are a direct function of baroreceptor responsiveness, since reflex activation of the vagus nerve controls the pattern of sinus rhythm. Several studies confirm that in low-risk patients with cardiovascular disease, after a ventricular premature beat, sinus rhythm exhibits a characteristic pattern of early acceleration and subsequent deceleration. By contrast, patients at high risk for cardiovascular events exhibit essentially a flat, nonvarying response to the ventricular premature beat, indicating inability to activate the vagus nerve and its cardioprotective effect. This method is an independent predictor of total mortality in patients with ischemic heart disease or heart failure (Schmidt et al. 1999; Bauer et al. 2008). Heart rate deceleration capacity is a related and even more comprehensive marker of autonomic control and may be of considerable clinical value in assessing overall autonomic regulation of the heart in patients with diverse types of cardiovascular disease (Bauer et al. 2006). Both heart rate turbulence and deceleration capacity could provide valuable insights into autonomic control in patients with epilepsy.

## AMBULATORY ELECTROCARDIOGRAM-BASED T-WAVE ALTERNANS TO ASSESS VULNERABILITY TO ARRHYTHMIAS AND RISK FOR SUDDEN CARDIAC DEATH

Extensive scientific evidence spanning more than a decade points to a fundamental link between TWA, a beat-to-beat fluctuation in the morphology of the T wave of the ECG, and susceptibility to malignant ventricular tachyarrhythmias (Verrier et al. 2009, 2011; Verrier and Ikeda 2013). This electrocardiographic phenomenon is an indicator of temporal–spatial heterogeneity of repolarization, a precondition for reentrant arrhythmias. TWA also detects derangements in intracellular calcium cycling, which is subject to the influences of both the autonomic nervous system and alterations in myocardial substrate, particularly ischemia and scar associated with infarction (Table 14.2). Similar mechanisms may operate in association with cardiac fibrosis, contraction band necrosis, or other types of myocardial injury that are known to occur in patients with epilepsy.

Diverse physiologic interventions have been shown to alter TWA magnitude in parallel with their influence on vulnerability to ventricular tachyarrhythmias. Specifically, these include elevations in heart rate, coronary artery occlusion and reperfusion, and sympathetic nerve stimulation (Nearing et al. 1991). In the chronically instrumented canine model developed to emulate anger (Verrier et al. 1987; Kovach et al. 2001), a pronounced increase in TWA was observed during behavioral arousal. A 3-minute period of coronary artery occlusion potentiated arrhythmia risk, more than doubling the magnitude of anger-induced TWA (Figure 14.5). The stress-related effects were significantly lessened by metoprolol, further implicating a major role of $beta_1$-adrenergic receptors in sympathetic nerve induction of cardiac vulnerability and TWA (Kovach et al. 2001). Vagus nerve stimulation, blockade of beta-adrenergic receptors, and sympathetic denervation, which reduce susceptibility to ventricular tachyarrhythmias, also decrease TWA magnitude (Verrier et al. 2009). These series of observations underscore

## TABLE 14.2
## Fundamental Concepts

• Basis for TWA's prediction is its reflection of the degree and extent of temporal–spatial heterogeneity of repolarization and perturbations in intracellular calcium handling.
• TWA is a trigger of arrhythmia as well as a marker of risk, as it sets the stage for unidirectional block and reentry and its containment is cardioprotective.
• TWA level indicates a continuum of risk for arrhythmic death that applies across disease states.
• TWA can serve as a target for therapy as it is within the causal pathway of arrhythmogenesis.
    –Medications or interventions that reduce TWA level also lower arrhythmia risk.
    –Conversely, proarrhythmic agents increase TWA.

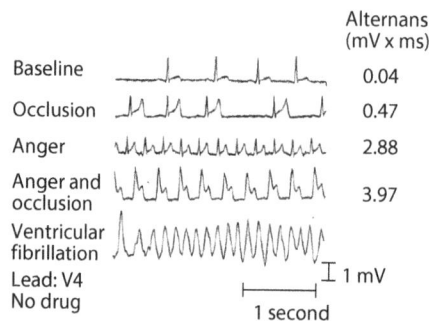

**FIGURE 14.5** Segments of electrocardiogram (ECG) tracings with measurements of maximum T-wave alternans (TWA) magnitude at baseline, during myocardial ischemia, during anger-like state, and with simultaneous anger-like state and myocardial ischemia in one dog that experienced ventricular fibrillation at 42 seconds after provocation of anger-like response was superimposed at 1 minute of coronary artery occlusion. (From Kovach, JA *J Am Coll Cardiol*, 37, 1719–1725, 2001. With permission.)

the fundamental link between TWA and vulnerability to lethal arrhythmias, which underlies the utility of this parameter in assessing propensity for life-threatening ventricular arrhythmias.

## CLINICAL EVIDENCE OF AMBULATORY ELECTROCARDIOGRAM-BASED T-WAVE ALTERNANS FOR THE PREDICTION OF SUDDEN CARDIAC DEATH

A time-domain method, termed Modified Moving Average analysis, was developed to quantify TWA during both routine exercise stress testing and ambulatory electrocardiographic monitoring (Nearing and Verrier 2002; Verrier et al 2011). The technique is based on the powerful noise rejection principle of recursive averaging (Figure 14.6), and respiration and motion artifacts have been further reduced by cubic alignment and other filters. Modified moving average analysis computes TWA level as the peak difference between A and B beats in an ABAB beat stream at any point between the J and T points of the ECG. This technique has been used in clinical studies enrolling >5000 patients that generated OR of 2.94 to 17.1 for cardiovascular death and 4.8 to 22.6 for sudden cardiac death (Verrier et al. 2011; Verrier and Ikeda 2013).

Ambulatory electrocardiographic monitoring of TWA was used to investigate the effects of physical activity (Verrier et al. 2003), circadian factors (Zanobetti et al. 2009), mental

stress (Kop et al. 2004; Lampert et al. 2009), and sleep states in arrhythmogenesis in patients with diverse conditions including myocardial ischemia, infarction, and heart failure (Verrier et al. 2011). Recently, in a prospective trial, Sakaki et al. (2009) demonstrated the remarkable predictive capacity of TWA in ambulatory ECGs to indicate risk for cardiovascular mortality and sudden cardiac death in patients with ischemic and nonischemic cardiomyopathy (Figures 14.7 and 14.8).

As mental stress has been implicated in seizure-induced risk, it is important to recognize that TWA has been shown to detect vulnerability to cardiac arrhythmias induced by mental arithmetic or anger recall in patients with implantable cardioverter defibrillators (ICDs). Kop et al. (2004) and Lampert et al. (2009) reported that during these routine challenges, patients with ICDs exhibited significant increases in TWA level compared to age-matched control subjects. Furthermore, Lampert et al. (2009) determined that the rise in TWA level appears to coincide with enhanced risk for life-threatening arrhythmias. Testing patients with epilepsy during simple mental tasks such as mental arithmetic could be used to disclose latent vulnerability to arrhythmias attributable to heightened adrenergic activity, behavioral state, or substrate changes, as manifest by elevated levels of TWA.

Strzelczyk et al. (2011) were the first investigators to report the effects of epilepsy on TWA. They found that patients with drug-resistant epilepsy exhibited significant increases in TWA to >140 μV for 15 minutes immediately following secondary generalized tonic–clonic seizures.

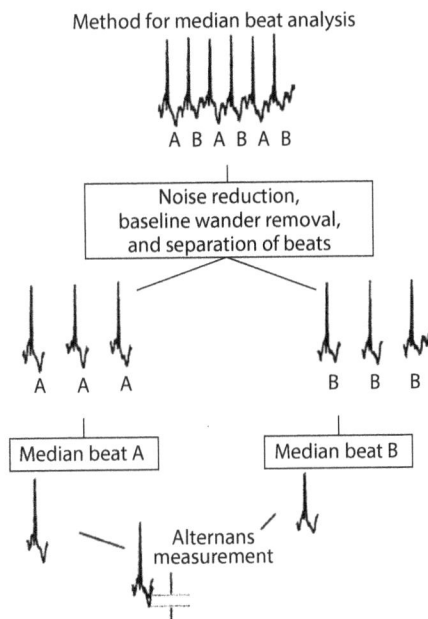

**FIGURE 14.6** Flow chart of the major components of the Modified Moving Average method of T-wave alternans analysis. The left ventricular endocardial ECG was obtained from a representative experiment in which coronary artery occlusion subsequently resulted in ventricular fibrillation. ECGs are filtered to reduce high frequency noise and to remove baseline wander. Ventricular and supraventricular premature beats as well as beats with a high noise level are removed. The even beats in the sequence are then assigned to Group A and the odd beats to Group B. Modified moving average computed beats of types A and B are computed continuously. The $n$th modified moving average computed beat is developed from the $n-1$th ECG beat and the $n-1$th modified moving average computed beat. The amplitude of the effect of any one heart beat on the modified moving average computed beat is also limited by the bounds on $\Delta A$ and $\Delta B$. The alternans estimate is determined as the maximum absolute difference between $A$ and $B$ modified moving average computed beats within the ST segment and T-wave region. The output period can be adjusted as desired. (From Nearing, BD and RL Verrier, *J Appl Physiol*, 92, 541–549, 2002. With permission.)

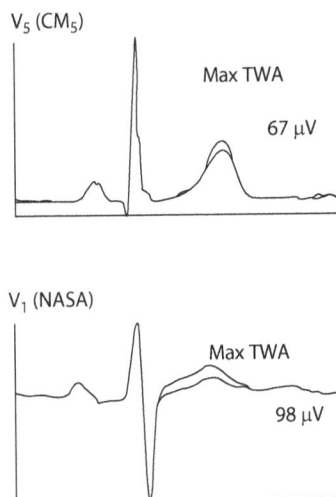

**FIGURE 14.7** An example of a positive Modified Moving Average (MMA) TWA test. Superimposed complexes from precordial leads V5 (CM5) and V1 (NASA) illustrate TWA. In this patient, TWA was determined to be positive because the peak TWA voltage was 98 μV in lead V1. (From Sakaki, K et al., *Heart Rhythm*, 6, 332–337, 2009. With permission.)

An HRV indicator of vagus nerve activity, namely, the standard deviation of N–N intervals (SDNN) declined in parallel. Furthermore, during preictal baseline, TWA was elevated to >70 μV in patients with either secondary generalized tonic–clonic seizures or complex partial seizures. This level of TWA is significantly greater than that exhibited by patients with cardiomyopathy (Sakaki et al. 2009) or by patients with cardiac disease who died suddenly (Verrier et al. 2003; Verrier and Ikeda 2013). This evidence of the prevalence of high levels of TWA in patients with epilepsy supports a role for cardiovascular mechanisms in SUDEP.

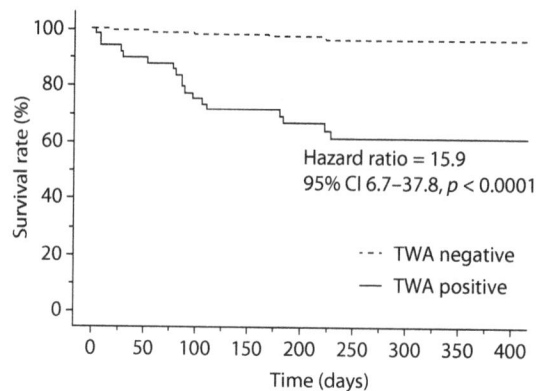

**FIGURE 14.8** Event-free curves for cardiac mortality using a peak TWA voltage from 24-hour ambulatory ECGs in either lead V1 or V5. (From Sakaki, K et al., *Heart Rhythm*, 6, 332–337, 2009. With permission.)

## VAGUS NERVE STIMULATION IN EPILEPSY

Experimentally, vagus nerve stimulation has been shown to protect against ventricular arrhythmias during myocardial ischemia. Myocardial infarction may damage nerve pathways by sustained reduction in supply of oxygen and nutrients to the nerve, thereby limiting its potential to be activated. SeizureZactivity causes local vasospasm and accumulation of microthrombi and could also thereby lead to impaired blood flow and damage to the nerve supply. Vanoli et al. (1991) demonstrated the antifibrillatory effect of vagus nerve stimulation during exercise-induced ischemia in canines with a healed myocardial infarction. Direct stimulation of the right cervical vagus nerve through a chronically implanted electrode at 15 seconds after onset of exercise-induced acute myocardial ischemia reduced the incidence of ventricular fibrillation by 92%. This effect was only partly due to the attendant heart rate reduction, as in half of the animals, the antiarrhythmic efficacy of vagus nerve stimulation persisted despite maintenance of constant heart rate by atrial pacing.

The potential for vagus nerve stimulation to elicit beneficial cardiac effects in patients with heart failure was recently explored by Schwartz et al. (2008), who demonstrated that this procedure is safe and well-tolerated, as indicated by some improvement in heart failure class and a decrease in left ventricular end-systolic volume. The exciting possibility that chronically implanted vagus nerve stimulation devices may suppress arrhythmias clinically remains to be explored. The potential for this form of therapy is underscored by the extensive experimental evidence and the clinical demonstration that vagomimetic maneuvers such as carotid sinus massage and administration of agents such as phenylephrine or edrophonium can terminate ventricular tachyarrhythmias (Waxman et al. 1994).

Vagus nerve stimulation has been approved by the Food and Drug Administration since 1997 for the adjunctive treatment of medically refractory partial seizures in patients over 12 years of age (Schachter 2009). Side effects related to stimulation are usually mild; include hoarseness, throat pain, coughing, shortness of breath, and tingling; and almost always resolve with adjustment in the stimulation settings. Although there are mixed reports of measurable autonomic effects of vagus nerve stimulation when used for epilepsy (Banzett et al. 1999; Binks et al. 2001; Schachter 2008; Wheeler et al. 2011), seizure rates were halved after >1 year of vagus nerve stimulation therapy from a rate of 1 per 150 person-years (Tomson et al. 2005; Englot et al. 2011; Elliott et al. 2011). Importantly, SUDEP rates were also halved after >2 years of treatment (Annegers et al. 2000). Therefore, the possibility exists but remains to be proven that vagus nerve stimulation may reduce cardiac arrhythmias and risk for sudden death, potentially mediated by the efferent cardiac vagus nerve (Vanoli et al. 1991; Verrier and Antzelevitch 2004; Schachter 2006). The capacity of vagus nerve stimulation to reduce TWA magnitude in patients with epilepsy (Schomer et al. 2014) provides additional evidence of its potential effectiveness in reducing SUDEP, as TWA magnitude is strongly associated with risk for cardiovascular death including sudden death (Verrier et al. 2011; Verrier and Ikeda 2013).

## CONCLUSIONS AND IMPLICATIONS

Extensive evidence implicates the interaction between autonomic factors and a vulnerable myocardial substrate in predisposing patients to life-threatening cardiac arrhythmias. Adrenergic influences constitute the primary trigger, and vagus nerve stimulation can antagonize the arrhythmogenic effect of catecholamines to exert a cardioprotective action. Recently, new ambulatory electrocardiographic tools have been developed to assess autonomic function and vulnerability to cardiac arrhythmias, namely, heart rate turbulence and TWA, respectively. Although these methodologies have been extensively tested in populations with ischemic and nonischemic heart disease, their use in patients with epilepsy has been limited. As it is likely that arrhythmic events result from an interaction between autonomic triggers and a vulnerable myocardial substrate, there is a great need for systematic longitudinal studies of ECG-based pathophysiologic markers including ST-segment changes, QRS interval duration, R-wave changes, and TWA to provide insights into the factors leading to SUDEP and to improve diagnosis and therapy in patients with epilepsy. The well-established capacity of TWA to indicate risk for lethal arrhythmias and cardiovascular mortality (Verrier et al. 2011; Verrier and Ikeda 2013) supports its use as a Cluster Identification variable in determining SUDEP mechanisms and potentially in patient management (Table 5.1).

Increasing use of implantable loop recorders in patients with epilepsy promises to expand the opportunity to understand disturbances in autonomic function and cardiac rhythm associated with ictal events (Zaidi et al. 2000; Rugg-Gunn et al. 2004; Ronkainen et al. 2006). Thus, in the future, these parameters could not only play a role in advancing our understanding of the underlying cardiac pathologies responsible for SUDEP but also enable evaluation of cardiac antiarrhythmic therapies as well as monitoring medical antiepileptic therapy for potential proarrhythmic effects. Such studies could lead to therapies designed to ameliorate cardiac effects of seizure.

Especially intriguing is the possibility that vagus nerve stimulation could not only reduce seizure activity but may also protect the heart, as activation of this neural pathway may be antiarrhythmic. Ambulatory ECG-based TWA can detect vagus nerve influences on vulnerability to arrhythmias, providing a tool for quantification of the potential cardioprotective effect of this intervention.

## DISCLOSURE

Dr. Verrier is coinventor of the Modified Moving Average method of T-wave alternans analysis, with patent assigned to Georgetown University and Beth Israel Deaconess Medical Center and licensed to GE Healthcare, Inc., and Medtronic, Inc.

## REFERENCES

Annegers JF, Coan SP, Hauser WA, Leestma J. Epilepsy, vagal nerve stimulation by the NCP system, all-cause mortality, and sudden, unexpected, unexplained death. *Epilepsia* 2000;41:549–53.

Annegers JF, Hauser WA, Shirts SB. Heart disease mortality and morbidity in patients with epilepsy. *Epilepsia* 1984; 25:699–704.

Ansakorpi H, Korpelainen JT, Huikuri HV, Tolonen U, Myllyla VV, Isojarvi JI. Heart rate dynamics in refractory and well controlled temporal lobe epilepsy. *J Neurol Neurosurg Psychiatry* 2002;72:26–30.

Armour JA. Myocardial ischaemia and the cardiac nervous system. *Cardiovasc Res* 1999;41:41–54.

Banzett RB, Guz A, Paydarfar D, Shea SA, Schachter SC, Lansing RW. Cardiorespiratory variables and sensation during stimulation of the left vagus in patients with epilepsy. *Epilepsy Res* 1999;35:1–11.

Bardai A, Lamberts RJ, Blom MT, Spanjaart AM, Berdowski J, van der Staal SR, Brouwer HJ, Koster RW, Sander JW, Thijs RD, Tan HL. Epilepsy is a risk factor for sudden cardiac arrest in the general population. *PLoS One* 2012;7(8):e42749.

Bauer A, Kantelhardt JW, Barthel P, Schneider R, Mäkikallio T, Ulm K, Hnatkova K, et al. Deceleration capacity of heart rate as a predictor of mortality after myocardial infarction: Cohort study. *Lancet* 2006;367:1674–81.

Bauer A, Malik M, Schmidt G, Barthel P, Bonnemeier H, Cygankiewicz I, Guzik P, et al. Heart rate turbulence: Standards of measurement, physiological interpretation, and clinical use: International

Society for Holter and Noninvasive Electrocardiology Consensus. *J Am Coll Cardiol* 2008;52:1353–65.

Billman GE, Schwartz PJ, Stone HL. Baroreceptor reflex control of heart rate: A predictor of sudden cardiac death. *Circulation* 1982;66:874–80.

Binks AP, Paydarfar D. Schachter SC, Guz A, Banzett RB. High strength stimulation of the vagus nerve in awake humans: A lack of cardiorespiratory effects. *Respirat Physiol* 2001;127:125–33.

Blum AS, Ives JR, Goldberger AL, Al-Aweel IC, Krishnamurthy KB, Drislane FW, Schomer DL. 2000. Oxygen desaturations triggered by partial seizures: Implications for cardiopulmonary instability in epilepsy. *Epilepsia* 41:536–41.

Blumhardt LD, Smith PEM, Owen L. Electrocardiographic accompaniments of temporal lobe epileptic seizures. *Lancet* 1986;8489:1051–6.

Brodde O-E. Beta$_1$- and beta$_2$-adrenoceptors in the human heart: Properties, function and alterations in chronic heart failure. *Pharmacol Rev* 1991;43:203–42.

Brotherstone R, Blackhall B, McLellan A. Lengthening of corrected QT during epileptic seizures. *Epilepsia* 2010;51:221–32.

Brotherstone R, McLellan A. Parasympathetic alteration during sub-clinical seizures. *Seizure* 2012;21:391–8.

Bruce RA, Kluge W. Defibrillatory treatment of exertional cardiac arrest in coronary disease. *JAMA* 1971; 216:653–8.

Dasheiff RM, Dickinson LJ. Sudden unexpected death of epileptic patient due to cardiac arrhythmia after seizure. *Arch Neurol* 1986; 43:194–6.

DeGiorgio CM, Miller P, Meymandi S, Chin A, Epps J, Gordon S, Gornbein J, Harper RM. RMSSD, a measure of vagus-mediated heart rate variability, is associated with risk factors for SUDEP: The SUDEP-7 inventory. *Epilepsy Behav* 2010;19:78–81.

Derry CP, Duncan S. Sleep and epilepsy. *Epilepsy Behav* 2013;26:394–404.

Devinsky O. Effects of seizures on autonomic and cardiovascular function. *Epilepsy Curr* 2004;4:43–6.

Devinsky O. Sudden unexpected death in epilepsy. *N Engl J Med* 2011;365:1801–11.

Drake ME, Andrews JM, Castleberry CM, Drake ME Jr. Electrophysiologic assessment of autonomic function in epilepsy. *Seizure* 1998;7:91–6.

Drake ME, Reider CR, Kay A. Electrocardiography in epilepsy patients without cardiac symptoms. *Seizure* 1993;2:63–5.

Dutsch M, Hilz MJ, Devinsky O. Impaired baroreflex function in temporal lobe epilepsy. *J Neurol* 2006;253:1300–8.

Earnest MP, Thomas GE, Eden RA, Hossack KF. The sudden unexplained death syndrome in epilepsy: Demographic, clinical, and postmortem features. *Epilepsia* 1992;33:310–6.

Elliott RE, Morsi A, Kalhorn SP, Marcus J, Sellin J, Kang M, Silverberg A, Rivera E, Geller E, Carlson C, Devinsky O, Doyle WK. Vagus nerve stimulation in 436 consecutive patients with treatment-resistant epilepsy: Long-term outcomes and predictors of response. *Epilepsy Behav* 2011;20:57–63.

Englot DJ, Chang EF, Auguste KI. Vagus nerve stimulation for epilepsy: A meta-analysis of efficacy and predictors of response. *J Neurosurg* 2011;115:1248–55.

Eriksson SH. Epilepsy and sleep. *Curr Opin Neurol* 2011;24:171–6.

Espinosa PS, Lee JW, Tedrow UB, Bromfield EB, Dworetzky BA. Sudden unexpected near death in epilepsy: Malignant arrhythmia from a partial seizure. *Neurology* 2009;72:1702–3.

Evrengul H, Tanriverdi H, Dursunoglu D, Kaftan A, Kuru O, Unlu U, Kilic M, et al. Time and frequency domain analyses of heart rate variability in patients with epilepsy. *Epilepsy Res* 2005;63:131–9.

Falconer B, Rajs J. Postmortem findings of cardiac lesions in epileptics: A preliminary report. *Forensic Sci* 1976;8:63–71.

Ferlisi M, Tomei R, Carletti M, Moretto G, Zanoni T. Seizure induced ventricular fibrillation: A case of near-SUDEP. *Seizure* 2013;22:249–51.

Gami AS, Howard DE, Olson EJ, Somers VK. Day-night pattern of sudden death in obstructive sleep apnea. *N Engl J Med* 2005;352:1206–14.

Glasscock E. Genomic biomarkers of SUDEP in brain and heart. *Epilepsy Behav* 2013; pii:S1525-5050(13)00485-X.

Glasscock E, Yoo JW, Chen TT, Klassen TL, Noebels JL. Kv1.1 potassium channel deficiency reveals brain-driven cardiac dysfunction as a candidate mechanism for sudden unexplained death in epilepsy. *J Neurosci* 2010;30:5167–75.

Hajsadeghi S, Afsharian S, Fereshtehnejad SM, Keramati MR, Mollahoseini R. Serum levels of cardiac troponin I in patients with uncomplicated epileptic seizure. *Arch Med Res* 2009;40:24–8.

Han J, Moe G. Nonuniform recovery of excitability in ventricular muscle. *Circ Res* 1964;14:44–60.

Hocker S, Prasad A, Rabinstein AA. Cardiac injury in refractory status epilepticus. *Epilepsia* 2013;54:518–22.

Jallon P. Mortality in patients with epilepsy. *Curr Opin Neurol* 2004;17:141–6.

Janse MJ, Wit AL. Electrophysiological mechanisms of ventricular arrhythmias resulting from myocardial ischemia and infarction. *Physiol Rev* 1989;69:1049–169.

Janszky I, Hallqvist J, Tomson T, Ahlbom A, Mukamal KJ, Ahnve S. Increased risk and worse prognosis of myocardial infarction in patients with prior hospitalization for epilepsy—The Stockholm Heart Epidemiology Program. *Brain* 2009;132(Pt 10):2798–804.

Johnson JN, Hofman N, Haglund CM, Cascino GD, Wilde AAM, Ackerman MJ. Identification of a possible pathogenic link between congenital long QT syndrome and epilepsy. *Neurology* 2009;72:224–231.

Johnson JN, Tester DJ, Bass NE, Ackerman MJ. Cardiac channel molecular autopsy for sudden unexpected death in epilepsy. *J Child Neurol* 2010;25:916–21.

Josephson CB, Rahey S, Sadler RM. Neurocardiogenic syncope: Frequency and consequences of its misdiagnosis as epilepsy. *Can J Neurol Sci* 2007;34: 221–4.

Kales A, Kales JD. Evaluation, diagnosis, and treatment of clinical conditions related to sleep. *JAMA* 1970;213:2229–32.

Kenneback G, Ericson M, Tomson T, Bergfeldt L. Changes in arrhythmia profile and heart rate variability during abrupt withdrawal of antiepileptic drugs. Implications for sudden death. *Seizure* 1997;6:369–75.

Kloster R, Engelskjøn T. Sudden unexpected death in epilepsy (SUDEP): A clinical perspective and a search for risk factors. *J Neurol Neurosurg Psychiatry* 1999;67:439–44.

Kop WJ, Krantz DS, Nearing BD, Gottdiener JS, Quigley JF, O'Callahan M, DelNegro AA, et al. Effects of acute mental stress and exercise on T-wave alternans in patients with implantable cardioverter defibrillators and controls. *Circulation* 2004;109:1864–9.

Kovach JA, Nearing BD, Verrier RL. An angerlike behavioral state potentiates myocardial ischemia-induced T-wave alternans in canines. *J Am Coll Cardiol* 2001;37:1719–25.

Kowey PR, Verrier RL, Lown B. Effect of alpha-adrenergic receptor stimulation on ventricular electrical properties in the normal canine heart. *Am Heart J* 1983;105:366–71.

La Rovere MT, Bigger JT Jr., Marcus FI, Mortara A, Schwartz PJ. Baroreflex sensitivity and heart-rate variability in prediction of total cardiac mortality after myocardial infarction. ATRAMI (Autonomic Tone and Reflexes after Myocardial Infarction) Investigators. *Lancet* 1998;351:478–84.

Lampert R, Shusterman V, Burg M., McPherson C, Batsford W, Goldberg A, Soufer R. Anger-induced T-wave alternans predicts future ventricular arrhythmias in patients with implantable cardioverter-defibrillators. *J Am Coll Cardiol* 2009;53:774–8.

Langan Y, Nashef L, Sander JW. Sudden unexpected death in epilepsy: A series of witnessed deaths. *J Neurol Neurosurg Psychiatry* 2000;68:211–3.

Langan Y, Nashef L, Sander JW. Case-control study of SUDEP. *Neurology* 2005;64:1131–3.

Lathers CM, Schrader PL. Stress and sudden death. *Epilepsy Behav* 2006;9:236–42.

Lathers CM, Schrader PL, Bungo MW. The mystery of sudden death: Mechanisms for risks. *Epilepsy Behav* 2008;12:3–24.

Lathrop DA, Spooner PM. On the neural connection. *J Cardiovasc Electrophysiol* 2001;12:841–4.

Leestma JE, Kalelkar MB, Teas SS, Jay GW, Hughes JR. Sudden unexpected death associated with seizures: Analysis of 66 cases. *Epilepsia* 1984;25:84–8.

Leestma JE, Walczak T, Hughes JR, Kalelkar MB, Teas SS. A prospective study on sudden unexpected death in epilepsy. *Ann Neurol* 1989;26:195–203.

Leutmezer F, Schernthaner C, Lurger S, Potzelberger K, Baumgartner C. Electrocardiographic changes at the onset of epileptic seizures. *Epilepsia* 2003;44:348–54.

Li P, Ghadersohi S, Jafari B, Teter B, Sazgar M. Characteristics of refractory vs. medically controlled epilepsy patients with obstructive sleep apnea and their response to CPAP treatment. *Seizure* 2012;21:717–21.

Linzer M, Grubb BP, Ho S, Ramakrishnan L, Bromfield E, Estes NA. Cardiovascular causes of loss of consciousness in patients with presumed epilepsy: A cause of the increased sudden death rate in people with epilepsy? *Am J Med* 1994;96:146–54.

Lombardi F. Clinical implications of present physiological understanding of HRV components. *Card Electrophysiol Rev* 2002;6:245–9.

Lombardi F, Verrier RL, Lown B. Relationship between sympathetic neural activity, coronary dynamics, and vulnerability to ventricular fibrillation during myocardial ischemia and reperfusion. *Am Heart J* 1983;105:958-65.

Lotufo PA, Valiengo L, Bensenor IM, Brunoni AR. A systematic review and meta-analysis of heart rate variability in epilepsy and antiepileptic drugs. *Epilepsia* 2012;53:272–82.

Lown B, Verrier RL, Corbalan R. Psychologic stress and threshold for repetitive ventricular response. *Science* 1973;182:834-6.

Massetani R, Strata G, Galli R, Gori S, Gneri C, Limbruno U, Di Santo D, Mariani M, Murri L. Alteration of cardiac function in patients with temporal lobe epilepsy: Different roles of EEG-ECG monitoring and spectral analysis of RR variability. *Epilepsia* 1997;38:363–9.

Mittleman MA, Maclure M, Sherwood JB, Mulry RP, Tofler GH, Jacobs SC, Friedman R, Benson H, Muller JE. Triggering of acute myocardial infarction onset by episodes of anger. *Circulation* 1995;92:1720–5.

Moseley B, Bateman L, Millichap JJ, Wirrell E, Panayiotopoulos CP. Autonomic epileptic seizures, autonomic effects of seizures, and SUDEP. *Epilepsy Behav* 2013;26:375–85.

Moseley BD, Wirrell EC, Nickels K, Johnson JN, Ackerman MJ, Britton J. Electrocardiographic and oximetric changes during partial complex and generalized seizures. *Epilepsy Res* 2011;95:237–45.

Mukherjee S, Tripathi M, Chandra PS, Yadav R, Choudhary N, Sagar R, Bhore R, Pandey RM, Deepak KK. Cardiovascular autonomic functions in well-controlled and intractable partial epilepsies. *Epilepsy Res* 2009;85:261–9.

Nashef L, Walker F, Allen P, Sander JW, Shorvon SD, Fish DR. Apnoea and bradycardia during epileptic seizures: Relation to sudden death in epilepsy. *J Neurol Neurosurg Psychiatry* 1996;60:297–300.

Natelson BH, Suarez RV, Terrence CF, Turizo R. Patients with epilepsy who die suddenly have cardiac disease. *Arch Neurol* 1998;55:857–860.

Nearing BD, Huang AH, Verrier RL. Dynamic tracking of cardiac vulnerability by complex demodulation of the T-wave. *Science* 1991;252:437–40.

Nearing BD, Verrier RL. Modified moving average method for T-wave alternans analysis with high accuracy to predict ventricular fibrillation. *J Appl Physiol* 2002;92:541–9.

Nearing BD, Verrier RL. Tracking heightened cardiac electrical instability by computing interlead heterogeneity of T-wave morphology. *J Appl Physiol* 2003;95:2265–72.

Nei M, Ho RT, Abou-Khalil BW, Drislane FW, Liporace J, Romeo A, Sperling MR. EEG and ECG in sudden unexplained death in epilepsy. *Epilepsia* 2004;45:338–45.

Nei M, Ho RT, Sperling MR. EKG abnormalities during partial seizures in refractory epilepsy. *Epilepsia* 2000;41:542–8.

Opeskin K, Thomas A, Berkovic SF. Does cardiac conduction pathology contribute to sudden unexpected death in epilepsy? *Epilepsy Res* 2000;40:17–24.

Opherk C, Coromilas J, Hirsch LJ. Heart rate and EKG changes in 102 seizures: Analysis of influencing factors. *Epilepsy Res* 2002;52:117–27.

Opie LH. *Heart physiology: From Cell to Circulation*, 4th edition. Philadelphia, PA: Lippincott Williams and Wilkins; 2004.

Partemi S, Cesale S, Pezzella M, Campuzano O, Paravidino R, Pascali VL, Zara F, et al. Loss-of-function KCNH2 mutation in a family with long QT syndrome, epilepsy, and sudden death. *Epilepsia* 2013;54:e112–6.

P-Codrea Tigaran S, Dalager-Pedersen S, Baandrup U, Dam M, Vesterby-Charles A. Sudden unexpected death in epilepsy: Is death by seizures a cardiac disease? *Am J Forensic Med Pathol* 2005;26:99–105.

Persson H, Kumlien E, Ericson M, Tomson T. Preoperative heart rate variability in relation to surgery outcome in refractory epilepsy. *Neurology* 2005;65:1021–5.

Persson H, Kumlien E, Ericson M, Tomson T. Circadian variation in heart-rate variability in localization-related epilepsy. *Epilepsia* 2007;48:917–22.

Petkar S, Hamid T, Iddon P, Clifford A, Rice N, Claire R, McKee D, Curtis N, Cooper P, Fitzpatrick AP. Prolonged implantable electrocardiographic monitoring indicates a high rate of misdiagnosis of epilepsy—REVISE study. *Europace* 2012;14:1653–60.

Poh M-Z, Loddenkemper T, Reinsberger C, Swenson NC, Goyal S, Madsen JR, Picard RW. Autonomic changes with seizures correlate with postictal EEG suppression. *Neurology* 2012;78:1868–76.

Ponnusamy A, Marques JL, Reuber M. Comparison of heart rate variability parameters during complex partial seizures and psychogenic nonepileptic seizures. *Epilepsia* 2012;53:1314–21.

Ramadan M, El-Shahat NA, Omar A. Gomaa M, Belal T, A Sakr S, Abu-Hegazy M, Hakim H, A Selim H, A Omar S. Interictal electrocardiographic and echocardiographic changes in patients with generalized tonic-clonic seizures. *Int Heart J* 2013;54:171–5.

Reddy PR, Reinier K, Singh T, Mariani R, Gunson K, Jui J, Chugh SS. Physical activity as a trigger of sudden cardiac arrest: The Oregon Sudden Unexpected Death Study. *Int J Cardiol* 2009;131:345-9.

Rocamora R, Kurthen M, Lickfett L, von Oertzen J, Elger CE. Cardiac asystole in epilepsy: Clinical and neurophysiologic features. *Epilepsia* 2003;44:179–85.

Ronkainen E, Korpelainen JT, Heikkinen E. Myllylä VV, Huikuri HV, Isojärvi JI. Cardiac autonomic control in patients with refractory epilepsy before and during vagus nerve stimulation treatment: A one-year follow-up study. *Epilepsia* 2006;47:556–62.

Rossenbacker T, Nuyens D, Van Paesschen W, Heidbuchel H. Epilepsy? Video monitoring of long QT syndrome-related aborted sudden death. *Heart Rhythm* 2007;4:1366–7.

Rugg-Gunn FJ, Simister RJ, Squirrell M, Holdright DR, Duncan JS. Cardiac arrhythmias in focal epilepsy: A prospective long-term study. *Lancet* 2004;364 (9452):2212–9.

Ryvlin P, Montavont A, Kahane P. Sudden unexpected death in epilepsy: From mechanisms to prevention. *Curr Opin Neurol* 2006;19:194–9.

Ryvlin P, Nashef L, Lhatoo SD, Bateman LM, Bird J, Bleasel A, Boon P, et al. Incidence and mechanisms of cardiorespiratory arrests in epilepsy monitoring units (MORTEMUS): A retrospective study. *Lancet Neurol* 2013;12:966–77.

Sakaki K, Ikeda T, Miwa Y. Miyakoshi M, Abe A, Tsukada T, Ishiguro H, Mera H, Yusu S, Yoshino H. Time-domain T-wave alternans measured from Holter electrocardiograms predicts cardiac mortality in patients with left ventricular dysfunction: A prospective study. *Heart Rhythm* 2009;6:332–7.

Schachter SC. Therapeutic effects of vagus nerve stimulation in epilepsy and implications for sudden unexpected death in epilepsy. *Clin Auton Res* 2006;16:29–32.

Schachter SC. Review of "Effects of vagus nerve stimulation on cardiovascular regulation in patients with epilepsy." *Journal Watch: Neurology* 2008;10:52.

Schachter SC. Vagal nerve stimulation. In: Shorvon S, Perucca E, J. Engle, editors. *The Treatment of Epilepsy*, 3rd edition. London, UK: Blackwell Publishing; 2009, pp. 1017–23.

Scheepers B, Clough P, Pickles C. The misdiagnosis of epilepsy: Findings of a population study. *Seizure* 1998;7:403–6.

Schmidt G, Malik M, Barthel P. Schneider R, Ulm K, Rolnitzky L, Camm AJ, Bigger JT Jr., Schömig A. Heart-rate turbulence after ventricular premature beats as a predictor of mortality after acute myocardial infarction. *Lancet* 1999;353:1390–6.

Schomer AC, Nearing BD, Schachter SC, Verrier RL. Vagus nerve stimulation reduces cardiac electrical instability assessed by quantitative T-wave alternans analysis in patients with drug-resistant focal epilepsy. *Epilepsia*, in press. doi: 10.1111/epi.12855.

Schwartz PJ, De Ferrari G, Sanzo A, Landolina M, Rordorf R, Raineri C, Campana C, Revera M, Ajmone-Marsan N, Tavazzi L, Odero A. Long term vagal stimulation in patients with advanced heart failure: First experience in man. *Eur J Heart Failure* 2008;10:884–91.

Sevcencu C, Struijk JJ. Autonomic alterations and cardiac changes in epilepsy. *Epilepsia* 2010;51:725–37.

Shaw TR. Recurrent ventricular fibrillation associated with normal QT intervals. *Q J Med* 1981;50:451–62.

Shorvon S, Tomson T. Sudden unexpected death in epilepsy. *Lancet* 2011;378:2028–38.

Smith D, Defalla BA, Chadwick DW. The misdiagnosis of epilepsy and the management of refractory epilepsy in a specialist clinic. *Q J Med* 1999;92:15–23.

Smith DC, Vieweg VR. Acute transmural myocardial infarction. Its occurrence in a young man without demonstrable coronary artery disease. *JAMA* 1974;229:811–3.

Somers VK, Dyken ME, Mark AL, Abboud FM. Sympathetic nerve activity during sleep in normal subjects. *N Engl J Med* 1993;328:303–7.

Stollberger C, Finsterer J. Cardiorespiratory findings in sudden unexplained/unexpected death in epilepsy (SUDEP). *Epilepsy Res* 2004;59:51–60.

Strzelczyk A, Adjei P, Scott CA, Bauer S, Rosenow F, Walker MC, Surges R. Postictal increase in T-wave alternans after generalized tonic-clonic seizures. *Epilepsia* 2011;52:2112–7.

Surges R, Adjei P, Kallis C. Erhuero J, Scott CA, Bell GS, Sander JW, Walker MC. Pathologic cardiac repolarization in pharmacoresistant epilepsy and its potential role in sudden unexpected death in epilepsy: A case-control study. *Epilepsia* 2010a;51:233–42.

Surges R, Henneberger C, Adjei P, Scott CA, Sander JW, Walker MC. Do alterations in inter-ictal heart rate variability predict sudden unexpected death in epilepsy? *Epilepsy Res* 2009;87: 277–80.

Surges R, Scott CA, Walker MC. Enhanced QT shortening and persistent tachycardia after generalized seizures. *Neurology* 2010b;74:421–6.

Surges R, Taggart P, Sander JW, Walker MC. Too long or too short? New insights into abnormal cardiac repolarization in people with chronic epilepsy and its potential role in sudden unexpected death. *Epilepsia* 2010c;51:738–44.

Swallow RA, Hillier CE, Smith PE. Sudden unexplained death in epilepsy (SUDEP) following previous seizure-related pulmonary oedema: Case report and review of possible preventative treatment. *Seizure* 2002;11:446–8.

Tigaran S, Molgaard H, McClelland R, Dam M, Jaffe AS. Evidence of cardiac ischemia during seizures in drug refractory epilepsy patients. *Neurology* 2003;60:492–5.

Tigaran S, Rasmussen V, Dam M, Pedersen S, Hogenhaven H, Friberg B. ECG changes in epilepsy patients. *Acta Neurol Scand* 1997;96:72–5.

Tomson T, Walczak T, Sillanpaa M, Sander J. Sudden unexpected death in epilepsy: A review of incidence and risk factors. *Epilepsia* 2005;46(Suppl 11):54–61.

Toth V, Hejjel L, Fogarasi A, Gyimesi C, Orsi G, Szucs A, Kovacs N, Komoly S, Ebner A, Janszky J. Periictal heart rate variability analysis suggests long-term postictal autonomic disturbance in epilepsy. *Eur J Neurol* 2010;17:780–7.

Tu E, Bagnall RD, Duflou J, Semsarian C. Postmortem review and genetic analysis of sudden unexpected death in epilepsy (SUDEP) cases. *Brain Pathol* 2011;21:201–8.

Tulppo MP, Makikallio TH, Takala TES, Seppanen T, Huikuri HV. Quantitative beat-to-beat analysis of heart rate dynamics during exercise. *Am J Physiol* 1996;271:H244–52.

Vanoli E, De Ferrari GM, Stramba-Badiale M, Hull SS Jr., Foreman RD, Schwartz PJ. Vagal stimulation and prevention of sudden death in conscious dogs with a healed myocardial infarction. *Circ Res* 1991;68:147–81.

Venkataraman V, Wheless JW, Willmore LJ, Motookal H. Idiopathic cardiac asystole presenting as an intractable adult onset partial seizure disorder. *Seizure* 2001;10:359–64.

Verrier RL. Central nervous system modulation of cardiac rhythm. In: Rosen MR, Palti Y, eds. *Lethal Arrhythmias Resulting from Myocardial Ischemia and Infarction*. Boston, MA: Kluwer Academic Publishers; 1988, pp. 149–64.

Verrier RL, Antzelevitch CA. Autonomic aspects of arrhythmogenesis: The enduring and the new. *Curr Opin Cardiol* 2004;19:2–11.

Verrier RL, Hagestad EL, Lown B. Delayed myocardial ischemia induced by anger. *Circulation* 1987;75:249–54.

Verrier RL, Harper RM. Central and autonomic mechanisms regulating cardiovascular function. In: Kryger MH, Roth T, Dement WC, eds. *Principles and Practice of Sleep Medicine*, 5th edition. Philadelphia, PA: WB Saunders; 2010.

Verrier RL, Ikeda T. Ambulatory ECG-based T-wave alternans monitoring for risk assessment and guiding medical therapy: Mechanisms and clinical applications. *Prog Cardiovasc Dis* 2013;56:172–85.

Verrier RL, Josephson ME. Cardiac arrhythmogenesis during sleep: Mechanisms, diagnosis, and therapy. In: Kryger MH, Roth T, Dement WC, eds. *Principles and Practice of Sleep Medicine*, 5th edition. Philadelphia, PA: WB Saunders; 2010.

Verrier RL, Klingenheben T, Malik M, El-Sherif N, Exner D, Hohnloser S, Ikeda T, et al. Microvolt T-wave alternans: Physiologic basis, methods of measurement, and clinical utility. Consensus guideline by the International Society for Holter and Noninvasive Electrocardiology. *J Am Coll Cardiol* 2011;44:1309–24.

Verrier RL, Kumar K, Nearing BD. Basis for sudden cardiac death prediction by T-wave alternans from an integrative physiology perspective. *Heart Rhythm* 2009;6:416–22.

Verrier RL, Mittleman MA. Life-threatening cardiovascular consequences of anger in patients with coronary heart disease. *Cardiol Clin* 1996;14:289–307.

Verrier RL, Mittleman MA. Sleep-related cardiac risk. In: Kryger MH, Roth T, Dement WC, eds. *Principles and Practice of Sleep Medicine*, 5th edition. Philadelphia, PA: WB Saunders; 2010.

Verrier RL, Nearing BD, LaRovere MT, Pinna GD, Mittleman MA, Bigger JT, Schwartz PJ. for the ATRAMI Investigators. Ambulatory ECG-based tracking of T-wave alternans in post-myocardial infarction patients to assess risk of cardiac arrest or arrhythmic death. *J Cardiovasc Electrophysiol* 2003;14:705–11.

Walker F, Fish DR. Recording respiratory parameters in patients with epilepsy. *Epilepsia* 1997;38(11 Suppl):S41–2.

Waxman MB, Cameron D, Wald RW. Vagal activity and ventricular tachyarrhythmias. In: Levy MN, Schwartz PJ, eds. *Vagal Control of the Heart*. Mt. Kisco, NY: Futura; 1994, pp. 579–612.

Wheeler M, De Herdt V, Vonck K, Gilbert K, Manem S, Mackenzie T, Jobst B, et al. Efficacy of vagus nerve stimulation for refractory epilepsy among patient subgroups: A re-analysis using the Engel classification. *Seizure* 2011;20:331–5.

Yildiz GU, Dogan EA, Dogan U, Tokgoz OS, Ozdemir K, Genc BO, Ilhan N. Analysis of 24-hour heart rate variations in patients with epilepsy receiving antiepileptic drugs. *Epilepsy Behav* 2011;20:349–54.

Zaidi A, Clough P, Cooper P, Scheepers B, Fitzpatrick AP. Misdiagnosis of epilepsy: Many seizure-like attacks have a cardiovascular cause. *J Am Coll Cardiol*. 2000;36:181–4.

Zanobetti A, Stone PH, Speizer FE, Schwartz JD, Coull BA, Suh H, Nearing BD, Mittleman MA, Verrier RL, Gold DR. T-wave alternans, air pollution and traffic in high-risk subjects. *Am J Cardiol* 2009;104:665–70.

Zhou S, Chen LS, Miyauchi Y. Kar S, Kangavari S, Fishbein MC, Sharifi B, Chen PS. Mechanisms of cardiac nerve sprouting after myocardial infarction in dogs. *Circ Res* 2004;95:76–83.

Zijlmans M, Flanagan D, Gotman J. Heart rate changes and ECG abnormalities during epileptic seizures: Prevalence and definition of an objective clinical sign. *Epilepsia* 2002;43:847–54.

# 15 Patient Management Using Cluster Risk Factor Identifiers

*Claire M. Lathers, Steven C. Schachter, Paul L. Schraeder, and Braxton B. Wannamaker*

## CONTENTS

The risk of sudden unexpected death in epilepsy (SUDEP) in patients with epilepsy can be assessed in a number of ways, one of which is with the Cluster Risk Factor Identifiers, which were introduced in Chapters 4 and 5. A SUDEP Cluster Identifier (Cluster ID) is defined as a patient-specific combination of all known risk factors and postmortem examination, if performed. Cases may be SUDEP or patients with epilepsy thought to be at risk for death. Data from our risk factor method of classification and identification for SUDEP will be analyzed to assess, predict, prevent, or minimize risks for occurrence of SUDEP and to develop new pharmacological therapies and other preventive strategies.

## STEPS 1–5: STEPS TO CONSTRUCT INDIVIDUALIZED RISK FACTORS USING SUDEP RISK FACTOR CLUSTER ID

This chapter outlines the steps by which clinicians can use the Cluster Risk Factor Identifiers classification. The process begins by determining each patient's SUDEP Risk Factor Cluster ID. Individual Risk IDs define risk factors for SUDEP, including those related to central and peripheral nervous system dysfunction. Related or similar clusters will identify the types of risk factors for people with similar risk Cluster IDs, which we believe will ultimately allow better medical management before, during, and after seizures, and which will be further evaluated using our forensic international SUDEP database, now under development.

Table 15.1 summarizes our suggestions for evaluating individual patients using SUDEP Risk Factor Cluster Identifiers. The discussion that follows expands each patient management item found in Table 15.1.

### STEP 1: CONSTRUCT INDIVIDUALIZED RISK FACTORS FOR SUDEP USING CLUSTER IDs

The underlying assumption for our method is that different mechanisms of SUDEP and/or combinations of mechanisms occur in different patients. The Cluster ID method is a new risk factor classification system developed with the goal of improving individual patient management via an individualized understanding of SUDEP risk factors/mechanisms, including central and peripheral physiological factors. To personalize a patient's profile, physiological and pharmacological factors and responses as well as other risk factors will be designated by Cluster IDs. We hypothesize that the individualized assessment that generates Cluster IDs for a given patient with epilepsy will predict physiological responses to seizures and/or other epilepsy-related factors, including prescribed AEDs, and more broadly will provide an overall risk for SUDEP. Cluster Risk Factor Identification for patients with epilepsy will help their clinicians take steps to lower the risk of SUDEP, as well as to decrease or eliminate the occurrence of unwanted treatment-related side effects, including those arising from the autonomic nervous system. As of the publication of this book, a total of 115 of 173 cases, SUDEP and living patients with epilepsy, respectively, have been classified with our unique Cluster ID method (Chapter 14). Cohort data for 3000 de-identified patients in Dr. Wannamaker's practice will be used to analyze our risk cluster ID data (Chapters 8 and 10). We need to increase the sample sizes for both groups, as well as healthy controls, and plan to do so using retrospective data mining and prospective data collection.

### STEPS 2 AND 3: COLLECT AND EVALUATE DATA RELATING TO FAMILY MEDICAL HISTORY

From each patient with epilepsy, we will collect and evaluate data relating to family medical history of sudden cardiac death, myocardial infarction, and exercise-induced cardiac changes. Risk Factors associated with SUDEP are in Table 15.1.

### STEP 4: SCORE OF INDIVIDUAL SUDEP RISK FACTOR CLUSTER IDs

Related clusters will identify the degree of risk for individuals. The risk cluster IDs will allow better personalized

## TABLE 15.1

### Summary Patient Evaluation with SUDEP Risk Factor Cluster Identifiers

1. Construct Individualized Risk Factor Clusters for SUDEP since different mechanisms of SUDEP are involved in different patients
2. Collect and evaluate data relating to family medical history of sudden cardiac death, myocardial infarction, and exercise-induced cardiac changes. Factors associated with SUDEP should be identified, including evidence of cardiac autonomic arrhythmogenic events, implanted cardio defibrillators, pacemaker implants, cardiac function changes of Long QT, Torsades de Pointes, AV block, postictal increase in T-wave alternans, post generalize tonic-clonic seizures, and other relevant risk factors in Table 5.1
3. Collect and evaluate genetic and indirect evidence for channelopathies (Herreros, ch. 19, Lathers et al. 2011, ch. 20, SUDEP book)
4. Score each person with epilepsy to determine individual SUDEP Risk Factor Cluster ID using Table 5.1
5. Use our SUDEP database to evaluate individual Cluster IDs to determine level of risk for those with similar Cluster IDs
6. Review recent human physiological studies (Poh et al. 2012 and Chapter 14 of this book). Use their technique prospectively to collect data for the individual risk factor Cluster ID
7. Review ambulatory ECG T-wave alternans analysis (Verrier and Schachter, this book, ch. 43, SUDEP 2011 book) and use this technique prospectively to collect data for the individual risk factor Cluster ID
8. Review and use self-study to apply SUDEP Classification to selected cases. Methods used to apply the cluster ID system in the patient management and in the classification of cases in prospective and/or retrospective SUDEP studies are found in this book (Chapter 6 Lathers, Schraeder, Koehler, Chapter 7 Schraeder and Lathers, Chapter 8 Lathers, Schraeder, Schachter, Verrier)
9. Review background information about SUDEP (Schraeder and Lathers 2011, ch. 59; Lathers and Schraeder 2011, chs. 60, 61)
10. Review compliance with and safety of antiepileptic drugs (AEDs), including lamotrigine, carbamazepine, and polypharmacy (Chapters 32 and 33 in this book; Lathers and Schraeder, [Lathers et al. 2011, chs. 47 through 49] Schraeder and Lathers, [Lathers et al. 2011, ch. 50] Lathers, [Lathers et al. 2011, ch. 54])

---

medical management in people with epilepsy while identifying those at risk to prevent the occurrence of SUDEP. Enhanced understanding of the risk factor Cluster IDs will allow better medical management of seizures and/or related heart and respiratory factors and other parameters that may lead to SUDEP. One goal is personalized medicine for people with epilepsy. Development of preventive strategies, best AED regimens, and new AEDs will occur through a better understanding of interrelated changes in the autonomic nervous system, cardiac arrhythmias, and respiratory system. These interrelated mechanisms contribute to the occurrence of SUDEP and will be studied. We believe an in-depth understanding of risk factors for and mechanisms of SUDEP will increase the number of preventive medical strategies available for individuals with epilepsy, define the best regimen of AEDs for each individual through a personal SUDEP Cluster Risk Factor ID profile, contribute to the development of new epilepsy therapies, and ultimately reduce the probability of death.

### STEP 5: USE OUR FORENSIC INTERNATIONAL SUDEP DATABASE FOR HUMANS TO EVALUATE CLUSTER ID RISK FOR SIMILAR IDS

A risk factor cluster ID score for each person with epilepsy will be constructed to determine individual SUDEP Risk Factor Cluster IDs. Once cluster risks for individuals are identified, similar data will be grouped and clusters of risk factors constructed. Cluster identifiers of risk factors allow future individuals to be evaluated to determine their individual cluster identifier for risk factors associated with epilepsy and SUDEP. Risk data are being prepared for statistical analysis by risk analyst Dr. Claycamp (Chapter 4).

### STEPS 6–10: STEPS IN DEVELOPING CLUSTER IDS FOR A GIVEN PATIENT OR SUDEP CASE

#### STEP 6

Table 15.1 Reviews recent human physiological studies recording autonomic parameters such as that of Poh et al. (2012), discussed in Chapter 14.

#### STEP 7

Review ambulatory ECG T-wave alternans analysis method described by Verrier and Schachter in Chapter 14, this book and in Lathers et al. 2011, ch. 43, since this parameter may indicate risk for SUDEP.

#### STEP 8

To understand how to apply the SUDEP Classification and Cluster ID system, "Hands on exercise" and "Self Study" are used first to educate how to review and apply the classification system to cases and, second, how to use it in patient management. This system teaches researchers how to apply the SUDEP Classification and Cluster IDs system for use in prospective or retrospective SUDEP studies. For each case in Chapters 7 through 9, cover up the Cluster ID and use the method and risk factors in Chapter 5 to score the case with a Cluster ID. The case in Chapter 9 (Leestma and Lathers) is excellent for a starter. Then try the cases in Chapter 7 (Schraeder and Lathers) and in Chapter 8 (Lathers, Schraeder, Schachter, Verrier, Wannamaker) of this book.

#### STEP 9

To gain detailed understanding of the features of SUDEP, refer to Chapters 59 through 61 in our 2011 SUDEP book, *Sudden in Epilepsy : Forensic and Clinical Issues.*

**TABLE 15.2**

**Steps the Practicing Physician Can Do to Help Advance SUDEP Research**

1. Contribute your time and/or SUDEP cases to help those building forensic international SUDEP databases and conduct studies
2. Provide SUDEP cases in your patient database to those conducting retrospective database studies to fill in risk factor gaps in our Cluster ID method
3. Agree to collaborate with clinical experts who are conducting prospective studies to fill in risk factor gaps in our Cluster ID method database
4. Report each and every SUDEP case in your clinical practice to help gain a better understanding of the true incidence of SUDEP and identify the risk factors

*Sources:* Schraeder PL et al., *Epilepsy Res* 68: 137–43, 2006; Schraeder PL et al., *Am J Forensic Med Path* 30:123–6, 2009; Lathers CM et al., eds., *Sudden Death in Epilepsy: Forensic and Clinical Issues*, chapter 6, Boca Raton, FL: CRC Press/Taylor & Francis, 2011; Lathers CM and Schraeder PL, *Epilepsy Behav* 14:573–6, 2009.

## STEP 10

A review of discussions of issues relating to compliance and safety of AEDs and poly pharmacy itself are found in Chapters 31, 32, 33, and by Lathers and Schraeder, chapters 47, 48, 49, Schraeder and Lathers, ch. 50, and Lathers, ch. 54, in our 2011 SUDEP book.

Table 15.2 and the subsequent discussion addresses the following steps the practicing physician can do to help advance SUDEP research.

## STEP 1: HELP THOSE BUILDING A FORENSIC INTERNATIONAL SUDEP DATABASE OF BOTH HUMAN AND ANIMAL STUDIES

Contribute your time and/or SUDEP cases to help those of us who are building these databases. Animal databases of models and studies have and will continue to identify risk factors in brain, heart, and the respiratory system, providing a framework for better understanding of possible mechanisms of SUDEP in humans. We have begun to build our SUDEP forensic risk factor Cluster ID databases to form a foundation to aid in the design of effective preventive medical methods with the goal of reducing and/or eliminating SUDEP. We will continue to add to these databases as new information and/or cases of SUDEP occur. Use of the Cluster ID classification criteria of SUDEP Syndromes in patients with epilepsy will allow physicians to determine the appropriate clinical steps/therapies to protect a given patient. Use of the Forensic SUDEP Clusters will allow better management of people with epilepsy and will identify the varying degrees of risk within people with epilepsy for SUDEP. By providing a potential cluster guide for practicing physicians to use, they will be able to determine where each new patient with epilepsy is categorized using the SUDEP Syndrome Cluster Identification and to then ascertain this patient's given risk of SUDEP using the risk/incidence data in the Cluster IDs. The ultimate goal of our work will result in improved individual patient management via better understanding of the relative risk of death in SUDEP and knowledge of its occurrence. Thus, we are covering the topic of SUDEP from a very new and different angle. This innovative method develops a new forensic classification system.

Neurologists and, hopefully, other physicians, who care directly for people with epilepsy, can use this system of risk factor classification in conjunction with our human database to determine where each patient is located in the risk gradients. This information should also be used to detect and identify patients with the highest risk of SUDEP and allow the physician to work to prevent its occurrence.

## STEP 2: PROVIDE SUDEP CASES IN YOUR PATIENT DATABASE FOR RETROSPECTIVE STUDIES

Human autopsy data will be mined using forensic (Chapters 6 and 7), and non-forensic sources (Chapters 8 and 10). The goal is to identify possible mechanisms of SUDEP and to identify risk factors associated with deaths from SUDEP using our new method for SUDEP Cluster mechanism and risk factor ID. Retrospective mining of data from previous studies will be used to establish baseline parameter values and risk factors of neurological, electroencephalographic, and cardiovascular measurements to form clusters to identify those at low, medium, or high risk of SUDEP. Previous studies include National Aeronautics and Space Administration's (NASA's) life science database, SUDEP databases (Leestma et al. 1997; Lathers et al. 2011), and CDC's SUDEP database.

## STEP 3: AGREE TO COLLABORATE WITH CLINICAL EXPERTS AND SCIENTISTS WHO ARE CONDUCTING PROSPECTIVE STUDIES TO IDENTIFY RISK FACTORS FOR SUDEP

Mechanisms of death and the role of neurotransmitters and central and peripheral autonomic nervous system changes as contributing risk factors in brain, cardiac, and respiratory systems will be studied in multiple animal models. Interrelated effects of interictal and ictal epileptogenic activity in the brain, arrhythmogenic actions in the heart as well as laryngeal and hypoxic respiratory effects on the pulmonary system will also be examined. Studies of in vivo and in vitro autonomic ganglia, hypoxemia and seizures, and the role of laryngeal spasms and related hypoxemia and autonomic activity will be conducted. We are targeting the problem utilizing animal models and human studies to ascertain risk factors relevant to the interrelated mechanistic sites resulting in SUDEP. One translational study will be conducted. Mechanistic SUDEP findings in basic animal laboratories will be evaluated to determine what types of translational studies will next be conducted to transition findings in animals to relevance for humans. One translational lock step study will be performed based on animal findings of Lathers et al. (1987): Synchronization of cardiac autonomic neural discharge with epileptogenic activity: The lock step phenomenon (LSP) and Stauffer et al. (1989). A mechanistic hypothesis was developed by Dr. Susumu Sato, while serving as Head Epilepsy NIH, with Dr. Hughes to translate the animal finding to a mechanism for SUDEP in humans. (Chapter 28 in this book; Lathers et al. 2011, ch. 23). Dr. Slater's work (ch. 31) offers techniques of simultaneous polysomnographic evaluation with Video EEG, Stereoelectroencephalography and Magnetoencephalography with ECG/TWA in Refractory Patients Pre- and PostSurgery (Chapter 29 in this book). The translational LSP experiments will shed light on possible mechanism(s) for death in people with epilepsy. Refractory patients, both pre- and postsurgery, will be studied to evaluate the role of LSP in ictal and interictal discharges associated with cardiac autonomic changes.

Physicians should work to conduct prospective studies in people with refractory epilepsy designed to collect central and peripheral risk factors for epilepsy using noninvasive autonomic methodologies employed by Verrier and Schachter (Lathers et al. 2011, ch. 43; Chapter 14 in this book; Poh et al. 2012). Risk factors can be prospectively studied using the technique of Poh et al. (2012). Custom-built wrist-worn sensors continuously record the sympathetically mediated electrodermal activity (EDA) of patients with refractory epilepsy admitted to the long-term video-EEG monitoring unit. Parasympathetic-modulated high-frequency power of heart rate variability was measured from concurrent EKG recordings. It was concluded that the magnitude of both sympathetic activation and parasympathetic suppression increases with duration of EEG suppression after tonic-clonic seizures. The results provided autonomic correlates of postictal EEG suppression and highlight a critical window of postictal autonomic dysregulation that may be relevant in the pathogenesis of SUDEP. Meyer and Strittmatter (2013) stated they support the findings of Poh et al. (2012), implicating autonomic dysfunction as a pathophysiologic correlate of postictal EEG suppression and SUDEP, noting it is important to add further data. One of the most important mechanisms of SUDEP is cardiac arrhythmia precipitated by seizure discharge acting via the autonomic nervous system. Generators of autonomic imbalance include the insula, anterior cingulate gyrus, and ventromedial prefrontal cortex. Previous studies have demonstrated hemispheric lateralization in control of the autonomic nervous system, which is in large part mediated by the right insular cortex. In addition, cardiac autonomic control is under particular control of the right cerebral hemisphere. Knowledge of lateralization anatomy and pathophysiology of the central nervous system may contribute to a better understanding of SUDEP and allow identification of those at particularly high risk for SUDEP. This investigational new autonomic device will be used as a potential SUDEP biomarker (Poh et al. 2012) and is supervised by Dr. Reisenberger and Dr. Loddenkemper, Harvard Medical School.

Stimulation of the vagus nerve is an adjunct treatment for refractory partial seizures (Schachter 2009). Drs. Verrier and Schachter described evaluation of T-wave alternans as a risk stratifier in patients with epilepsy (Chapter 15, this book). Vagus nerve stimulation reduces T-wave alternans magnitude in people with epilepsy (Schomer et al. 2013), suggesting that it may be effective in reducing cardiac arrhythmias and risk of SUDEP. T-wave alternans is a beat-to-beat change in the morphology of the T-wave on the ECG. It is an indicator of temporal-spatial heterogeneity of repolarization, which may set up reentrant arrhythmias, and its magnitude predicts the likelihood of ventricular tachyarrhythmias (Verrier et al. 2009, 2011). T-wave alternans reflect changes in intracellular calcium cycling, autonomic nervous system activity, and myocardial substrate, including ischemia and infarction. See detailed discussion by Verrier and Schachter in Chapter 15, this book.

We have identified 53 national and international PIs, CO-I, and consultants who are all actively interested in and working on basic, translational, and clinical studies of SUDEP. Many of our collaborators have worked on basic science and clinical issues of SUDEP for over 25 or 35 years. Most of the world's recognized leaders in SUDEP are within our group of experts and have established long-time collaborations with each other. Their expertise will help train today's students to use our unique techniques to become leaders of tomorrow in the world of SUDEP preventive strategies.

## STEP 4: REPORT EACH AND EVERY SUDEP CASE IN YOUR CLINICAL PRACTICE, INCLUDING CASES EXAMINED BY MEDICAL EXAMINERS

Better reporting of the incidence of SUDEP is needed. There is a problem in defining the occurrence of SUDEP. The diagnosis of SUDEP in the United States is underutilized, caused mainly by the fact that primary physicians, forensic pathologists, and the forensic community in general, do not use the term on the death certificate. SUDEP worldwide is found to be more prevalent than assumed (Schraeder and So 2006, 2009; Schraeder et al. 2011). Clinical practices, neurologists, physicians, and the forensic community (medical examiners' and coroners' offices) globally must understand the importance of accurately identifying cases of SUDEP and citing the immediate cause of death as SUDEP in the death certificate. There is a gap in the reporting of SUDEP cases and the true number of deaths from SUDEP resulting in an underreporting of SUDEP (Lathers and Schraeder 2009). SUDEP refers to the sudden death of an individual with a clinical history of epilepsy. Evidence of terminal seizure activity may not be present. To find solutions to a clinical problem, one must understand how the clinical problem is defined. To prevent sudden death in people with epilepsy, one must first understand the risk factors associated with the condition, discover the mechanisms associated with the risks, and finally ascertain the interrelated mechanism(s) that cause SUDEP. One of the major problems in determining the frequency of sudden death in people with epilepsy (SUDEP) is that the diagnosis of SUDEP in the United States is underutilized as a cause of death on death certificates. Therefore, the incidence rate cited for SUDEP in studies that utilize death certificate information is most likely underreporting the rate of SUDEP. The occurrence of SUDEP worldwide is found to be more prevalent than assumed. Third-world countries, where data are even more limited than in Europe and North America, and where autopsy capability is limited, underreport SUDEP as a cause of death in people with epilepsy. For example, a "SUDEP underreporting" problem has been reported in Nigeria, where most deaths of individuals with epilepsy occur at home and no autopsies are conducted to determine the cause of death. Thus, the majority of these SUDEP cases are missed and never reported. As early as 1994, Coyle et al. commented that the incidence of SUDEP might be difficult to ascertain due to variations within the forensic investigation conducted by coroner's offices. There is great variation among coroners' offices related to the type and level of the investigation, the level of training of the death investigators, and the knowledge of SUDEP. These factors, along with others, lead to an underreporting of SUDEP deaths. To obtain an accurate profile of individuals at risk for SUDEP, the words "epilepsy" and especially "SUDEP" must appear on the death certificate.

## CONCLUSION

Books and reviews of Lathers et al. (1990, 2008, 2011, and this book, and Lathers 2009) have begun to address and identify possible mechanisms and risk factors for SUDEP. These works also explore the interaction among the central and peripheral autonomic nervous systems and the cardiopulmonary systems. Included are discussions of the potential interactive role of genetically determined subtle cardiac risk factors for arrhythmias with a predisposition for seizure-related cardiac arrhythmias. Finally, speculations about potential preventive measures to minimize the risk of SUDEP are also presented. This current text has begun ground-breaking work addressing patient management for people with epilepsy and the best preventive measures. Answers are long overdue. The Risk Factor Cluster ID will help to address gaps in our knowledge about causes of SUDEP. We began with the understanding that SUDEP is a syndrome with several, if not many, potentially interrelated underlying causes and pathophysiological mechanisms, and that some risk factors are relevant to some cases but not others. Clusters identify varying degrees of risk for each person, and risk cluster IDs will allow better medical management before, during, and after brain, cardiac, and/or respiratory changes in parameters that precede SUDEP. Clinical use of Risk Cluster IDs will reduce or eliminate unwanted risk factors for SUDEP, including central and peripheral autonomic changes associated with seizures in people with epilepsy.

## REFERENCES

CDC SUDEP Database. Centers for Disease Control and Prevention, National Center for Health Statistics. Compresses Mortality File 1979-1998 and 1999-2010. Accessed at http://wonder.cdc.gov/.

Coyle HP, Baker-Brian N, Brown SW. Coroners' autopsy reporting of sudden unexplained death in epilepsy (SUDEP) in the UK. *Seizure* 1994;3:247–54.

Herreros B. Cardiac channelopathies and sudden death. Chapter 19 In: Lathers CM, Schraeder PL, Bungo MW, Leestma JE, eds. *Sudden Death in Epilepsy: Forensic and Clinical Issues.* Boca Raton, FL: CRC Press/Taylor & Francis; 2011, pp. 285–302.

Hughes JD, Sato S. Sudden death in epilepsy: Relationship to sleep-wake circadian cycle and fractal physiology. In: Lathers CM, Schraeder PL, Bungo MW, Leestma JE, eds. *Sudden Death in Epilepsy: Forensic and Clinical Issues.* Boca Raton, FL: CRC Press/Taylor & Francis; 2011, pp.333–46.

Lathers CM. Sudden death. Personal reflections global call for action. *Epilepsy Behav* 2009;15(3):269–77.

Lathers CM, Koehler SA, Wecht CH, Schraeder PL. Forensic antiepileptic drug levels in autopsy cases of epilepsy. *Epilepsy Behav* 2011;22(4):778–85.

Lathers CM, Schraeder PL. eds. *Epilepsy and Sudden Death.* New York, NY: Marcel Dekker;1990.

Lathers CM, Schraeder PL. Verbal autopsies and SUDEP. *Epilepsy Behav* 2009;14:573–6.

Lathers CM, Schraeder PL. Antiepileptic Drugs. Benefit/risk clinical pharmacology: Possible role in cause and/or prevention of SUDEP Chapter 47. In: Lathers CM, Schraeder PL, Bungo MW, Leestma JE, eds. *Sudden Death in Epilepsy: Forensic and Clinical Factors.* Boca Raton, FL: CRC Press/Taylor & Francis; 2011, pp. 755–788.

Lathers CM, Schraeder PL. Antiepileptic Drugs. Benefit/risk clinical pharmacology: Possible role in cause and/or prevention of SUDEP Chapter 47. In: Lathers CM, Schraeder PL, Bungo MW, Leestma JE, eds. *Sudden Death in Epilepsy: Forensic and Clinical Factors.* Boca Raton, FL: CRC Press/Taylor & Francis; 2011, pp. 789–800.

Lathers CM, Schraeder PL. Experience-based teaching of therapeutics and clinical pharmacology of antiepileptic drugs. Sudden unexplained death in epilepsy: Do antiepileptic drugs have a role? Chapter 49 In: Lathers CM, Schraeder PL, Bungo MW, Leestma JE, eds. *Sudden Death in Epilepsy: Forensic and Clinical Factors.* Boca Raton, FL: CRC Press/Taylor & Francis; 2011, pp. 801–826.

Lathers CM, Schraeder PL. Clinical pharmacology problem solving unit: Clinical pearls about the perils of Patty Chapter 50 In: Lathers CM, Schraeder PL, Bungo MW, Leestma JE, eds. *Sudden Death in Epilepsy: Forensic and Clinical Factors.* Boca Raton, FL: CRC Press/Taylor & Francis; 2011, pp. 827–844.

Lathers CM, Schraeder PL. Could beta blocker antiarrhythmic and antiseizure activity help prevent SUDEP? Chapter 54 In: Lathers CM, Schraeder PL, Bungo MW, Leestma JE, eds. *Sudden Death in Epilepsy: Forensic and Clinical Factors.* Boca Raton, FL: CRC Press/Taylor & Francis; 2011, pp. 877–886.

Lathers CM, Schraeder PL, Bungo MW. The mystery of sudden death: Mechanisms for risks. *Epilepsy Behav* 2008; 12(1):3–24.

Lathers CM, Schraeder PL, Bungo MW, Leestma JE, eds. *Sudden Death in Epilepsy: Forensic and Clinical Issues.* Boca Raton, FL: CRC Press/Taylor & Francis; 2011.

Lathers CM, Schraeder PL, Weiner FL. Synchronization of cardiac autonomic neural discharge with epileptogenic activity: The lock step phenomenon. *Electroencephalogr Clin Neurophysiol* 1987;67(3):247–59.

Leestma JE, Annegers JF, Brodie MJ, Brown S, Schraeder P, Siscovick D, Wannamaker BB et al. Sudden unexplained death in epilepsy: Observations from a large clinical development program. *Epilepsia* 1997;47–55.

Meyer S, Strittmatter M. Comment on Poh et al. 2012. Autonomic changes with seizures correlate with postictal EEG suppression. *Neurology* 2013;80:1538–9.

NASA Life Science Data Archives LSDA.

Poh MZ, Loddenkemper T, Reinsberger C, Swenson NC, Goyal S, Madsen JR, Picard RW. Autonomic changes with seizures correlate with postictal EEG suppression. *Neurology* 2012;78(23):1868–76.

Schachter SC. Vagal nerve stimulation. In: Shorvon S, Perucca E, Engle J, eds. *The Treatment of Epilepsy,* 3rd edition, London, UK: Blackwell Publishing; 2009, pp.1017–23.

Schraeder PL, Delin K, McClelland RL, So EL. Coroner and medical examiner documentation of SUDEP. *Epilepsy Res* 2006;68:137–43.

Schraeder PL, Delin K, McClelland RL, So EL. A nationwide survey of the extent of autopsy examination in SUDEP. *Am J Forensic Med Path* 2009;30:123–6.

Schraeder PL, So EL, Lathers CM. Forensic case identification In: Lathers CM, Schraeder PL, Bungo MW, Leestma JE, eds. *Sudden Death in Epilepsy: Forensic and Clinical Issues*. Boca Raton, FL: CRC Press/Taylor & Francis; 2011, pp.95–108.

Schomer AC, Nearing BD, Schachter S, Shafer PO, Sundstrom D, Verrier RL. Protective effects of vagus nerve stimulation on cardiac electrical instability assessed by T-wave alternans in patients with drug-resistant epilepsy [abstract]. *Epilepsia* 2013;54:136.

Stauffer AZ, Dodd-O J, Lathers CM. The relationship of the lockstep phenomenon and precipitous changes in mean arterial blood pressure. *Electroencephalogr Clin Neurophysiol* 1989;72(4):340–5.

Verrier RL, Klingenheben T, Malik M, El-Sherif N, Exner D, Hohnloser S, Ikeda et al. Microvolt T-wave alternans: Physiologic basis, methods of measurement, and clinical utility. Consensus guideline by the International Society for Holter and Noninvasive Electrocardiology. *J Am Coll Cardiol* 2011;44:1309–24.

Verrier RL, Kumar K, Nearing BD. Basis for sudden cardiac death prediction by T-wave alternans from an integrative physiology perspective. *Heart Rhythm* 2009;6:416–22.

Verrier RL, Schachter SC. Neurocardiac interactions in sudden unexpected death in epilepsy: Can ambulatory electrocardiogram-based assessment of autonomic function and T-wave alternans help to predict risk? Chapter 43 In: Lathers CM, Schraeder PL, Bungo MW, Leestma JE, eds. *Sudden Death in Epilepsy: Forensic and Clinical Issues*. Boca Raton, FL: CRC Press/Taylor & Francis; 2011, pp.693–710.

# 16 Future Clinical and Animal Studies

*Claire M. Lathers, Steven C. Schachter, and Paul L. Schraeder*

## CONTENTS

This chapter summarizes 10 needed clinical studies or surveys of risk factors for and mechanisms of sudden unexpected death in epilepsy (SUDEP). It will be important to fill in the gaps in our knowledge and to then apply the SUDEP Syndrome Cluster ID method to allow for individualized risk factor profiles and personalized preventives.

## NEED TO DESIGN STUDIES AND SURVEYS TO DELINEATE RISK FACTORS FOR AND MECHANISMS OF SUDEP

1. Sympathetic/parasympathetic function/dysfunction: neural, continuous EKG (electrocardiogram) and EEG (electroencephalogram) monitoring, lockstep phenomenon. Power spectral analysis. Dr. Lathers asks if a given person with epilepsy who is otherwise normal can be designated or classified as having predominately sympathetic vs. predominately parasympathetic nervous system activity while in a normal resting, sitting position? If the answer is yes, then does one of these two categories place this patient at a greater risk from death via SUDEP? Investigation should center on people with epilepsy, preferably near miss SUDEP and/or refractory patients. Baseline data for normal subjects will be obtained from bed rest candidates selected from the general population and will not be highly fit candidates such as the astronauts themselves.

2. Clinical study for SUDEP and β-blockers and/or other new AED medicines: Dr. Lathers asks if there is a protective/preventive role of pharmacological agents such as β-adrenergic receptor blockers, including timolol and propranolol. The study will not be limited to the class of β-blockers. Dr. Schachter is studying other potential AED herbal ingredients.

3. TWA (T-Wave Alternans) in patients with epilepsy to identify risk for SUDEP: Drs. Verrier and Schachter raise the question of whether ambulatory electrocardiogram-based assessment of autonomic function and TWA will help to evaluate the risk for SUDEP in a given patient.

4. Respiratory changes in people with epilepsy contributing to SUDEP. Dr. Lathers.

5. How to use SUDEP Syndrome Clusters in clinical practice and classification system in prospective or retrospective SUDEP studies. Summary. Dr Lathers.

6. Summary clinical design for future AED and SUDEP studies. Review current literature, consider formats for future reports, and guide the readers in considering another generation and needed answers for clinical management of patients thought to be at risk for SUDEP. Dr. Schraeder.

7. Targeting magnesium levels and efficacy of membrane stabilizer. Dr. Schraeder. Consideration in therapy of seizures related to eclampsia and migraine.

8. Uniform method to screen patients with epilepsy and ascertain the family history. Dr. Schraeder. Questionnaire to be designed for use by all practitioners.

9. What is the best approach to patient/family education about SUDEP? Dr. Schraeder.

10. SUDEP autopsy evidence of the role of brain and heart is needed. Dr. Lathers.

To fill in data gaps and construct SUDEP Syndrome Cluster Identifications. Ten clinical suggestions follow with discussion on supporting animal data where pertinent:

1A. Clinical study SUDEP. Sympathetic/parasympathetic function/dysfunction: neural, continuous EKG and EEG monitoring, lockstep phenomenon. Power spectral analysis.
   A. Two questions raised by Dr. Lathers are as follows:
      1. Can individuals, either normal or those with epilepsy, be designated or classified as having "predominately" sympathetic vs. "predominately" parasympathetic nervous system activity while in a normal resting, sitting position?
      2. If yes, then does one of these two categories place a person with epilepsy at a greater risk from death via SUDEP?

B. People with epilepsy should be studied, preferably those with near miss SUDEP and/or refractory epileptics. Baseline data for normal subjects will be obtained from bed rest candidates selected from the general population and will not be highly fit candidates such as the astronauts themselves.

1B. Animal Studies. Sympathetic/parasympathetic dysfunction and arrhythmia induction as potential factors in SUDEP Risk Stratification in sudden death animal models. Use of animal models allows scientists to address questions in a controlled experimental setting. Ultimately, these data are extrapolated to clinical issues to allow treatment of symptoms and/or design of clinical regimens to prevent the occurrence of SUDEP. Numerous preclinical animal studies (in cat, dog, pig, and rat) have been conducted as a model for cardiac sudden death (see Chapter 1 and 17 thorough 21). Studies showed that sympathetic nerve stimulation, arrhythmic doses of ouabain, or coronary artery occlusion increased temporal dispersion of recovery of ventricular myocardium and thereby induced arrhythmia and/or sudden death. Cardiac arrhythmias in the animal model for ouabain-included toxicity were associated with sympathetic neural nonuniform autonomic dysfunction (Lathers and Schraeder 1982; Lathers et al. 1977a, b), i.e., predisposing to cardiac arrhythmia and sudden death. Stimulation of the sympathetic ventrolateral cardiac nerve produced a shift in the origin of the pacemaker and tachyarrhythmias because the nerve is not uniformly distributed to the various regions of the heart but is localized to the atrioventricular junctional and ventricular regions, as studied by Randall et al. (1978). This nonuniform distribution of sympathetic nerves also contributed to initiation of arrhythmia as a nonuniform neural discharge occurred (Lathers 1980; Lathers et al. 1986a, b; Lathers et al. 1974, 1978, 1988b, 1990; Lathers and Roberts 1980). Application of this sudden death animal model to studies of epileptogenic activity and SUDEP (Carnel et al. 1980; Lathers and Schraeder 1982, 1990; Lathers and Schraeder 2011; Schraeder and Lathers 1980, 1983) allowed examination of physiology and pharmacology in multiple animal models. Details are found in the animal studies presented Chapters 1 and 17 through 21. (Lockstep phenomenon. Lathers and Schraeder [2011, ch. 28, 447–8]. Lathers, Schraeder, and Weiner 1987).

Lathers et al. (1983) and Lathers and Schraeder (1987) first reported that cardiac sympathetic and vagal neural discharges were intermittently synchronized 1:1 with epileptogenic discharge, i.e., the lockstep phenomenon (Lathers et al. ch. 28, 2011a). This relationship was designated as real when it was locked 1:1 and semilocked when the relationship was almost 1:1. The abnormal cardiac neural discharge and cardiac arrhythmias were associated with subconvulsant interictal activity. It was suggested that if cardiac arrhythmias provoke SUDEP, then the lockstep phenomenon may be a factor in people with epilepsy who exhibited no overt seizure activity at the time of demise (Lathers et al. 1987). Stauffer et al. (1989, 2011) found that a higher mean proportion of time was spent in precipitous changes in blood pressure, i.e., <23 mmHg per 10-second interval, in association with an unstable lockstep phenomenon pattern. An unstable lockstep phenomenon pattern was defined as all time intervals of 10 seconds or more during which the lockstep phenomenon existed but the interspike intervals were not constant. Dodd-O and Lathers (1990) also noted that when stable lockstep phenomenon was lost, both precipitous mean arterial blood pressure changes and the incidence of ECG (electrocardiogram) changes occurred more frequently. They suggested that development of the abnormal rhythmic activity of the unstable lockstep phenomenon may alter neurotransmitter release and initiate autonomic dysfunction, thereby potentially contributing to SUDEP. The importance of central neuronal outflow in altering the peripheral efferent discharge to the heart is well recognized as is the observation that efferent sympathetic discharge can initiate abnormalities in the electrocardiogram (Lathers et al. 1977a,b; Lathers et al. 1978). Development of lockstep phenomenon may precede occurrence of changes in the ECG or vice versa. All of these lockstep phenomenon studies (Dodd-O and Lathers 1990; Lathers et al. 1983, 1987; Lathers and Schraeder 1990, 2010; O'Rourke and Lathers 1990, 2011; Stauffer et al. 1989, 1990) suggest that at least four mechanisms can be postulated through which lockstep phenomena may be related to arrhythmia and SUDEP. Experiments are needed to verify the following possibilities as being operative as possible mechanisms of SUDEP:

1. Excessive stimulation of a previously damaged electrically unstable heart.
2. Occurrence of nonuniform postganglionic cardiac sympathetic discharge or an imbalance between sympathetic and parasympathetic neural innervation of the heart.
3. Sinus arrest and bradycardia associated with seizures and induced by parasympathetic nervous system hyperactivity.
4. Development of abnormally precipitous blood pressure changes.

Studies have demonstrated a lockstep phenomenon (Dodd-O and Lathers 2011, ch. 29, 465) of temporal synchronization between ECoG (electrocorticogram) activity and intrathoracic cardiac postganglionic sympathetic discharge during both ictal and interictal epileptogenic states (Lathers et al. 1987). Using diverse models, different investigators have shown evidence of intrinsic activity at various levels in the nervous system. Cortical rhythms, controlled by subcortical neurons (Kiloh et al. 1972b), thought by many to be located in the thalamus (Kiloh et al. 1972a), are the basis for the alpha (8–13 Hz), beta (20–22 Hz), delta (3–4 Hz), etc., rhythms of electroencephalography. Basar (1976) used stereotaxic procedures to demonstrate spontaneous activities from medial geniculate nuclei, inferior colliculus, mesencephalic reticular formation, and dorsal hippocampus. Numerous studies (Barman and Gebber 1980, 1981; Gebber and Barman 1981) suggest the existence of an inherent rhythm of sympathetic nerve discharge, possibly originating from the hypothalamus (Barman and Gebber 1982). The results of numerous studies (Barman and Gebber 1980, 1981, 1984; Gebber and Barman 1980, 1981) indicate that a temporal relationship exists between the intrinsic rhythms of the central and the autonomic nervous systems. Lathers et al. (1977a, b, 1978) reported that changes in the rate of autonomic discharge from postganglionic cardiac sympathetic branches may contribute to cardiac arrhythmias. Thus, it is quite plausible that the association between epileptogenic activity and autonomic dysfunction evidenced in both animal (Lathers and Schraeder 1982; Meldrum and Brierley 1973; Meldrum and Horton 1973; Wasterlain 1974) and human (Jay and Leestma 1981; Van Buren 1958) studies may be a manifestation of the disruption of a normal pattern of temporally related intrinsic cortical and autonomic discharges and may be one mechanistic cause of SUDEP (Dodd-O and Lathers 2011, ch. 29, 465).

2A. Clinical study for SUDEP. β-Blocking and other pharmacological agents.

   A. Dr. Lathers questions if there is a protective/preventive role of pharmacological agents such as the class of β-blockers, including timolol and propranolol, in people with epilepsy that may decrease the likelihood of SUDEP?

   B. The study will not be limited to the class of β-blockers. Other possible AED medicines should be studied.

2B. Animal studies. The concept that β-blocking agents may possess anticonvulsant action is not new and is discussed in depth by Lathers et al. (2011, ch. 34) (Bose et al. 1963; Conway et al. 1978; Papanicolaou et al. 1982). The studies of Dashputra et al. (1985), Jaeger et al. (1979), Murmann et al. (1966), and Tocco et al. (1980) demonstrated that propranolol possesses anticonvulsant actions. Mueller and

Dunwiddie (1983) showed that timolol selectively blocked the proconvulsant activity of 2-fluoro-norepinephrine and 1-isoproterenol in in vitro hippocampal slice preparations superfused with penicillin and elevated levels of potassium. Louis et al. (1982) reported that propranolol or timolol (0.25 µg/kg, i.c.v.) produced an anticonvulsant action when PTZ (pentylenetetrazol) was used to induce convulsions in rats. The anticonvulsant action of timolol reported here in swine is similar to the anticonvulsant action of diazepam when employed in the same experimental model (Lathers et al. 1987; Spivey et al. 1987).

The anticonvulsant action of β-blocking agents is commonly ascribed to a membrane-stabilizing effect, although exceptions have been reported (Lints and Nyquist-Battie 1985). Other proposed anticonvulsant mechanisms include decreased central serotonergic (Conway et al. 1978) and monoamine oxidase activity (Bose et al. 1963). An additional possible antiepileptic mechanism of the β-blocking agents may include β-adrenoceptor blockade, especially of $\beta_2$-receptors in the central nervous system (Papanicolaou et al. 1982). Although norepinephrine is generally believed to be anticonvulsant, studies suggest that norepinephrine may exacerbate seizure activity via activation of β-receptors. The state of abnormal seizure susceptibility, but not severity, in rats with a genetic propensity to epilepsy may be determined by norepinephrine deficits in the hypothalamus/thalamus (Dailey and Jobe 1986). Both severity and susceptibility can be determined by norepinephrine deficits in telencephalon, midbrain, and pons-medulla, while seizure severity but not susceptibility may be determined by norepinephrine abnormalities in the cerebellum. Noradrenergic effects may not be uniform throughout the hippocampus; thus, selective activation of α- or β-receptors by norepinephrine in the brain areas such as the hippocampus might produce either anticonvulsant or proconvulsant effects, respectively (Mueller and Dunwiddie 1983). β-Blocking agents can increase norepinephrine concentration in cerebral spinal fluid (Tackett et al. 1981) and potentiate the effects of exogenously administered norepinephrine on vas deferens contraction (Patil et al. 1968). If a similar action occurred in this study, the establishment of β blockade with timolol would increase the central norepinephrine concentration. The increased norepinephrine activity at the central postsynaptic $\alpha_1$-receptor sites may account for the anticonvulsant effects of β-blocking agents (Goldman et al. 1987). Thus, the protective mechanism for timolol against seizures induced by PTZ may be due to a selective blockade of seizure-inducing β-receptors, allowing available norepinephrine to stimulate the central $\alpha_1$-receptors that exert an anticonvulsant action. In addition to the possibility that the central $\alpha_1$-receptors may be involved in the anticonvulsant action of $\beta$-blocking agents, the role of central postsynaptic $\alpha_2$-receptors must be evaluated. Activation of $\alpha_2$-receptors decreases the excitability of CA1 pyramidal neurons (Mueller et al. 1981). Clonidine and 1-*m*-norepinephrine are more selective for $\alpha_2$ than for $\alpha_1$-receptors and inhibit epileptiform activity at low concentrations; the $\alpha_1$ agonist 1-phenylephrine was ineffective at much higher concentrations. These data suggest that central postsynaptic $\alpha_2$-receptors may play a greater role than $\alpha_1$-receptors in the anticonvulsant action of timolol observed in the present study.

Timolol exhibited anticonvulsant and antiarrhythmic activity. It has been theorized that pharmacological agents capable of suppressing epileptiform activity and the sympathetic component of cardiac arrhythmias may be the best regimens to prevent interictal activity and the associated cardiac arrhythmias that may contribute to SUDEP (Carnel et al. 1985; Lathers and Schraeder 1982; Lathers et al. 1984; Schraeder and Lathers 1983). In the experimental setting, the pharmacological agent timolol possesses components of both of these capabilities. Blockade of cardiac $\beta$-receptors, a cardiac neurodepressant effect, and/or membrane depressant actions of $\beta$-blocking agents are thought to contribute to the antiarrhythmic action of $\beta$-blocking agents (Lathers and Spivey 1987). PTZ has been used to induce seizure activity in humans (Franz 1980; Van Buren 1958), study seizure mechanisms (Faingold and Berry 1973; Krall et al. 1978; Langeluddeke 1936; Swinyard 1972), examine autonomic dysfunction associated with epileptogenic activity (Lathers and Schraeder 1982; Onuma 1957; Orihara 1952; Schraeder and Lathers 1983; Van Buren 1958; Van Buren and Ajmone-Marsan 1960), and screen anticonvulsant agents (Carnel et al. 1985; Faingold and Berry 1973; Lathers et al. 1984). Because it is accepted that PTZ is a convulsive model and that many drugs capable of suppressing the PTZ-induced epileptiform activity are anticonvulsant agents, the results of this study suggest that timolol exhibited an anticonvulsant action. Timolol's capacity to reverse the effects of PTZ on the brain does not necessarily imply intrinsic anticonvulsant properties. Additional studies in other experimental models of epilepsy are needed. In particular, it would be important to evaluate the capability of timolol to suppress interictal discharges and cardiac arrhythmias in other in vivo experimental models not involving PTZ (Lathers et al. 2011, ch. 34, 562–3).

Use of $\beta$-blockers such as timolol or propranolol to prevent SUDEP? A potential therapeutic role for $\beta$-adrenergic blockade with timolol, propranolol, or another agent in SUDEP prophylaxis in high-risk categories of people with epilepsy and supporting data are discussed. Evaluation of other pharmacological agents, including propranolol, should be considered in clinical studies or trials.

Sympathetic innervation and cardiac $\beta$-receptor density in association with sudden cardiac death. In a series of animal experiments, Lathers et al. (1985, 1986b, 1988a, 1990) examined sympathetic $\beta$-adrenergic receptor density gradient as a measure of cardiac sympathetic innervation in the cat heart. $\beta$-Receptor density was determined by the binding of $^3$H-dihydroalprenolol (Lathers et al. 1986b). As discussed by Lathers and Levin (2011, ch. 33), receptor density of the right atria was significantly lower than that of the left atria; the $\beta$-receptor density of the right ventricle was significantly lower than the density of the left ventricle. The density of the receptors in the ventricles was higher than in the atria. The $\beta$-receptor density of the distal distribution of the left anterior descending coronary artery was significantly higher than the proximal distribution. These regional differences in $\beta$-adrenoceptor densities are related to cardiac contractile strength of the different areas of the heart. Acute, abrupt, and irreversible coronary artery occlusion of the left anterior descending coronary artery did not significantly alter the $\beta$-adrenergic receptor density and resulted in death in $5.8 \pm 3.6$ minutes. The effect of timolol (5 mg/kg, PO, for 1, 2, or 8 weeks prior to acute, abrupt, and irreversible coronary occlusion) on the response of the cat heart to coronary occlusion was determined for the following parameters: postganglionic cardiac sympathetic neural discharge, blood pressure, heart rate and $\beta$-receptor density (Lathers et al. 1988a). After 1 week of timolol treatment, there were no significant changes in the $\beta$-adrenergic receptor density in any area. After 2 weeks, the densities of $\beta$-receptors increased in the left atria, left ventricle, and septum. By 8 weeks of treatment, the receptor densities in all areas increased. Heart rate did not vary before timolol and was decreased after all doses of timolol. Timolol increased the mean times to coronary artery occlusion-induced death. Timolol did not prevent postganglionic cardiac sympathetic neural discharge associated with arrhythmia. Timolol may increase $\beta$-receptor density and decrease synaptic norepinephrine, causing decreased release per cardiac sympathetic nerve impulse. Alternatively, molecules of timolol may accumulate in nerve endings and be released in greater concentrations at the receptors. This possibility could explain the protection against coronary artery occlusion-induced arrhythmia and death (Lathers et al. 1988a). Timolol pretreatment resulted in an increase in the $\beta$-adrenergic receptor density of all areas of the heart, and coronary occlusion had no significant effect on β-receptor density or on the response to timolol. Also, similar to the previous studies, distribution differences remained throughout the heart.

Stimulation of the sympathetic ventrolateral cardiac nerve produced a shift in the origin of the pacemaker and tachyarrhythmias because the nerve is not uniformly distributed to the various regions of the heart but is localized to the atrioventricular junctional and ventricular regions (Randall 1977, 1984). Such nonuniform distribution of sympathetic nerves also contributes to initiation of arrhythmia as nonuniform neural discharge occurs. Sympathetic innervation and its role in normal and abnormal cardiac function require further investigation (Lathers et al. l977a, b, 1978). Application of this animal model to studies of epileptogenic activity and SUDEP examined the physiology and pharmacology of the role in sympathetic innervation associated with autonomic cardiac neural nonuniform discharge, cardiac arrhythmias, and sudden death (Lathers and Schraeder 1982, Lathers and Schraeder 1983, 1995; Lathers et al.1986a, 1988b, 1989). Use of this animal model has allowed questions to be raised such as whether disease states alter the function of this neural discharge and if the sympathetic postganglionic neural discharge represents one site of action for pharmacological agents to prevent nonuniform neural discharge (Lathers et al. l977a, b, 1978; Lathers and Schraeder 1982; Schraeder and Lathers 1983). A postmortem study of postganglionic cardiac sympathetic innervation in patients with chronic temporal lobe epilepsy by Druschky et al. (2001) reported sympathetic dysfunction in the form of altered postganglionic cardiac sympathetic innervation in patients with chronic temporal lobe epilepsy and suggested that the altered postganglionic cardiac sympathetic innervation may increase risk of cardiac abnormalities and/or SUDEP. The exact role of innervation in arrhythmogenesis and developmental and regulatory mechanisms determining density and pattern of cardiac sympathetic innervation remain unclear. This clinical study of Druschky et al. (2001), conducted in humans, confirms the results and conclusions of the animal studies conducted by Lathers et al. in which the relationship of postganglionic cardiac sympathetic neural discharge was associated with arrhythmias and/or sudden death.

Question of whether regulation of cardiac nerves is a "new paradigm" in the management of sudden cardiac death. Ieda et al. (2006, 2007, 2008), as in the earlier studies by Lathers et al. (1977a, b, 1978) and Lathers and Schraeder (1982), addressed whether regulation of cardiac nerves is a new paradigm in the management of sudden cardiac death, as the heart is extensively innervated and its performance is regulated by the autonomic nervous system. Innervation density is high in the subepicardium and the central conduction system. In diseased hearts, cardiac innervation density varies, a condition that may lead to sudden cardiac death. After myocardial infarction, sympathetic denervation is followed by reinnervation within the heart, leading to unbalanced neural activation and lethal arrhythmia (Lathers et al. 1986b, 1988a, 1990). In the case of diabetic sensory neuropathy, silent myocardial ischemia may occur, associated with loss of pain perception during myocardial ischemia, a major cause of sudden cardiac death in diabetes mellitus (Ieda et al. 2008). To date, molecular mechanisms underlying innervation density are not well understood. Ieda et al. (2008) demonstrated that cardiac sympathetic innervation is determined by the balance of neural chemoattraction and chemorepulsion. Nerve growth factor, a potent chemoattractant, is synthesized by cardiomyocytes and is induced by endothelin-l upregulation in the heart. In contrast, Sema3a, a neural chemorepellent, is expressed strongly in the trabecular layer in early-stage embryos and at a lower level after birth and causes epicardial-to-endocardial transmural sympathetic innervation pattern. Cardiac nerve growth factor downregulation is a factor in diabetic neuropathy. Nerve growth factor supplementation rescues silent myocardial ischemia in diabetic neuropathy. Both Sema3a-deficient and Sema3a-overexpressing mice showed sudden death or lethal arrhythmias due to disruption of innervation patterning (Ieda et al. 2008). All of these regulatory mechanisms involved in neural development in the heart and their critical roles in cardiac performance need to be examined to determine relevance to methods for future use to decrease the risk of SUDEP.

Direct correlation between β-adrenergic receptor sensitivity, level of arrhythmia and mortality following coronary artery occlusion. The greater the sensitivity to β-adrenergic agonists, whether from hormones, exercise, or genetics, the greater the level of arrhythmia and mortality (Lujan et al. 2007; Billman et al. 1997, 2006; Houle et al. 2001; Du et al. 2000). β-Blocking agents may counteract these effects.

3A. Clinical study for SUDEP. TWA as a potential factor in SUDEP Risk Stratification. Verrier and Schachter (2011, ch. 43) raise the question of whether ambulatory ECG-based assessment of autonomic function and TWA will help to evaluate the risk for SUDEP in a given patient. The possible pathologic bases for SUDEP are diverse. To the extent that seizure activity enhances adrenergic state or affects the cardiac substrate to give rise to cardiac electrical instability and lethal arrhythmias, TWA may provide a valuable marker of risk in determining risk for SUDEP.

In general populations and in patients with cardiovascular disease, the utility of TWA in risk stratification for cardiovascular mortality and sudden cardiac death has been demonstrated in prospective studies enrolling >12,000 patients. Hazard ratios ranged from 2.1 to 23.5 for arrhythmic events in individuals with elevated TWA. The utility of TWA to stratify risk beyond standard clinical variables for cardiovascular disease, including demographic factors (e.g., age, sex, and race) and traditional cardiovascular risk markers (e.g., smoking, blood pressure, history, medications, and left ventricular ejection fraction) is confirmed in multivariate analyses (Verrier et al. 2011). Importantly, TWA is capable of indicating both antiarrhythmic and proarrhythmic effects of cardiac and noncardiac medications (Verrier and Nieminen 2010). The capacity of TWA to stratify risk for SUDEP in patients with epilepsy is, however, untested (Verrier and Schachter 2011, ch. 43). The availability of means to monitor TWA level from ambulatory ECGs is expected to allow significant progress.

3B. Animal studies. See Dr. Verrier's chapter discussion of non-SUDEP large animal experimental models of TWA as risk predictor for sudden cardiac death.

4A. Clinical study for SUDEP. Respiratory changes in people with epilepsy contributing to SUDEP.

4B. Animal studies. DBA mice as models of SUDEP. Published clinical observations from the laboratory of Faingold indicate that a major proposed cause for SUDEP patients is respiratory arrest that is commonly associated with a generalized convulsive seizure. DBA mice were known to exhibit generalized convulsive seizures in response to high-intensity acoustic stimuli that lead to respiratory arrest, whereas recent data indicate that the ECG of these mice remains active for several minutes beyond respiratory arrest onset. These data have led to the proposal that DBA/2 mice are a useful model of respiratory arrest–mediated SUDEP. They documented prevention of SUDEP in >90% of DBA/2 mice by rapid intervention with mechanical respiratory support, allowing multiple testing of individual mice for investigating possible preventative measures. The susceptibility of DBA/1 mice to respiratory arrest can be blocked, both acutely and following semichronic (5-day) treatment, with a selective serotonin reuptake inhibitor (fluoxetine, Prozac), with the mice subsequently returning to respiratory arrest susceptibility. These findings indicate the potential usefulness of DBA/1 and DBA/2 mice as models of human SUDEP. Agents such as selective serotonin reuptake inhibitors and selective 5-HT receptor agonists that have proved effective in preventing respiratory arrest in these mice have the potential to be effective preventative agents for human SUDEP (Faingold et al 2011a, b).

5A. Clinical study for SUDEP. How to use SUDEP Syndrome Clusters in clinical practice and Classification System in prospective or retrospective SUDEP studies. Summary. This information is presented in Chapters 5 through 10, 12, 15, 34.

5B. Animal studies. How to use SUDEP Syndrome Clusters. See Chapter 17.

6. Clinical study for SUDEP. Develop an effective summary clinical design for AED (antiepileptic drug) and SUDEP studies of the future. Dr. Schraeder asks what literature exists now and what should be the literature in the future. Effective clinical designs for future studies should be developed to generate needed answers for clinical management of patients thought to be at risk for SUDEP.

7. Clinical study for SUDEP. Question of magnesium levels in patient and efficacy of membrane stabilizer. Magnesium OTC preparation injected is effective against eclampsia-related seizures. There is anecdoctal evidence on migraine treatment from two or three patients with side effects associated with higher therapeutic levels of standard AEDs.

8. Clinical study for SUDEP. Need to develop a uniform method to screen patients with epilepsy to ascertain family history. Initial questions are as follows: who died, when and of what causes? A questionnaire should be designed for use by all practitioners.

9. Clinical study for SUDEP. What is the best approach to patient/family education about SUDEP? See chapter 57 by Hanna and Panelli in our 2011 SUDEP book and Chapter 33 in this book.

SUDEP Syndrome Clusters allow better identification of patients at higher and highest risk for death from SUDEP and management of people with epilepsy. An initial consideration is whether SUDEP risk is a function of medications or a measure of severity of seizure disorder. The incidence and risk factors will be added to the SUDEP Syndrome Clusters based on pathological mechanisms. Use of the SUDEP Syndrome Clusters will allow discussion of the relative risk for SUDEP by age group, etiology of seizures, and location of origin of seizures and type and number of AEDs used, allowing identification of people with epilepsy at higher and highest risk for death of SUDEP and better management of people with epilepsy.

Lathers et al. (2011c, ch. 6) examined AED levels detected in postmortem toxicological analysis in seven cases. Four of seven had subtherapeutic AED levels, two had therapeutic levels, and only one victim of SUDEP had levels above the therapeutic range. Five cases had no detectable AED levels. AED levels at autopsy were either absent or subtherapeutic in 9 of 10 SUDEP cases, findings consistent with the likelihood of poor AED compliance. Subtherapeutic levels of AEDs may be a risk factor for SUDEP that could contribute to increased inter-ictal and/or ictal epileptiform activity with associated autonomic dysfunction leading to disturbance of heart rate, heart rhythm, and/or blood pressure. If needed, the AED information was subpoenaed from the hospital where the victim died, collected from pill bottles at the home of the victim, or learned through contacting the physician. If the patient died in the hospital, medical history was obtained from the next of kin. We did not analyze frequency of drug changes or new AEDs unless the information was found in the medical record. No recent changes in the types of the AEDs prescribed or in the doses prescribed for the victims in our study were presumed. Only chemical drug names were noted, not brand names or generic AED products (Lathers and Schraeder 2002).

The role of AEDs and compliance in cause and/or prevention of SUDEP is not clear (Lathers 2011b). Each patient, each AED, and combination of AEDs require examination to individualize benefit/risk ratios. Drug therapies may increase or decrease SUDEP risk. The advantage of newer AEDs is less adverse sedation, which may minimize noncompliance. Many new AEDs also have less frequent drug interactions, leading to improved tolerability. Compliance with AEDs and maintenance of stable therapeutic drug levels is crucial in avoiding SUDEP. Noncompliance with AED medication may be the most important (Hughes 2009) or one of the important risk factors for SUDEP (Lathers and Schraeder 2011b). Clinical pharmacology questions to be asked after death include evaluation of the AED dose, the actual AED or combination, possible drug–drug interactions, lower level of quantification of the assay method postmortem, and whether there was a recent change in the AED dose or AEDs prescribed. Additional details are found in the article by Lathers (2011) (Global Discussion SUDEP).

The SUDEP Cluster Identifiers should strengthen and allow for greater pharmacological personalization of AEDs for a given person, especially when the genetic propensities are known along with information of which types of AEDs seem to work best for individuals located in a given cluster group.

Lamotrigine. Leestma et al. (1997) reviewed deaths in patients receiving lamotrigine. It must be considered whether this interpretation remains valid or if the data indicate a negative role for lamotrigine in some patients.

10. Clinical study of SUDEP. SUDEP autopsy of brain and heart in causes of death.

It is important to look for evidence of the roles of the brain and the heart in the cause of death when conducting an autopsy on a person with epilepsy who has died suddenly. Neuronal clusters, increased perivascular oligodendroglia, gliosis, cystic gliotic lesions, decreased myelin, cerebellar Bergmann's glosis, and folial atrophy were found to be present in a higher percentage of the brains of SUDEP victims compared to brains from age- and sex-matched control subjects. Additional autopsy results are needed to clarify the role of changes in the heart in SUDEP. There is a need for clinical studies to focus on the contribution of cardiac autonomic dysfunction and/or AEDs, with or without other drugs, to the development of cardiac abnormalities to gain an understanding of the mechanism of death in people with epilepsy (Lathers and Schraeder 1982). Disturbance of function of the autonomic nervous system may contribute (Lathers et al. 2008), but the process is unknown. The occurrence of seizures is often associated with minimal changes in cardiac conduction and rhythm. Chin et al. (2004) reported myocardial infarction following brief convulsive seizures. Chin et al. (2005) described the occurrence of postictal neurogenic stunned myocardium. Natelson et al. (1998) found irreversible pathological changes in the form of subendocardial perivascular and interstitial fibrosis in four of seven hearts of SUDEP victims. These unanswered questions pertaining to the role of changes in the heart tissue in SUDEP emphasize the need to educate the coroner's and medical examiners' staff about the importance of obtaining such information in deaths of people with a history of epilepsy (Lathers et al. 2011). Likewise, evidence of the role of pulmonary systems in SUDEP must be investigated.

## CONCLUSION

### PATIENT MANAGEMENT USING SUDEP SYNDROME CLUSTERS

It is important to apply SUDEP Syndrome Cluster Classification to cases selected to educate readers about the use of clusters in patient management and classification system in prospective or retrospective SUDEP studies (Koehler et al. 2011). Details are found in Chapters 6 through 10. It is also important that data available from family histories, such as sudden cardiac death, be collected along with information of myocardial infarctions, exercise fitness of family members, or other relevant risk factors associated with SUDEP. Table 5.1 in Chapter 5 lists multiple risk factors to be considered when developing cluster IDs for people with epilepsy and/or for those who have died of SUDEP. One must remember to search for direct or indirect evidence of channelopathies. Recent relevant human physiological studies can be performed using new autonomic measurement techniques such as that of Poh et al. (2012). The main goal is to develop Individualized Risk Factors because different SUDEP mechanisms operate in different patients. Individualized Risk Factors for SUDEP will ultimately allow for personalized medicine for people with epilepsy.

## REFERENCES

Barman SM, Gebber GL. Sympathetic nerve rhythm of brain stem origin. *Am J Physiol* 1980;239:R42–7.

Barman SM, Gebber GL. Brain stem neuronal types with activity patterns related to sympathetic nerve discharge. *Am J Physiol* 1981;242:R335–41.

Barman SM, Gebber, GL. Hypothalamic neurons with activity patterns related to sympathetic nerve discharge. *Am J Physiol* 1982;242:R34–R43.

Barman SM, Gebber GL. Spinal interneurons with sympathetic nerve-related activity. *Am J Physiol* 1984;247:R761–67.

Basar E. Abstract methods of general systems analysis. In: Basar E, ed. *Biophysical and Physiological Systems Analysis*. Reading, MA: Addison-Wesley;1976, pp. 23–47.

Billman GE, Castillo LC, Hensley J, Hohl CM, Altschuld RA. Beta2-adrenergic receptor antagonists protect against ventricular fibrillation: In vivo and in vitro evidence for enhanced sensitivity to beta2-adrenergic stimulation in animals susceptible to sudden death. *Circulation* 1997;96:1914–22.

Billman GE, Kukielka M, Kelley R, Moustafa-Bayoumi M, Altschuld RA. Endurance exercise training attenuates cardiac beta2-adrenoceptor responsiveness and prevents ventricular fibrillation in animals susceptible to sudden death. *Am J Physiol Heart Circ Physiol* 2006;290:H2590–9.

Bose BC, Saifi AQ, Sharma S. Studies on anticonvulsant and antifibrillatory drugs. *Arch Int Pharmacodyn* 1963;146:106–13.

Carnel SB, Schraeder PL, Lathers CM. Autonomic dysfunction in epilepsy II: Cardiovascular changes associated with pentylenetetrazol induced seizures. *Clin Res* 1980;28:609A.

Carnel SB, Schaeder PL, Lathers CM. Effect of Phenobarbital pretreatment on cardiac neural discharge and pentylenetetrazol-induced epileptogenic activity in the cat. *Pharmacology* 1985;30(4):225–40.

Chin PS, Branch KR, Becker KJ. Myocardial infarction following brief convulsive seizures. *Neurology* 2004;63:2453–4.

Chin PS, Branch KR, Becker KJ. Postictal neurogenic stunned myocardium. *Neurology* 2005;64(11):1977–8.

Conway J, Greenwood DT, Middlemiss DN. Central nervous actions of ß-adrenoceptor antagonists. *Clin Sci Molec Med* 1978;54:119–24.

Dashputra PG, Patki VP, Hemnani TJ. Antiepileptic action of beta-adrenergic blocking drugs: Pronethal and propranolol. *Mater Med Pol* 1985;2:88–92.

Dailey JW, Jobe PC. Indices of noradrenergic function in the central nervous system of seizure-naive genetically epilepsy-prone rats. *Epilepsia* 1986 Nov-Dec;27(6):665–70.

Dodd-O JM, Lathers CM. A characterization of the lockstep phenomenon in phenobarbital-pretreated cats. Chapter 13 In: Lathers CM and Schraeder PL, eds. *Epilepsy and Sudden Death*. New York, NY: Marcel Dekker; 1990, pp. 199–220.

Dodd-O JM, Lathers CM. Characterization of the lockstep phenomenon in phenobarbital-pretreated cats. Chapter 29 In: Lathers CM, Schraeder PL, Bungo, MW, Leestma JE, eds. *Sudden Death in Epilepsy: Forensic and Clinical Issues*. Boca Raton, FL: CRC Press/Taylor & Francis Group; 2011, pp. 465–80.

Druschky A, Hiltz MJ, Hopp P, Platsch G, Radespiel-Tröger M, Druschky K, Kuwert T, Stefan H, Neundörfer B. Interictal cardiac autonomic dysfunction in temporal lobe epilepsy demonstrated by [ (123) I]metaiodobenzylguanidine-SPECT. *Brain* 2001;124(Pt 12):372–82.

Du XJ, Gao XM, Jennings GL, Dart AM, Woodcock EA. Preserved ventricular contractility in infarcted mouse heart overexpressing beta 2 adrenergic receptors. *Am J Physiol Heart Circ Physiol* 2000;279(5):H2456–63.

Faingold CL, Berry CA. Quantitative evaluation of the pentylenetetrazol-anticonvulsant interaction on the EEG of the cat. *Eur J Pharmacol*1973;24:381–8.

Faingold CL, Tupal S, Mhaskar Y, Uteshev VV. DBA mice as models of sudden unexpected death in epilepsy. In: Lathers CM, Schraeder PL, Bungo MW, Leestma JE, eds. *Sudden Death in Epilepsy: Forensic and Clinical Issues*. Boca Raton, FL: CRC Press/Taylor & Francis Group; 2011a, pp. 659–78.

Faingold CL, Tupal S, Randall M. Prevention of seizure-induced sudden death in a chronic SUDEP model by semichronic administration of a selective serotonin reuptake inhibitor. *Epilepsy Behav* 2011b;22(2):186–90.

Franz DN. *The Pharmacological Basis of Therapeutics*. New York, NY: Macmillan; 1980.

Gebber GL, Barman SM. Basis for 2-6 cycle/s rhythm in sympathetic nerve discharge. *Am J Physiol*1980;239:R48–R56.

Gebber GL, Barman SM. Sympathetic-related activity of brain stem neurons in baroreceptor-denervated cats. *Am J Physiol* 1981;240:R348–55.

Goldman BD, Stauffer AZ, Lathers CM. Beta blocking agents and the prevention of sudden unexpected death in the epileptic person: Possible mechanisms. *Fed Proc* 1987;46:705.

Hanna J, Panelli R. Challenges in overcoming ethical, legal and communication barriers in SUDEP. Chapter 57 In: Lathers CM, Schraeder PL, Bungo, MW, Leestma JE, eds. *Sudden Death in Epilepsy: Forensic and Clinical Issues*. Boca Raton, FL: CRC Press/Taylor & Francis Group; 2011, pp. 915–36.

Houle MS, Altschuld RA, Billman GE. Enhanced in vivo and in vitro contractile responses to beta (2)-adrenergic receptor stimulation in dogs susceptible to lethal arrhythmias. *J Appl Physiol* 2001;91:1627–37.

Hughes JR. A review of sudden unexpected death in epilepsy: Prediction of patients at risk. *Epilepsy Behav* 2009;14:280–7

Ieda M, Kanazawa H, Ieda Y, Kimura K, Matsumura K, Tomita Y, Yagi T et al. Nerve growth factor is critical for cardiac sensory innervations and rescues neuropathy in diabetic hearts. *Circulation* 2006;114:2351–63.

Ieda M, Kanazawa H, Kimura K, Hattori F, Ieda Y, Taniguchi M, Lee JKet al. Sema3a maintains normal heart rhythm through sympathetic innervation patterning. *Nat Med* 2007;13: 604–12.

Ieda M, Kimura K, Kanazawa H, Fukuda K. Regulation of cardiac nerves: A new paradigm in the management of sudden cardiac death? *Curr Med Chem* 2008;15:1731–6.

Jaeger V, Esplin B, Capek R. The anticonvulsant effects of propranolol and beta-adrenergic blockade. *Experientia* 1979;35:8081.

Jay GW, Leestma JE. Sudden death in epilepsy. A comprehensive review of the literature and proposed mechanisms. *Acta Neurol Scand* 1981;63(Suppl. 82):1–66.

Kiloh LG, McComas AJ, Osselton JW. The neural basis of the EEG. In: Kiloh LG, McComas AJ, Osselton JW, eds. *Clinical Encephalography*. London, UK: Butterworths; 1972a, pp. 21–34.

Kiloh LG, McComas AJ, Osselton JW. Normal findings. In: Kiloh LG, McComas AJ, Osselton JW, eds. *Clinical Encephalography*. London, UK: Butterworths; 1972b, pp. 52–70.

Koehler SA, Schraeder PL, Lathers CM, Wecht CH. One-year postmortem forensic analysis of deaths in persons with epilepsy. In: Lathers CM, Schraeder PL, Bungo MW, Leestma JE, eds. *Sudden Death in Epilepsy: Forensic and Clinical Issues.* Boca Raton, FL: CRC Press/Taylor & Francis Group; 2011, pp. 145–59.

Krall RL, Perry JK, White BG, Kupferberg HJ, Swinyard EA. Antiepileptic drug development. II. Anticonvulsant drug screening. *Epilepsia* 1978;19:409–28.

Langeluddeke A. Die diagnostische Bedeutung experimentell erzeugter Krampfe. Dsch Med Wehnschr 1936;62:1588–90.

Lathers CM. Effect of timolol on autonomic neural discharge associated with ouabain-induced arrhythmia. *Eur J Pharmacol* 1980;64(2–3):95–106.

Lathers CM. Animal model for sudden cardiac death: Autonomic cardiac sympathetic nonuniform neural discharge. Chapter 27 In: Lathers CM, Schraeder PL, Bungo, MW, Leestma JE, eds. *Sudden Death in Epilepsy: Forensic and Clinical Issues.* Boca Raton, FL: CRC Press/Taylor & Francis Group; 2011a, pp. 427–36.

Lathers CM. Antiepileptic drugs, compliance and SUDEP. In: Chapman D, Panelli R, Hanna J, Jeffs T, eds. *Unexpected Death in Epilepsy: Continuing the Global Conversation.* Camberwell, Australia: Epilepsy Australia Ltd; 2011b, pp. 72–3.

Lathers CM. Sudden death: Animal models to examine nervous system sites of action for disease and pharmacological intervention. Chapter 25 In: Lathers CM, Schraeder PL, Bungo, MW, Leestma JE, eds. *Sudden Death in Epilepsy: Forensic and Clinical Issues.* Boca Raton, FL: CRC Press/Taylor & Francis Group; 2011c, pp. 363–94.

Lathers CM. Could beta blocker antiarrhythmic and antiseizure activity help prevent SUDEP? Chapter 54, In: Lathers CM, Schraeder PL, Bungo, MW, Leestma JE, eds. *Sudden Death in Epilepsy: Forensic and Clinical Issues.* Boca Raton, FL: CRC Press/Taylor & Francis Group; 2011d; pp. 877–86.

Lathers CM, Jim KF, Spivey WH, Khan C, Dolce K, Matthews WD. Antiepileptic activity of beta blocking drugs. Chapter 34 In: Lathers CM, Schraeder PL, Bungo MW, Leestma JE, eds. *Sudden Death in Epilepsy: Forensic and Clinical Issues.* Boca Raton, FL: CRC Press/Taylor & Francis Group; 2011a, pp. 551–66.

Lathers CM, Kelliher GJ, Roberts J, Beasley AB. Nonuniform cardiac sympathetic nerve discharge: Mechanism for coronary occlusion and digitalis-induced arrhythmia. *Circulation* 1978;57:1058–65. Young Investigator Award, American College of Cardiology, February 24, 1976.

Lathers CM, Kelliher G, Roberts J, Beasley AB. Role of the adrenergic nervous system in arrhythmia produced by acute coronary artery occlusion. Myocardial Ischemia Symposium, Philadelphia Physiological Society, May 6, 1976. In: Lefer A, Kelliher G, Rovetto M, eds. *Pathophysiology and Therapeutics of Myocardial Ischemia.* New York, NY: Spectrum Publications; 1977a, pp.123–47.

Lathers CM, Koehler SA, Wecht CH, Schraeder PL. Forensic antiepileptic drug levels in autopsy cases of epilepsy. *Epi Behav* 2011b;22(4):778–85.

Lathers CM, Levin RM. Animal model for sudden cardiac death: Sympathetic innervation and myocardial beta receptor densities. Chapter 33 In: Lathers CM, Schraeder PL, Bungo, MW, Leestma JE, eds. *Sudden Death in Epilepsy: Forensic and Clinical Issues.* Boca Raton, FL: CRC Press/Taylor & Francis Group; 2011, pp. 539–50.

Lathers CM, Levin RM, Spivey WH. Regional distribution of myocardial beta-adrenoceptors in the cat. *Eur J Pharmacol* 1986a;130:111–7.

Lathers CM, Roberts J. Digitalis cardiotoxicity revisited. *Life Sci* 1980;27(19):1713–33

Lathers CM, Roberts J, Kelliher GJ. Relationship between the effect of ouabain on arrhythmia and interspike intervals (ISI) of cardiac accelerator nerves. *Pharmacologist* 1974;16:201.

Lathers CM, Roberts J, Kelliher GJ. Correlation of ouabain-induced arrhythmia and nonuniformity in the histamine-evoked discharge of cardiac sympathetic nerves. *J Pharmacol Exp Ther* 1977b;203(2):467–79.

Lathers CM, Schraeder PL. Autonomic dysfunction in epilepsy III: Characterization of autonomic cardiac neural discharge associated with pentylenetetrazol induced seizures. *Clin Res* 1980;28:615A.

Lathers CM, Schraeder PL. Autonomic dysfunction in epilepsy: Characterization of autonomic cardiac neural discharge associated with pentylenetetrazol-induced epileptogenic activity. *Epilepsia* 1982;23(6):633–47.

Lathers CM, Schraeder PL, eds. *Epilepsy and Sudden Death.* New York, NY: Marcel Dekker; 1990.

Lathers CM, Schraeder PL. Clinical pharmacology: Drugs as a benefit and/or risk in sudden unexpected death in epilepsy? *J Clin Pharmacol* 2002;42(2):123–36.

Lathers CM, Schraeder PL, Bungo MW. The mystery of sudden death: Mechanisms for risks. *Epilepsy Behav* 2008;12:3–24.

Lathers CM, Schraeder PL. Experience-based teaching of therapeutics and clinical pharmacology of antiepileptic drugs. Sudden unexplained death in epilepsy. Do antiepileptic drugs have a role? *J Clin Pharmacol* 1995;35:573–87.

Lathers CM, Schraeder PL. Animal model for sudden unexpected death in persons with epilepsy. Chapter 28 In: Lathers CM, Schraeder PL, Bungo MW, Leestma JE, eds. *Sudden Death in Epilepsy: Forensic and Clinical Issues.* Boca Raton, FL: CRC Press/Taylor & Francis Group; 2011a, pp. 437–64.

Lathers CM, Schraeder PL. Antiepileptic drugs benefit/risk clinical pharmacology: Possible role in cause and/or prevention of SUDEP. Chapter 47 In: Lathers CM, Schraeder PL, Bungo MW, Leestma JE, eds. *Sudden Death in Epilepsy: Forensic and Clinical Issues.* Boca Raton, FL: CRC Press/Taylor & Francis Group; 2011b, pp. 755–89

Lathers CM, Schraeder PL, Carnel SB. Neural mechanisms in cardiac Arrhythmias associated with epileptogenic activity: The effect of phenobarbital in the cat. *Life Sci* 1984;34:1919–36.

Lathers CM, Schraeder PL, Bungo MW, Leestma JE, eds. *Sudden Death in Epilepsy.* Boca Raton, FL: CRC Press/Taylor & Francis Group; 2011c.

Lathers CM, Schraeder PL, Weiner FL. Synchronization of cardiac autonomic neural discharge with epileptogenic activity: The lockstep phenomenon. *Electroencephalogr Clin Neurophysiol* 1987;67(3):247–59.

Lathers CM, Spivey WH. The effect of beta blockers on cardiac neural discharge associated with coronary occlusion in the cat. *J Clin Pharmacol* 1987;27(8):582–92.

Lathers CM, Spivey WH, Levin RM. The effect of chronic timolol in an animal model for myocardial infarction. *J Clin Pharmacol* 1988a;28:736–45.

Lathers CM, Spivey WH, Levin RM, Tumer N. The effect of dilevalol on cardiac autonomic neural discharge, plasma catecholamines, and myocardial beta receptor density associated with coronary occlusion. *J Clin Pharmacol* 1990;30(3):241–53.

Lathers CM, Spivey WH, Suter LE, Lerner JP, Tumer N, Levin RM. The effect of acute and chronic administration of timolol on cardiac sympathetic neural discharge, arrhythmia, and beta adrenergic receptor density associated with coronary occlusion in the cat. *Life Sci* 1986b;39(22):2121–41.

Lathers CM, Spivey WH, Tumer N. The effect of timolol given five minutes after coronary occlusion on plasma catecholamines. *J Clin Pharmacol* 1988b;28:289–99.

Lathers CM, Stauffer AZ, Turner N, Kraras CM, Goldman BD. Anticonvulsant and antiarrhythmic actions of the beta blocking agent timolol. *Epilepsy Res* 1989 4:42–54.

Lathers CM, Weiner FL, Schraeder PL. Synchronization of cardiac autonomic neural discharge with epileptogenic activity: The locked step phenomenon. *Circ Res* 1983;31:630A.

Leestma JE, Annegers JF, Brodie MJ, Brown S, Schraeder P, Siscovick D Wannamaker B et al.: Sudden unexplained death in epilepsy (SUDEP) in a large clinical development program. *Epilepsia* 1997;38:47–55.

Lints CE, Nyquist-Battie C. A possible role for beta-adrenergic receptors in the expression of audiogenic seizures. *Pharmacol Biochem Behav* 1985;22:711–16.

Louis WJ, Papanicolaou J, Summers RJ, Vajda FJE. Role of central beta adrenoceptors in the control of pentylenetetrazol-induced convulsions in rats. *Br J Pharmacol* 1982;75:441–6.

Lujan HL, Kramer VJ, DiCarlo SE. Sex influences the susceptibility to reperfusion-induced sustained ventricular tachycardia and beta-adrenergic receptor blockade in conscious rats. *Am J Physiol Heart Circ Physiol* 2007;293:H2799–2808.

Meldrum BS, Brierley JB. Prolonged epileptic seizures in primates. *Arch Neurol* 197328:10–7.

Meldrum BS, Horton RW. Physiology of status epilepticus in primates. *Arch Neurol* 1973;28:1–9.

Mueller AL, Dunwiddie TV. Anticonvulsant and proconvulsant actions of alpha- and beta-noradrenergic agonists on epileptiform activity in rat hippocampus in vitro. *Epilepsia* 1983;24:51–64.

Mueller AL, Hoffer BJ, Dunwiddie TV. Noradrenergic responses in rat hippocampus: Evidence for mediation by alpha and beta receptors in the in vitro slice. *Brain Res* 1981;214:113–26.

Murmann W, Almirante L, Saccani-Gueli M. Central nervous system effects of four beta-adrenergic receptor blocking agents. *J Pharm Pharmacol* 1966;18:317–8.

Natelson BH, Suarez RV, Terrence CF, Turizo R. Patients with epilepsy who die suddenly have cardiac disease. *Arch Neurol* 1998;55:857–60.

Onuma T. Relationships of the predisposition to convulsions with the action potentials of the autonomic nerves and the brain. II. Changes in action potential of the autonomic nerves and the brain under conditions for increasing the predisposition to convulsions. *Tohoku J Exp Med* 1957;65:121–9.

Orihara O. Comparative observations of the action potential of autonomic nerve with EEC *Tohoku J Exp Med* 1952;57: 43–54.

O'Rourke D, Lathers CM. Interspike interval histogram characterization of synchronized cardiac sympathetic neural discharge and epileptogenic activity in electrocorticogram of cat. Chapter 15 In: Lathers CM and Schraeder PL, eds. *Epilepsy and Sudden Death*. New York, NY: Marcel Dekker; 1990, pp. 239–260.

O'Rourke DK, Lathers CM. Interspike interval histogram characterization of synchronized cardiac sympathetic neural discharge and epileptogenic activity in electrocorticogram of cat. In: Lathers CM, Schraeder PL, Bungo, MW, Leestma JE, eds. *Sudden Death in Epilepsy: Forensic and Clinical Issues*. Boca Raton, FL: CRC Press/Taylor & Francis Group; 2011, pp. 495–512.

Papanicolaou J, Vajda FJ, Summers RJ, Louis WJ. Role of beta-adrenoreceptors in the anticonvulsant effect of propranolol on leptazol–induced convulsions in rats. *Pharm Pharmacol* 1982;34:124–5.

Patil PN, Tye A, May C, Hetey S, Miyagi S. Steric aspects of adrenergic drugs. XI. Interactions of dibenamine and beta adrenergic blockers. *J Pharmacol Exp Ther* 1968;163:309–19.

Poh MZ, Loddenkemper T, Reinsberger C, Swenson NC, Goyal S, Madsen JR, Picard RW. *Neurology* 2012;78(23):1868–76.

Randall, WC, ed. *Neural Regulation of the Heart*. New York, NY: Oxford University Press; 1977, pp.1–440.

Randall, WC. ed. *Nervous Control of Cardiovascular Function*. New York, NY: Oxford University Press; 1984, pp. 1–476.

Randall WC, Thomas JX, Euler DE, Rozanski GJ. Cardiac dysrhythmias associated with autonomic nervous system imbalance in the conscious dog. In: Schwartz PJ, Brown AM, Malliani A, Zanchetti A, eds. *Perspectives in Cardiovascular Research, vol 2, Neural Mechanisms in Cardiac Arrhythmias*. New York, NY: Raven Press; 1978, pp. 123–38.

Schraeder PL, Lathers CM. Autonomic dysfunction in epilepsy I: A proposed animal model for unexplained sudden death in epilepsy. *Clin Res* 1980;28:618A.

Schraeder PL, Lathers CM. Cardiac neural discharge and epileptogenic activity in the cat: An animal model for unexplained death. *Life Sci* 1983;32:1371–82.

Schraeder PL, So EL, Lathers CM. Forensic case identification. Chapter 6 In: Lathers CM, Schraeder PL, Bungo MW, Leestma JE, eds. *Sudden Death in Epilepsy: Forensic and Clinical Issues*. Boca Raton, FL: CRC Press/Taylor & Francis Group; 2011, pp. 95–108.

Spivey WH, Lathers CM. Effect of timolol on the sympathetic nervous system in coronary occlusion in cats. *Ann Emerg Med* 1985;14:939–44.

Spivey WH, Unger HD, Lathers CM, McNamara RM. Intraosseous diazepam suppression of pentylenetetrazol-induced epileptogenic activity in pigs. *Ann Emergency Med* 1987;16:156–9.

Stauffer AZ, Dodd-O J, Lathers CM. The relationship of the lock-step phenomenon and precipitous changes in mean arterial blood pressure. *Electroencephalogr Clin Neurophysiol* 1989;72(4):340–5.

Stauffer AZ, Dodd-O JM, Lathers CM. Relationship of lock step phenomenon and precipitous changes in blood pressure. Chapter 14. In: Lathers CM and Schraeder PL, eds. *Epilepsy and Sudden Death*. New York, NY: Marcel Dekker; 1990, pp. 221–238.

Stauffer AZ, Dodd-O JM, Lathers CM. Relationship of the lock-step phenomenon and precipitous changes in blood pressure. In: Lathers CM, Schraeder PL, Bungo MW, Leestma JE, eds. *Sudden Death in Epilepsy: Forensic and Clinical Issues*. Boca Raton, FL: CRC Press/Taylor & Francis Group; 2011, pp. 481–94.

Swinyard EA. Assay of antiepileptic drug activity in experimental animals: Standard tests. In: *Anticonvulsant Drugs International Encyclopedia of Pharmacology and Therapeutics*. Oxford, UK: Pergamon Press, Section 19.1; 1972: pp. 47–65.

Tackett RL, Webb JG, Privitera PJ. Cerebroventricular propranolol elevates cerebrospinal fluid norepinephrine and lowers blood pressure. *Science* 1981;213:911–3.

Tocco DJ, Clineschmidt BV, Duncan AEW, Deluna FA, Baer JR.Uptake of the beta-adrenergic blocking agents propranolol and timolol by rodent brainhelationship to central pharmacological action. *J Cardiovasc Res* 2:133–43.

Van Buren JM. Some autonomic concomitants of ictal autonomism. *Brain* 1958;81:505–28.

Van Buren JM, Ajmone-Marsan C. Correlations of autonomic and EEG components in temporal lobe epilepsy. *Arch Neurol* 1960;3:683–703.

Verrier RL, Klingenheben T, Malik M, El-Sherif N, Exner D, Hohnloser S, Ikeda Tet al. Microvolt T-wave alternans: Physiologic basis, methods of measurement, and clinical utility. Consensus guideline by the International Society for Holter and Noninvasive Electrocardiology. *J Am Coll Cardiol* 2011;44:1309–24.

Verrier RL, Nieminen T. T-wave alternans as a therapeutic marker for antiarrhythmic agents. *J Cardiovasc Pharmacol* 2010;55:544–54.

Verrier RL, Schachter SC. Neurocardiac interactions in sudden unexpected death in epilepsy: Can ambulatory electrocardiogram-based assessment of autonomic function and T-wave alternans help to predict risk? Chapter 43 In: Lathers CM, Schraeder PL, Bungo MW, Leestma JE, eds. *Sudden Death in Epilepsy: Forensic and Clinical Issues*. Boca Raton, FL: CRC Press/Taylor & Francis Group; 2011, pp. 693–710.

Wasterlain CG. Mortality and morbidity from serial studies. An experimental study. *Epilepsia* 1974;15:155–76.

# 17 Animal Model Cluster IDs
## Mechanisms and Risk Factors for SUDEP

*Claire M. Lathers*

## CONTENTS

In 1902 Spratling reported on the causes and manner of death in epilepsy, including sudden unexpected death. For the next 100 years, examinations of mechanisms of sudden unexpected death in epilepsy (SUDEP) in controlled animal experiments were few. Published human case reports or epidemiology studies with conjectures about the mechanisms of sudden death did appear in the literature. None of these human reports could concretely address mechanisms of and risk factors for SUDEP due to limitations of conducting explorative, definitive studies in humans. Research funding for animal studies were almost nonexistent with many focused on the concerns about raising the issue of sudden death when talking with people with epilepsy, their family and friends. It was not until ~2008–2013 that National Institutes of Health with strong encouragement by the American Epilepsy Society, Citizens United for Research in Epilepsy (CURE), and other organizations funded studies about SUDEP. Their most recent call for proposals finally addressed the need for and lack of animal studies to address mechanisms of and risk factors for SUDEP.

Dr. Lathers' developed surgical techniques in whole-animal experimental studies at the Medical School, University at Buffalo, where she recorded from single muscle spindle afferent and efferent spinal nerves to study the effect of alcohol on muscle motor gait control (Lathers and Smith 1976). Surgical animal studies conducted by Dr. Lathers in her laboratory at the Medical College of Pennsylvania used animal models to induce disease to mimic myocardial infarction and digitalis toxicity and set the stage and knowledge base for subsequent studies of experimental epilepsy and sudden death (Figure 17.1). Studies of sudden cardiac death and ouabain toxicity experiments conducted from 1973 to 1979 were published (Lathers et al. 1977a,b; Lathers et al. 1978; Lathers 1980, 1981). Autonomic nonuniform neural discharge in postganglionic cardiac sympathetic nerves innervating the heart was associated with changes in autonomic parameters of cardiac rate and rhythm, blood pressure, and death. These studies became the foundation for SUDEP experiments initiated by Lathers and Schraeder in 1979, published as abstracts in 1980 and as full research publications (Lathers and Schraeder 1982a,b; Schraeder and Lathers 1983). Interictal and ictal electroencephalography (EEG) changes were associated with autonomic nonuniform neural discharge. Autonomic neural imbalance within and between the sympathetic and parasympathetic cardiac nerves, the lockstep phenomenon, cardiac arrhythmias, and death occurred. SUDEP mechanisms, prevention of these mechanisms, and drugs to be used or avoided were expanded in numerous studies. From 1972 throughout 1988, many medical and graduate students; postdoctoral fellows; residents in emergency medicine, neurosurgery, and cardiovascular surgery; faculty in anatomy, cardiology, and pathology; and scientists at different medical schools and pharmaceutical companies worked in Dr. Lathers' laboratory in the Medical College of Pennsylvania and/or with her to expand the findings of mechanistic causes of sudden death in those with cardiac diseases or epilepsy.

The above animal model findings provided knowledge about SUDEP mechanisms, prevention and useful therapeutic drugs but did not provide a method to predict the likelihood of SUDEP. However, these animal experiments have become the starting point for application of our new SUDEP Risk Factor Cluster Identification (ID) methodology to delineate types of experimental data and to predict risk factors for the possibility of SUDEP occurring in a given individual. Knowledge of a given animal model Risk Factor Cluster ID will allow a given laboratory to select an appropriate animal model(s) to study mechanisms of and risk factors for SUDEP to determine how best to prevent its occurrence. Examples of how to score animal models for our SUDEP Risk Factor Cluster IDs are found in this chapter and Figure 17.1 and

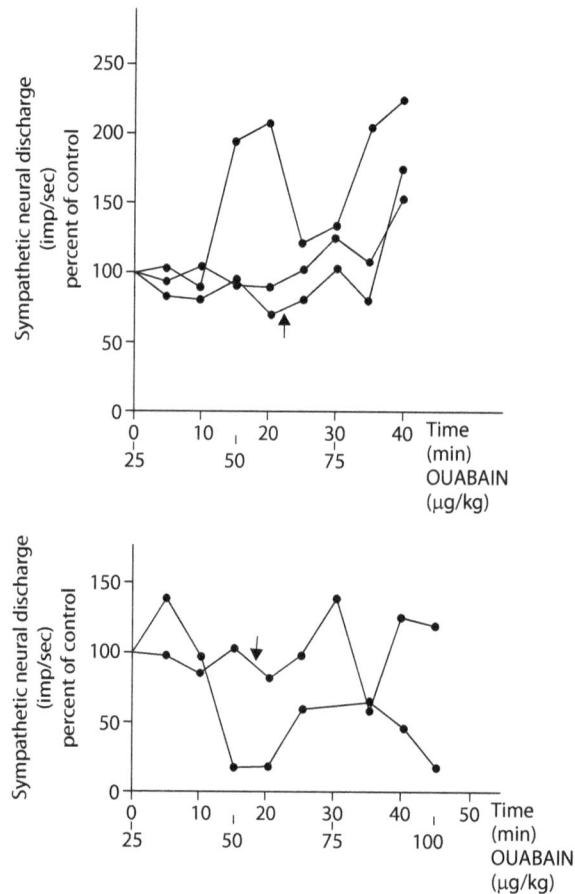

**FIGURE 17.1** The effect of ouabain (25 μg/kg i.v.) on postganglionic cardiac sympathetic neural discharge (impulses/second). The data are graphed as a function of time in minutes. In the upper graph, three nerves were monitored in one cat. In the lower graph, two postganglionic cardiac nerves were monitored in another cat. (From Lathers, Cm, *Eur J Pharmacol*, 64(2–3), 95–106, 1980. With permission.)

in Dr. Verrier's animal model discussion in Chapter 9. The SUDEP Risk Factor method itself is found in Chapters 4 and 5. Mechanistic risk factors for death via SUDEP are based on pathophysiological mechanisms of brain, heart, and/or respiratory systems with assigned numbers of 1, 2, or 3, respectively. Category 4 is for unknown mechanisms. Subcategories include risk factors of A–E etiology, origin, type, severity of seizures, and age of onset of epilepsy; F cardiac autonomic arrhythmogenic findings such as ventricular fibrillation or asystole, G cardiac function, H respiratory and hypoxia pathology, I syncope, J genetics, Q age group, etc. Cluster Identifier K for subcategory of AEDs, if determined, indicates if levels were found to be therapeutic, subtherapeutic, above the therapeutic range, or absent. Question: Is risk related to the antiepileptic drug (AED) used or tapering of AED and is increased risk related to the number of AEDs, types of comedications, and/or alcohol (L1a4) or illicit drug (L1a5) use? Variable M is concomitant diagnosed diseases, whether contributory to cause of death, progressive pathology such as a tumor, which contributed to death in a person with epilepsy but not SUDEP. Mc2 and Mc14 are variables of intracranial and intraocular pressures, vision, and optic nerve. Psychological diseases N, with subcategories of stress N1, anxiety N2, depression N3, and bipolar disease N4 are included. Unusual factors of climate, temperature, omega-3

fatty acids, lunar phase, time of year, traffic, etc., are in cluster identifier O. Sex is Cluster Identifier P, age at time of death is Q, R indicates if a person was a smoker while S is incidence/occurrence of SUDEP as reported or determined for a given study, if known. S1 identifies U.S. states/counties of death and S2 designates foreign countries. Cluster Identifier T1 and T2 indicate data from humans and animals, respectively. U is race/ethnicity and the V ID is postmortem examination.

## OUABAIN TOXICITY/DEATH MODEL

(See Figure 17.1) Lathers developed two different animal models to examine the role of autonomic cardiac neural discharge in the production of cardiac arrhythmias and/or death. Anesthetized cats were studied by performing a right thoracotomy in animals on a respirator to allow recordings of neural discharge from postganglionic cardiac sympathetic nerves (Lathers 1980; Lathers et al. 1974, 1977a, 1977b). Blood gases were maintained within the physiological range during the surgical procedure. In the first model, ouabain was administered intravenously (i.v.) every 15 minutes until arrhythmias were elicited and continued until death occurred. Neural discharge in the minute prior to the onset of arrhythmia was simultaneously increased in one nerve, decreased in another, and decreased to a lesser extent in the third nerve (reproduced with permission from Lathers (1980; Figure 17.1 upper graph). Immediately prior to ouabain-induced arrhythmia, neural discharge was slightly increased in one postganglionic cardiac sympathetic nerve and depressed in the other postganglionic cardiac sympathetic nerve branch recorded from a second animal (lower graph) (Lathers 1980). This discharge pattern was designated "nonuniform" (Lathers 1980; Lathers et al. 1974; Lathers et al. 1977a; Lathers et al. 1977b). In contrast, when the neural discharge in each of three postganglionic sympathetic branches was increased, this was a "uniform" neural discharge. Neural discharge was also designated "uniform" when all neural activity was decreased or unchanged. The uniform postganglionic cardiac sympathetic neural discharge was hypothesized to be necessary at the cardiac myocardial junctions to maintain normal electrical excitability and automaticity, i.e., normal sinus rhythm. In contrast, a "nonuniform" neural discharge occurred when activity in one sympathetic branch was increased and that in a second was decreased, while discharge was not altered in a third (Lathers 1980). Nonuniform neural discharge was hypothesized to be manifested in the heart as inhomogeneity of myocardial electrical excitability and conduction patterns as demonstrated by Han and Moe (1964). They found that myocardial nonuniformity could cause ventricular arrhythmias, including death via ventricular fibrillation.

## CORONARY OCCLUSION SUDDEN DEATH MODEL

The second animal model developed by Lathers (2011, ch. 27, p. 427) in her laboratory mimicked the cardiac arrhythmias occurring in victims of sudden death associated with an acute myocardial infarction. Abrupt acute coronary occlusion of the left anterior descending coronary artery was done in anesthetized cats. The resulting cardiac arrhythmias and death were also associated with a nonuniform cardiac sympathetic neural discharge (Lathers 1980, 1981; Lathers et al. 1977a, 1977b,1978). The associated arrhythmia was suppressed by cardiac-selective beta-adrenergic blocking agents (Spivey and Lathers 1985; Lathers and Spivey 1987; Lathers et al. 1988a,b).

## EPILEPTOGENIC SUDDEN DEATH MODEL

The data obtained in these animal models for digitalis, ouabain or digoxin, toxicity and coronary occlusion raised the question of whether a new animal model of neural nonuniformity and arrhythmias could be developed to investigate experimental mechanisms of sudden unexplained death in persons with epilepsy. Six years after Lathers developed the above two animal models to study the role of the autonomic nervous system in causing arrhythmias and death due to digitalis toxicity and coronary occlusion, these models were modified in collaboration with Dr. Schraeder to study the effects of epileptogenic activity on autonomic cardiac neural discharge and risk for potentially fatal arrhythmias (Lathers

and Schraeder 2011, ch. 28, p. 437; Lathers and Schraeder 1982a,b; Lathers and Schraeder 1990a,b,c; Schraeder and Lathers 1983).

The modified cat model was used to investigate reported cardiac neural autonomic dysfunction and cardiac arrhythmias. Further, this model would help examine relationships of epileptogenic activity, autonomic nervous system, and the cardiopulmonary system to identify possible mechanisms of SUDEP. We found subconvulsant, interictal discharges were associated with autonomic cardiac neural nonuniform discharge and cardiac arrhythmias. These studies established that cortical seizure discharges were associated with neural activity characterized by increases, decreases, or no change in the discharge of simultaneously recorded postganglionic cardiac sympathetic activity. The findings were similar to ouabain induced and/or coronary occlusion models of cardiac arrhythmia. The observation of cardiac sympathetic neural nonuniform discharges in association with seizure discharges was congruent with those of Han and Moe (1964). Further, the studies demonstrated that cardiac sympathetic neural disturbance, whether secondary to direct sympathetic nerve stimulation, ouabain toxicity, or coronary occlusion, increased temporal dispersion of recovery of ventricular excitability. This underlying electrical instability predisposes the ventricular myocardium to arrhythmia. Some experiments also monitored vagal cardiac neural discharge with the sympathetic cardiac neural discharge. Dysfunction of both was evident at the time of occurrence of the dysfunctions and cardiac arrhythmias. Splanchnic nerve activity was monitored as an indicator of catecholamine release from the adrenal medulla. It was concluded that occurrence of cardiac arrhythmias and/or death was associated with autonomic neural dysfunction within sympathetic neural branches to the heart or within the parasympathetic nervous system. In other words, cardiac arrhythmias and/or death may be the manifestation of an imbalance between the two divisions of the autonomic nervous system, i.e., the parasympathetic and sympathetic nervous system (Lathers et al. 1977a,b, 1978).

### IMBALANCE IN SYMPATHETIC AND PARASYMPATHETIC CARDIAC NEURAL DISCHARGE, INTERICTAL AND ICTAL ACTIVITY, AND ARRHYTHMIA

In addition to the effect of ictal discharges on sympathetic and parasympathetic cardiac neural discharges, subconvulsant interictal cortical discharges induced by pentylenetetrazol (PTZ) were also associated with autonomic cardiac neural nonuniform discharges and cardiac conduction and rhythm changes (Lathers and Schraeder 1980, 1982a,b, 1983; Schraeder and Lathers 1980, 1983, 1989; Carnel et al. 1985). Subsequent studies examined the relationship of the effect of interictal activity, arrhythmias, and death with altered autonomic nonuniform postganglionic cardiac and sympathetic and parasympathetic postganglionic cardiac neural discharge. Other experiments examined the effect of pretreatment with phenobarbital (PB), finding a delay in the onset time of interictal and ictal activity but no protective effect on the associated autonomic neural changes once the epileptiform discharges were established (Lathers et al. 1984; Carnel et al. 1985). The same observations were extant in a model of focal epilepsy using injection of penicillin into the hippocampus of the cat (Tumer et al. 1993; Lathers and Schraeder 1990a; Lathers et al. 1993).

Another series of experiments (Lathers et al. 1983,1987; Lathers and Schraeder 1990a,b,c; Lathers and Schraeder 2011, ch. 28; Stauffer et al. 1989; Stauffer et al. 1990 and 2011, ch. 30; O'Rourke and Lathers 1990, ch. 15; O'Rourke and Lathers 2011, ch. 31) explored the lockstep phenomenon, i.e., the synchronization of interictal cortical discharges with postganglionic cardiac sympathetic and parasympathetic neural discharges and changes of blood pressure, cardiac conduction, and rhythm, including the effects of PB on this phenomenon (Dodd-O and Lathers 1990). Timolol (intracerebroventricular [i.c.v.] injection) exhibited an anticonvulsant effect (Lathers et al. 1989a). Subsequent experiments by Mameli et al., using hemispherectomized rats, induced epilepsy with penicillin applied to the rat hypothalamus. In this model, both interictal and ictal activity induced cardiac arrhythmias. These data were confirmatory of the data documenting the arrhythmogenic potential of epileptiform discharges obtained in the cat model. (Please see relevant comments by Lathers and colleagues, Schraeder, Carnel, Weiner, Suter, Kraras, Tumer, Jim, Spivey, Stauffer, Dodd-O, O'Rourke, Goldman, Schoffstall, and Levin in this chapter and in Chapters 18, 19, 20, and 21).

## MODULATION OF PRESYNAPTIC GAMMA-AMINOBUTYRIC ACID (GABA) RELEASE

Experimental evidence supports the possibility that GABA release is modulated by prostaglandin E 2 and enkephalins in autonomic dysfunction characterized by nonuniform discharge (Suter and Lathers 1984; Kraras et al. 1987; Lathers et al. 1988c; Lathers 1990; Schwartz and Lathers 1990). Lathers and colleagues (Kraras et al. 1987; Lathers et al. 1988c; Schwartz and Lathers 1990) inquired into whether enkephalins elicit epileptogenic activity by inhibiting the release of GABA and result in associated autonomic dysfunction and cardiac arrhythmias. A prolonged elevation of immunoreactive methionine (met)-enkephalin content in the septum, hypothalamus, amygdala, and hippocampus of rats occurred after PTZ-induced convulsions (Vindrola et al. 1984). Increased concentrations of met-enkephalins were associated with a greater percent inhibition of potassium-stimulated GABA release (Brennan et al. 1980). Snead and Bearden (1980) found that leucine-enkephalin in the central nervous system may induce epileptogenic activity.

## CARDIAC BETA-RECEPTOR DENSITY

Again, the importance of the gradation of beta receptors with increasing density from base to apex appeared to be its relationship with cardiac contractile function. Timolol

decreased heart rate and blood pressure prior to occlusion. The mean times to arrhythmia and death were not significantly increased by any dosing regimen of timolol, although there was a trend for an increase in the time to death after 1 week of timolol pretreatment. Also there was an increase in the time to arrhythmia and death after 14 days of pretreatment. When compared with data obtained in control cats administered only saline, chronic timolol produced minimal changes in postganglionic cardiac sympathetic neural discharge. Timolol given chronically (p.o.) or acutely (5 mg/kg, i.v. given 15 minutes prior to occlusion) also did not prevent the cardiac sympathetic discharge associated with the development of arrhythmia. The time to arrhythmia and death in the acutely treated cats was increased, but not significantly. Since cardiac sympathetic neural discharge increased as blood pressure fell in the control period but did not increase after occlusion in the timolol-treated animals, the combination of timolol and occlusion may have modified neural discharge via an action on the baroreceptor mechanism. Chronic treatment with timolol produced an occlusion-induced decrease in beta-adrenergic receptor density that was not observed in cats in which only occlusion was done but not timolol was given.

Both the ouabain toxicity and coronary occlusion studies (Lathers, Roberts et al 1977a,b, 1978) and subsequent SUDEP studies (Lathers and Schraeder 1982, Ieda 2007) provide evidence that dysregulation of cardiac nerves contributes significantly to sudden cardiac death. Innervation density is high in the subepicardium and the central conduction system. In diseased hearts, cardiac innervations density varies, a condition that may lead to sudden cardiac death. After myocardial infarction, sympathetic denervation is followed by reinnervation within the heart, leading to unbalanced neural activation and lethal arrhythmia (Lathers et al. 1986b, 1988a, 1990).

## POSTGANGLIONIC CARDIAC SYMPATHETIC NONUNIFORM NEURAL DISCHARGE

Use of the modified sudden death coronary occlusion animal model (Lathers et al. 1977a; Lathers et al. 1977b; Lathers et al. 1978; Lathers 1980) has provided answers to two questions: (1) Do disease states alter function of this neural discharge and (2) Does the sympathetic postganglionic cardiac neural discharge represents one site for action of pharmacological agent to modify function by preventing the nonuniform neural discharge (ouabain or coronary occlusion—Lathers et al. 1974; Lathers et al. 1977a; Lathers et al. 1977b; Lathers et al. 1978; Lathers 1980) (epilepsy—Lathers and Schraeder 1982a,b; Schraeder and Lathers 1983). These two questions have been answered just recently for persons with epilepsy. A study has been conducted for postganglionic cardiac sympathetic innervations in patients with chronic temporal lobe epilepsy. Druschky et al. (2001) found sympathetic dysfunction in the form of altered postganglionic cardiac sympathetic innervation in persons with chronic temporal lobe epilepsy and commented that autonomic dysfunction is associated with the risk of cardiac abnormalities and/or SUDEP. The exact role of neural innervation in arrhythmogenesis, as well as in regulatory mechanisms determining density and pattern of cardiac sympathetic innervation, have been studied by Lathers et al. (1986), Lathers et al. (1988a), Lathers et al. (1990), and Lathers laboratory coauthors, and are discussed by Lathers and Levin (2011, ch. 33). The clinical study of Druschky et al. (2001) conducted in humans confirms the numerous animal studies conducted by Lathers, Roberts, Kelliher, Schraeder, and colleagues over the years.

## AED ACTIVITY OF BETA-BLOCKING AGENTS

Experiments were designed to explore the ability of beta-blocking agents to suppress seizures induced by PTZ in two species, the cat and the pig. (Lathers et al. 1989a; Lathers et al. 2011a, ch. 34, pp. 563–4). Cats were anesthetized with alpha-chloralose and PTZ (10–20 mg i.c.v.) was administered to elicit epileptiform activity, including both interictal and ictal discharges. Timolol 10, 100, 500 µg/kg i.c.v. and 1, 5, 10, and/or 20 mg/kg i.v. was then administered at 5-minute intervals to determine whether it suppressed the epileptiform activity. After the administration of PTZ, mean arterial blood pressure and heart rate increased and epileptiform activity developed. All doses of timolol caused a decrease in the blood pressure and heart rate elevated by PTZ. The administration of timolol also suppressed the epileptiform activity and associated cardiac rhythm changes. Similar findings were obtained in cats that received the same doses of timolol administered at different time intervals. Both anticonvulsant and antiarrhythmic actions of the beta-blocking agent timolol were demonstrated after central administration in cats.

Domestic swine (13–20 kg) were prepared for recordings of arterial blood pressure, electrocardiography, and electrocortical activity. Seizure activity was induced by PTZ (100 mg/kg i.v.). Sixty seconds after the onset of seizure activity, the animals received either no drug (control) or propranolol (2.5 mg/kg i.v.). A transient increase in the mean arterial blood pressure was observed following PTZ administration. Intravenous propranolol significantly suppressed the seizure duration (seconds per minute interval) at 1 minute following drug administration: seizure duration for control, 36.3 ± 4.8 versus i.v. propranolol, 12.3 ± 5.1. Intravenous propranolol also produced a maximal decrease of 32–38% in the basal heart rate and reduced the transient increase in mean arterial blood pressure elicited by PTZ, with no significant effect on the basal mean arterial blood pressure. Plasma propranolol levels were found to be 6.07 ± 1.43 µg/mL at 1 minute after administration, falling to 1.10 ± 0.27 µg/mg over the following 19 minutes of the experiment (Lathers et al. 1989b). The data demonstrate that propranolol via the intraosseous or i.v. routes possesses anticonvulsant activity against PTZ-induced seizures in both the pig and the cat, respectively, and that timolol exhibited anticonvulsant and antiarrhythmic activity in the cat. Valium and lorazepam (Jim et al. 1989) also exhibited anticonvulsant activity in the pigs similar to that of propranolol (Lathers et al. 1989b). Also see discussion of beta-blockers in animal models of seizure by Lathers in this chapter and Lathers et al., Chapter 37, in this book.

*An Example of How To Score Animal Models For Our SUDEP Risk Factor Cluster IDs* follows and is also summarized in Figure 17.1; in Dr. Verrier's animal model discussion, Chapter 9, and in Dr. Faingold's model below and in his Chapter 31, in this book. The SUDEP Risk Factor method itself is found in Chapters 4 and 5, this book.

## CAT MODELS SUDEP/SUDDEN DEATH: CONFIRMING HUMAN DATA 15–22 YRS LATER

### PENTYLENETETRAZOL, I.V., LATHERS AND SCHRAEDER (1982A,B). PHENOBARBITAL (PB) LATHERS ET AL. (1984), CARNEL ET AL. (1985)

1, 2, A11a1, A11a2, A11b, or A11c, C1, C2, C3, F1, F1a, F2, F2a, F2b, G1, K1a1, PB, T2, V2b (lung)

*Cluster Number 1.* Brain. EEG interictal, brief ictal, and ictal activity as contributory mechanisms for SUDEP can be studied in this animal model.

*Cluster Number 2.* Cardiac autonomic neural discharge and associated arrhythmias and/or death as contributory mechanisms for SUDEP may be studied using this animal model.

*Cluster Number 3.* Respiratory and hypoxia mechanisms of SUDEP may not be studied using this model because a respirator is required to ventilate the cat after open chest surgery to record postganglionic cardiac sympathetic and vagal neural discharge. In these experiments, blood gases were monitored during the period before the administration of PTZ alone or Pb pretreatment followed by PTZ to maintain pH, pO2, and pCO2 levels. Future experiments could monitor blood gas values throughout the entire experiment rather than during only the period before administration of PTZ and/or PB to determine if the method of artificial respiration used does or does not prevent hypoxia, hypercarbia, and alteration in acid–base balance, all factors which may additionally contribute to alterations in autonomic parameters monitored in the model. A postmortem external autopsy revealed lung pathology, including pulmonary edema.

Cluster Numbers 1 and 2 can be studies as contributory mechanisms for SUDEP

A. Epilepsy Localization Categories
   A11a Left hemisphere
   A11a1 Temporal
   A11a2 Frontal
   A11b Right hemisphere
   A11c Both hemispheres, nonlateralized
   C1 Interictal, subconvulsant discharges
   C2 Brief ictal
   C3 Ictal
   F Cardiac arrhythmogenic includes subcategories:
   F Autonomic (ANA) neural
   F1 Sympathetic (Sym)
   F1a Fibrillation

F2 Parasympathetic (PNS)

F2a Asystolic

F2b Ictal bradycardia

G1 Function, long QT, AV block

K1a1 Phenobarbital

T2 Animal data

V Postmortem examination

V2b (lung) Nondecomposed body: External examination only without toxicological analysis

## DBA MICE AS MODELS OF SUDDEN UNEXPECTED DEATH IN EPILEPSY

### SUDEP Syndrome Cluster Identifier: 1, (2 maybe), 3 A, H, J, T2

The dilute brown non-Agouti (DBA/2) mouse has been proposed as a model of SUDEP (Venit et al. 2004; Tupal and Faingold 2006, Faingold et al. 2011 a,b). DBA mice are genetically susceptible to generalized convulsive seizures evoked by acoustic stimulation (audiogenic seizures) that results in sudden death. Significant evidence indicates that the sudden death in the DBA/2 mice is caused by generalized convulsive seizure-associated respiratory arrest with a role for serotonin. See Dr. Faingold et al., Chapter 31 of this book for full details of this mouse model. *Cluster Number 1.* Brain. EEG interictal, brief ictal, and ictal activity as contributory mechanisms for SUDEP can be studied in this animal model. *Cluster Number 2.* Cardiac autonomic neural discharge and associated arrhythmias and/or death as contributory mechanisms for SUDEP may or may not be studied using this animal model, depending on the experimental design. *Cluster Number 3.* Respiratory and hypoxia mechanisms of SUDEP may be studied in this model.

## CONCLUSIONS

Animal models are presented for investigator selection to study mechanisms of and risk factors for SUDEP. How to score animal models for our SUDEP Risk Factor Cluster IDs is described. Data from these animal models will become part of our animal database to push forward knowledge of SUDEP. Data from these animal models will become part of our animal database to push forward knowledge of SUDEP in autopsy studies like that of Lathers et al. 2011b.

## REFERENCES

Brennan MJ, Cantrill RC, Wylie BA. Modulation of synaptosomal GABA release by enkephalin. *Life Sci* 1980;27:1097–101.

Carnel SB, Schaeder PL, Lathers CM. Effect of Phenobarbital pretreatment on cardiac neural discharge and pentylenetetrazol-induced epileptogenic activity in the cat. *Pharmacology* 1985;30(4):225–40.

Dodd-O J, Lathers CM. A characterization of the lockstep phenomenon in phenobarbital pretreated cats. In: Lathers CM, Schraeder PL, eds. *Epilepsy and Sudden Death.* New York: Marcel Dekker; 1990, pp. 199–220.

Druschky A, Hiltz MJ, Hopp P, Platsch G, Radespiel-Trőger M, Druschky K, Kuwert T, Stefan H, Neundörfer B. Interictal cardiac autonomic dysfunction in temporal lobe epilepsy demonstrated by [ (123) I-meta I-odobenzylguanidine-SPECT. *Brain* 2001;124(Pt 12):372–82.

Faingold CL, Tupal S, Mhaskar Y, Uteshev VV. DBA mice as models of sudden unexpected death in epilepsy. Chapter. 41 In: Lathers CM, Schraeder PL, Bungo MW, Leestma JE, eds. *Sudden Death in Epilepsy: Forensic and Clinical Issues.* Boca Raton, FL: CRC Press/Taylor & Francis Group; 2011a, pp. 659–78.

Faingold CL, Tupal S, Randall M. Prevention of seizure-induced sudden death in a chronic SUDEP model by semichronic administration of a selective serotonin reuptake inhibitor. *Epilepsy Behav* 2011b Oct;22(2):186-90.

Han J, Moe GK. Nonuniform recovery of excitability in ventricular muscle. *Circ Res* 1964 Jan;14:44–60.

Ieda M, Kanazawa H, Kimura K, Hattori F, Ieda Y, Taniguchi M, Lee JK, Matsumura K, Tomita Y, Miyoshi S, et al. Sema3a maintains normal heart rhythm through sympathetic innervation patterning. *Nat Med* 2007;13(5):604–12.

Jim KF, Lathers CM, Farris VL, Pratt LF, Spivey WH. Suppression of pentylenetetrazol elicited seizure activity by intraosseous lorazepam in pigs. *Epilepsia* 1989;30:480–6.

Kraras CM, Tumer N, Lathers CM. The role of enkephalins in the production of epileptogenic activity and autonomic dysfunction: origin of arrhythmia and sudden death in the epileptic patient? *Med Hypotheses* 1987;23(1):19–31.

Lathers CM. Effect of timolol on postganglionic cardiac and preganglionic splanchnic sympathetic neural discharge associated with ouabain-induced arrhythmia. *Eur J Pharmacol* 1980;64(2–3):95–106.

Lathers CM. *Induced disease. Myocardial Infarction. Mammalian Models for Research on Aging.* Washington, DC: National Academy of Science, National Academy Press; 1981, pp. 224–8.

Lathers CM. Role of neuropeptides in the production of epileptogenic activity and arrhythmias. In: Lathers CM, Schraeder PL, eds. *Epilepsy and Sudden Death.* New York: Marcel Dekker; 1990, pp. 309–27.

Lathers CM. Epilepsy and sudden death. Personal reflections and global call for action. *Epilepsy Behav* 2009;15(3):269–77.

Lathers CM. Animal model for sudden cardiac death: autonomic cardiac sympathetic nonuniform neural discharge. In: Lathers CM, Schraeder PL, Bungo, MW, Leestma JE, eds. *Sudden Death in Epilepsy: Forensic and Clinical Factors.* Boca Raton, FL: CRC Press/Taylor & Francis Group; 2011, pp. 427–36.

Lathers CM, Jim KF, High WB, Spivey WH, Matthews WD, Ho T. An investigation of the pathological and physiological effects of intraosseous sodium bicarbonate in pigs. *J Clin Pharmacol* 1989a;29(4):354–9.

Lathers CM, Jim KF, Spivey WH. A comparison of intraosseous and intravenous routes of administration for antiseizure agents. *Epilepsia* 1989b;30(4):472–9.

Lathers CM, Jim KF, Spivey WH, Khan C, Dolce K, Matthews WD. Antiepileptic activity of beta blocking drugs. In: Lathers CM, Schraeder PL, Bungo MW, Leestma JE, eds. *Sudden Death in Epilepsy: Forensic and Clinical Factors.* Boca Raton, FL: CRC Press/Taylor & Francis Group; 2011a; pp. 551–66.

Lathers CM, Kelliher GJ, Roberts J, Beasley AB. Nonuniform cardiac sympathetic nerve discharge: Mechanism for coronary occlusion and digitalis-induced arrhythmia. *Circulation* 1978;57:1058–65.

Lathers CM, Kelliher G, Roberts J, Beasley AB. Role of the adrenergic nervous system in arrhythmia produced by acute coronary artery occlusion. Myocardial Ischemia Symposium,

Philadelphia Physiological Society, May 6, 1976. In: Lefer A, Kelliher G, Rovetto M, eds. *Pathophysiology and Therapeutics of Myocardial Ischemia*. New York: Spectrum Publications; 1977a, pp. 123–47.

Lathers CM, Koehler SA, Wecht CH, Schraeder PL. Forensic antiepileptic drug levels in autopsy cases of epilepsy. *Epilepsy Behav* 2011b, 22:778–85.

Lathers CM, Levin RM. Animal model for sudden cardiac death. Sympathetic innervations and myocardial beta-receptor densities. In: Lathers CM, Schraeder PL, Bungo MW, Leestma JE, eds. *Sudden Death in Epilepsy: Forensic and Clinical Factors*. Boca Raton, FL: CRC Press/Taylor & Francis Group; 2011, pp. 539–50.

Lathers CM, Levin RM, Spivey WH. Regional distribution of myocardial beta receptors in the cat. *Eur J Pharmacol* 1986;130(1–2):111–7.

Lathers CM, Lipka LJ. Cardiac arrhythmia, sudden death, and psychoactive agents. *J Clin Pharmacol* 1987;27(1):1–14.

Lathers CM, Roberts J, Kelliher GJ. Relationship between the effect of ouabain on arrhythmia and interspike intervals (ISI) of cardiac accelerator nerves. *Pharmacologist* 1974;16:201.

Lathers CM, Roberts J, Kelliher GJ. Correlation of ouabain-induced arrhythmia and nonuniformity in the histamine-evoked discharge of cardiac sympathetic nerves. *J Pharmacol Exp Ther* 1977b;203(2):467–79.

Lathers, CM, Schraeder PL. Autonomic dysfunction in epilepsy III: Characterization of autonomic cardiac neural discharge associated with pentylenetetrazol-induced seizures. *Clin Res* 1980;28:616A.

Lathers CM, Schraeder PL. Autonomic dysfunction in epilepsy: Characterization of autonomic cardiac neural discharge associated with pentylenetetrazol-induced epileptogenic activity. *Epilepsia* 1982a;23(6):633–47.

Lathers CM, Schraeder PL. Autonomic dysfunction in epilepsy: Characterization of autonomic cardiac neural discharge associated with pentylenetetrazol-induced epileptogenic activity. *Epilepsia* 1982b;23(6):633–48.

Lathers CM, Schraeder PL. Autonomic dysfunction, cardiac arrhythmias, and epileptogenic activity. 15th Epilepsy International Symposium and Am Epilepsy Soc Meeting. Unexpected, Unexplained Death in Epileptic Persons *Symposium*, 15, 13; 1983.

Lathers CM, Schraeder PL. Arrhythmias associated with epileptogenic activity elicited by penicillin. In: Lathers CM, Schraeder PL, eds. *Epilepsy and Sudden Death*. New York: Marcel Dekker; 1990a, pp. 157–67.

Lathers CM, Schraeder PL, eds. *Epilepsy and Sudden Death*. New York: Marcel Dekker; 1990b.

Lathers CM, Schraeder PL. Synchronized cardiac neural discharge and epileptogenic activity, The Lockstep Phenomenon: Correlation with cardiac arrhythmias. In: Lathers CM, Schraeder PL, eds. *Epilepsy and Sudden Death*. New York: Marcel Dekker; 1990c, pp. 187–97.

Lathers CM, Schraeder PL. Verbal autopsies and SUDEP. *Epilepsy Behav* 2009;14(4):573–6.

Lathers CM, Schraeder PL. Animal model for sudden unexpected death in persons with epilepsy. Chapter. 28 In: Lathers CM, Schraeder PL, Bungo, MW, Leestma JE, eds. *Sudden Death in Epilepsy: Forensic and Clinical Factors*. Boca Raton, FL: CRC Press/Taylor & Francis Group; 2011, pp. 437–64.

Lathers CM, Schraeder PL, Bungo MW. Letter to the Editor: Unanswered Questions SUDEP. *Epilepsy Behav* 2008a; 13:265–9.

Lathers CM, Schraeder PL, Bungo, MW. Sudden death: neurocardiologic mystery. In: Sher L, ed. *Psychological Factors and Cardiovascular Disorders: Role of Stress and Psychosocial Influences*. New York: Nova Biomedical Books; 2008b, pp. 263–311.

Lathers CM, Schraeder PL, Carnel SB. Neural mechanisms in cardiac arrhythmias associated with epileptogenic activity: The effect of phenobarbital in the cat. *Life Sci* 1984;34(20):1919–36.

Lathers CM, Schraeder PL, Tumer N. The effect of phenobarbital on autonomic function and epileptogenic activity induced by the hippocampal injection of penicillin in cats. *J Clin Pharmacol* 1993;33(9):837–44.

Lathers CM, Schraeder PL, Weiner FL. Synchronization of cardiac autonomic neural discharge with epileptogenic activity: the lock step phenomenon. *Electroencephalogr Clin Neurophysiol* 1987;67(3):247–59.

Lathers CM, Smith CM. Ethanol effects on muscle spindle afferent activity and spinal reflexes. *J Pharmacol Exp Therapeutics* 1976;126–34.

Lathers CM, Spivey WH. The effect of beta blockers on cardiac neural discharge associated with coronary occlusion in the cat. *J Clin Pharmacol* 1987;27(8):582–92.

Lathers CM, Spivey WH, Levin RM. The effect of chronic timolol in an animal model for myocardial infarction. *J Clin Pharmacol* 1988a;28(8):736–45.

Lathers CM, Spivey WH, Levin RM, Tumer N. The effect of dilevalol on cardiac autonomic neural discharge, plasma catecholamines, and myocardial beta receptor density associated with coronary occlusion. *J Clin Pharmacol* 1990;30(3): 241–53.

Lathers CM, Spivey WH, Suter LE, Lerner JP, Tumer N, Levin RM. The effect of acute and chronic administration of timolol on cardiac sympathetic neural discharge, arrhythmia, and beta receptor density associated with coronary occlusion in the cat. *Life Sci* 1986;39(22):2121–41.

Lathers CM, Spivey WH, Tumer N. The effect of timolol given five minutes post coronary occlusion on plasma catecholamines. *J Clin Pharmacol* 1988b;28(4):289–9.

Lathers CM, Stauffer AZ, Tumer N, Kraras CM, Goldman BD. Anticonvulsant and antiarrhythmic actions of the beta blocking agent timolol. *Epilepsy Res* 1989a;4(1):42–54.

Lathers CM, Tumer N, Kraras CM. The effect of intracerebroventricular D-ALA²-methionine enkephalinamide and naloxone on cardiovascular parameters in the cat. *Life Sci* 1988c;43(26):2287–98.

Lathers CM, Tumer N, Schoffstall JM. Plasma catecholamines, pH, and blood pressure during cardiac arrest in pigs. *Resuscitation* 1989b;18(1):59–74.

Lathers CM, Weiner FL, Schraeder PL. Synchronization of cardiac autonomic neural discharge with epileptogenic activity. *Cir Res* 1983;31:630A.

O'Rourke DK, Lathers CM. Interspike interval histogram characterization of synchronized cardiac sympathetic neural discharge and epileptogenic activity in the electrocorticogram of the cat. In: Lathers CM, Schraeder PL, eds. *Epilepsy and Sudden Death*. New York: Marcel Dekker; 1990, pp. 239–59.

O'Rourke D, Lathers CM. Interspike interval histogram characterization of synchronized cardiac sympathetic neural discharge and epileptogenic activity in electrocorticogram of cat. In: Lathers CM, Schraeder PL, Bungo MW, Leestma JE, eds. *Sudden Death in Epilepsy: Forensic and Clinical Issues*. Boca Raton, FL: CRC Press/Taylor & Francis Group; 2011, pp. 495–512.

Schraeder PL, Lathers CM. Cardiac neural discharge and epileptogenic activity in the cat: An animal model for unexplained death. *Life Sci* 1983;32:1371–82.

Schraeder PL, Lathers CM. Paroxysmal autonomic dysfunction and epileptogenic activity and sudden death. *Epilepsy Res* 1989;3(1):55–62.

Schwartz RD, Lathers CM. GABA neurotransmission, epileptogenic activity, and cardiac arrhythmias. In: Lathers CM, Schraeder PL, eds. *Epilepsy and Sudden Death* New York: Marcel Dekker; 1990, pp. 293–307.

Snead OC III, Bearden LJ. Anticonvulsants specific for petit mal antagonize epileptogenic effect of leucine enkephalin. *Science* 1980;210(4473):1031–3.

Spivey WH, Lathers CM. Effect of timolol on the sympathetic nervous system in coronary occlusion in cats. *Ann Emerg Med* 1985. 14: 939–44.

Spratling WT. The causes and manner of death in epilepsy. *Med News* 1902;80:1225–7.

Stauffer AZ, Dodd-O J, Lathers CM. The relationship of the lock-step phenomenon and precipitous changes in mean arterial blood pressure. *Electroencephalogr Clin Neurophysiol* 1989;72(4):340–5.

Stauffer AZ, Dodd-O J, Lathers CM. Relationship of the lock-step phenomenon and precipitous changes in blood pressure. In: Lathers CM, Schraeder PL, eds. *Epilepsy and Sudden Death.* New York: Marcel Dekker; 1990, pp. 221–38.

Stauffer AZ, Dodd-O JM, Lathers CM. Relationship of lock step phenomenon and precipitous changes in blood pressure. In: Lathers CM, Schraeder PL, Bungo MW, Leestma JE, eds. *Sudden Death in Epilepsy: Forensic and Clinical Issues.* Boca Raton, FL: CRC Press/Taylor & Francis Group; 2011, pp. 481–94.

Suter L, Lathers CM. Modulation of presynaptic gamma amino-butyric acid release by prostaglandin E2: Explanation for epileptogenic activity and dysfunction in autonomic cardiac neural discharge leading to arrhythmias. *Med Hypotheses* 1984;15(1):15–30.

Tumer N, Schraeder PL, Lathers CM. The effect of phenobarbital upon autonomic function and epileptogenic activity induced by the hippocampal injection of penicillin in cats. *J Clin Pharmacol* 1993;33(9):837–44.

Tupal S, Faingold CL. Evidence supporting a role of serotonin in modulation of sudden death induced by seizures in DBA/2 mice. *Epilepsia* 2006;47:21–6.

Venit EL, Shepard BD, Seyfried TN. Oxygenation prevents sudden death in seizure-prone mice. *Epilepsia* 2004;45:993–6.

Vindrola O, Asai M, Zubieta M, Talavera E, Rodriguez E, Linares G. Pentylenetetrazol kindling produces a long-lasting elevation of IR-Met-enkephalin but not IR-Leu-enkephalin in rat brain. *Brain Res* 1984;297(1):121–5.

# Section II

## SUDEP Animal Models

*Mechanisms of Risks*

# 18 Sudden Death Animal Models to Study Nervous System Sites of Action for Disease and Pharmacological Intervention

*Claire M. Lathers*

## CONTENTS

## INTRODUCTION

How does one unravel the mystery of sudden unexpected death in persons with epilepsy (SUDEP)? Physicians must identify the persons with epilepsy who are at risk for SUDEP and use all available preventive medical and lifestyle measures, gleaning as much information as possible about the deaths of SUDEP victims by talking with medical examiners and coroners, reviewing autopsy reports (Schraeder et al. 2006, 2009, 2010), and obtaining verbal autopsy information provided by family members and close friends of the victim. The latter technique will help to fill in details missing from the physical autopsy or when no autopsy is done (Lathers and Schraeder 2009). It is also important to utilize in vivo and in vitro models of SUDEP to investigate risk factors, mechanisms, and preventive measures (Lathers et al. 2008; Scorza et al. 2008). Animal models allow us to focus on the details of one or more of the contributing mechanisms of risk for SUDEP. Use of experimental animals allows us to examine the contributing mechanisms of risk for SUDEP, with functional positive and negative feedback systems operating to maintain the normal physiology before experimental modifications, and then to study the effect of dysfunction induced by experimental manipulation of the intact physiological system. Techniques may be applied to various animal models to glean information about the molecular and genetic mechanisms of risks for SUDEP. The various animal models described in this chapter are relevant to the induction of cardiac arrhythmias by various mechanisms and shed light and provide understanding of the problem of sudden death, whether of cardiac or epileptogenic origin.

Application of the principles of clinical pharmacology when using animal models will provide two beneficial effects for persons at risk of sudden death. First, these models will provide the foundation for understanding the factors involved in the origin of arrhythmogenesis and in the future will contribute to the development of new categories of drugs that have both antiarrhythmic and antiepileptic effects. Second, application of the principles of clinical pharmacology when using animal models will allow development of techniques for better drug administration (e.g., introduction of the intraosseous route for pediatric seizing patients in whom a traditional intravenous line cannot be rapidly established in the emergency room in a life and death situation) (Spivey et al. 1985; Lathers et al. 1989c). Application of clinical pharmacology principles to animal models will provide a better understanding of the mechanisms of the origin of cardiac arrhythmias and changes in the nervous system associated with epileptogenic activity and ultimately guiding the development of preventative pharmacological measures.

Nervous system sites of action for disease and/or pharmacological intervention are numerous. Animal models have been designed to mimic diseases such as coronary occlusion and myocardial or digitalis toxicity. The symptoms observed in both models are associated with the development of cardiac arrhythmias and/or sudden death (Lathers 1981). Cardiac arrhythmias that may trigger sudden death in patients originate from three primary sites of action, namely, directly in the heart, in the peripheral autonomic nervous system, or in the central autonomic nervous system and from combinations of some or all of these factors (Lathers et al. 1977, 1978). The central and peripheral autonomic nervous systems are connected, unless a patient has had a cardiac transplant.

In the following sections, various animal models are presented and the information included for each method is followed by possible applications to the problem of SUDEP. The discussion is a brief overview of models that can be used to study mechanisms of action for initiation of sudden death, whether for cardiac sudden death or sudden death in persons with epilepsy. Information obtained using these models,

## TABLE 18.1

### Selected Action Sites for Disease and Drugs

1. Central or peripheral autonomic nervous systems, including afferent and efferent neural activity

2. Superior cervical ganglia

3. Preganglionic nerve

4. Stellate ganglia

5. Postganglionic nerve

6. Baroreceptors

7. Heart

8. Preganglionic splanchnic nerve

9. Adrenal glands, release of circulating catecholamines

with appropriate modification, will provide insights into the mechanisms of sudden death. The data obtained from animal models will not only indicate physiological sites of action for disease but also indicate pharmacological sites of action for antiepileptic drugs (AEDs) or antiarrhythmic drugs to prevent sudden death, as described in Table 18.1.

## IN VITRO ANIMAL MODELS

### RAT/MOUSE HIPPOCAMPAL SLICES

Synaptic plasticity is a long-lasting change in the efficacy of synaptic transmission resulting from patterned activities of the presynaptic nerve (Alkadhi et al. 2005). One type of synaptic plasticity is designated long-term potentiation and is an activity-dependent marked increase in synaptic efficacy. In the central nervous system area of the hippocampus, long-term potentiation is thought to be a cellular correlate of attention, learning, and memory (Sarvey et al. 1989), studying synaptic transmission and synchronous activity in in vitro hippocampal slices obtained from rats (Dahl and Sarvey 1989; Lathers and Sarvey 1989; Sarvey et al. 1989). The hippocampal slice preparation is a tool to study the pharmacological effects of various drugs because the slice is viable and stable for several hours, allowing known concentrations of drugs to be added to the bathing medium and then washed out. The effects of norepinephrine and the β-blocking agent propranolol on long-term potentiation were examined. Norepinephrine (20 μM for 30 minutes) induced a long-lasting potentiation modified by propranolol (Figure 18.1).

Norepinephrine induced an activity-independent long-lasting depression of synaptic transmission in the lateral perforant path input to dentate granule cells, whereas high-frequency stimulation induced activity-dependent long-term potentiation. Bramham et al. (1997) investigated the role of endogenous activation of β-adrenergic receptors in long-term potentiation of the lateral and medial perforant paths under conditions affording selective stimulation of these pathways in the rat hippocampal slice. Propranolol (1 μM), a β-receptor antagonist, blocked long-term potentiation induction of both

lateral and medial perforant path-evoked field excitatory postsynaptic potentials. It was concluded that there is a broad requirement for norepinephrine in different types of synaptic plasticity, including activity-independent depression and activity-dependent long-term potentiation in the lateral perforant path.

A concentration-dependent long-lasting potentiation of the evoked population spike in the dentate gyrus of rat hippocampal slices was elicited by bath application of the GABAB receptor agonist baclofen (Burgard and Sarvey 1991). High-concentration baclofen also produced a loss of inhibition, which manifested as the appearance of epileptiform, multiple-evoked population spikes. Data suggested that baclofen produces a selective disinhibitory effect in the granule cell layer of the dentate gyrus by inhibiting the activity of GABAergic interneurons. High concentrations of baclofen appeared to produce a long-lasting potentiation most likely due to a loss of inhibition.

Lea and Sarvey (2003) reported modulation of epileptiform burst frequency by the metabotropic glutamate receptor subtype mGluR3. This receptor modulates high potassium (10 mM), low calcium (0.5 mN) induced spontaneous epileptic burst activity in acute rat hippocampal slice dentate granule cells. Activation of the group II metabotropic glutamate receptor subtype 3 induced an increase in spontaneous burst duration, while inhibition reversibly reduced the spontaneous burst frequency. The number of spikes per burst was not altered. Nevertheless, this type of neuronal activity does induce spontaneous epileptiform burst frequency. This method is one model that may be explored to further understand mechanisms for and prevention of spontaneous epileptiform activity in the hippocampus. Recent data indicate that a deficit in glutamatergic synaptic transmission recorded in hippocampal slices obtained from aged mice, but not γ-aminobutyric acid (GABA)-mediated synchronous network activity, may be coupled with alterations in synchronous network activity that could lead to deficient information process (Brown et al. 2005). This type of hippocampal activity may also be altered by epileptic discharges and/or AEDs administered to patients with epilepsy resulting in an impairment of cognitive function. Definitive studies need to be conducted to evaluate this possibility.

### ISOLATED AUTONOMIC GANGLIA

Isolated superior cervical ganglia and stellate ganglia have been studied. The stellate ganglia and/or left stellate nerve activity become target sites for drug action and/or disease and may be studied in vitro (Alkadhi and McIsaac 1973, 1974; McIsaac 1978) and in vivo (Alzoubi et al. 2010). New studies are needed to examine the role of this site of action for both the induction and prevention of SUDEP. In vitro experiments are needed to examine the effects of anticonvulsant drugs. Data obtained in vitro should be compared with those obtained in vivo (see discussion later). A phenomenon similar to long-term potentiation in the hippocampus was identified in sympathetic ganglia even earlier

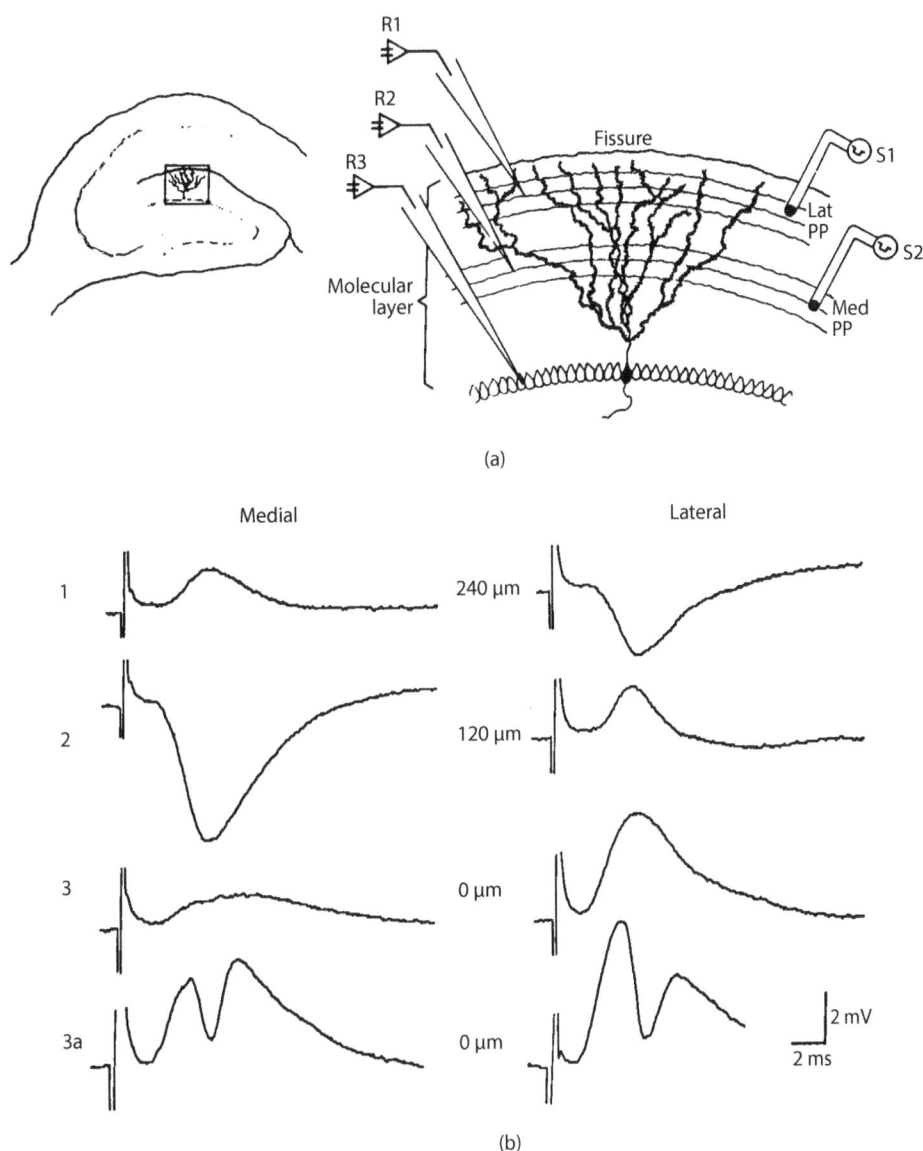

**FIGURE 18.1**    Scheme of a hippocampal rat slice showing the dentate gyrus and projections of the lateral and medial PPs, the respective stimulating electrodes (S1 and S2) and recording electrodes (R1, R2, and R3) in the outer molecular (R1), midmolecular (R2), and granule cell (R3) layers. (From Dahl, D. and JM Sarvey, *Proc Natl Acad Sci USA*, 86 (12), 4776–80, 1989. With permission.)

than its definition in the hippocampus (Alkadhi et al. 2005). Ganglionic long-term potentiation of the nicotinic pathway is a long-lasting increase in synaptic effectiveness induced in autonomic ganglia after a brief train of relatively high-frequency stimulation of the preganglionic nerve and occurs in mammalian, amphibian, and avian species. Stress is a risk factor for sudden cardiac death and sudden death in persons with epilepsy (Pickworth et al. 1990; Lathers and Schraeder 2006). Sustained enhancement in ganglionic transmission occurs in chronic mental stress and may affect activity of autonomic functions of heart rate, arrhythmias, and blood pressure (Alkadhi and Alzoubi 2007). Superior cervical ganglia from rats that developed hypertension as a result of chronic psychosocial stress express ganglionic long-term potentiation in vivo (Alzoubi et al. 2008). Synaptic plasticity

in sympathetic ganglia may involve a molecular cascade similar to that of long-term potentiation in the hippocampal CA1 region. Future studies should be done to examine molecular changes in levels of phosphorylated CAMKII, total CaMKII, nitric oxide synthase, and calmodulin in superior cervical ganglia obtained from animals studied in models in which epilepsy is induced.

Exposure to adrenergic agonists, as well as neuroactive peptides and cyclic nucleotides, may produce long-lasting increases in synaptic effectiveness. Thus, one would predict that a β-blocking agent would prevent this long-lasting increase in synaptic effectiveness and could exhibit an antiepileptic activity for β blockers via an action on the preganglionic nerve and/or the autonomic ganglia. Understanding how to manipulate the mechanisms of induction and maintenance of ganglionic long-term potentiation in persons with epilepsy who may be at risk for sudden death is most important as the ganglionic long-term potentiation response is dependent on serotonin for both its induction and maintenance (Alkadhi et al. 2005). See Chapter 17 (Faingold et al. 2010; Paterson 2010), for discussions on the possible role of serotonin in SUDEP or sudden infant death.

The aging process itself is thought to involve a decrease in the ability of humans and animals to respond to stress (Alzoubi et al. 2008). Old animals have an exaggerated sympathetic activity associated with increased morbidity and mortality. In vivo expression of long-term potentiation in the superior cervical ganglion of aged animals may contribute to the moderate hypertension observed in aged subjects. Alzoubi et al. (2008) found elevations in molecular signals required for expression of long-term potentiation in sympathetic ganglia in obese Zucker rats in vivo. They also demonstrated that synaptic plasticity in sympathetic ganglia may involve a molecular cascade similar to long-term potentiation of the brain hippocampal area CA1. Additional studies of the role of these molecular signals in animal models of epilepsy are required to obtain a better understanding of the molecular mechanisms and of how to manipulate them to prevent sudden death.

Long-term depression is a use-dependent decrease in synaptic efficacy and is a type of synaptic plasticity related to cognitive function in the central nervous system (Alkadhi et al. 2008). Long-term depression has been demonstrated in rat superior cervical ganglia and suggests that expression of ganglionic long-term depression involves activation of 5-HT (3) receptors.

## LANGENDORFF PREPARATION TO STUDY ISOLATED CAT, RAT, OR MOUSE HEARTS

Langendorff established the isolated perfused mammalian heart preparation in 1897, a method still valid today (Skrzypiec-Spring et al. 2007). Crystalloid perfusates or blood enter the heart via a cannula in the ascending aorta at constant pressure or constant flow. Leaflets of the aortic valve are closed by the retrograde flow in the aorta. This action allows all of the perfusate to enter the coronary arteries via the ostia at the aortic root. The perfusate passes through coronary circulation and drains into the right atrium via the coronary sinus. The method allows direct measurement of cardiac contractile function and coronary flow without interference from changes in the systemic circulation (Grover and Singh 2007). Use of this method provided the basis for understanding heart physiology, including the roles of temperature, oxygen and calcium ions for heart contractile function, origin of cardiac electrical activity in the atrium, negative chronotropic effect of vagus stimulation, and chemical transmission of impulses in the vagus nerve by acetylcholine (Skrzypiec-Spring et al. 2007). The preparation is used to study ischemia-reperfusion injuries, cell-based therapy, and donor heart preservation for transplant and may be used to study vascular reactivity (Reichelt et al.

2009). Snyder et al. (1994) examined the decrease in norepinephrine release from cardiac adrenergic nerve terminal after ischemia and reperfusion, whereas Vasilets et al. (1989) prevented reperfusion-induced arrhythmias by $Na^+/H^+$ exchange block. Hearts with the right cardiac sympathetic nerve intact can be isolated and perfused and used to study the effect of β blockers such as propranolol on presynaptic β2 receptor–mediated response in the rat heart (Mortimer et al. 1991), the role of calcium in adrenergic neurochemical transmission in the aging heart (Roberts et al. 1990), and gender differences (Tumer et al. 1992). Lathers et al. (1981, 1982) used in vivo animal data and compared/contrasted findings obtained in the Langendorff preparations in rats to study the contributory role of the autonomic nervous system to cardiac arrhythmias and/or death. The central and peripheral autonomic nervous system inputs are not present in the Langendorff isolated beating heart preparation. Therefore, this preparation is used to examine effects of drugs on the heart, independent of autonomic neural input and independent of circulating substances such as catecholamines both of which may trigger cardiac arrhythmias and/or death in in vivo preparations. Langendorff hearts were obtained from animals denervated chemically by pretreatment with reserpine, bretylium, or 6-hydroxydopamine or from rats whose hearts were surgically denervated, and the effect of arrhythmic doses of digitalis glycosides were studied. In cats, pharmacological denervation with bretylium pretreatment (2 µg/kg/min, i.v., until death) or with surgical denervation 2 weeks prior to 6-hydoxydopamine (20 mg/kg, i.v., 3 or 14 days before ouabain infusion to toxicity and death) revealed that the protective action of only bretylium versus ouabain toxicity was eliminated by pretreatment with 6-OH dopamine (Lathers et al. 1982). Neither surgical denervation 2 weeks prior to the experiment nor 6-OH dopamine given 3 or 14 days before ouabain infusion protected against the arrhythmogenic actions of ouabain. As 6-OH dopamine and surgical denervation prevented the action of bretylium on ouabain-induced ventricular arrhythmia, bretylium action appears to be on the adrenergic nerve terminal. Bretylium, which acts on the adrenergic nerve terminal to leave it structurally intact but not functional and protected against ouabain-induced arrhythmia and death, differed from the effect of procedures that cause degeneration of the adrenergic nerve terminal (i.e., 6-OH dopamine and surgical denervation). The data suggest that for the protective effect of sympathectomy against ouabain-induced arrhythmia to develop, the adrenergic nerve terminal must be present, although not functional, as far as adrenergic neurotransmission is concerned. Neither a change in heart rate nor a change in blood pressure appeared to be a factor in the protective effect of bretylium. Thus, comparison of data from these various animal models using both in vitro and in vivo data allowed conclusions to be made regarding the role of the actual heart rate in the initiation of cardiac arrhythmias and/or sudden death.

In another laboratory, mean heart rates were compared in vivo and in an isolated ex vivo preparation (Langendorff preparation) using hearts from rats with epilepsy (Colugnati et al. 2005). Differences occurred in the mean heart rate in vivo, but no differences were found in the heart rate ex vivo, suggesting a central nervous system modulation on the heart that could lead to SUDEP. This conclusion was based on the fact that as the Langendorff preparation is an isolated heart preparation, it is devoid of input from the central nervous system. Thus, use of various in vitro and in vivo experimental designs will allow clarification of the role of autonomic innervation and the influence of central and peripheral nervous systems in relation to epileptogenic activity, heart rate, arrhythmias, and sudden death.

## CANINE PURKINJE FIBER PREPARATION

Chlorpromazine, 10 μg/mL, in Tyrode's solution decreased $V_{max}$ and time to 50% repolarization (Lipka and Lathers 1987). No consistent change in the time to 95% repolarization was found. Chlorpromazine action on calcium-mediated slow response produced by canine Purkinje fibers superfused with 12 mM KCl and 0.2 mg/L isoproterenol in Tyrode's solution demonstrated that chlorpromazine prolonged the upstroke of the slow response and increased the duration of the stimulus necessary to produce the slow response. Data were interpreted to mean that chlorpromazine alters cardiac conduction to induce arrhythmia. The pharmacological agent may be acting to initiate arrhythmia by altering the cardiac slow response (Lipka et al. 1988).

## IN VIVO ANIMAL MODELS

### CANINE AND FELINE MODELS TO INDUCE MYOCARDIAL INFARCTION, ARRHYTHMIAS, AND SUDDEN DEATH

Dog and cat models are used to study myocardial infarction, arrhythmias, and sudden death as they induce sequelae similar to those observed in humans. Mechanisms of arrhythmia development, role of imbalance in autonomic neural discharge, altered electrophysiology of the myocardium, size and location of ischemic and/or infracted areas, biochemical and molecular changes, presence of coronary collaterals, pathophysiology of myocardial perfusion, and drug effects on the sequelae of coronary occlusion may be examined in various in vivo animal models. Myocardial infarction can be induced readily in dogs and cats (Lathers 1981). Many techniques are used to occlude coronary arteries to produce symptoms comparable to those observed in humans. See Table 18.2. Use of these models contributed to progress made in the diagnosis and treatment of human myocardial infarction.

The technique of acute coronary ligation has been used for more than 100 years (Cohnheim and von Schultess-Rechberg 1981; Lathers 1981). Many research laboratories used this model in the 1960s and 1970s (Ceremuzynski et al. 1969; Gillis 1971; Lathers et al. 1977, 1978; Bissett et al. 1979) and continued to use this model in subsequent years (Lathers 1975, 1979, 1980a, 1980b, 1981; Lathers et al. 1976, 1978, 1988a; Spivey and Lathers 1985). In contrast to acute

---

**TABLE 18.2**

**Techniques for Producing Myocardial Infarction in Dogs and Cats**

1. Acute coronary ligation in anesthetized, thoracotomized animals

2. Two-stage coronary ligation in anesthetized, thoracotomized animals

3. Gradual coronary occlusion using various types of materials implanted in anesthetized, thoracotomized animals

4. Use of selective catheterization to deliver emboli to coronary arteries in unanesthetized, closed-chest dogs

*Source:* Lathers, CM, *Mammalian Models for Research on Aging,* National Academy Press, Washington, DC, 224–8, 1981.

---

coronary ligation, the two-stage coronary occlusion method developed in the dog by Harris (1950) results in a larger number of animals surviving occlusion. First, a partial coronary occlusion is done, followed by complete coronary occlusion in an anesthetized, thoracotomized dog. Twenty-four hours after the dog has recovered from anesthesia, various types of experiments may be initiated (Harris et al. 1971; Gillis et al. 1973; Heng et al. 1978; Reynolds et al. 1979; Ritchie et al. 1979; Hashimoto et al. 1979). Techniques of gradual occlusion are used because they allow development of collateral circulation, mimicking the prompt development of collaterals when human coronary blood flow is restricted in advanced coronary atherosclerosis (Baroldi et al. 1956). One limitation of all the aforementioned methods of coronary ligation is that thoracotomy, done to expose and manipulate the coronary artery, alters neural and lymphatic pathways while opening the pericardium, and surgical follow-up procedures are more difficult. The resulting infarction is dependent on many factors, including size of the artery, site and speed of occlusion, anatomy and preexisting state of other major arteries and myocardium, distribution, extent of collateral circulation (Jobe 1967), and whether anesthesia has been used. Anesthesia itself may exert a protective influence (Bland and Lowenstein 1976) and decrease the probability of fatal ventricular fibrillation.

Closed-chest techniques of occlusion have evolved and may employ selective catheterization to deliver multiple small emboli to the coronary arteries using lycopodium spores, glass or plastic beads, and clots (Agress et al. 1952; Guzman et al. 1962). As one would predict, these techniques did produce obstruction of small vessels, but the changes were unpredictable and dissimilar to lesions observed in humans. Injection of autologous clots into the left anterior descending coronary arteries of dogs has been used to induce embolization until infarction or arrhythmia developed (Baumstark et al. 1978). Likewise, use of wire conductors to induce thrombus formation with electrical or thermal energy was reported (Salazar 1961). Roswell et al. (1965) tried the infusion of adenosine diphosphate into major coronary arteries to produce occlusive platelet aggregation and myocardial infarction. All of these techniques made it difficult to regulate the size and location of the obstruction. Thus, the technique of coronary latex microsphere (25-μm diameter) embolization was developed to study postinfarction arrhythmias. These latex microspheres were used to examine pharmacological alterations of different parts of the coronary circulation to further elucidate the hemodynamic relationships between collateral and nutritive microcirculation (Wichmann et al. 1978) changes in collateral blood flow and development of myocardial necrosis (Reimer and Jennings 1979) and the time events of ischemic cell death and ability of pharmacological agents to limit the size of the infarction (Jugdutt et al. 1979). Data using these techniques especially provided information about changes occurring early after the occurrence of infarction (i.e., often in the time interval when patients do not survive long enough to reach a hospital).

Using dog and cat models, techniques have been developed to study the ability of pharmacological agents to limit the area of necrosis post infarction (Maroko et al. 1972; Reimer et al. 1973; Lucchesi et al. 1976; Powell et al. 1976) and to develop new techniques to measure size. Drugs such as practolol (Libby et al. 1973; Marshall and Parratt 1974; Lathers et al. 1976), methylprednisolone (Spath et al. 1974; Busuttil et al. 1975; Lathers 1979), and metoprolol (Sivam and Seth 1978; Lathers 1980b) were studied early on. Techniques to measure infarct size included 99m technetium pyrophosphate scans (Bonte et al. 1974; Willerson et al. 1979), thallium-201 myocardial perfusion imaging (Ritchie et al. 1979), indium-111 γ-emitting radionuclide labeling (Thakur et al. 1979), iodine-131 labeled antibody (Fab) 2 fragment imaging (Khaw et al. 1978a,b), computerized axial tomography scans (Siemers et al. 1978), intravenous administration of diatrizoate meglumine and sodium (Renografin-76) (Higgins et al. 1979), reduced nicotinamide adenine dinucleotide fluorescence photography (Barlow and Chance 1976), serial creatinine phosphokinase technique (Shell et al. 1971), nitroblue tetrazolium test (Nachlas and Shnitka 1963), and two-dimensional echocardiography (Meltzer et al. 1979).

Both dogs and cats have been studied to evaluate the role of the autonomic nervous system in the production of acute coronary occlusion-induced arrhythmias (Constantin 1963; Malliani et al. 1969; Gillis 1971; Rotman et al. 1972; Webb et al. 1972; Levitt et al. 1976; Gillis et al. 1976). These species have also been used to examine mechanisms by which antiarrhythmic agents act on autonomic neural discharge (Lathers 1975; Kupersmith 1976; Levitt et al. 1976). Altered sympathetic neural discharge to the heart and/or an imbalance between the sympathetic and parasympathetic nervous systems is thought to be involved in the production of ventricular arrhythmias after occlusion (Webb et al. 1972; Levitt et al. 1976; Schwartz et al. 1976; Lathers et al. 1977, 1978; Wehrmacher et al. 1979). Other factors involved in cardiac susceptibility to ventricular arrhythmias include extent and intensity of ischemia, severity of metabolic alteration within the ischemic area, perfusion gradient between the nonischemic and ischemic cardiac muscles, and extent of coronary vascular collateralization (Corday et al. 1977). The autonomic nervous system directly affects the first three factors. Pharmacological or surgical interventions that correct

regional ischemia to decrease extent of ischemic injury may also decrease the incidence of ventricular fibrillation. Lown et al. (Lown and Wolf 1971; Lown et al. 1977) reviewed the data supporting the role of altered sympathetic discharge and acute myocardial ischemia in sudden cardiac death after myocardial infarction. At that time, a number of experiments were ongoing in Dr. Lathers' laboratory (Lathers et al. 1977, 1978), resulting in an animal model to monitor neural discharge in two or three postganglionic cardiac nerves simultaneously (see later). Nerve activity was monitored before and after initiation of arrhythmias and/or death. Several years later, this model was adapted to monitor electroencephalogram (EEG) and the role of cardiac neural discharge in this animal model of sudden death associated with interictal and ictal activity.

## Cat Postganglionic Cardiac Sympathetic, Preganglionic Splanchnic Sympathetic, and Vagal Nerve Recordings Simultaneously with EKG Recordings after Acute Coronary Occlusion or Ouabain Toxicity–Induced Arrhythmias and/or Death

In two in vivo animal models, altered postganglionic cardiac sympathetic discharge induced cardiac arrhythmias and/or death (Lathers et al. 1977, 1978). Acute occlusion of the left anterior descending coronary artery in cats anesthetized with α-chloralose and pretreated with atropine induced arrhythmia within 3 minutes. Some of these animals died in ventricular fibrillation (Lathers et al. 1978). In the animals with arrhythmia, postganglionic cardiac neural discharge became nonuniform (i.e., spontaneous discharge increased in nine nerves, decreased in five nerves, and showed no change in one nerve). The nonuniform neural discharge was associated with development of arrhythmia after occlusion. In some cats, neural discharge did not change within the first 3 minutes after coronary artery occlusion and arrhythmia did not occur. In a different set of animals, ouabain toxicity was initiated by giving bolus injections of ouabain (25 μg/kg, i.v.) every 15 minutes until death. Development of ouabain-induced arrhythmia was also accompanied by a nonuniform pattern in the neural discharge (Lathers et al. 1977). This nonuniform neural discharge may alter ventricular excitation and conduction to produce arrhythmia in the manner described by Han and Moe (1964). They demonstrated nonuniform recovery of excitability in cardiac ventricular muscle. The nonuniform postganglionic cardiac sympathetic neural discharge may be, in part, one mechanism involved in the production of coronary occlusion or ouabain-induced arrhythmias. In a different series of studies, Lathers (1980a) examined the effect of pretreatment with the β-blocking agent timolol (5 mg/kg, i.v., infused at a rate of 0.5 mg/kg/min for 10 minutes). Postganglionic cardiac and preganglionic splanchnic sympathetic and vagal neural discharge, ouabain-induced arrhythmia, heart rate, and mean arterial blood pressure were monitored. The first bolus injection of ouabain was given 15 minutes after the timolol infusion. Timolol increased the time to ouabain-induced arrhythmia and death from $23 \pm 3$ to $48 \pm 7$ and $46 \pm 3$ to $76 \pm 9$ minutes, respectively ($p < .05$). Heart rate and mean arterial blood pressure decreased from $137 \pm 4$ to $104 \pm 6$ beats/min and $133 \pm 6$ to $103 \pm 7$ mmHg, respectively ($p < .05$). Ouabain did not reverse the decreases. The infusion of timolol did not significantly alter the neural activity monitored from the vagus and the postganglionic cardiac and preganglionic splanchnic sympathetic nerves. Ouabain after timolol did not alter splanchnic nor vagal discharge. Postganglionic cardiac sympathetic neural discharge exhibited both increases and decreases (i.e., a nonuniform neural discharge, with development of ouabain-induced arrhythmia). The ouabain-induced nonuniformity did not occur in animals pretreated with timolol. The protective effect of timolol may be due, in part, to prevention of the nonuniform postganglionic cardiac sympathetic neural discharge and to prevention of ouabain-induced increases in vagal discharge. Establishment of β-blockade and a direct negative inotropic action may also contribute to the antiarrhythmic action of timolol. This animal model (Lathers et al. 1977, 1978) was modified to simultaneously monitor EEG to develop a new animal model for sudden explained death in persons with epilepsy (Lathers and Schraeder 1982; Schraeder and Lathers 1983).

## CAT POSTGANGLIONIC CARDIAC SYMPATHETIC NERVE RECORDINGS SIMULTANEOUSLY WITH SYNCHRONIZED EKG AND EEG RECORDINGS

A new animal model was developed to examine mechanisms for risk of sudden death in persons with epilepsy (Lathers and Schraeder 1982). Epileptic activity was induced with pentylenetetrazol. Electrocorticogram, postganglionic cardiac sympathetic discharge, lead II EKG, and mean arterial blood pressure were monitored. Autonomic dysfunction was characterized by several findings: the autonomic cardiac nerves did not always respond in a predictable manner to changes in blood pressure, a marked increase in variability of the mean autonomic cardiac sympathetic and parasympathetic neural discharge occurred, and a very large increase occurred in the variability of the discharge rate of parasympathetic nerves after 50 mg/kg pentylenetetrazol but did not develop until 100 mg/kg in the sympathetic nerves. While pentylenetetrazol (10 mg/kg) induced interictal epileptogenic activity, at higher doses the duration of ictal activity increased and the interictal discharges, if present, were of shorter duration. Autonomic imbalance occurred with both interictal and ictal discharges. Interictal epileptogenic activity was associated with nonuniform autonomic cardiac postganglionic neural discharge and by an imbalance of postganglionic cardiac sympathetic and vagal discharges causing cardiac arrhythmias (ventricular fibrillation or asystole) and/or sudden death. This model is discussed in depth in ch. 28 (Lathers and Schraeder 2009).

Using this animal model, the lockstep phenomenon was detected. The lockstep phenomenon is the occurrence of postganglionic cardiac sympathetic and vagal discharges intermittently synchronizing one for one with both ictal and interictal cortical discharges in a time-locked fashion. The incidence of lockstep was less often detected with cardiac vagal neural discharge (Lathers and Schraeder 1987; Lathers et al. 1987; Stauffer et al. 1989, 1990). Premature ventricular contractions, ST/T changes, conduction blocks, and precipitous changes in blood pressure occurred concomitantly with the onset of interictal activity associated with the lockstep phenomenon. The duration of each lockstep phenomenon pattern was examined. Autonomic dysfunction with epileptogenic activity causing cardiac arrhythmias has been postulated as a cause of sudden unexplained death in persons with epilepsy. The lockstep phenomenon and associated patterns as related to precipitous changes in mean arterial pressure and/or occurrence of arrhythmias are indicators of changes in autonomic function. One potential mechanism for SUDEP is considered to be the development of the lockstep phenomenon. Understanding the autonomic changes, as indicated by postganglionic cardiac sympathetic and vagal discharges associated with the lockstep phenomenon, may contribute to the prevention of sudden death in persons with epilepsy. See Chapter 28 for details of the lockstep phenomenon (Lathers and Schraeder 2010).

## CONSCIOUS SHEEP AND CARDIAC SYMPATHETIC NERVE ACTIVITY

The aforementioned animal models utilized anesthetized cats. Currently, a conscious sheep model has been developed to examine cardiac sympathetic nerve activity and ventricular fibrillation during acute myocardial infarction (Jardine et al. 2005, 2007). Electrodes were glued into the thoracic cardiac nerves, allowing conscious cardiac sympathetic nerve activity recordings to be obtained before and after myocardial infarction. Mean arterial blood pressure and heart rate were also recorded. An early increase in cardiac sympathetic nerve activity burst size indexes occurred before 60 minutes postmyocardial infarction, mediated by an excitatory sympathetic reflex (Jardine et al. 2007). The authors concluded that this mechanism was important in the genesis of ventricular fibrillation or sustained ventricular tachycardia. In another study, cardiac sympathetic nerve activity increased within 1 hour of the onset of myocardial infarction (Jardine et al. 2005). Cardiac sympathetic nerve activity burst frequency increased from baseline 2 hours post myocardial infarction and remained elevated for 2 days. Cardiac sympathetic nerve activity burst area also increased and was sustained for 7 days after myocardial infarction. Baroreflex slopes for pulse interval and cardiac sympathetic nerve activity did not change. In a third study (Charles et al. 2008), urocortin 1, an entity that works with the sympathetic nervous system to participate in cardiac and circulatory regulation, was studied. Urocortin 1 reduced cardiac sympathetic nerve activity, with significant decreases in a dose-related response for burst frequency, burst incidence, and burst area compared with time-matched control data. Urocortin 1 induced significant rises in heart rate and cardiac output and reduced peripheral resistance with no effect on mean arterial blood pressure. It was recommended that urocortin 1 be evaluated as a potential therapeutic application in acute myocardial injury and heart disease. Lathers et al. (Lathers et al. 1987; Lathers and Schraeder 1987) found that the lockstep phenomenon is associated with interictal and ictal activity and the occurrence of cardiac arrhythmias and/or death. The conscious sheep model should be studied after implanting chronic EEG electrodes and monitoring before and after induction of epileptogenic activity with an agent such as pentylenetetrazol. Potential new anticonvulsant drugs should also be evaluated in this model.

## Neurogenic Cardiac Arrhythmias in Anesthetized Rabbits

Another animal model used to study the role of the sympathetic nervous system in the genesis of neurogenic cardiac arrhythmias is an in vivo halothane-anesthetized rabbit model (Poisson et al. 2000). Chronic bipolar electrodes can be implanted within the posterior hypothalamus of halothane-anesthetized rabbits. Every 15 days, after three 10-minute interval control electrical stimulations, the effects of techniques to induce interictal and ictal epileptogenic activity with the intravenous or central administration of pentylenetetrazol or the central application of penicillin or the induction of cardiac arrhythmias via acute coronary occlusion can be studied. In the rabbit model, the effects of procedures or pharmacological agents may be studied on parameters of blood pressure, heart rate, and EKG. EKG effects to be monitored include the number of extrasystoles and abnormal complexes and whether a pharmacological agent exhibits antiarrhythmic activity. This model can also be used to examine the action of AEDs on EEG and EKG and the associated effects, if any, as antiarrhythmic agents.

## Cat Triceps Sura Muscle Preparation, Afferent and Efferent Electrophysiological Recordings, and/or C1 Spinal Cord Transection

Zipes (2008) emphasized that substantial evidence exists for a neural component in sudden cardiac death. Because sympathetic nerve injury promotes cardiac arrhythmia and sudden death, one method to protect against death is to modulate autonomic tone to decrease risk of ventricular arrhythmias. Indeed, spinal cord stimulation provides protection against ventricular tachycardia/ventricular fibrillation when tested in animal models of postinfarction heart failure. Stimulation of the thoracic spinal cord may be one treatment for refractory angina. One animal model to examine the effect of spinal afferent and efferent changes is the cat triceps sura muscle preparation. When developing new anticonvulsant drugs, one must ask the question of whether AEDs alter motor coordination, and if so is the action occurring via an action in the spinal cord and/or in the central nervous system and/or via a peripheral action? Observations of AED effects in unanesthetized animals,

while also obtaining blood levels of new AEDs, will reveal if mild to marked motor incoordination is elicited by the investigational AED and will demonstrate at what blood level this effect occurs.

Sir John Eccles and coauthors (1975a,b,c,d) and Armstrong et al. (1968) used various electrophysiological versions of an elegant animal model, the cat triceps sura muscle preparation, to study the electrophysiological effects of drugs on afferent and efferent (spinal reflexes) and their central actions. This anesthetized cat model was used by Lathers and Smith (1976) to study pharmacological action of drugs such as ethanol on muscle spindle afferent activity and on the mono- and polysynaptic spinal reflexes. Mean phasic and static discharge frequency responses were examined. Supramaximal single shocks to the muscle nerve allows one to record drug-induced changes from control in the mean amplitudes of the mono- and polysynaptic reflexes in spinal animals. Using this model, one could determine if spindle afferent excitation is involved in the motor effects of new anticonvulsant drugs. Likewise, use of this animal model in a separate series of studies in spinal animals (C1 spinal cord transection) will demonstrate if new anticonvulsant drugs induce actions occurring at peripheral and spinal sites and/or if AED actions are modified by supraspinal sites in terms of impairment of skeletomotor function. Data obtained from the use of this animal model can be embellished by simultaneously recording EEG changes. The model may be studied in cats with and without C1 spinal section to separate central versus peripheral effects. Likewise, this cat model was used by Lathers and Smith (1976) to examine changes in the burst patterns of spinal afferent nerve discharge by measuring interspike intervals before and after the administration of drugs such as succinylcholine and ethanol. Future studies using this animal model are needed and will contribute to our knowledge of central, spinal, and peripheral actions of AEDs.

## C1 Spinal Cord Transection or Bilateral Adrenal Vein Ligation Effect on Thioridazine-Induced Arrhythmia and Death in the Anesthetized Cat

Some psychoactive agents may induce autonomic dysfunction, cardiac arrhythmias, and/or sudden death. To explore whether the cardiotoxic and/or sudden death actions of the phenothiazine drug thioridazine is due to an action on the central nervous system or via release of catecholamines from the adrenal glands, the effect of C1 spinal cord transection or bilateral adrenal vein ligation may be studied using various experimental designs. Thioridazine 1 mg/kg/min was infused intravenously into three groups of cats: (1) thioridazine only, (2) after bilateral adrenal ligation, and (3) after spinal cord section at the atlanto-occipital junction (C1) (Lathers et al. 1986). Times to arrhythmia and death with thioridazine alone or after bilateral adrenal ligation or after spinal cord section were not significantly different. Thus, the data suggest that neither adrenomedullary catecholamines nor the central sympathetic component above C1 plays a significant role in acute thioridazine-induced arrhythmia. The action of thioridazine to induce arrhythmia in spite of transection of the spinal cord or bilateral adrenal vein ligation suggests that its cardiotoxicity is a result of a direct myocardial effect. Thioridazine depressed blood pressure without producing the sustained reflex tachycardia normally seen with hypotension, indicating that this drug may modify the baroreceptor reflex arc. In the future, with the addition of EEG electrodes, this animal model may be used to examine the effect of C1 spinal cord transection to separate central, from spinal, from peripheral effects in animal models with epileptogenic activity. Also, this cat model, with simultaneous recording of the EEG, may be used to explore the role of adrenal catecholamines in the initiation of cardiac arrhythmias and/or death associated with epileptogenic activity.

The effect of another phenothiazine drug, chlorpromazine, was studied using two different models (Lathers and Lipka 1986). Dial-urethane-anesthetized cats were studied to determine times to ouabain-induced arrhythmia and death. Data were compared with data obtained in dial-urethane cats with no ouabain. Doses of chlorpromazine (5, 10, 20, 30, 40, or 60 mg/kg, i.v.) were found to be neither arrhythmogenic nor antiarrhythmic in the ouabain toxicity model. In animals receiving just chlorpromazine at a rate of 1 mg/kg/min (i.v.), bilateral adrenal vein ligation to eliminate the action of adrenal catecholamines decreased, rather than increased, the dose of chlorpromazine necessary to produce arrhythmia and death. Thus, adrenal catecholamines did not appear to contribute to chlorpromazine-induced arrhythmia, although the procedure of bilateral adrenal vein ligation was deleterious in combination with chlorpromazine. In all experimental models, chlorpromazine did depress the blood pressure but did not produce the reflex tachycardia normally observed with hypotension, suggesting chlorpromazine, like thiordazine, may alter baroreceptor reflex arc activity. Chlorpromazine-induced death occurred via cardiovascular collapse. Because chlorpromazine modifies the autonomic parameters of blood pressure, heart rate, and cardiac electrophysiology, sudden unexplained death in persons taking this medication may be due to drug-induced arrhythmias.

## C1 SPINAL CORD TRANSECTION OR 6-HYDROXYDOPAMINE OR INTRACEREBROVENTRICULAR TREATMENT IN ANESTHETIZED CATS

In another series of experiments, the role of the central nervous system in the production of phenothiazine-induced arrhythmia and death versus direct drug action on the heart was examined (Lipka et al. 1988). Spinal cords were transected at the atlanto-occipital junction prior to the 1 mg/kg/min intravenous infusion of chlorpromazine or thioridazine. No protection against drug-induced arrhythmia or death was found. These data were compared to data obtained in other cats in which 6-OH-dopamine was utilized to develop an in situ denervated heart preparation. The 6-OH-dopamine was administered prior to intravenous injection of atropine and infusion of chlorpromazine, 1 mg/kg/min. In the preparations treated with 6-OH-dopamine, no protection against chlorpromazine-induced arrhythmia or death occurred. In another group of animals, 0.5 mg of chlorpromazine was administered intracerebroventricularly to α-chloralose anesthetized cats. This central administration of chlorpromazine did not induce arrhythmia or death, although the blood pressure was initially decreased. It was concluded that neither chlorpromazine nor thioridazine appeared to produce arrhythmia or death via a central locus. These phenothiazine drugs may be acting directly on myocardial conduction to produce arrhythmia and death (Lipka 1987; Lipka et al. 1988).

In the future, with the addition of EEG electrodes to cats, the model may be used to differentiate central nervous sites of action from direct cardiac actions in animals with interictal and ictal activity, with and without the occurrence of arrhythmias or death. Comparison of these in vivo data with those obtained using in vitro canine Purkinje fibers, although two different species, again suggested that chlorpromazine acts on cardiac conduction to induce arrhythmia and may trigger arrhythmias by altering the cardiac slow response (Lipka 1987). Classically, data obtained in animal models are examined for evidence that may be provided for use when treating humans. Lipka and Lathers (1987) discuss the fact that major tranquilizers as well as antidepressant agents have been associated with clinical seizures, although the incidence is low if the doses are therapeutic. Animal model data indicate that phenothiazines act as anticonvulsant drugs at higher doses and are convulsants at lower doses. Antidepressants exert anticonvulsant actions at low doses and convulsant action with high doses. Obviously, drugs of lower seizure production potential should be substituted for those with greater potential in treating epileptic patients for psychiatric disorders. The problem of a possible comorbid role for psychotropic drugs in sudden death in epileptic persons must be considered. Some psychoactive agents have been associated with sudden death as well as cardiac arrhythmia and seizure production. Therefore, administration of psychoactive agents to a person with epilepsy should be approached with caution. Psychoactive agents that have a minimal risk of altering cardiac rhythm or seizure threshold should be used if such drugs are required.

## Intracerebroventricular Anticonvulsant and Antiarrhythmic Pharmacological Actions

α-Chloralose-anesthetized cats received pentylenetetrazol, 10 and/or 20 mg, intracerebroventricularly to induce interictal and ictal activity (Lathers et al. 1989a). Timolol (10, 100, and 500 mg/kg) was administered intracerebroventricularly, or doses of 1, 5, 10, and/or 20 mg/kg were given intravenously. The central dosing of timolol reversed the epileptiform activity of pentylenetetrazol in the brain and suppressed associated increases in blood pressure, heart rate, and cardiac arrhythmias. Kraras et al. (1987) hypothesized that since D-alanine2 met-enkephalin induced a centrally mediated vasopressor response and attenuation of the baroreceptor reflex in conscious cats (Yukimura et al. 1981), possibly leading to autonomic imbalance, the latter may precipitate arrhythmias and sudden death in persons with epilepsy. They concluded that resolution of the question of whether enkephalins elicit epileptogenic activity and autonomic dysfunction via inhibition of GABA release is important as an understanding of this mechanism should eventually allow for the design of pharmacological agents that prevent epileptogenic activity, autonomic dysfunction, and the associated risk of SUDEP.

Studies were conducted to determine if D-ALA2 methionine enkephalinamide (DAME) contributed, at least in part, to initiation of autonomic dysfunction. Lathers and Schraeder (1982) established autonomic dysfunction associated with epileptogenic activity induced by pentylenetetrazol, and Vindrola et al. (1983) reported increased DAME levels in rat brain after pentylenetetrazol-induced epileptogenic activity. A series of experiments studied the effects of intracerebroventricular DAME and naloxone in the cat to determine what changes occurred in autonomic cardiovascular parameters (Lathers et al. 1988b). The data suggest that DAME may induce epileptogenic activity and cardiovascular changes via an action on central opiate receptors. The authors hypothesized that increased levels of DAME inhibit the release of GABA and this then increases vagal bradycardia and hypotension. The latter event causes an imbalance in peripheral autonomic cardiac neural discharge that may initiate arrhythmias and/or sudden unexplained death in the individual with epilepsy. Additional studies are needed to explore this hypothesis and possible mechanism to determine the potential role in cause of sudden death (Kraras et al. 1987). It is of interest to note that a few years later Asai et al. (1994) found that valproic acid induced rapid changes in the levels of striatal methionine-enkephalin levels in rat brain and suggested that there may be an association with its anticonvulsant activity. The role of enkephalins in the induction of seizures and SUDEP and how drugs may modify this effect need further study.

## Central Hippocampal Penicillin Induced Epileptogenic Activity in Anesthetized Cats

Focal hippocampal administration of penicillin G in cats is another animal model to study autonomic dysfunction in blood pressure and heart rate and rhythm associated with induced epileptiform activity (Lathers and Schraeder 1990; Lathers et al. 1993). The delay in onset of epileptiform activity at the site of injection ranged from 1 second to 16 minutes and consisted of interictal discharges or ictal discharges. Blood pressure and heart rate increased significantly from control ($p < .05$) with the onset of epileptiform activity. Electrocardiogram (ECG) changes were found and included P–R interval changes, increased P-wave amplitude, QRS complex changes, T-wave inversion, and ST elevation. Phenobarbital (20 mg/kg, i.v.) suppressed epileptogenic activity and depressed the blood pressure and heart rate below control levels ($p < .05$). In another series of experiments, penicillin G injected into the right hippocampus

of cats produced epileptiform activity and increased the blood pressure and heart rate significantly from control levels ($p < .05$). Phenobarbital (20 mg/kg, i.v., and 40 mg/kg, i.v.) also prevented the penicillin-induced epileptiform activity. Phenobarbital (40 mg/kg, i.v.) reversed the effect of penicillin on blood pressure and heart rate, to levels below control ($p < .05$). Phenobarbital decreased both epileptiform activity and autonomic dysfunction. Changes in autonomic function induced by hippocampal penicillin were similar to those induced by the intravenous administration of pentylenetetrazol.

## INTRAOSSEOUS DRUGS IN A CARDIAC ARREST MODEL DURING RESUSCITATION IN ANESTHETIZED SWINE

Obtaining venous access is a difficult problem faced by a physician caring for the pediatric patient in cardiac arrest. The intraosseous route (through the bone via an 18-gauge spinal needle placed in the right proximal tibia) was established as a rapid and effective alternative for venous access in a cardiac arrest model (Spivey et al. 1985). Domestic swine (15–26 kg) were anesthetized with ketamine 20 mg/kg (i.m.) and α-chloralose 25 mg/kg (i.v.), given gallamine (4 mg/kg, i.v.) to prevent muscle fasciculations, and ventilated with a respirator. Catheters were placed in the right ventricle, left ventricle, and femoral arteries for mean arterial blood pressure recordings and blood pH sampling every 2 minutes. Ventricular fibrillation and cardiac arrest were induced by endocardial stimulation with a Grass S88 stimulator. Five-minute postarrest resuscitation was initiated with a mechanical resuscitator. Ten-minute postarrest sodium bicarbonate 1 mEq/kg was administered by the peripheral intravenous, central, or intraosseous route. Blood pH was sampled every 2 minutes for 30 minutes from the right ventricle, left ventricle, and femoral artery. Analysis of variance revealed that central and intraosseous routes were significantly different ($p < .05$) from the peripheral group. All three groups were significantly different ($p < .05$) from control. Pathology studies revealed only minor damage to bone when sodium bicarbonate was administered intraosseously (Lathers et al. 1989c). In a different series of experiments using the same methods, ventricular fibrillation was induced in anesthetized domestic swine (Lathers et al. 1989b). After the cardiac arrest was induced postarrest resuscitation was initiated 5 minutes later, and at 10 minutes after arrest sodium bicarbonate 1 mEq/kg was given via the peripheral intravenous, central, or intraosseous route. Controls did not receive bicarbonate. Catecholamine samples were taken from the femoral artery every 2 minutes. Two-way analysis of variance did not reveal any difference in mean arterial pressures in the four groups. In all groups, blood pH from the femoral artery demonstrated a respiratory alkalosis, peaking at pH 7.48, 5 minutes after initiation of mechanical resuscitation. In groups receiving sodium bicarbonate, respiratory alkalosis peaked at pH $7.77 \pm 0.09$ central and pH $7.65 \pm 0.06$ peripheral 2 minutes post infusion and at pH $7.71 \pm 0.06$ intraosseous 8 minutes post infusion. Analysis of variance revealed that the central and intraosseous routes were significantly different ($p < .05$) from the peripheral group. All three groups were different ($p < .05$) from control. Plasma epinephrine and norepinephrine concentrations at 0, 6, 10, 12, 20, and 30 minutes post arrest in the control group were 3 and 10, 94 and 327, 119 and 329, 92 and 234, 33 and 135, and 127 and 62 ng/mL, respectively. All three groups receiving sodium bicarbonate demonstrated similar patterns and were not different from control. The value of the rapid onset of the intraosseous route versus the peripheral route was confirmed. Today, the use of the intraosseous route as an alternative venous access for drug administration has greatly increased and is used in every emergency room in the United States. Modification of this cardiac arrest/resuscitation intraosseous model in anesthetized swine by adding EEG recording electrodes was also studied in Dr. Lathers' laboratory. The studies examined the effect of anticonvulsant drugs administered via the intraosseous route for rapid treatment/control of convulsing pediatric patients in the emergency room when a traditional intravenous line cannot be established (see discussion in the following section).

## INTRAOSSEOUS DRUG ADMINISTRATION OF ANTICONVULSANT EPILEPSY DRUGS IN ANESTHETIZED SWINE

Intravenous access for AED administration may be difficult and time consuming in an actively seizing infant. The intraosseous route was established to be a rapid and effective alternative for diazepam administration (Spivey et al. 1987). Domestic swine were anesthetized with ketamine (20 mg/kg, i.m.) and α-chloralose (80 mg/kg, i.v.) and given gallamine (4 mg/kg, i.v.) to prevent muscle fasciculations. Tracheostomies were performed, and the animals were ventilated with a respirator. The left femoral vein was cannulated, and pentylenetetrazol (100 mg/kg) was injected to elicit epileptogenic activity in swine that had undergone craniotomies for electrocortical recording. Diazepam (0.1 mg/kg) was administered intravenously or intraosseously; control animals received no drug. Epileptogenic activity was suppressed below control levels within 1 minute in the intravenous group and within 2 minutes in the intraosseous group. Two-way analysis of variance did not show a significant difference between the intravenous and the intraosseous routes. Both were different ($p < .05$) when compared to control. There was no significant difference in plasma diazepam levels between the two groups at 1, 2, 5, 10, 15, and 20 minutes. The validity of the use of the intraosseous route to control seizures in pediatric patients when an intravenous line cannot be established was established by this study.

DL-Propranolol, a β-adrenoceptor antagonist, exhibits antiepileptic activity in various animal seizure models. Another study assessed the efficacy of intraosseous propranolol in suppressing pentylenetetrazol-induced seizure activity in pigs (Jim et al. 1989). Domestic swine were prepared for recordings of arterial blood pressure, ECG, and electrocortical activity. Seizure activity was induced by pentylenetetrazol (100 mg/kg, i.v.). Sixty seconds after onset of seizure activity, animals received either no drug (control) or propranolol (intravenous or intraosseous). A transient increase (16.3%–50.0%) in mean arterial blood pressure was observed following pentylenetetrazol administration. Both intraosseous and intravenous propranolol significantly suppressed seizure duration (s/min interval) 1 minute following drug administration; seizure duration control, 36.3 ± 4.8; intravenous propranolol, 12.3 ± 5.1; intraosseous propranolol, 18.3 ± 6.0. Intravenous and intraosseous propranolol produced a maximal decrease of 32%–38% in basal heart rate and reduced the transient increase in mean arterial blood pressure elicited by pentylenetetrazol, with no significant effect on basal mean arterial blood pressure. Another series compared the effects of propranolol with diazepam (Lathers and Sarvey 1989). Sixty seconds after the onset of epileptogenic activity, the animals received saline or diazepam (0.1 mg/kg) or propranolol (2.5 mg/kg) intravenously or via the intraosseous route. Both diazepam and propranolol were effective in suppressing epileptogenic activity via intravenous or intraosseous route. Thus, the intraosseous route is a rapid and effective alternative route for administration of AEDs when an intravenous route cannot be readily established. In a third series of experiments by Jim et al. (1989), 60 seconds after onset of seizure activity, animals received no drug (control) or lorazepam (1.0 mg/kg) administered intravenously or intraosseously. Both intraosseous and intravenous lorazepam significantly suppressed duration of seizure activity (second per minute interval) within 1 minute following administration: duration of seizure activity control, 46.2 ± 3.6; intravenous lorazepam, 25.0 ± 5.1; intraosseous (18-gauge) lorazepam, 27.6 ± 6.0; and intraosseous (13-gauge) lorazepam, 24.0 ± 2.4. Seizure activity was essentially abolished at 1 minute following lorazepam infusion. Both intravenous and intraosseous lorazepam did not have significant effects on basal heart rate and mean arterial blood pressure. The data demonstrate that in swine the intraosseous route is an effective alternative venous access for lorazepam administration and the size of the spinal needles used did not affect the antiepileptic efficacy of the intraosseous infusion of lorazepam.

## SYMPATHETIC NERVE SPROUTING AND ELECTRICAL REMODELING IN DOGS: MECHANISMS OF SUDDEN CARDIAC DEATH

A positive correlation between nerve density and a clinical history of ventricular arrhythmia has been found in studies of cardiac nerves in explanted native hearts of transplant recipients. Sympathetic stimulation is important in the generation of sudden cardiac death. Chen et al. (2001) hypothesized that myocardial infarction results in nerve injury, followed by sympathetic nerve sprouting and regional (heterogeneous) myocardial hyperinnervation. Coupling between augmented sympathetic nerve sprouting with electrically remodeled myocardium results in ventricular tachycardia, ventricular fibrillation, and sudden cardiac death.

If nerve sprouting can be modified, arrhythmia control may result. Nerve growth factor augmented myocardial sympathetic nerve sprouting. This hypothesis was based on studies in dogs with complete atrioventricular (AV) block and myocardial infarction in which the nerve growth factor infusion to the left stellate ganglion facilitated development of ventricular tachycardia, ventricular fibrillation, and sudden cardiac death.

Electrical stimulation is a method to elicit nerve sprouting (Swissa et al. 2004). Subthreshold electrical stimulation of the left stellate ganglia induced cardiac nerve sprouting and sympathetic hyperinnervation and facilitated development of this canine model of ventricular arrhythmia and sudden cardiac death.

## LEFT AND RIGHT STELLATE GANGLION INFUSIONS IN DOGS WITH MYOCARDIAL INFARCTION AND COMPLETE HEART BLOCK

In vivo, the stellate ganglia and left stellate nerve activity become target sites for drug action and/or disease. A high incidence of sudden cardiac death occurs in dogs with myocardial infarction, complete AV block, and nerve growth factor infusion into the left stellate ganglion (Zhou et al. 2001). Nerve growth factor infusion into the right stellate ganglion is antiarrhythmic, in contrast to the proarrhythmic effect observed when nerve growth factor is infused into the left stellate ganglion (Zhou et al. 2005). The effect on the QT intervals was studied after osmotic pump infusion of nerve growth factor over a 5-week period to the stellate ganglia (Zhou et al. 2001). Heart rhythm and QT and R–R intervals were monitored via implantable cardiac defibrillator ECG recordings. A time-dependent increase of QTc intervals occurred in the left stellate ganglia animals and a time-dependent decrease of QTc intervals in the right stellate ganglia dogs. Nerve growth factor infusion to the left and right stellate ganglia causes left and right ventricular sympathetic nerve sprouting and hyperinnervation, respectively. Nerve growth factor infusion to the left stellate ganglion in dogs with myocardial infarct and complete AV block increased QT interval and incidence of ventricular tachycardia, ventricular fibrillation, and sudden cardiac death, whereas infusion to the right stellate ganglion shortened the QT interval and reduced the incidence of ventricular tachycardia. The QT interval prolongation was causally related to the occurrence of ventricular arrhythmia in dogs with nerve sprouting, myocardial infarction, and complete AV block.

Nerve growth factor infusion into the left stellate ganglia significantly increased β (3)-AR immunoreactivity in dogs and significantly decreased β (3)-AR immunoreactivity when infused into the right stellate ganglia when control dogs were compared with dogs with myocardial infarction and complete AV block (Zhou et al. 2005). Thus, nerve growth factor infusion into the right versus the left stellate ganglia induced differential β-adrenoceptor expression in the left ventricular myocardium.

## SPONTANEOUS STELLATE GANGLION NERVE ACTIVITY AND VENTRICULAR ARRHYTHMIA AND/OR SUDDEN DEATH IN A CANINE MODEL

Simultaneous continuous long-term recordings of left stellate ganglion nerve activity in dog with nerve growth factor infusion to the left stellate ganglion, AV block, and myocardial infarction included low-amplitude burst discharge activity and high-amplitude spike discharge activity, and both were associated with an increase in heart rate (Zhou et al. 2008). Most ventricular tachycardia (86.3%) and sudden death were preceded within 15 seconds by either of the two types of neural discharge. The closer the time to onset of ventricular tachycardia, the more the neural discharge that occurs. Much of the high-amplitude neural discharge was followed by ventricular arrhythmia (21%) or by changes in QRS morphology (65%). Actual electrical stimulation of the left stellate ganglia increased transmural heterogeneity of repolarization (T peak-end intervals) and induced either ventricular tachycardia or fibrillation. Increase in synaptogenesis and nerve sprouting was confirmed after nerve growth factor infusion to the left stellate ganglion. Experiments are needed in which in vivo animal models of sudden death are used and spontaneous stellate ganglion nerve activity is monitored to correlate changes in arrhythmias and/or the occurrence of sudden death. Lathers et al. (Lathers and Schraeder 1987; Stauffer et al. 1989) reported changes in the burst patterns of postganglionic cardiac sympathetic neural burst discharge patterns accelerated with changes in EEG and/or arrhythmias and/or death and termed this the lockstep phenomenon. Similar changes seem to occur in spontaneous discharge of the stellate ganglion nerves.

## CARDIAC REMODELING POST MYOCARDIAL INFARCTION IN MICE

Another experimental model of myocardial infarction uses mice undergoing ligation of the left coronary artery and then treated for 30 days post infarction with vehicle or with a transforming growth factor-β, a key cytokine that both initiates and terminates tissue repair (Ellmers et al. 2008). Sustained production of transforming growth factor-β underlies development of tissue fibrosis, particularly after myocardial infarction. This progressive ventricular remodeling results in a deterioration of cardiac function. An orally active specific inhibitor of the transforming growth factor-β receptor 1 (SD-208) was demonstrated to reduce mean arterial pressure. It also produces a trend for reduced ventricular and renal gene expression of transforming growth factor-β activated kinase-1, a downstream modulator of transforming growth factor-β signaling. It caused a significant decrease in collagen 1 and a marked decrease in cardiac mass. Decreased circulating levels of plasma renin activity and downregulating components of cardiac and renal renin–angiotensin system (angiotensinogen, angiotensin converting enzyme, and angiotensin II type I receptor) occurred. The data indicate that block of the transforming growth factor-β signaling pathway did produce a significant amelioration of the deleterious cardiac remodeling post infarction. Application of this mouse model for sudden death allows one the option to use genetically altered mice to study various molecular aspects of sudden death. In addition, application of simultaneous EEG monitoring will reveal associated changes in epileptogenic activity and may provide a better understanding of cardiac changes in persons with epilepsy who have previously experienced arrhythmias and whose hearts are found on autopsy to exhibit increased mass.

## DIGENIC MOUSE MODEL: COMBINATION OF TWO EPILEPSY GENES TO MASK EPILEPSY

Glasscock et al. (2007) combined two epilepsy-associated ion channel mutations with mutually opposing excitability defects and overlapping subcellular localization to generate a digenic mouse mode of human idiopathic epilepsy. Increasing membrane excitability occurred by removing Shaker-like K$^+$ channel, which is encoded by the *Kcna1* gene. This masked the absence of epilepsy caused by a P/Q-type Ca (2+) channelopathy due to a missense mutation in the *Cacna1a* gene. A decrease in network excitability via impairment of the function of *Cacna1a* Ca (2+) channels attenuated limbic seizures and sudden death in *Kcna1*-null mice. The authors recommend additional experiments to be done to improve the accuracy of genetic risk assessment of this complex disease.

## PRIMATE MODELS FOR SEIZURE AND SUDEP

That primates exhibit seizures has been reported as early as 1918 by Sherrington (1918) for the adult *Macaca fulignosus*. Autopsy revealed no gross lesions, but histological studies were not done. Reports of epilepsy are reported to occur in macaque, red, and patas monkeys, and in lemurs and baboons. Emotion or noise may trigger the response. Epileptic symptoms may be observed in monkeys, less frequently in chimpanzees and orangutans, and can be Jacksonian or generalized tonic-clonic seizures (van Bogaert and Innes 1962). A few unexpected deaths may occur in convulsive seizures and have been reported for monkeys in which seizures had not been observed previously during life. Autopsy often revealed purulent or nonpurulent meningoencephalitis. Cases of unexplained cachexia may be associated with rare epileptic seizures and lymphocytic meningoencephalitis. Some cases of clinical epilepsy may also exhibit paraplegia not explained by pathological findings. Epilepsies in monkeys do occur after cranial fractures. Meningoencephalitic scars of variable localization and age may be noted in some monkeys. In monkeys that die from acute clinical disease, it may be impossible to relate age or significance of the location of meningoencephalitic scars. The exact trigger factors for spontaneous epilepsies in monkeys or apes are not known.

Very recently, Szabo et al. (2009) examined causes of death in 46 epileptic baboons and 78 nonepileptic controls because the baboon is a model of primary generalized epilepsy. A complete pathological examination was conducted

at the Southwest Foundation for Biomedical Research in San Antonio, Texas. Baboons with seizures died at a younger age than controls ($p < .001$). Almost all of the epileptic baboons that died suddenly without an apparent cause were found to have pulmonary congestion or edema but not evidence of trauma, systemic illness, or heart disease compared to nine control baboons (12%) ($p < .001$). Most of the control baboons demonstrated evidence of a concurrent illness. Serosanguinous bronchial secretions were found in 15 of the seizure baboons (58%), but only in 3 controls (4%) ($p < .001$). Chronic multifocal fibrotic changes in myocardium were noted in three (12%) of the seizure baboons and in one control baboon. The authors conclude that untreated seizures appear to reduce the life expectancy of captive baboons and that sudden unexpected death in epilepsy may be a common cause of natural death in epileptic baboons.

When speculating on the results of the autopsies, one must be very careful to note that the findings of pulmonary congestion and/or edema may still have occurred secondarily to the occurrence of a cardiac arrhythmia that would not be detected on autopsy. Thus, one may not 100% conclude that respiratory changes were the initial trigger for the death event. Furthermore, the finding of multifocal fibrotic changes in the myocardium of three of the seizure baboons suggests that cardiac arrhythmias may indeed have occurred. A future study with a larger number of baboons is needed.

One may speculate that the stress of captivity may exert a negative effect on some of the baboons to a greater effect than on others. This question could be answered by conducting a comparative study of these animals with those found living in the wild. Nevertheless, conducting a postmortem examination of these baboons does help us to focus on mammals in the species phylum very close to humans. It will be of help to expand the number of animals in the study of Szabo et al. (2009).

## OTHER ANIMAL MODELS

Due to space limitations, other animal models have not been discussed. For example, Goodman et al. (1990, 2010) have studied the acute cardiovascular response during kindled seizures in rats. The reader is presented with a few final, abbreviated facts about different models and study findings and is encouraged to examine this information when designing laboratory studies to delineate mechanisms and prevention of arrhythmias and/or sudden death in persons with epilepsy. One unresolved question is the role of serotonin in the initiation of arrhythmia and sudden death. The actions of serotonin (5-hydroxytryptamine) are multifactoral and appear to vary in different parts of the central nervous system. The effect of serotonin on excitatory postsynaptic currents has been studied using whole-cell recordings from superficial dorsal horn neurons in neonatal rat spinal cord slices (Hori et al. 1996). It was concluded that serotonin can induce long-lasting facilitation of evoked excitatory postsynaptic currents and spontaneous release of excitatory transmitter at superficial dorsal horn synapses of the rat spinal cord. This effect appears to be modulated by the protein kinase C inhibitor calphostin C, which appears to link to the serotonin 2 receptor and to directly activate the exocytotic machinery. Whole-cell patch-clamp recordings from projection neurons and interneurons of the rat basolateral amygdala have been done to examine the effects of serotonergic modulation of neurotransmission. Rainnie (1999) concluded that acute serotonin release directly activates GABAergic interneurons of the basolateral amygdala, via activation of serotonin 2 receptors, and increases the frequency of inhibitory synaptic events in projection neurons. Chronic serotonin release, or high levels of serotonin, reduce the excitatory drive onto interneurons and may act as a feedback mechanism to prevent excess inhibition within the nucleus. The entorhinal cortex is thought to be involved in the generation of temporal lobe epilepsy (Deng and Lei 2008). The entorhinal cortex receives serotonergic innervations from the raphe nuclei in the brain stem. Cellular and molecular mechanisms involved in the facilitation of GABAergic transmission and depression of epileptic activity in the superficial layers of the entorhinal cortex were studied. Serotonin was found to increase GABA release in rat entorhinal cortex by inhibiting interneuron TASK-3 $K^+$ channels. The authors concluded that serotonin-mediated depression of neuronal excitability and increased GABA release contribute to its antiepileptic effects in the entorhinal cortex. Studies are needed to identify the role of not only serotonin in sudden death but also other transmitters such as GABA, catecholamines, neuropeptides, and so on. Tupal and Faingold (2006) and Faingold et al. (2010, ch. 41) have published evidence supporting a role of serotonin in modulation of sudden death induced by seizures in DBA/2 mice. Future studies are needed to identify sites of action for disease and/or pharmacological interventions.

The earlier discussion, although not all inclusive, presents in vitro and in vitro models that can be used to study mechanisms of action for initiation of sudden death and physiological sites for AEDs or antiarrhythmic drugs to act to prevent sudden death. The discussion provides insights into potential in vitro and in vivo models, which when used in conjunction with molecular methods and genetic animal models will ultimately lead to a better understanding of sudden death and how to prevent sudden death with selected use of current or yet-to-be developed pharmacological agents. Study of genetically designed mice with congenital and acquired long QT syndrome will provide a better understanding of sudden cardiac death originating from ventricular arrhythmogenesis, one of the major causes of mortality in the developed world (Killeen et al. 2008). Readers are also referred to additional relevant animal models found in published papers and in this book. Specifically, Bealer et al. (2010) has examined chronic alterations in cardiac sympathovagal balance induced by status epilepticus in rats (Metcalf et al. 2009). Saito et al. (2006) discuss repeatable focal seizure suppression using a rat preparation to examine the effect of seizure activity after urethane anesthesia and reversible carotid artery occlusion. McCloskey et al. (2006) used stereological methods to examine the robust size and stability of ectopic hilar granule

cells after pilocarpine-induced status epilepticus in rats. Discussing the neurobiology of epilepsy, Scharfman (2007) notes, using temporal lobe epilepsy as an example, that genes, developmental mechanisms, and neuronal plasticity play a major role in creating a state of underlying hyperexcitability. However, the critical control points or emergence of chronic seizures in temporal lobe epilepsy and their persistence, frequency, and severity have yet to be clearly understood. Misonou et al. (2004) have examined the biochemical regulation of ion channel localization and phosphorylation by neuronal activity in the kainite model of continuous seizures in rats as it relates to excitatory neurotransmission and the intrinsic excitability of pyramidal neurons.

Nutritional and lifestyle factors (including factors such as stress [Lathers and Schraeder 2006]) have been suggested to play a role in sudden death (Scorza et al. 2008). Lathers et al. (2008) proposed mechanistic factors in SUDEP, listing risk categories of arrhythmogenic factors, respiratory factors and hypoxia, and psychological factors and mechanisms for risks associated with each category. See Tables 1.1 through 1.8. Scorza et al. (2008) noted that clarification of risk factors and establishment of the mechanism of SUDEP are important to establish preventative measures for SUDEP. They emphasized the need to strive for full seizure control and the importance of encouraging patients with epilepsy worldwide to receive nonmedical, lifestyle-modifying interventions that have generally accepted public health benefits, even though there is as yet no consensus that they may or may not prevent sudden death. Both animal studies and clinical studies are needed to definitely address risk factors of ω-3 fatty acids, cold temperatures, exercise, and heart rate to the development of cardiac arrhythmias and/or sudden death in persons with epilepsy. The reader is referred to the works of Lathers et al. (2008), Scorza et al. (2008), and Lathers et al. (2010) for an in-depth discussion on risk factors for SUDEP. Prospective studies of patients need to be done to determine how we can identify which persons with epilepsy are at risk for SUDEP.

## CONCLUSIONS

Valuable insights are obtained from both in vitro and in vivo animal models, just as valuable data are obtained from using animal models in many different species to examine a clinical problem observed in humans. When both in vitro and in vivo models are used, one must evaluate the data obtained from an in vitro model and then compare results obtained from in vivo models to clearly understand how to interpret the composite data. Use of multiple animal models will shed light on mechanisms and risks associated with the problem of sudden unexplained death in persons with epilepsy by revealing physiological sites of actions for drugs to act. Use of multiple animal models will also demonstrate beneficial effects of pharmacological interventions. Researchers must use the best combination of research tools available to them to elucidate the mechanisms of risk for sudden death whether in persons with epilepsy or in persons with heart disease. Of course, one must realize that, in general, no one animal model for disease completely mimics the symptoms and findings of the disease state in humans. When possible, risk factors and all supporting medical information must be obtained for persons with epilepsy or persons with cardiac disease who are thought to be potential candidates for sudden death in an effort to prevent the sudden death event.

## REFERENCES

Agress CM, Rosenberg MJ, Jacobs HI, Binder MJ, Schneiderman A, Clark WG. Protracted shock in the closed-chest dog following coronary remobilization with graded microspheres. *Am J Physiol* 1952;170:536–49.

Alkadhi KA, Alzoubi KH, Aleisa AM. Plasticity of synaptic transmission in autonomic ganglia. *Prog Neurobiol* 2005;75(2):83–108.

Alkadhi KA, Alzoubi KH. Role of long-term potentiation of sympathetic ganglia (gLTP) in hypertension. *Clin Exp Hypertens* 2007;29:267–86.

Alkadhi KA, McIsaac RJ. Non-nicotinic transmission during ganglionic block with chlorisondamine and nicotine. *Eur J Pharmacol* 1973;24(1):78–85.

Alkadhi KA, McIsaac RJ. Effect of preganglionic nerve stimulation on sensitivity of the superior cervical ganglion to nicotinic blocking agents. *Br J Pharmacol* 1974;51 (4):533–39.

Alkadhi KA, Al-Hijailan RS, Alzoubi KH. Long-term depression in the superior cervical ganglion of the rat. *Brain Res* 2008;1234:25–31.

Alzoubi KH, Aleisa AM, Alkadhi KA. Expression of gLTP in sympathetic ganglia of obese Zucker rats in vivo: Molecular evidence. *J Mol Neurosci* 2008;35(3):297–306.

Alzoubi KH, Aleisa AM, Alkadhi KA. In vivo expression of ganglionic long-term potentiation in superior cervical ganglia from hypertensive aged rats. *Neurobiol Aging* 2010;31(5):805–12.

Armstrong DM, Eccles JC, Harvey RJ, Matthews PB. Responses in the dorsal accessory olive of the cat to stimulation of hind limb afferents. *J Physiol* 1968;194(1):125–45.

Asai M, Talavera E, Massarini A, Zubieta M, Vindrola O. Valproic acid-induced rapid changes of met-enkephalin levels in rat brain. Probable association with abstinence behavior and anticonvulsant activity. *Neuropeptides* 1994;27(3):203–10.

Barlow CH, Chance B. Ischemic areas in perfused rat hearts: Measurement by NADH fluorescence photography. *Science* 1976;193(4256):909–10.

Baroldi GO, Mantero O, Scomazzoni G. The collaterals of the coronary arteries in the normal pathologic hearts. *Circ Res* 1956;4:223–29.

Baumstark AE, Levin DC, Fishbein MC. Experimental myocardial infarction in dogs with normal coronary arteries. Angiographic resolution of coronary arterial emboli. *Radiology* 1978;128(1):31–5.

Bealer SL, Metcalf CS, Little JG, Vatta M, Brewster A, Anderson A. Sympathetic nervous system dysregulation of cardiac function and myocyte potassium channel remodeling in rodent seizure models: Candidate mechanisms for SUDEP. In: Lathers CM, Schraeder P, Bungo MW, Leestma J, eds. *Sudden Death in Epilepsy: Forensic and Clinical Factors*. Boca Raton, FL: CRC Press/Taylor & Francis Group; 2010.

Bissett JK, Watson JW, Scovil JA, Schmidt N, McConnell JR, Kane J. Changes in myocardial refractory periods following ischemia in the porcine heart. *J Electrocardiol* 1979;12(1):35–40.

Bland JH, Lowenstein E. Halothane-induced decrease in experimental myocardial ischemia in the non-failing canine heart. *Anesthesiology* 1976;45(3):287–93.

Bonte FJ, Parkey RW, Graham KD, Moore J, Stokely EM. A new method for radionuclide imaging of myocardial infarcts. *Radiology* 1974;110(2):473–74.

Bramham CR, Bacher-Svendsen K, Sarvey JM. LTP in the lateral perforant path is beta-adrenergic receptor-dependent. *Neuroreport* 1997;8(3):719–24.

Brown JT, Richardson JC, Collingridge GL, Randall AD, Davies CH. Synaptic transmission and synchronous activity is disrupted in hippocampal slices taken from aged TAS10 mice. *Hippocampus* 2005;15(1):110–7.

Burgard EC, Sarvey JM. Long-lasting potentiation and epileptiform activity produced by GABAB receptor activation in the dentate gyrus of rat hippocampal slice. *J Neurosci* 1991;11(5):1198–209.

Busuttil RW, George WJ, Hewitt RL. Protective effect of methylprednisolone on the heart during ischemic arrest. *J Thorac Cardiovasc Surg* 1975;70(6):955–65.

Ceremuzynski L, Staszewska-Barczak J, Herbaczynska-Cedro K. Cardiac rhythm disturbances and the release of catecholamines after acute coronary occlusion in dogs. *Cardiovasc Res* 1969;3(2):190–7.

Charles CJ, Jardine DL, Nicholls MG, Rademaker MT, Richards AM. Urocortin 1 exhibits potent inhibition of cardiac sympathetic nerve activity in conscious sheep. *J Hypertens* 2008;26(1):53–60.

Chen PS, Chen LS, Cao JM, Sharifi B, Karagueuzian HS, Fishbein MC. Sympathetic nerve sprouting, electrical remodeling and the mechanisms of sudden cardiac death. *Cardiovasc Res* 2001;50(2):409–16.

Cohnheim J, von Schultess-Rechberg A. Uber de folgen der Kranzarterienschliessung fur das Herz. *Virchow's Arch Pathol Anat* 1981;85:503.

Colugnati DB, Gomes PA, Arida RM, de Albuquerque M, Cysneiros RM, Cavalheiro EA, Scorza FA. Analysis of cardiac parameters in animals with epilepsy: Possible cause of sudden death? *Arq Neuropsiquiatr* 2005;63(4):1035–41.

Constantin L. Extracardiac factors contributing to the hypotension during coronary occlusion. *Am J Cardiol* 1963;11:205–17.

Corday E, Heng MK, Meerbaum S, Lang TW, Farcot JC, Osher J, Hashimoto K. Derangements of myocardial metabolism preceding onset of ventricular fibrillation after coronary occlusion. *Am J Cardiol* 1977;39(6):880–9.

Dahl D, Sarvey JM. Norepinephrine induces pathway-specific long-lasting potentiation and depression in the hippocampal dentate gyrus. *Proc Natl Acad Sci U S A* 1989;86(12):4776–80.

Deng PY, Lei S. Serotonin increases GABA release in rat entorhinal cortex by inhibiting interneuron TASK-3 K+ channels. *Mol Cell Neurosci* 2008;39(2):273–84.

Eccles JC, Rosen I, Scheid P, Taborikova H. The differential effect of cooling on responses of cerebellar cortex. *J Physiol* 1975a;249(1):119–38.

Eccles JC, Scheid P, Taborikova H. Responses of red nucleus neurons to antidromic and synaptic activation. *J Neurophysiol* 1975b;38(4):947–64.

Eccles JC, Nicoll RA, Schwarz WF, Taborikova H, Willey TJ. Reticulospinal neurons with and without monosynaptic inputs from cerebellar nuclei. *J Neurophysiol* 1975c;38(3):513–30.

Eccles JC, Rantucci T, Scheid P, Taborikova H. Somatotopic studies on red nucleus: Spinal projection level and respective receptive fields. *J Neurophysiol* 1975d;38(4):965–80.

Ellmers LJ, Scott NJ, Medicherla S, Pilbrow AP, Bridgman PG,. Yandle TG, Richards AM, Protter AA, Cameron VA. Transforming growth factor-beta blockade down-regulates the renin–angiotensin system and modifies cardiac remodeling after myocardial infarction. *Endocrinology* 2008;149(11):5828–34.

Faingold CL, Tupal S, Mhaskar Y, Uteshev V. DBA mice as models of sudden unexpected death in epilepsy. Chapter 41 In: Lathers CM, Schraeder PL, Bungo MW, Leestma JE, eds. *Sudden Death in Epilepsy: Forensic and Clinical Factors.* Boca Raton, FL: CRC Press/Taylor & Francis Group; 2010.

Gillis RA. Role of the nervous system in the arrhythmias produced by coronary occlusion in the cat. *Am Heart J* 1971;81(5):677–84.

Gillis RA, Levine FH, Thibodeaux H, Raines A, Standaert FG. Comparison of methyllidocaine and lidocaine on arrhythmias produced by coronary occlusion in the dog. *Circulation* 1973;47(4):697–703.

Gillis RA, Corr PB, Pace DG, Evans DE, DiMicco J, Pearle DL. Role of the nervous system in experimentally induced arrhythmias. *Cardiology* 1976;61(1):37–49.

Glasscock E, Qian J, Yoo JW, Noebels JL. Masking epilepsy by combining two epilepsy genes. *Nat Neurosci* 2007;10(12):1554–8.

Goodman JH, Homan RW, Crawford IL. Acute cardiovascular response during kindled seizures. Chapter 11 In: Lathers CM, SchraederP, eds. *Epilepsy and Sudden Death.* New York, NY: Marcel Dekker; 1990.

Goodman JH, Homan RW, Crawford IL. Acute cardiovascular response during kindled seizures. Chapter 40 In: Lathers CM, Schraeder P, Bungo MW, Leestma JE, eds. *Sudden Death in Epilepsy: Forensic and Clinical Factors.* Boca Raton, FL: CRC Press/Taylor & Francis Group; 2010.

Grover GJ, Singh R. The isolated, perfused pseudo-working heart model. *Methods Mol Med.* 2007;139:145–50.

Guzman SV, Swenson E, Jones M. Intercoronary reflex. Demonstration by coronary angiography. *Circ Res* 1962; 10:739–45.

Han J, Moe GK. Nonuniform recovery of excitability in ventricular muscle. *Circ Res* 1964;14:44–60.

Harris AS. Delayed development of ventricular ectopic rhythms following experimental coronary occlusion. *Circulation* 1950;1(6):1318–28.

Harris AS, Otero H, Bocage AJ. The induction of arrhythmias by sympathetic activity before and after occlusion of a coronary artery in the canine heart. *J Electrocardiol* 1971;4(1):34–43.

Hashimoto K, Tsukada T, Matsuda H, Nakagawa Y, Imai S. Antiarrhythmic effects of bupuranolol against canine ventricular arrhythmias induced by halothane-adrenaline or two-stage coronary ligation. *J Cardiovasc Pharmacol* 1979;1(2):205–17.

Heng MK, Norris RM, Peter T, Nisbet HD, Singh BN. The effect of glucose-insulin-potassium on experimental myocardial infarction in the dog. *Cardiovasc Res* 1978;12(7):429–35.

Higgins CB, Sovak M, Schmidt W, Siemers PT. Differential accumulation of radiopaque contrast material in acute myocardial infarction. *Am J Cardiol* 1979;43(1):47–51.

Hori Y, Endo K, Takahashi T. Long-lasting synaptic facilitation induced by serotonin in superficial dorsal horn neurones of the rat spinal cord. *J Physiol* 1996;492 (Pt 3):867–76.

Jardine DL, Charles CJ, Frampton CM, Richards AM. Cardiac sympathetic nerve activity and ventricular fibrillation during acute myocardial infarction in a conscious sheep model. *Am J Physiol Heart Circ Physiol* 2007;293(1):H4339.

Jardine DL, Charles CJ, Ashton RK, Bennett SI, Whitehead M, Frampton CM, Nicholls MG. Increased cardiac sympathetic nerve activity following acute myocardial infarction in a sheep model. *J Physiol* 2005;565 (Pt 1):325–33.

Jim KF, Lathers CM, Farris VL, Pratt LF, Spivey WH. Suppression of pentylenetetrazol-elicited seizure activity by intraosseous lorazepam in pigs. *Epilepsia* 1989;30(4):480–6.

Jobe CL. Selection and development of animal models of myocardial infarction. Paper read at the Symposium on Animal Models for Biomedical Research, July 10, Dallas, TX; 1967.

Jugdutt BI, Becker LC, Hutchins GM. Early changes in collateral blood flow during myocardial infarction in conscious dogs. *Am J Physiol* 1979;237(3):H371–80.

Khaw BA, Beller GA, Haber E. Experimental myocardial infarct imaging following intravenous administration of iodine-131 labeled antibody (Fab′)2 fragments specific for cardiac myosin. *Circulation* 1978a;57(4):743–50.

Khaw BA, Gold HK, Leinbach RC, Fallon JT, Strauss W, Pohost GM, Haber E. Early imaging of experimental myocardial infarction by intracoronary administration of [131]I-labelled anticardiac myosin (Fab′)2 fragments. *Circulation* 1978b;58(6):1137–42.

Killeen MJ, Thomas G, Sabir IN, Grace AA, Huang CL. Mouse models of human arrhythmia syndromes. *Acta Physiol (Oxf)* 2008;192(4):455–69.

Kraras CM, Tumer N, Lathers CM. The role of enkephalins in the production of epileptogenic activity and autonomic dysfunction: Origin of arrhythmia and sudden death in the epileptic patient? *Med Hypotheses* 1987;23(1):19–31.

Kupersmith J. Antiarrhythmic drugs: Changing concepts. *Am J Cardiol* 1976;38(1):119–21.

Lathers CM. Effect of practolol and stalol on ouabain-induced nonuniform adrenergic nerve activity. *Pharmacologist* 1975;34:745.

Lathers CM. The effect of methylprednisolone on autonomic neural discharge associated with acute coronary occlusion in the cat. *Pharmacologist* 1979;21:201.

Lathers CM. Effect of timolol on autonomic neural discharge associated with ouabain-induced arrhythmia. *Eur J Pharmacol* 1980a;64(2–3):95–106.

Lathers CM. The effect of metoprolol on coronary occlusion-induced arrhythmia and autonomic neural discharge. *Fed Proc* 1980b;39:771.

Lathers CM. Induced disease. Myocardial infarction in dogs and cats. In: *Mammalian Models for Research on Aging.* Washington, DC: National Academy Press; 1981, pp. 224–8.

Lathers CM, Sarvey JM. Effect of the beta blocking agent propranolol on longer term potentiation induced by norepinephrine in rat hippocampal slices. Research conducted in Dr. Sarvey's laboratory; 1989.

Lathers CM, Kelliher GJ, Roberts J, Teres AJ, Beasley AB. Effect of practolol and coronary anatomy on occlusion-induced arrhythmia and the associated nonuniform neural discharge. *Clin Res* 1976;24:617.

Lathers CM, Schraeder PL. Arrhythmias associated with epileptogenic activity elicited by penicillin. Chapter 9 In: Lathers CM, Schraeder P, eds. *Epilepsy and Sudden Death.* New York, NY: Marcel Dekker; 1990.

Lathers CM, Schraeder PL, Bungo MW. Sudden death: Neurocardiologic mystery. Chapter 13 In Sher L, ed. *Psychological Factors and Cardiovascular Disorders.* Hauppauge, NY: Nova Science; 2008.

Lathers CM, Schraeder P, Bungo MW, Leestma J. *Sudden Death in Epilepsy: Forensic and Clinical Factors.* Boca Raton, FL: CRC Press/Taylor & Francis Group; 2010.

Lathers CM, Schraeder PL. Verbal autopsies. *Epilepsy Behav* 2009;14:573–6.

Lathers CM, Kelliher GJ, Roberts J, Beasley AB. Nonuniform cardiac sympathetic nerve discharge: Mechanism for coronary occlusion and digitalis-induced arrhythmia. *Circulation* 1978;57(6):1058–65.

Lathers CM, Gerard-Ciminera JL, Baskin SI,. Krusz JC, Kelliher GJ, Roberts J. The action of reserpine, 6-hydroxydopamine, and bretylium on digitalis-induced cardiotoxicity. *Eur J Pharmacol* 1981;76(4):371–9.

Lathers CM, Gerard-Ciminera JL, Baskin SI, Krusz JC, Kelliher GJ, Goldberg PB, Roberts J. Role of the adrenergic nerve terminal in digitalis-induced cardiac toxicity: A study of the effects of pharmacological and surgical denervation. *J Cardiovasc Pharmacol* 1982;4(1):91–8.

Lathers CM, Roberts J, Kelliher GJ. Correlation of ouabain-induced arrhythmia and nonuniformity in the histamine-evoked discharge of cardiac sympathetic nerves. *J Pharmacol Exp Ther* 1977;203(2):467–79.

Lathers CM, Stauffer AZ, Tumer N, Kraras CM, Goldman BD. Anticonvulsant and antiarrhythmic actions of the beta blocking agent timolol. *Epilepsy Res* 1989a;4(1):42–54.

Lathers CM, Jim KF, High WB, Spivey WH, Matthews WD, Ho T. An investigation of the pathological and physiological effects of intraosseous sodium bicarbonate in pigs. *J Clin Pharmacol* 1989b;29(4):354–9.

Lathers CM, Jim KF, Spivey WH. A comparison of intraosseous and intravenous routes of administration for antiseizure agents. *Epilepsia* 1989c;30(4):472–9.

Lathers CM, Lipka LJ. Chlorpromazine: Cardiac arrhythmogenicity in the cat. *Life Sci* 1986;38(6):521–38.

Lathers CM, Schraeder PL, Weiner FL. Synchronization of cardiac autonomic neural discharge with epileptogenic activity: The lockstep phenomenon. *Electroencephalogr Clin Neurophysiol* 1987;67(3):247–59.

Lathers CM, Schraeder PL, Bungo MW. The mystery of sudden death: Mechanisms for risks. *Epilepsy Behav* 2008;12(1):3–24.

Lathers CM, Schraeder PL, Tumer N. The effect of phenobarbital on autonomic function and epileptogenic activity induced by the hippocampal injection of penicillin in cats. *J Clin Pharmacol* 1993;33(9):837–44.

Lathers CM, Schraeder PL. Autonomic dysfunction in epilepsy: Characterization of autonomic cardiac neural discharge associated with pentylenetetrazol-induced epileptogenic activity. *Epilepsia* 1982;23(6):633–47.

Lathers CM, Schraeder PL. Review of autonomic dysfunction, cardiac arrhythmias, and epileptogenic activity. *J Clin Pharmacol* 1987;27(5):346–56.

Lathers CM, Schraeder PL. Stress and sudden death. *Epilepsy Behav* 2006;9(2):236–42.

Lathers CM, Flax RF, Lipka LJ. The effect of C1 spinal cord transection or bilateral adrenal vein ligation on thioridazine-induced arrhythmia and death in the cat. *J Clin Pharmacol* 1986;26(7):515–23.

Lathers CM, Spivey WH, Levin RM. The effect of chronic timolol in an animal model for myocardial infarction. *J Clin Pharmacol* 1988a;28(8):736–45.

Lathers CM, Tumer N, Kraras CM. The effect of intracerebroventricular d-ALA2 methionine enkephalinamide and naloxone on cardiovascular parameters in the cat. *Life Sci* 1988b;43(26):2287–98.

Lathers CM, Smith CM. Ethanol effects on muscle spindle afferent activity and spinal reflexes. *J Pharmacol Exp Ther* 1976;197(1):126–34.

Lea IV, PM, Sarvey JM. Modulation of epileptiform burst frequency by the metabotropic glutamate receptor subtype mGluR3. *Epilepsy Res* 2003;53(3):207–15.

Levitt B, Cagin N, Kleid J, Somberg J, Gillis R. Role of the nervous system in the genesis of cardiac rhythm disorders. *Am J Cardiol* 1976;37(7):1111–3.

Libby P, Maroko PR, Covell JW, Malloch CI, Ross Jr. J, Braunwald E. Effect of practolol on the extent of myocardial ischaemic injury after experimental coronary occlusion and its effects of ventricular function in the normal and ischaemic heart. *Cardiovasc Res* 1973;7(2):167–73.

Lipka LJ. Mechanisms involved in the production of cardiac arrhythmias by chlorpromazine and other psychoactive agents. PhD Thesis. Research conducted in Dr. Lathers' Laboratory. Pharmacology, Medical College of Pennsylvania, Philadelphia, PA; 1987.

Lipka LJ, Lathers CM, Roberts J. Does chlorpromazine produce cardiac arrhythmia via the central nervous system? *J Clin Pharmacol* 1988;28(11):968–83.

Lipka LJ, Lathers CM. Psychoactive agents, seizure production, and sudden death in epilepsy. *J Clin Pharmacol* 1987;27(3):169–83.

Lown B, Wolf M. Approaches to sudden death from coronary heart disease. *Circulation* 1971;44(1):130–42.

Lown B, Verrier RL, Rabinowitz SH. Neural and psychologic mechanisms and the problem of sudden cardiac death. *Am J Cardiol* 1977;39(6):890–902.

Lucchesi BR, Burmeister WE, Lomas TE, Abrams GD. Ischemic changes in the canine heart as affected by the dimethyl quaternary analog of propranolol, UM-272 (SC-27761). *J Pharmacol Exp Ther* 1976;199(2):310–28.

Malliani A, Schwartz PJ, Zanchetti A. A sympathetic reflex elicited by experimental coronary occlusion. *Am J Physiol* 1969;217(3):703–9.

Maroko PR, Libby P, Bloor CM, Sobel BE, Braunwald E. Reduction by hyaluronidase of myocardial necrosis following coronary artery occlusion. *Circulation* 1972;46(3):430–37.

Marshall RJ, Parratt JR. Proceedings: The effects of practolol in the early stages of experimental myocardial infarction. *Br J Pharmacol* 1974;52(1):124.

McCloskey DP, Hintz TM, Pierce JP, Scharfman HE. Stereological methods reveal the robust size and stability of ectopic hilar granule cells after pilocarpine-induced status epilepticus in the adult rat. *Eur J Neurosci* 2006;24(8):2203–10.

McIsaac RJ. Post-tetanic enhancement of stimulus-induced muscarinic after discharge in the rat superior cervical ganglion. *J Pharmacol Exp Ther* 1978;207(1):72–82.

Meltzer RS, Woythaler JN, Buda AJ, Griffin JC, Harrison WD, Martin RP, Harrison DC, Popp RL. Two dimensional echocardiographic quantification of infarct size alteration by pharmacologic agents. *Am J Cardiol* 1979;44(2):257–62.

Metcalf CS, Radwanski PB, Bealer SL. Status epilepticus produces chronic alterations in cardiac sympathovagal balance. *Epilepsia* 2009;50 (4):747–54.

Misonou H, Mohapatra DP, Park EW, Leung V, Zhen D, Misonou K, Anderson AE, Trimmer JS. Regulation of ion channel localization and phosphorylation by neuronal activity. *Nat Neurosci* 2004;7(7):711–8.

Mortimer ML, Tumer N, Johnson MD, Roberts J. Effect of age on presynaptic beta2 receptor mediated responses in the rat heart. *Mech Ageing Dev* 1991;59(1–2):17–25.

Nachlas MM, Shnitka TK. Macroscopic identification of early myocardial infarcts by alterations in dehydrogenase activity. *Am J Pathol* 1963;42:379–405.

Paterson DS. Medullary serotonergic abnormalities in sudden infant death syndrome: Implications in SUDEP. Chapter 5 In: Lathers CM, Schraeder PL, Bungo MW, Leestma JE, eds. *Sudden Death in Epilepsy: Forensic and Clinical Factors*. Boca Raton, FL: CRC Press/Taylor & Francis Group; 2010.

Pickworth WB, Gerard-Ciminara J, Lathers CM. Stress, arrhythmias, and seizures. Chapter 22 In: Lathers CM, Schraeder P, eds. *Epilepsy and Sudden Death*. New York, NY: Marcel Dekker; 1990.

Poisson D, Christen MO, Sannajust F. Protective effects of I (1)-antihypertensive agent moxonidine against neurogenic cardiac arrhythmias in halothane-anesthetized rabbits. *J Pharmacol Exp Ther* 2000;293(3):929–38.

Powell Jr, WJ, DiBona DR, Flores J, Leaf A. The protective effect of hyperosmotic mannitol in myocardial ischemia and necrosis. *Circulation* 1976;54(4):603–15.

Rainnie DG. Serotonergic modulation of neurotransmission in the rat basolateral amygdala. *J Neurophysiol* 1999;82(1):69–85.

Reichelt ME, Willems L, Hack BA, Peart JN, Headrick JP. Cardiac and coronary function in the Langendorff-perfused mouse heart model. *Exp Physiol* 2009;94(1):54–70.

Reimer KA, Rasmussen MM, Jennings RB. Reduction by propranolol of myocardial necrosis following temporary coronary artery occlusion in dogs. *Circ Res* 1973;33(3):353–63.

Reimer KA, Jennings RB. The changing anatomic reference base of evolving myocardial infarction. Underestimation of myocardial collateral blood flow and overestimation of experimental anatomic infarct size due to tissue edema, hemorrhage and acute inflammation. *Circulation* 1979;60(4):866–76.

Reynolds RD, Kelliher GJ, Ritchie DM, Roberts J, Beasley AB. Comparison of the arrhythmogenic effect of myocardial infarction in the cat and dog. *Cardiovasc Res* 1979;13(3):152–9.

Ritchie DM, Kelliher GJ, MaLathersillan A, Fasolak W, Roberts J, Mansukhani S. The cat as a model for myocardial infarction. *Cardiovasc Res* 1979;13(4):199–206.

Roberts J, Mortimer ML, Ryan PJ, Johnson MD, Tumer N. Role of calcium in adrenergic neurochemical transmission in the aging heart. *J Pharmacol Exp Ther* 1990;253(3):957–64.

Roswell HC, Mustard JF, Packham MA, Dodds WJ. The hemostatic mechanism and its role in cardiovascular disease of swine. Paper read at The Swine in Biomedical Research, July 19–22, Richland, WA; 1965.

Rotman M, Wagner GS, Wallace AG. Bradyarrhythmias in acute myocardial infarction. *Circulation* 1972;45(3):703–22.

Saito T, Sakamoto K, Koizumi K, Stewart M. Repeatable focal seizure suppression: A rat preparation to study consequences of seizure activity based on urethane anesthesia and reversible carotid artery occlusion. *J Neurosci Methods* 2006;155(2):241–50.

Salazar AE. Experimental myocardial infarction. Induction of coronary thrombosis in the intact closed-chest dog. *Circ Res* 1961;9:1351–6.

Sarvey JM, Burgard EC, Decker G. Long-term potentiation: Studies in the hippocampal slice. *J Neurosci Methods* 1989;28(1–2):109–24.

Scharfman HE. The neurobiology of epilepsy. *Curr Neurol Neurosci Rep* 2007;7(4):348–54.

Schraeder PL, Lathers CM. Cardiac neural discharge and epileptogenic activity in the cat: An animal model for unexplained death. *Life Sci* 1983;32(12):1371–82.

Schraeder PL, Delin K, McClelland RL, So EL. Coroner and medical examiner documentation of sudden unexplained deaths in epilepsy. *Epilepsy Res* 2006;68(2):137–43.

Schraeder PL, Delin K, McClelland RL, So EL. A nationwide survey of the extent of autopsy in sudden unexplained death in epilepsy. *Am J Forensic Med Pathol* 2009;30 (2):123–6.

Schraeder PL, So EL, Lathers CM. Forensic case identification. Chapter 6 In: Lathers CM, Schraeder PL, Bungo MW, Leestma JE, eds. *Sudden Death in Epilepsy: Forensic and Clinical Factors*. Boca Raton, FL: CRC Press/Taylor & Francis Group; 2010.

Schwartz PJ, Stone HL, Brown AM. Effects of unilateral stellate ganglion blockade on the arrhythmias associated with coronary occlusion. *Am Heart J* 1976;92(5):589–99.

Scorza FA, Arida RM, Cavalheiro EA. Preventive measures for sudden cardiac death in epilepsy beyond therapies. *Epilepsy Behav* 2008;13(1):263–4; author reply 265.

Shell WE, Kjekshus JK, Sobel BE. Quantitative assessment of the extent of myocardial infarction in the conscious dog by means of analysis of serial changes in serum creatine phosphokinase activity. *J Clin Invest* 1971;50(12):2614–25.

Sherrington CS. Stimulation of the motor cortex in a monkey subject to epileptiform seizures. *Brain* 1918;41:48–9.

Siemers PT, Higgins CB, Schmidt W, Ashburn W, Hagan P. Detection, quantitation and contrast enhancement of myocardial infarction utilizing computerized axial tomography: Comparison with histochemical staining and 99mTc-pyrophosphate imaging. *Invest Radiol* 1978;13(2):103–09.

Sivam SP, Seth SD. Metoprolol—A new cardioselective beta adrenoceptor antagonist in experimental cardiac arrhythmias. *Indian J Med Res* 1978;68:176–82.

Skrzypiec-Spring M, Grotthus B, Szelag A, Schulz R. Isolated heart perfusion according to Langendorff—Still viable in the new millennium. *J Pharmacol Toxicol Methods* 2007;55(2):113–26.

Snyder DL, Gao E, Johnson MD, Roberts J. Decrease in norepinephrine release from cardiac adrenergic nerve terminals after ischemia and reperfusion. *Ann N Y Acad Sci* 1994;723:389–91.

Spath Jr. JA, Lane DL, Lefer AM. Protective action of methylprednisolone on the myocardium during experimental myocardial ischemia in the cat. *Circ Res* 1974;35(1):44–51.

Spivey WH. Lathers CM. Effect of timolol on the sympathetic nervous system in coronary occlusion in cats. *Ann Emerg Med* 1985;14(10):939–44.

Spivey WH, Lathers CM, Malone DR, Unger HD, Bhat S, McNamara RN, Schoffstall J, Tumer N. Comparison of intraosseous, central, and peripheral routes of sodium bicarbonate administration during CPR in pigs. *Ann Emerg Med* 1985;14(12):1135–40.

Spivey WH, Unger HD, Lathers CM, McNamara RM. Intraosseous diazepam suppression of pentylenetetrazol-induced epileptogenic activity in pigs. *Ann Emerg Med* 1987;16(2):156–9.

Stauffer AZ, Dodd-O J, Lathers CM. The relationship of the lockstep phenomenon and precipitous changes in mean arterial blood pressure. *Electroencephalogr Clin Neurophysiol* 1989;72(4):340–5.

Stauffer AZ, Dodd-O J, Lathers CM. Relationship of the lockstep phenomenon and precipitous changes in blood pressure. Chapter 14 In: Lathers CM, Schraeder P, eds. *Epilepsy and Sudden Death*. New York, NY: Marcel Dekker; 1990.

Swissa M, Zhou S, Gonzalez-Gomez I, Chang CM, Lai AC, Cates AW, Fishbein MC, Karagueuzian HS, Chen PS, Chen LS. Long-term subthreshold electrical stimulation of the left stellate ganglion and a canine model of sudden cardiac death. *J Am Coll Cardiol* 2004;43(5):858–64.

Szabo CA, Knape KD, Leland MM, Feldman J, McCoy KJ, Hubbard GB, Williams JT. Mortality in captive baboons with seizures: A new model for SUDEP? *Epilepsia* 2009;50(8):1995–8.

Thakur ML, Gottschalk A, Zaret BL. Imaging experimental myocardial infarction with indium-111-labeled autologous leukocytes: Effects of infarct age and residual regional myocardial blood flow. *Circulation* 1979;60(2):297–305.

Tumer N, Mortimer ML, Roberts J. Gender differences in the effect of age on adrenergic neurotransmission in the heart. *Exp Gerontol* 1992;27(3):301–7.

Tupal S, Faingold CL. Evidence supporting a role of serotonin in modulation of sudden death induced by seizures in DBA/2 mice. *Epilepsia* 2006;47(1):21–6.

van Bogaert L, Innes JRM. Neurologic diseases of apes and monkeys. Chapter IV. In: Innes JRM, Saunders LZ, editors. *Comparative Neuropathology*. New York, NY: Academic Press; 1962.

Vasilets LA, Mokh VP, Khodorov BI. Prevention of reperfusion-induced arrhythmia by Na+/H+ exchange block. *Kardiologiia* 1989;29(2):91–4.

Vindrola O, Asai M, Zubieta M, Linares G. Brain content of immunoreactive [Leu5]enkephalin and [Met5]enkephalin after pentylenetetrazol-induced convulsions. *Eur J Pharmacol* 1983;90(1):85–9.

Webb SW, Adgey AA, Pantridge JF. Autonomic disturbance at onset of acute myocardial infarction. *Br Med J* 1972;3(5818):89–92.

Wehrmacher WH, Talano JV, Kaye MP, Randall WC. The unbalanced heart. Animal models of cardiac dysrhythmias. *Cardiology* 1979;64(2):65–74.

Wichmann J, Loser R, Diemer HP, Lochner W. Pharmacological alterations of coronary collateral circulation: Implication to the steal-phenomenon. *Pflugers Arch* 1978;373(3):219–24.

Willerson JT, Parkey RW, Buja LM, Bonte FJ. Technetium-99m stannous pyrophosphate 'hot spot' imaging to detect acute myocardial infarcts. *Cardiovasc Clin* 1979;10(2):139–48.

Yukimura T, Stock G, Stumpf H, Unger T, Ganten D. Effects of [dAla2]-methionine-enkephalin on blood pressure, heart rate, and baroreceptor reflex sensitivity in conscious cats. *Hypertension* 1981;3(5):528–33.

Zhou S, Jung BC, Tan AY, Trang VQ, Gholmieh G, Han SW, Lin SF, Fishbein MC, Chen PS, Chen LS. Spontaneous stellate ganglion nerve activity and ventricular arrhythmia in a canine model of sudden death. *Heart Rhythm* 2008;5(1):131–9.

Zhou S, Cao JM, Tebb ZD, Ohara T, Huang HL, Omichi C, Lee MH et al. Modulation of QT interval by cardiac sympathetic nerve sprouting and the mechanisms of ventricular arrhythmia in a canine model of sudden cardiac death. *J Cardiovasc Electrophysiol* 2001;12(9):1068–73.

Zhou S, Paz O, Cao JM, Asotra K, Chai NN, Wang C, Chen LS, Fishbein MC, Sharifi B, Chen PS. Differential beta-adrenoceptor expression induced by nerve growth factor infusion into the canine right and left stellate ganglia. *Heart Rhythm* 2005;2(12):1347–55.

Zipes DP. Heart-brain interactions in cardiac arrhythmias: Role of the autonomic nervous system. *Cleve Clin J Med* 2008;75(Suppl 2):S94–6.

# 19 A Characterization of the Lockstep Phenomenon in Phenobarbital-Pretreated Cats

*Jeffrey M. Dodd-O and Claire M. Lathers*

## CONTENTS

## INTRODUCTION

Sudden unexplained death (SUD) was defined by Jay and Leestma (1981) as "non-traumatic death occurring in an individual within minutes or hours of the onset of the final illness or ictus." These patients are not previously known to be suffering from any illness that would normally be expected to cause sudden death, and no pathologic explanation for their death has been found. Up to a 13% incidence of SUD has been reported in persons with epilepsy, with the epileptic population most at risk for SUD being the young person with a mean age of 32 years (Jay and Leestma 1981; Krohn 1977). Many causes for SUD have been postulated, including autonomic dysfunction and its relation to epileptogenic discharge (Jay and Leestma 1981).

Using diverse models, different investigators have shown evidence of intrinsic activity at various levels in the nervous system. Cortical rhythms, controlled by subcortical neurons (Kiloh et al. 1972b) thought by many to be located in the thalamus (Kiloh et al. 1972a), are the basis for the alpha (8–13 Hz), beta (20–22 Hz), delta (3–4 Hz), etc., rhythms of electroencephalography. Basar (1976) used stereotaxic procedures to demonstrate spontaneous activities from medial geniculate nuclei, inferior colliculus, mesencephalic reticular formation, and dorsal hippocampus. Numerous studies (Barman and Gebber 1980, 1981; Gebber and Barman 1981) suggest the existence of an inherent rhythm of sympathetic nerve discharge, possibly originating from the hypothalamus (Barman and Gebber 1982). The results of Gebber and Barman (1981, 1984) indicate that a temporal relationship exists between the intrinsic rhythms of the central and the autonomic nervous systems. Lathers et al. (1977, 1978) reported that changes in the rate of autonomic discharge from postganglionic

cardiac sympathetic branches may contribute to cardiac dysrhythmias. Thus, it is quite plausible that the association between epileptogenic activity and autonomic dysfunction evidenced in both animal (Lathers and Schraeder 1982; Meldrum and Brierley 1973; Meldrum and Horton 1973; Wasterlain 1974) and human (Jay and Leestma 1981; Van Buren 1958) studies may be a manifestation of the disruption of a normal pattern of temporally related intrinsic cortical and autonomic discharges.

Studies in this laboratory have demonstrated a temporal synchronization between electrocorticogram (ECoG) activity and intrathoracic cardiac postganglionic sympathetic discharge during both ictal and interictal epileptogenic states (Lathers et al. 1987). The purpose of this chapter is to describe this phenomenon in phenobarbital-pretreated cats undergoing epileptogenic activity induced by pentylenetetrazol (PTZ). This relationship between the central nervous system discharges and the autonomic nervous system may prove important in explaining the high incidence of SUD in epilepsy.

## METHOD

Nine cats were anesthetized with 80 mg/kg intravenous (i.v.) α-chloralose. Tracheostomy was performed, and the femoral artery and vein were cannulated. Ventilation was maintained using a small-animal respirator, with intravenous gallamine (4 mg/kg doses, intermittently) being used to maintain paralysis. Arterial blood gases were monitored, and ventilation was altered to maintain the $pO_2$, $pCO_2$, and pH values within an acceptable physiological range. A bilateral frontal craniectomy was performed, and the dura was resected to record ECoG activity. A thoracotomy and a right partial pneumonectomy were performed to expose the cardiac post-ganglionic and right cardiac vagal nerves near the heart. The former were identified as sympathetic by their discharge response to blood pressure drop produced by intravenous injection of 5 g/kg histamine (Lathers et al. 1978). These nerves were desheathed, and nerve activity was recorded in one or more small nerve branches. Mean arterial blood pressure, electrocardiogram (ECG) (lead II of the ECG), heart rate, and rectal temperature were monitored continuously throughout the experiment. Rectal temperature was maintained between 37.5°C and 38.5°C.

A 10-minute control period was monitored before beginning infusion of phenobarbital (20 mg/kg i.v.) over 10 minutes. One hour after completing the phenobarbital infusion, six doses of PTZ (10, 20, 50, 100, 200, and 2000 mg/kg) were administered intravenously at 10-minute intervals. The half-life of this drug in the cat is unknown (Knoll Laboratories, pers. comm., 1979) but has been shown to be 1.4 hours in the dog (Jun 1976). If one assumes the half-life to be similar in the cat, these doses of PTZ administered were probably cumulative.

Epileptiform discharges were categorized in three degrees, according to duration of discharge. Polyspike discharges continuing for 10 seconds or longer were designated as prolonged ictal. Repetitive polyspike bursts of less than 10-second duration interrupted by brief periods of baseline cerebral activity were classified as brief ictal. These types of ictal activity are analogous to those seen in the electro-encephalogram (EEG) during clinical seizures. Interictal spikes were those bilateral discrete paroxysmal spikes and/or polyspike and wave discharges analogous to the nonictal epileptogenic activity seen routinely in the interictal EEG of patients with a seizure disorder.

In distinguishing interictal discharges from brief ictal activity, spikes occurring more frequently than 3.3 per second were not counted as interictal discharges. This maximal rate was decided on after determining that each oscillation of the polygraph pen required at least 100 ms to occur. A 200-ms return to baseline activity was considered evidence distinguishing a series of consecutive interictal spikes from one continuous brief ictal discharge. Spikes occurring more frequently than 3.3 per second (or 300 ms between the beginnings of any two consecutive spikes) were classified as part of the same polyspike discharge activity.

An interictal ECoG spike was considered to be time locked to a sympathetic discharge only if the latter began within 200 ms of the beginning of the interictal ECoG spike. Each brief ictal discharge was analyzed as a single unit along with its corresponding autonomic activity. The brief ictal and autonomic discharges were considered time locked only if the autonomic activity depicted a single polyspike discharge whose first spike began after the brief ictal discharge began, and whose last spike began before the end of the final spike composing the brief ictal discharge. When the ECoG displayed prolonged ictal activity, the autonomic and ECoG discharge during this time period was not considered to be time locked.

When sympathetic and ECoG spikes were time locked for an uninterrupted time period ≥ 10 seconds, the total duration of this event was measured. Time-locked discharges were considered to depict the lockstep phenomenon (LSP) when (1) at least two episodes of time-locked autonomic and epileptogenic activities occurred during the 10-second interval and (2) sympathetic activity occurred more frequently than ECoG activity, or vice versa. In the latter criterion, no more than one discharge from the less frequent component was allowed to exist without being time locked. If the sympathetic and ECoG spikes were not consistently time locked over a period of at least 10 seconds (uninterrupted), these spikes were not considered to be exhibiting LSP. If the discharges were time locked for more than 10 seconds and then interrupted for 4.5 seconds or less, the time-locked discharges were classified as uninterrupted LSP. Interruptions longer than 4.5 seconds indicated that LSP had ended.

The amount of LSP was quantified in terms of incidence and duration. To quantify incidence, the number of time-locked ECoG and autonomic spikes exhibiting LSP was determined for the 10-minute interval following each dose of PTZ. Next, the total numbers of sympathetic and ECoG spikes were determined for each of the nine cats for each of the six doses of PTZ. Also listed were the number of LSP discharges per total number of sympathetic discharges (LSP/S) and ECoG discharges (LSP/E). The value LSP/S is a measure of the proportion of all sympathetic spikes that are locked to ECoG spikes under the conditions of LSP. Likewise, the value LSP/E is a measure of the proportion of all ECoG spikes that are locked to sympathetic spikes under the conditions of LSP.

To quantify duration, the total time (in seconds) that each cat spent in or out of LSP was determined. This was further classified to depict one of the following situations:

1. The duration of LSP during each minute following administration of PTZ. In this case, all doses of PTZ were grouped together and time spent in LSP was determined only as a function of the latency period following the administration of PTZ.
2. The duration of LSP during each dose of PTZ administered. In this case, duration of LSP was determined for each dose of PTZ regardless of the delay between administration of the drug and beginning of LSP.

One-factor analysis of variance (ANOVA) with repeated measures on time compared the mean proportions of total time that cats displayed LSP following the administration of PTZ. Means were collapsed across doses. A post hoc Student Newman–Keuls test ($\alpha$ = 0.050) was performed when indicated.

Analogous tests compared the observed frequency of LSP during each dose of PTZ. The mean proportions of total time that cats displayed LSP during each 10-minute interval following the administration of each dose of PTZ were examined.

To determine whether the observed incidence of LSP could be due to chance alone, two multiple regressions were performed. In these analyses, the dependent variables were LSP/S and LSP/E. The independent variables were the number of sympathetic and ECoG spikes.

Each ECoG spike was associated with two other ECoG spikes, one preceding it by 2.8 seconds and one following it by 2.8 seconds, a repeated ECoG interval observed in all cats. The 2.8-second interval could contain other episodes of ECoG activity. Frequently, each episode of ECoG activity contained within this 2.8-second interval was itself associated with two other ECoG spikes, one preceding it by 2.8 seconds and one following it by 2.8 seconds. The number of spikes contained within this 2.8-second interval varied greatly. However, the 2.8-second repeated ECoG interval was not considered to be present whenever it contained more than one other ECoG discharge within these borders.

Figure 19.1 shows a diagram of these criteria for classification of presence or absence of the repeated ECoG interval. The ordinate displays the amplitude of the spike, and the abscissa displays the time interval between spikes. Tracing I in Figure 19.1 displays the basic 2.8-second interval. This interval is actually the duration of the latency period from the end of one spike to the beginning of a spike with which it is associated. All spikes labeled A are related by this 2.8-second latency period. In tracing II, each pair of A spikes related by a 2.8-second interval envelops another B spike. Each B spike is itself related to two other B spikes by a 2.8-second interval. In tracing III, each pair of A spikes related by a 2.8-second repeated ECoG interval envelops two additional (B and C) spikes. Tracing HI violates our criteria for categorization as the presence of repeated ECoG interval.

Determination was made of the total time (seconds) for which the repeated ECoG interval was observed. If the repeated ECoG interval (defined earlier) was present before

being interrupted for 4.5 seconds or less, it was considered to be present without interruption, because interruptions longer than 4.5 seconds marked the end of the repeated ECoG interval.

Sympathetic ECoG activity was classified based on both LSP (presence vs. absence) and the repeated ECoG interval (presence or absence). The four patterns are as follows: (1) LSP present with repeated ECoG interval present, (2) LSP present with repeated ECoG interval absent, (3) LSP absent with repeated ECoG interval present, and (4) LSP absent with repeated ECoG interval absent.

The cats were evaluated for all doses of LSP, excluding the 2000 mg/kg dose. If artifact-rendered segments of either the sympathetic or the ECoG printout were unreadable, this segment was deleted.

A paired t test was used to compare time spent in LSP with repeated ECoG interval present with time spent in LSP with repeated ECoG interval absent. A second paired t test was performed to compare time spent in LSP with repeated ECoG interval present with time spent with LSP absent with repeated ECoG interval present.

An ANOVA with repeated measures on time and dose and a post hoc Student Neuman–Keuls test ($\alpha = 0.050$) were performed for each of the following six patterns of ECoG-sympathetic activity: (1) LSP present with repeated ECoG interval present, (2) LSP present with repeated ECoG interval absent, (3) total LSP, (4) LSP absent with repeated ECoG interval present, (5) LSP absent with repeated ECoG interval absent, and (6) total LSP absent.

Precipitous, rather than gradual, changes in mean arterial pressure were measured to highlight any possible changes in the character of LSP coincident with a change in mean arterial blood pressure. The mean arterial blood pressure changes occurring in all nine cats were reviewed during the control, phenobarbital infusion, and PTZ treatment periods.

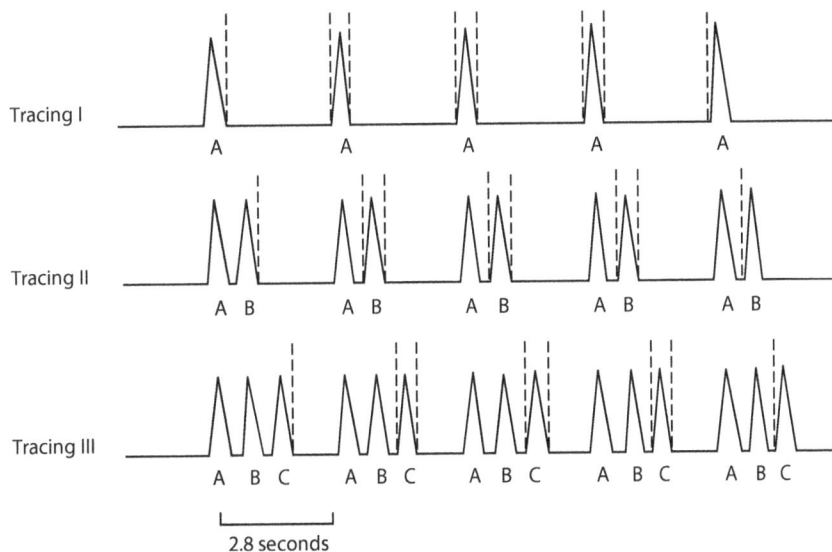

FIGURE 19.1 Repeated 2.8-second interval in the electrocorticogram. Tracing I, basic 2.8-second repeated interval. Tracing II, acceptable variation of the 2.8-second repeated interval. Tracing III, unacceptable variation. A, B, and C show each separate subset of interrelated spikes.

Systolic changes greater than 23 mm Hg over a 10-second interval were never seen during the control period; thus, changes greater than 23 mm Hg over a 10-second interval were defined as precipitous. A total of 89 such episodes were analyzed after administration of all doses of PTZ except 2000 mg/kg. This dosage led to death in all cats.

The incidence of precipitous change in mean arterial blood pressure was analyzed using two different methods. Ninety-five percent confidence intervals were constructed around the incidences of precipitous mean arterial blood pressure changes for each minute following the administration of all doses of PTZ. Ninety-five percent confidence intervals were also constructed around the incidences of precipitous mean arterial blood pressure changes at each dose of PTZ.

The ECG of each cat was analyzed during the control period to find any abnormality intrinsic to that particular cat. These were discarded, and any new abnormalities occurring after the administration of PTZ were evaluated. Each change was classified according to the time interval and dose during which it occurred. The ECG parameters examined were (1) T wave changes, (2) P wave changes, (3) changes in the QRS complexes, (4) appearance of a Q wave, (5) premature ventricular contractions, and (6) ventricular tachycardia.

Ninety-five percent confidence intervals were constructed around the incidences of ECG changes for each minute following dosing with PTZ and for each dose of PTZ administered.

## RESULTS

As depicted in Figure 19.2, no ECoG spikes were time locked to a sympathetic discharge in the control period (Figure 19.2, I) or in the period during the infusion of phenobarbital before the administration of PTZ (Figure 19.2, II). Interictal ECoG spikes were time locked to the sympathetic discharge in Figure 19.2 (III) and were designated as LSP.

The latency period varied, but the ECoG discharge always preceded the corresponding sympathetic discharge. Sympathetic discharge was observed less frequently than ECoG discharge. However, in 93% of the time periods during which sympathetic activity was present, the proportion of these discharges that were time locked to ECoG spikes was 0.85 or greater. Further analysis using multiple regressions and bivariate correlations suggested that the incidence of observed LSP was limited more by the incidence of observed sympathetic discharge than by the incidence of observed ECoG discharge.

Table 19.1 compares, for each cat, the percentage of time that LSP was present (with or without the repeated ECoG interval) with the percentage of time absent. In eight of nine cats, LSP was observed to be present during at least 55%

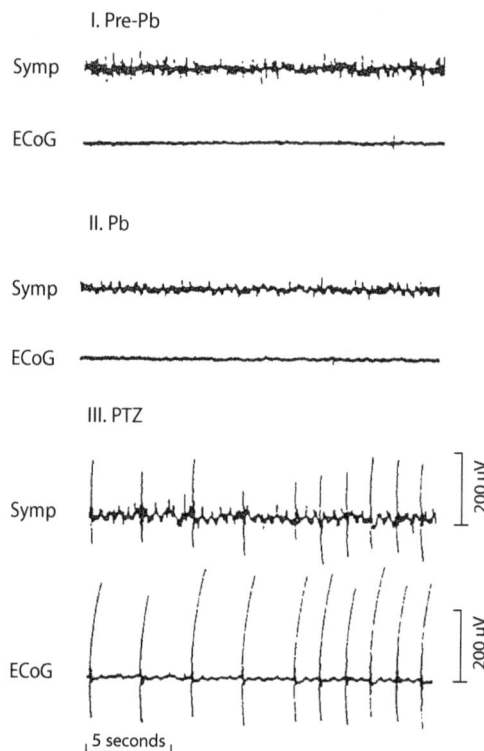

**FIGURE 19.2** Occurrence of sympathetic and electrocorticogram discharges in a time-locked manner, i.e., lockstep phenomenon. Traces in I, II, and III are three different time periods from the same cat: I, during prephenobarbital (Pre-Pb) control period; II, 9 minutes, 50 seconds into phenobarbital (Pb) control period; III, 8 minutes, 50 seconds into 200 mg/kg PTZ dosage. Symp, cardiac sympathetic postganglionic neurons. Horizontal calibration is 5 cm/s in all cases. Vertical calibration is 200 μV/cm in all cases. Mean arterial blood pressures (not shown)–electrocardiogram patterns–mean heart rates were (I) 120–normal–131, (II) 54–normal–112, and (III) 98–normal–152.

**TABLE 19.1**

**Contingency Table Displaying the Presence or Absence of the LSP versus the Presence or Absence of the Repeated Electrocortical Interval**

| Cat No. | LSP Present, Repeated ECoG Interval Present (% Total for Cat) | LSP Present, Repeated ECoG Interval Absent (% Total for Cat) | LSP Absent, Repeated ECoG Interval Present (% Total for Cat) | LSP Absent, Repeated ECoG Interval Absent (% Total for Cat) |
|---|---|---|---|---|
| 1 | 68 | 13 | 15 | 5 |
| 2 | 40 | 12 | 18 | 31 |
| 3 | 13 | 1 | 18 | 68 |
| 4 | 60 | 1 | 14 | 26 |
| 5 | 41 | 3 | 24 | 33 |
| 6 | 63 | 3 | 5 | 29 |
| 7 | 42 | 0 | 26 | 32 |
| 8 | 46 | 7 | 24 | 22 |
| 9 | 67 | 3 | 9 | 21 |
| Average | 49 | 5 | 17 | 30 |

of the experiment (LSP present being defined as LSP present with repeated ECoG interval present and with repeated ECoG interval absent). In all cats following all doses of PTZ, LSP was present 66% of the time on average.

The proportion of time each cat demonstrated each pattern is shown in Table 19.1. As an example, cat 4 demonstrated the pattern LSP present with repeated ECoG interval present for 60% of the time. This was determined by dividing the total number of seconds evaluated (3000 seconds) into the total time the pattern was observed (1801 seconds). Similarly, this cat demonstrated the pattern LSP present with repeated ECoG interval absent 1% of the time, pattern LSP absent with repeated ECoG interval present 14% of the time, and pattern LSP absent with repeated ECoG interval absent 26% of the time.

Note that for the one cat in which LSP was not present during at least 55% of the experiment, the data contained long recording periods that were technically inadequate for quantitative description of the relationship between ECoG and sympathetic spikes. Observation of these periods in cat 8 revealed that they were usually composed of global increases in ECoG activity associated with global increases in sympathetic activity.

Table 19.2 lists the incidences of sympathetic spikes (No. Symp) and ECoG spikes (No. ECoG) for the 10-minute period following the administration of a dose of PTZ for each cat. Also listed, in decimal form, are measures of (1) the proportion of sympathetic spikes that occurred time locked to ECoG spikes (TL/S) and (2) the proportion of ECoG spikes that occurred time locked to sympathetic spikes (TL/E). In 40 of the 45 (89%) measured time intervals, ECoG discharges occurred more frequently than sympathetic discharges. Also, in 43 of 45 (93%) of the measured time periods, the ratio TL/S was greater than 0.85. This high incidence of ECoG activity occurring more frequently than sympathetic activity, combined with the high proportion (>0.85) of observed sympathetic spikes being time locked to ECoG spikes in 93% of the measured time periods, suggests that the incidence of

observed sympathetic firings was the limiting factor in the total number of times when time-locked activity (and, secondarily, LSP) was observed.

Further evidence that the incidence of LSP is limited by the frequency of sympathetic discharge was that (1) multiple regressions showed no significant predictor where TL/S is dependent, (2) multiple regressions showed that TL/E was related to No. Symp and No. ECoG (multiple $r = 0.86$ significant to 0.00005), and (3) bivariate correlation of No. Symp (0.55, step 1, proportion of variance = 0.30) and No. ECoG (0.01, step 2, proportion of variance = 0.73) suggested that ECoG becomes a factor in increasing the predictability of ECoG time locked only after sympathetic activity has made its impact.

A certain stability to the neural activity and a high incidence of LSP were associated with the presence of the repeated 2.8-second interval in ECoG. Disruption of this rhythm was associated with a degeneration of LSP. When LSP was present, it was associated an average 74% of the time ($p < .01$) with a 2.8-second repeated ECoG interval (13,131 seconds of LSP present with repeated ECoG interval present divided by [13,131 + 4,545] seconds of LSP present with and without a repeated ECoG interval present). Furthermore, when the repeated ECoG interval was present LSP was absent 9% of the time (1,268 seconds of repeated ECoG interval present with LSP absent divided by [13,131 + 1,268] seconds of repeated ECoG interval present with and without LSP present) ($p < .01$). When the repeated ECoG interval was absent, LSP was absent more frequently than present (average 17% LSP without ECoG vs. average 30% LSP absent without ECoG).

The relative prevalence (in seconds) of each sympathetic ECoG pattern following the administration of PTZ was examined. Figure 19.3 shows that as the time period after the administration of the most recent dose of PTZ increased (1) the mean proportion of time that LSP was present with repeated ECoG interval present increased regularly (Figure 19.3a), (2) mean proportion of time that LSP was present

**TABLE 19.2**

**Proportion of Sympathetic and Electrocortical Spikes and Proportions of Each in the LSP**

| | PZT 10 mg/kg | | | | PZT 20 mg/kg | | | | PZT 50 mg/kg | | | |
|---|---|---|---|---|---|---|---|---|---|---|---|---|
| Cat. No. | No. Symp | No. ECoG | LSP S | LSP E | No. Symp | No. ECoG | LSP S | LSP E | No. Symp | No. ECoG | LSP S | LSP E |
| 1 | 253 | 313 | 1.0000 | 0.8083 | 354 | 356 | 0.9972 | 0.9916 | 451 | 450 | 0.9956 | 0.9978 |
| 2 | 48 | 161 | 0.9583 | 0.2857 | 340 | 465 | 0.9882 | 0.7225 | 471 | 582 | 0.9915 | 0.9193 |
| 3 | — | — | — | — | 73 | 308 | 0.5753 | 0.1364 | 224 | 302 | 0.8036 | 0.5960 |
| 4 | — | — | — | — | 204 | 396 | 0.5887 | 0.3682 | 358 | 368 | 0.9915 | 0.9511 |
| 5 | — | — | — | — | 219 | 227 | 1.0000 | 0.9648 | 129 | 641 | 1.0000 | 0.2012 |
| 6 | — | — | — | — | 256 | 390 | 0.9883 | 0.6477 | 337 | 352 | 0.9941 | 0.9517 |
| 7 | — | — | — | — | 239 | 260 | 1.0000 | 0.9192 | 345 | 359 | 1.0000 | 0.9610 |
| 8 | 139 | 9 | 0.0504 | 0.7778 | 276 | 301 | 0.9746 | 0.8937 | 304 | 310 | 0.9901 | 0.9710 |
| 9 | — | — | — | — | 346 | 374 | 0.9942 | 0.9198 | 298 | 346 | 0.9933 | 0.8555 |

| | PZT 100 mg/kg | | | | PZT 200 mg/kg | | | | PZT 2000 mg/kg | | | |
|---|---|---|---|---|---|---|---|---|---|---|---|---|
| Cat. No. | No. Symp | No. ECoG | LSP S | LSP E | No. Symp | No. ECoG | LSP S | LSP E | No. Symp | No. ECoG | LSP S | LSP E |
| 1 | 441 | 429 | 0.9728 | 1.0000 | 318 | 306 | 0.9245 | 0.9608 | 10 | 10 | 1.0000 | 1.0000 |
| 2 | 290 | 335 | 1.0000 | 0.8657 | 124 | 284 | 0.9919 | 0.4331 | 48 | 48 | 1.0000 | 1.0000 |
| 3 | 110 | 125 | 0.8727 | 0.7680 | 262 | 255 | 0.8588 | 0.8824 | — | — | — | — |
| 4 | 399 | 430 | 1.0000 | 0.9279 | 392 | 402 | 0.9974 | 0.9726 | — | — | — | — |
| 5 | 238 | 328 | 0.9958 | 0.7226 | 211 | 285 | 0.8720 | 0.6456 | 22 | 24 | 0.9091 | 0.8333 |
| 6 | 359 | 395 | 0.9944 | 0.9038 | 225 | 277 | 0.9956 | 0.8087 | 7 | 13 | 1.0000 | 0.5385 |
| 7 | 444 | 443 | 0.9752 | 0.9774 | 347 | 352 | 0.9337 | 0.9204 | — | — | — | — |
| 8 | 376 | 432 | 0.9947 | 0.8657 | 158 | 364 | 1.0000 | 0.4341 | 18 | 36 | 1.0000 | 0.5000 |
| 9 | 403 | 398 | 0.9876 | 1.0000 | 359 | 372 | 0.9972 | 0.9624 | 46 | 47 | 1.0000 | 0.9787 |

with repeated ECoG interval absent decreased irregularly (Figure 19.3b), and (3) mean proportion of time that LSP was present with or without repeated ECoG interval present increased gradually (Figure 19.3c). Similarly, Figure 19.3d, e, and f shows that as the time period after the administration of the most recent dose of PTZ increased (1) the mean proportion of time that LSP was absent with repeated ECoG interval present increased irregularly over the first 7 minutes, then decreased; these changes were not statistically significant; (2) the mean proportion of the time that LSP was absent with repeated ECoG interval absent decreased steadily over the first 5 minutes, then increased somewhat; minute 1 was significantly greater than all others; and (3) the mean proportion of time that LSP was absent with or without the repeated ECoG interval present decreased progressively, minutes 1 and 2 being significantly greater than the others. Overall, the presence of LSP was directly related to the duration of the time interval after the administration of the most recent dose of PTZ. This relationship is fairly consistent from minute to minute. Similarly, the presence of the repeated ECoG interval was directly related to the duration of the time interval after the administration of the most recent dose of PTZ. This relationship was somewhat inconsistent from minute to minute.

Using repeated-measure ANOVA and Student Newman–Keuls test, the relative prevalence of each sympathetic ECoG pattern in all cats during the entire 10-minute period following the administration of each dose of PTZ was examined.

In one sympathetic ECoG pattern, LSP absent with repeated ECoG interval present, the mean proportions of time that the pattern existed following each of the five doses of PTZ were statistically comparable. Figure 19.4a shows the pattern LSP present with repeated ECoG interval present. Two distinct groups were separated, with prevalence following the first dose eliciting none or only minimal interictal epileptogenic activity, significantly less than following any of the subsequent three doses. Prevalence during the final dose, which induced almost no ictal activity and very little interictal activity, was not significantly different from either of the other groups ($p < .05$). In a similar manner, the other four ECoG-sympathetic patterns showing varying prevalence are seen in Figure 19.4 as a function of dose of PTZ administered, i.e., as a function of increasing amounts of epileptogenic activity consisting of more ictal activity and less interictal discharges.

In Figure 19.5a, the incidence of precipitous changes in mean arterial blood pressure for epileptiform discharges induced by all doses of PTZ in all cats was recorded as a function of the time interval after the last administration of PTZ. It showed that a statistically greater ($p < .05$) incidence of these changes occurred during minute 1. It held fairly constant during minutes 2 through 10, inclusive.

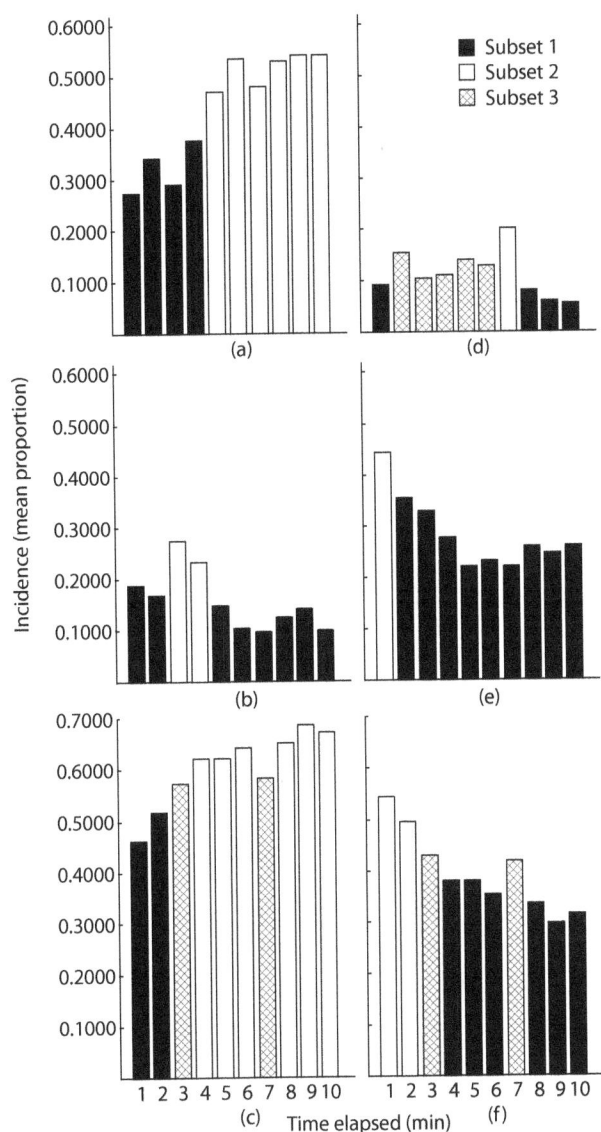

**FIGURE 19.3** Histograms representing the results of the Student Newman–Keuls test for each of the six sympathetic electrocortico-gram (ECoG) patterns as a function of time interval following the administration of pentylenetetrazol (PTZ). (a) Lockstep phenomenon (LSP) present with repeated 2.8-second ECoG interval present, (b) LSP present with repeated 2.8-second ECoG interval absent, (c) LSP present whether repeated 2.8-second ECoG interval is present or absent, (d) LSP absent with repeated 2.8-second interval present, (e) LSP absent with repeated 2.8-second ECoG interval absent, and (f) LSP absent whether repeated 2.8-second ECoG interval is present or absent. Ordinate displays the mean proportion (for nine cats) of each 1-minute interval following administration of all doses of PTZ during which the sympathetic ECoG pattern in question was observed. Abscissa displays the time-elapsed interval (in minutes) following administration of PTZ in all cats. Patterns within bars distinguish the subsets (minutes) having statistically comparable mean proportions of time during which sympathetic ECoG pattern was observed. Subset 1 consists of 1-minute intervals having statistically similar mean proportions of time during which sympathetic ECoG pattern was observed. Subset 2 consists of 1-minute intervals having statistically similar mean proportions of time during which sympathetic ECoG pattern was observed. Subset 3 consists of 1-minute intervals having mean proportions of time during which sympathetic ECoG pattern was observed, which is not distinct from either of other two groups.

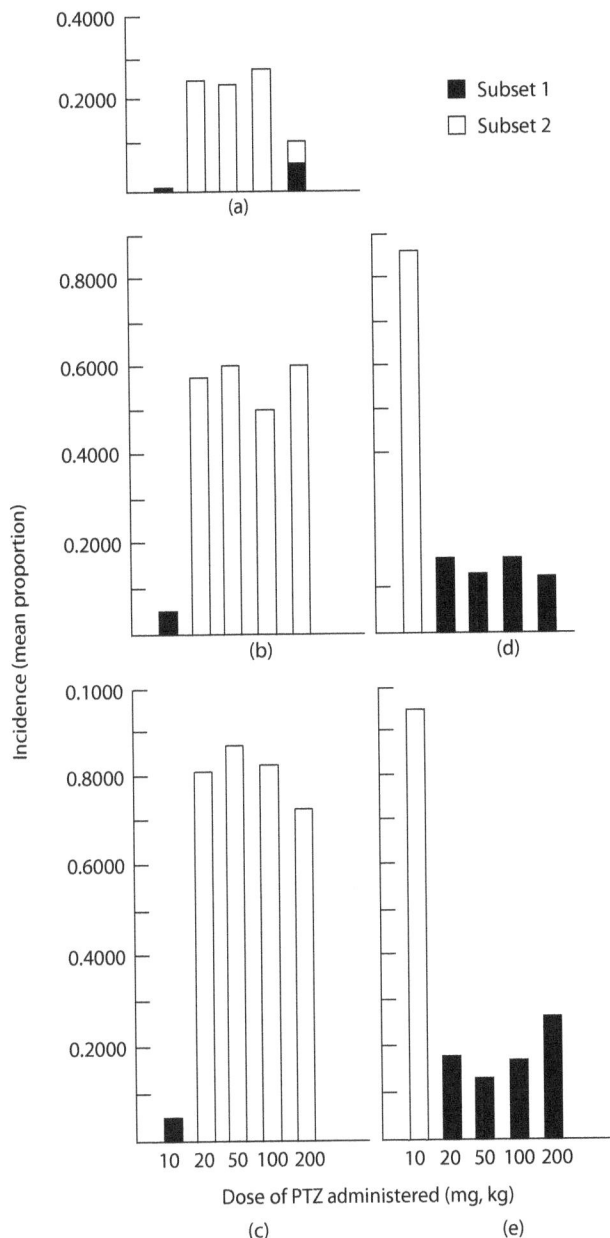

**FIGURE 19.4** Histograms representing results of Student Newman–Keuls test for each of five sympathetic ECoG patterns as a function of dose of pentylenetetrazol (PTZ) administered. (a) Lockstep phenomenon (LSP) present with repeated 2.8-second ECoG interval present, (b) LSP present with repeated 2.8-second ECoGinterval absent,(c) LSP present whether repeated 2.8-second ECOG interval is present or absent, (d) LSP absent with repeated 2.8-second ECoG interval absent, and (e) LSP absent whether repeated 2.8-second ECoG interval is present or absent. Ordinate displays the mean proportion (for nine cats) of the 10-minute period following administration of a given dose of PTZ during which the sympathetic ECoG pattern in question was observed. The abscissa displays dose of PTZ administered. Patterns within bars distinguish subsets (minutes) having statistically comparable mean proportions of time during which sympathetic ECoG pattern was observed. Subset 1 consists of 1-minute intervals having statistically similar mean proportions of time during which sympathetic ECoG pattern was observed. Subset 2 consists of 1-minute intervals having statistically similar mean proportions of time during which sympathetic ECoG pattern was observed.

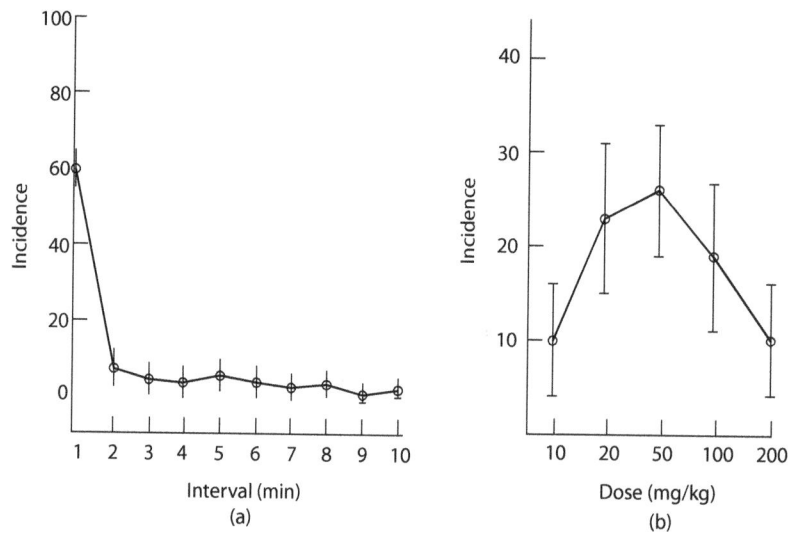

**FIGURE 19.5** Total incidence of mean arterial blood pressure changes for all nine cats both as a function of time interval since administration of most recent doses of pentylenetetrazol (PZT) and as a function of dose PZT administered. (a) Total incidence of mean arterial blood pressure changes for all cats versus minute time interval since most recent administration of PTZ. Vertical bars indicate 95% confidence intervals. No confidence interval can be determined for the values in minute 9. (b) Total incidence of mean arterial blood pressure changes for all cats versus dose of PTZ administered. Vertical bars indicate 95% confidence intervals.

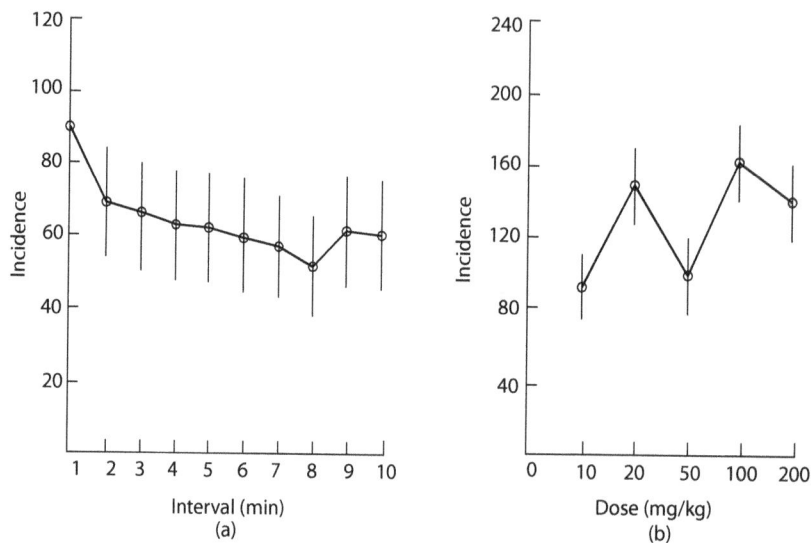

**FIGURE 19.6** Total incidence of electrocardiogram (ECG) changes for all nine cats both as a function of time interval since administration of most recent doses of pentylenetetrazol (PTZ) and as a function of dose of PZT administered. (a) Total incidence of ECG changes for all cats versus minute interval since the most recent administration of PZT. Vertical bars indicate 95% confidence intervals. (b) Total incidence of ECG changes for all cats versus dose of PTZ administered. Vertical bars indicate 95% confidence intervals.

The incidence of mean arterial blood pressure changes for increasing amounts of epileptogenic activity induced by the increasing doses of PTZ displayed a bell-shaped distribution (Figure 19.5b) with a peak following PTZ at 50 mg/kg dose. Ninety-five percent confidence intervals showed this incidence to be higher than that following either the 10 or 200 mg/kg dose of PTZ.

The incidence of changes in the ECG decreased during the first 8 minutes inclusive following the administration of PTZ (Figure 19.6a). This difference was statistically significant ($p < .06$) during minute 1 compared to minute 7 or 8.

The occurrence of changes in the ECG was least frequent following 10 mg/kg PTZ than following any other dose. This dose of PTZ elicited little or no interictal activity in most cats and almost no ictal activity. This was a statistically significant difference from the prevalence following all other doses except 50 mg/kg PTZ. This dose of PTZ elicited primarily ictal activity.

The mean proportion of each minute during which LSP was present and the mean proportion of each minute during which the repeated ECoG interval was observed were directly proportional to the time interval elapsed after the administration of all doses of PTZ. When parameters of autonomic dysfunction were examined as a function of the time interval since the administration of all doses of PTZ, the incidence of blood pressure change was significantly greater (95% confidence interval) during the first minute following the epileptogenic activity induced by the administration of all doses of PTZ than during any other minute. Furthermore, the blood pressure became more stable with increasing time after each dose. Likewise, the incidence of ECG changes decreased over the first 8 minutes following the administration of PTZ and was statistically greater following minute 1 than following minute 7 or 8, when epileptiform activity decreased. When this stable LSP was lost, both precipitous mean arterial blood pressure changes and incidence of ECG changes occurred more frequently.

Just as the mean proportion of time during which LSP was observed was statistically greater after the PTZ dose of 50 mg/kg when maximal numbers of epileptiform discharges were induced, the incidence of mean arterial pressure change was significantly greater after this dose than after the 10 and 200 mg/kg PTZ doses, which were less epileptogenic than the 50 mg/kg dose. No relationship between incidence of ECG changes and LSP, as a function of PTZ dosage, could be found; rather, there seemed to be a correlation with the doses inducing the greatest degree of epileptiform discharge.

## DISCUSSION

We examined the temporal synchronization between ECoG and sympathetic spikes that was observed in a PTZ animal model of epilepsy, pretreated with the antiepileptic drug phenobarbital. These temporally synchronized spikes were designated LSP when they occurred consistently over a period of 10 or more uninterrupted seconds. The administration of PTZ to phenobarbital-pretreated cats converted the normal baseline state of desynchronized sympathetic discharges and phenobarbital spindles into a state of hypersynchronized cortical and sympathetic activities.

This laboratory has frequently used PTZ treatment of cats to create an experimental model of epileptogenic activity (Lathers et al. 1978, 1984, 1987; Schraeder and Lathers 1983). The dosing regimen has been developed to produce all degrees of subconvulsant and convulsant activities (Schraeder and Lathers 1983). In this way, the full spectrum of cortical epileptiform activity can be examined. Phenobarbital was used by this laboratory as an anticonvulsant in this animal model.

The possibility that this observed temporal synchronization of ECoG and sympathetic spikes represents artifact, originating from either outside or within the cat, was examined first. Possible mechanical artifact from the respirator or the 60-Hz alternating current used to power the polygraph was dismissed for two reasons. First, other experiments undertaken with the same equipment in the same room in the same time period produced no such artifact. Second, these potential sources would produce artifact at a constant rate throughout the entire experiment. Sympathetic spikes, ECoG spikes, and LSP were not observed at a constant rate

throughout the entire experiment. In addition, neither sympathetic nor ECoG spikes were observed during either control period.

The possibility of intrinsic artifact from cardiac or skeletal muscle contractions was considered. However, neither the ECoG nor sympathetic spikes bore relationship to the incidence of changes in the ECG. Furthermore, the use of gallamine effectively blocked spontaneous muscle contractions. Analysis with multiple regression showed that the time-locked occurrence of ECoG spikes and sympathetic spikes was not random. This analysis suggested that the incidence of LSP was directly related to the incidence of sympathetic spikes.

Epileptogenic activity induced by PTZ appears to be necessary to allow this phenomenon to express itself. Although, in eight of the nine cats LSP was present more often than absent (>55% of time in seconds) while the cat was under the influence of PTZ, this phenomenon was not found in any cat during the control period. Epileptogenic activity induced by PTZ is an experimental model of primary generalized epilepsy. The method of action of this drug, however, is uncertain (Stone 1972). There are three proposed methods of action of PTZ, which would allow the LSP to express itself: (1) spatial and temporal summation of neuronal discharges in a subcortical center producing a stimulus strong enough to overcome the cortical and ganglionic threshold (Hahn 1960); (2) increased synaptic recruitment, resulting in the amplification of subcortical stimuli along their path so that, on reaching the cortex and sympathetic ganglion, they are capable of causing these neurons to discharge; and (3) increased irritability of all neurons so that subcortical impulses could stimulate cortical and ganglionic neurons (Hahn 1960). In each case, PTZ effectively creates a hyperirritable state of epileptogenic electrical activity present in the central and autonomic nervous systems. Although phenobarbital can act to minimize this irritability, the effect of this pharmacological agent in this study was eventually overcome by increased epileptogenic activity.

The 2.8-second repeated ECoG interval, a type of latency period between the end of one spike and the beginning of another associated spike, appeared to convey a stabilizing effect on the presence of LSP. When this repeated ECoG interval was present, LSP was present a significantly greater percentage of time than when LSP was absent. When the repeated ECoG interval was not present, LSP was much less common and the distinct ECoG spikes often degenerated into prolonged ictal activity. Our analysis minimized the degree of association between the repeated ECoG interval and the presence of LSP. Our definition of a repeated ECoG interval excludes periods when two or more additional ECoG spikes are contained within the 2.8-second interval, even if these additional ECoG spikes are time locked to sympathetic spikes. A more liberal definition would result in a more frequent association between LSP and repeated ECoG interval.

The mean proportion of each minute during which LSP was present was directly proportional to the time interval elapsed following the administration of PTZ. The direct relationship reflects the fact that episodes of epileptogenic activity, and particularly prolonged ictal activity, are most frequently observed shortly after PTZ is administered. Similarly, the incidence of precipitous blood pressure change was significantly greater ($p < .05$) during the first minute following the administration of all doses of PTZ than during any other minute. Likewise, the incidence of ECG changes decreased over the first 8 minutes following administration of all doses of PTZ, with minute 1 containing a significantly higher incidence compared to minute 7 or 8. Thus, the possibility arises of a relationship between the presence of LSP and both a stable mean arterial pressure and a normally functioning autonomic nervous system.

## SUMMARY

The concept of rhythmic neuronal activity being associated with normal central and autonomic nervous system activities is not new. Normal and abnormal cortical patterns are the basis of the clinical use of electroencephalography. Sympathetic nerve discharge patterns have been characterized by others (Barman and Gebber 1980; Gebber and Barman 1980). A temporal relationship between discharge patterns of the central and autonomic nervous systems has also been shown previously (Gebber and Barman 1981). Loss of this rhythmic stability can alter neurotransmitter release (Birks 1978; Birks et al. 1981) and initiate autonomic dysfunction (Lathers and Schraeder 1982; Lathers et al. 1977). This chapter characterizes LSP and supports the idea of closely related central and autonomic rhythmic activity, which is important in maintaining homeostasis. The data showed that when a stable LSP was lost, both precipitous mean arterial blood pressure changes and the incidence of ECG changes occurred more frequently. This suggests that the LSP, either by its mere presence or by the rhythm at which it occurs, may play a role in the origin of autonomic dysfunction, contributing to the rise of SUD in epilepsy.

## ACKNOWLEDGMENTS

The authors gratefully acknowledge Dr. Adele Kaplan for her statistical expertise and critical review of the manuscript. We are indebted to Dr. Paul L. Schraeder for his discussions.

## REFERENCES

Barman SM, Gebber GL. Sympathetic nerve rhythm of brain stem origin. *Am J Physiol (Regul Integr Comp Physiol)* 1980;239(8):R42–7.

Barman SM, Gebber GL. Brain stem neuronal types with activity patterns related to sympathetic nerve discharge. *Am J Physiol (Regul Integr Comp Physiol)* 1981;242(11):R335–41.

Barman SM, Gebber GL. Hypothalamic neurons with activity patterns related to sympathetic nerve discharge. *Am J Physiol (Regul Integr Comp Physiol)* 1982;242(11):R34–43.

Barman SM, Gebber GL. Spinal interneurons with sympathetic nerve-related activity. *Am J Physiol (Regul Integr Comp Physiol)* 1984;247(16):R761–7.

Basar E. Abstract methods of general systems analysis. In: Basar E, ed. *Biophysical and Physiological Systems Analysis*. Reading, MA: Addison-Wesley; 1976, pp. 23–47.

Birks RI. Regulation by patterned preganglionic neural activity of transmitter stores in a sympathetic ganglion. *J Physiol* 1978;280:559–72.

Birks RI, Laskey W, Polosa C. The effect of burst patterning of preganglionic input on the efficacy of transmission at the cat stellate ganglion. *J Physiol* 1981;318:531–9.

Gebber GL, Barman SM. Basis for 2–6 cycle/s rhythm in sympathetic nerve discharge. *Am J Physiol (Regul Integr Comp Physiol)* 1980;239(8):R48–56.

Gebber GL, Barman SM. 1981. Sympathetic-related activity of brain stem neurons in baroreceptor-denervated cats. *Am J Physiol (Regul Integr Comp Physiol)* 1981;240(9):R348–55.

Hahn F. Analeptics. *Pharmacol Rev* 1960;12:447–530.

Jay GW, Leestma JE. Sudden death in epilepsy. A comprehensive review of the literature and proposed mechanisms. *Acta Neurol Scand* 1981;63(Suppl 82):1–66.

Jun, H. W. 1976. Pharmacokinetic studies of pentylenetetrazol in dogs. *J Pharmacol Sci* 65:1038–41.

Kiloh LG, McComas AJ, Osselton JW. The neural basis of the EEG. In: Kiloh LG, McComas AJ, Osselton JW, eds. *Clinical Encephalography*. London: Butterworths; 1972a, pp. 21–34.

Kiloh LG, McComas AJ, Osselton JW. Normal findings. In: Kiloh LG, McComas AJ, Osselton JW, eds. *Clinical Encephalography*. London: Butterworths; 1972b, pp. 52–70.

Krohn W. Causes of death among epileptics. *Epilepsia* 1977;4:315–21.

Lathers CM, Kelliher GJ, Roberts J, Beasley AB. Nonuniform cardiac sympathetic nerve discharge. Mechanisms for coronary occlusion and digitalis-induced arrhythmia. *Circulation* 1978;57:1058–65.

Lathers CM, Roberts J, Kelliher GJ. Correlation of ouabain-induced arrhythmia and nonuniformity in the histamine-evoked discharge of cardiac sympathetic nerves. *J Pharmacol Exp Ther* 1977;203:467–79.

Lathers CM, Schraeder PL. Autonomic dysfunction in epilepsy: Characterization of autonomic cardiac neural discharge associated with pentylenetetrazol-induced epileptogenic activity. *Epilepsia* 1982;23:633–47.

Lathers CM, Schraeder PL, Camel SB. Neural mechanism in cardiac arrhythmia associated with epileptogenic activity: The effect of phenobarbital in the cat. *Life Sci* 1984;34:1919–36.

Lathers CM, Schraeder PL, Weiner FL. Synchronization of cardiac autonomic neural discharge with epileptogenic activity: The lockstep phenomenon. *Electroencephalogr Clin Neurophysiol* 1987;67:247–59.

Meldrum BS, Brierley JB. Prolonged epileptic seizures in primates. *Arch Neurol* 1973;28:10–7.

Meldrum BS, Horton RW. Physiology of status epilepticus in primates. *Arch Neurol* 1973;28:1–9.

Schraeder PL, Lathers CM. Cardiac neural discharge and epileptogenic activity in the cat: An animal model for unexplained death. *Life Sci* 1983;32:1371–82.

Stone WE. Systemic chemical convulsants and metabolic derangements. In: Purpura DP, Perry JK, Tower D, Woodbury DM, Walter R, eds. *Experimental Models of Epilepsy. A Manual for the Laboratory Worker*. New York, NY: Raven Press; 1972, pp. 407–33.

Van Buren JM. Some autonomic concomitants of ictal automatism. A study of temporal lobe attacks. *Brain* 1958;81:505–28.

Wasterlain CG. Mortality and morbidity from serial studies. An experimental study. *Epilepsia* 1974;15:155–76.

# 20 Relationship of the Lockstep Phenomenon and Precipitous Changes in Blood Pressure

*Amy Z. Stauffer, Jeffrey M. Dodd-O, and Claire M. Lathers*

## CONTENTS

## INTRODUCTION

Sudden unexplained death (SUD) is defined as "nontraumatic death occurring in an individual within minutes or hours of the onset of the final illness or ictus" (Jay and Leestma 1981). No anatomic cause of death can be demonstrated at autopsy. The prevalence of SUD in persons with epilepsy has been estimated to be between 1 death in 525 epileptic persons and 1 per 2100 (Leestma et al. 1984). Autonomic dysfunction occurring in conjunction with epileptogenic activity and causing fatal cardiac arrhythmia and/or arrest has been postulated as an explanation for the increased prevalence of SUD in persons with epilepsy (Leestma et al. 1984).

Lathers and Schraeder (Lathers and Schraeder 1982; Schraeder and Lathers 1983) demonstrated that autonomic dysfunction occurs during ictal and interictal epileptogenic activity induced by pentylenetetrazol (PTZ). Lathers et al. (1987) defined the lockstep phenomenon (LSP), during which postganglionic cardiac sympathetic neural discharge occurs as if time locked to electrocorticographic epileptiform discharges (Figure 20.1). The purpose of this study is to determine whether LSP in any of its patterns is related to sudden alterations in autonomic function as manifested by precipitous changes in mean arterial blood pressure. A better understanding of LSP and how it correlates with changes in physiological parameters such as mean arterial blood pressure, cardiac neural discharge, and cardiac rate and rhythm will help to delineate mechanisms that may contribute to sudden death in the epileptic person. Such an understanding should then allow one to develop better drugs and/or combination of drugs to prevent the physiologic changes that may result in a fatal event.

## METHOD

Nine cats were intravenously (i.v.) anesthetized with 80 mg/kg α-chloralose. Tracheostomies were performed, and the femoral arteries and veins were cannulated. The animals were ventilated with a small-animal respirator, maintaining $pO_2$, $pco_2$, and pH within an acceptable physiological range. Intermittent doses of gallamine (2 mg/kg i.v.) maintained paralysis. After bilateral frontal craniectomy, the dura was resected to allow placement of electrodes for recording of the electrocardiogram (ECoG). A thoracotomy and a right partial pneumonectomy were performed to expose the cardiac postganglionic sympathetic and right cardiac vagal nerves. Sympathetic nerves were identified by their response to a blood pressure drop induced by histamine (5 μg/kg i.v.). The activity of sympathetic nerves, ECoG, ECG (lead II), and the mean arterial blood pressure were recorded and stored on magnetic tape. Rectal temperature was maintained at 37.5°C–38.5°C.

Each cat received 20 mg/kg intravenous phenobarbital infused over 10 minutes after a 10-minute control period. One hour after completion of the infusion of phenobarbital, the animals received six doses (10, 20, 50, 100, 200, and 2000 mg/kg) of PTZ intravenously at 10-minute intervals. Although the half-life of PTZ in the cat is unknown (Knoll Laboratories, personal communication), it has been shown to be 1.4 hours in the dog (Jun 1976). If the assumption is made that the half-life of PTZ in the cat is similar to that in the dog, then the doses of PTZ were cumulative.

Three categories of epileptiform discharges were defined according to duration. Polyspike discharges of 10 or more seconds were classified as prolonged ictal. Repetitive polyspike discharges less than 10-second duration that were

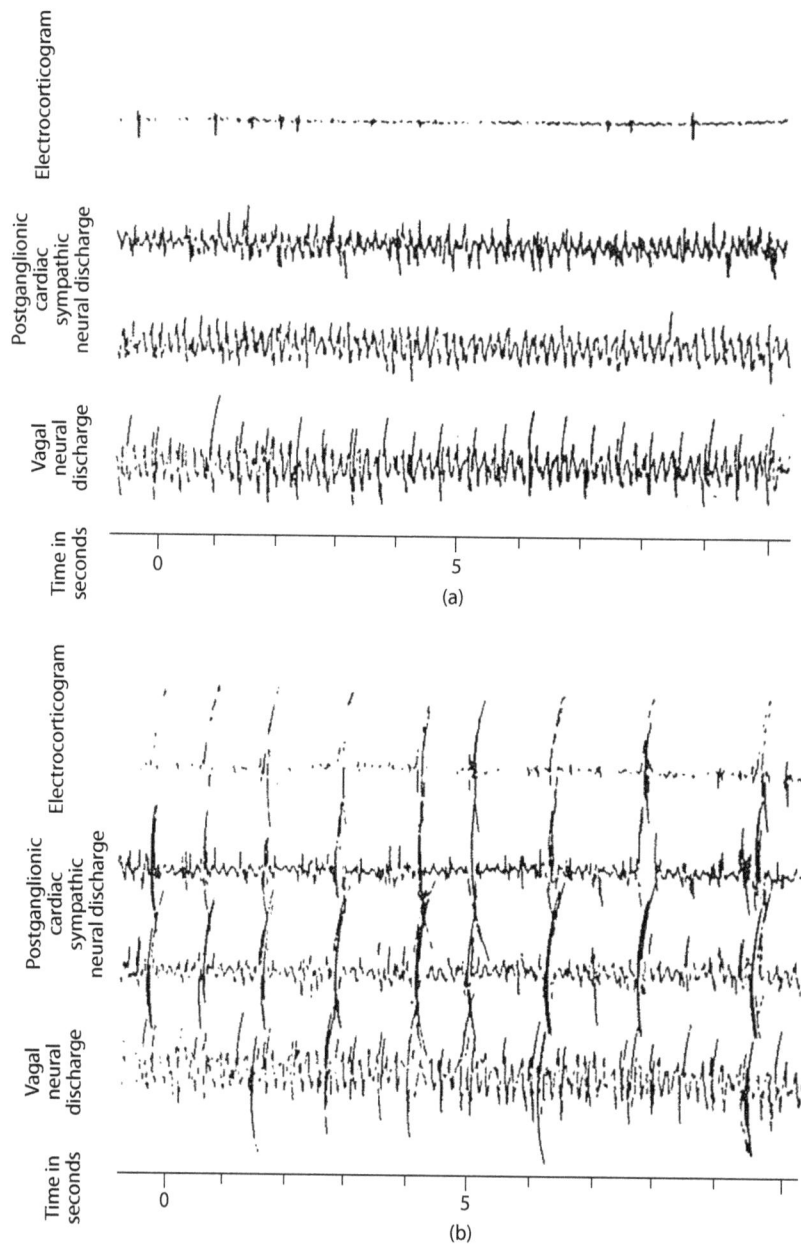

**FIGURE 20.1** Electrocorticographic and autonomic cardiac neural discharge monitored in one cat. The records in each panel, from top to bottom, illustrate the electrocardiogram and neural discharge for two sympathetic postganglionic and the vagal cardiac nerves, respectively. (a) Data obtained during the control period; (b) data recorded 43 seconds after the administration of pentylenetetrazol of 10 mg/kg (intravenously). (From Lathers, CM et al., *Electroencephalogr Clin Neurophysiol*, 67, 247–59, 1987. With permission.)

interrupted by periods of depression of cerebral activity were classified as brief ictal. Prolonged ictal and brief ictal activities are analogous to the activity seen in the electroencephalogram (EEG) during clinical seizures. Discrete paroxysmal spikes and/or polyspikes and wave discharges, which are analogous to the nonictal epileptogenic activity seen in the interictal EEG of patients with a seizure disorder, were classified as interictal spikes.

The term "lockstep phenomenon" is used to describe the occurrence of sympathetic postganglionic discharge and various types of epileptogenic ECoG activity in a time-locked

fashion (Dodd-O and Lathers, this book, Chapter 19; Lathers et al. 1987). In the present experiment, the parameters used to define the occurrence of LSP are those utilized by Dodd-O and Lathers. When an interictal ECoG spike occurred, it was said to be time locked to a sympathetic spike only if the sympathetic spike began within 200 ms of the beginning of the interictal ECoG spike. If the ECoG activity was brief ictal in type, it was considered as a single event and was analyzed with the sympathetic neural activity occurring during the corresponding time interval. The LSP was said to exist if and only if the first spike of the sympathetic polyspike discharge began after the corresponding brief ictal discharge began, and if the last spike of the sympathetic polyspike discharge began before the final spike of the brief ictal discharge ended. Time periods during which the ECoG displayed prolonged ictal activity were not considered to contain LSP.

The total amounts of time that the LSP was present and absent were analyzed. The LSP was considered to be present only when the previously mentioned criteria were fulfilled for an uninterrupted time interval of 10 or more seconds. During this 10-second interval, at least two episodes of time-locked sympathetic postganglionic and ECoG discharges had to exist. When the incidences of sympathetic and ECoG discharges were not equal over the 10-second interval, a closer look was taken at the characteristics of the less frequently occurring discharge. If more than one of the less frequently occurring discharges appeared alone, the LSP was considered to be absent. If the LSP was interrupted after being present for an uninterrupted time interval of greater than 10 seconds, the LSP was considered to have ended if the period of interruption was greater than 4.5 seconds. If, however, the interruption in LSP lasted 4.5 seconds or less, the LSP was considered to exist without interruption.

The repeated 2.8-second ECoG interval is the interspike time interval found in a previous study to exist most frequently between ECoG spikes when LSP was present (Dodd-O and Lathers, this book, Chapter 19). The time interval is measured from the end of one ECoG spike to the beginning of another ECoG spike. Contained within this 2.8-second interval may be another ECoG spike. This third ECoG spike need not be related to either of the spikes that bind the 2.8-second interval in question. This third spike is, however, related to another ECoG spike that begins 2.8 seconds after the third ECoG spike ends.

The duration of time (in seconds) that the 2.8-second interval was present was determined as follows. To be considered to exist, the foregoing criteria had to be fulfilled for at least three consecutive 2.8-second intervals. Once present, the 2.8-second interval was considered to be present without interruption only if it continued without any interval of disruption lasting more than 4.5 seconds. If the repeated 2.8-second interval was present but was interrupted for more than 4.5 seconds, the repeated 2.8-second interval was said to have ended.

In an effort to explore the importance of LSP stability in maintaining blood pressure, a more specific classification of LSP was developed. First, four categories of LSP were created. The first of these, no LSP, included all of the time intervals in which the ECoG-sympathetic discharge pattern was such that conditions for the existence of LSP were not fulfilled. If the condition for LSP were present, the rate of LSP was classified as either stable or unstable. The term stable LSP was used to describe all uninterrupted time periods of 10 or more seconds during which the time interval between sympathetic spikes was unchanged. If the interspace interval was constant but then changed for no more than one interspike interval, stability was considered to be maintained. Two categories of stable LSP were observed: (1) stable LSP in which the repeated 2.8-second interval was present and (2) stable LSP in which the repeated 2.8-second interval was absent.

If the interspike interval was altered on two consecutive occasions, stability of LSP was considered to be lost. The term unstable LSP was used to describe all time intervals of 10 or more seconds during which LSP existed but the criteria for "stable LSP" were absent. The four categories (no LSP, stable LSP with 2.8-second interval, stable LSP without 2.8-second interval, and unstable LSP) were analyzed, and the unstable category was divided into unstable LSP with increasing rate and unstable LSP with decreasing rate. The term unstable LSP with increasing rate was used to describe periods of unstable LSP in which the duration of interspike interval decreased between consecutive spikes. The term "unstable LSP with decreasing rate" was used to describe those periods of unstable LSP in which the duration of the interspike interval increased between consecutive spikes. These two types of unstable LSP were analyzed along with the other three LSP patterns (no LSP, stable LSP with 2.8-second interval, and stable LSP without 2.8-second interval) to determine if direction, i.e., an increasing or decreasing rate, had any effect on blood pressure changes. In summary, the LSP patterns were

1. LSP absent
2. Stable LSP with 2.8-second interval
3. Stable LSP without 2.8-second interval
4. Unstable LSP (a) with increasing rate and (b) with decreasing rate

Mean arterial blood pressure changes were reviewed. After examination of the control period and the PTZ treatment period, it was found that mean arterial blood pressure changes of 23 mm Hg over a 10-second interval never occurred during the control period. This rate of change, i.e., 23 mm Hg over a 10-second period, was termed a precipitous blood pressure change. The occurrence and incidence of such changes were examined in all cats after the administration of each dose of PTZ except for the dose of 2000 mg/kg. This dose led to death in all the cats, and thus it was decided not to analyze characterization of this event with the rest of the experiment.

## STATISTICAL ANALYSIS

For all cats, the amount of time in seconds that was spent in each LSP pattern was recorded. The number of precipitous blood pressure changes was also determined. Since each precipitous blood pressure change occurred over a 10-s period, the amount of time in seconds that was spent in precipitous blood pressure changes is equal to the number of precipitous blood pressure changes multiplied by 10.

For each LSP pattern (no LSP, stable LSP with 2.8-second interval, stable LSP without 2.8-second interval, and unstable LSP), the proportion of time spent in precipitous blood pressure changes was calculated by dividing the amount of time spent in precipitous blood pressure changes by the total amount of time spent in that LSP pattern. This was done for each cat. To determine if any of the LSP patterns were associated with a significantly higher mean proportion of time in precipitous blood pressure changes, a one-way repeated-measures analysis of variance (ANOVA) was performed. LSP pattern was used as the independent variable, and mean proportion of time spent in precipitous blood pressure changes was used as the dependent variable. The Biomedical Program Package was used. To determine which of the LSP patterns was significantly different from the others, a post hoc Newman–Keuls test was performed if a significance of the $F$ ratio ($p < .05$) was found. Because the observations for each cat were proportions, the variances and means of the comparison groups were not independent of one another. Therefore, square root transformation ($X = \sqrt{x + 10}$) was applied to all data points before analysis. This strategy is suggested by Winer (1971) to stabilize the variances. The log transformation $X' = \log (x + 1.0)$ was also applied (Winer 1971). Neither strategy made a significant impact on variance heterogeneity. Since equal-sized groups weaken the impact of variance heterogeneity on $\alpha$, the untransformed values were used; however, Huynh–Feldt degrees of freedom were applied to correct for heterogeneity of variance.

To determine if any significant differences existed between unstable LSP with increasing rate and unstable LSP with decreasing rate, the unstable LSP category was divided into unstable LSP with increasing rate and unstable LSP with decreasing rate. The previous analysis was repeated.

The next question was whether a significantly different mean proportion of precipitous blood pressure changes occurred during any of the LSP patterns. For each LSP pattern, the number of precipitous blood pressure changes occurring with that LSP pattern was divided by the total number of precipitous blood pressure changes in that cat. To adjust for the fact that more time was spent in some LSP patterns than in others, this proportion was divided by the proportion of time spent in that LSP pattern, i.e., the amount of time spent in that

LSP pattern divided by the total time analyzed for that cat. This adjustment was done separately for each of the nine cats. A one-way repeated-measures ANOVA was performed, using LSP pattern as the independent variable and proportion of precipitous blood pressure changes as the dependent variable. The unstable LSP category was then divided into unstable LSP with increasing rate and unstable LSP with decreasing rate. The analysis was repeated to determine if there was a significant difference between unstable LSP with increasing rate, unstable LSP with decreasing rate, LSP absent, stable LSP with a 2.8-second interval, and stable LSP without a 2.8-second interval in terms of mean proportion of precipitous blood pressure changes. The difference between this analysis and the previous one lies in the fact that this analysis was limited to the time during which there were precipitous blood pressure changes, whereas the previous analysis took into account all time analyzed for each cat.

## RESULTS

### LSP Pattern versus Mean Proportion of Time Spent in Precipitous Blood Pressure Changes

In comparing the mean proportion of time spent in precipitous blood pressure changes for each LSP pattern, the one-way repeated-measures ANOVA showed borderline significance of the $F$ ratio (Huynh–Feldt probability $p = .056$). This indicates that a significantly different mean proportion of time was spent in precipitous blood pressure changes in one or more of the LSP patterns. The post hoc Newman–Keuls test showed that the unstable LSP pattern was significantly higher than all of the other LSP patterns in terms of mean proportion of time spent in precipitous blood pressure changes (Figure 20.2).

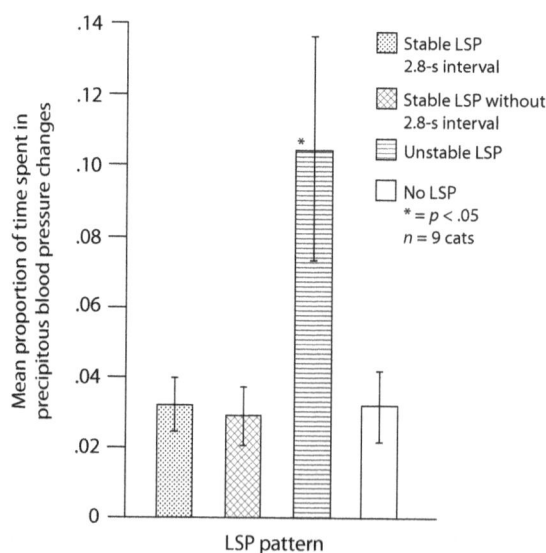

**FIGURE 20.2**   Mean proportion of time spent in precipitous blood pressure changes as a function of the lockstep phenomenon (LSP) pattern ($n = 9$ cats). The one-way repeated-measures analysis of variance showed borderline significance of the $F$ ratio (Huynh–Feldt probability $p = .056$), indicating that a significantly different mean proportion of time was spent in precipitous pressure changes in one or more of the LSP patterns. The post hoc Newman–Keuls test showed that the unstable LSP pattern was significantly higher than all other patterns in terms of mean proportion of time spent in precipitous blood pressure changes.

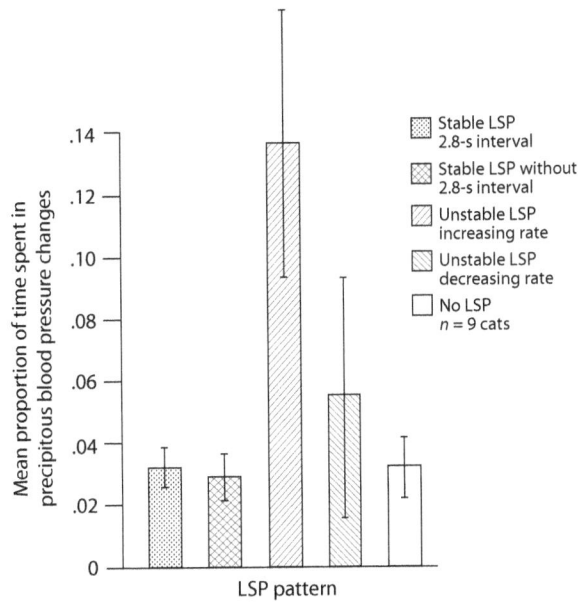

**FIGURE 20.3** Mean proportion of time spent in precipitous blood pressure changes as a function of LSP pattern ($n = 9$ cats). This analysis is identical to the one presented in Figure 20.2, except that the unstable LSP category is divided into unstable LSP with increasing rate and unstable LSP with decreasing rate. Although there were no statistically significant differences among the LSP patterns (Huynh–Feldt probability $p = .068$), the observed pattern was that unstable LSP with increasing rate contributed the highest mean proportion of time in precipitous blood pressure changes.

When the unstable LSP category was divided into unstable LSP with increasing rate and unstable LSP with decreasing rate and the analysis was repeated, the corrected (Huynh–Feldt) probability was .068. The observed pattern was that unstable LSP with increasing rate contributed the highest mean proportion of time in precipitous blood pressure changes, but the difference was not great enough to achieve statistical significance (Figure 20.3).

## LSP PATTERN VERSUS MEAN PROPORTION OF PRECIPITOUS BLOOD PRESSURE CHANGES

When comparing the mean proportions of precipitous blood pressure changes occurring during each of the LSP patterns (no LSP, stable LSP with 2.8-second interval, stable LSP without 2.8-second interval, and unstable LSP), the one-way repeated-measures ANOVA was not significant (Huynh–Feldt probability $p = .0926$). This indicated that there were no statistically significant differences among the LSP patterns in terms of mean proportion of precipitous blood pressure changes. However, the observation can be made (Figure 20.4) that the unstable LSP pattern had the highest mean proportion of precipitous blood pressure changes, although this difference was not statistically significant.

When the unstable LSP category was divided into unstable LSP with increasing rate and unstable LSP with decreasing rate, the ANOVA was also not significant (Huynh–Feldt probability $p = .2105$). Although there were no statistically

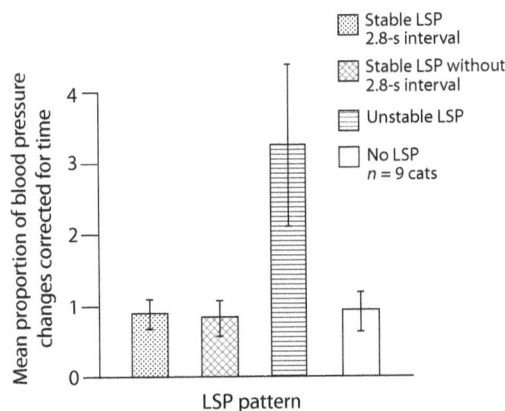

**FIGURE 20.4** Mean proportion of precipitous blood pressure changes (corrected for time) as a function of LSP pattern ($n = 9$ cats). The one-way repeated-measures analysis of variance was not significant (Huynh–Feldt probability $p = .093$), indicating that there were no statistically significant differences among the LSP patterns in terms of mean proportion of precipitous blood pressure changes. The observation can be made, however, that unstable LSP had the highest mean proportion of precipitous blood pressure changes.

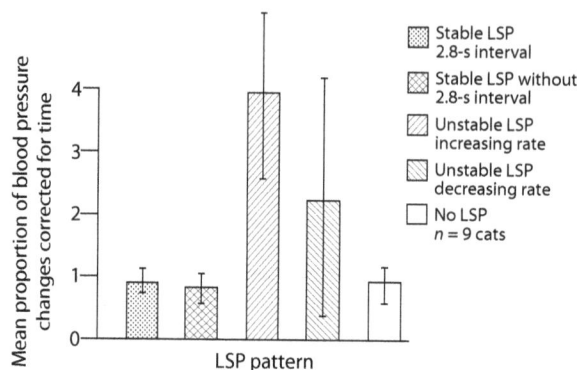

**FIGURE 20.5** Mean proportion of precipitous blood pressure changes (corrected for time) as a function of LSP pattern. Unstable LSP is divided into unstable LSP with increasing rate and unstable LSP with decreasing rate. The one-way repeated-measures analysis of variance showed no statistically significant differences among the LSP patterns in terms of mean proportion of precipitous blood pressure changes (Huynh–Feldt probability, $p = .2105$), but it can be observed that unstable LSP with increasing rate contributed the highest mean proportion of precipitous blood pressure changes. It can also be seen that the mean proportion of precipitous blood pressure changes for unstable LSP with decreasing rate was higher than the other three patterns.

significant differences among the LSP patterns in terms of mean proportion of precipitous blood pressure changes, it can be observed that unstable LSP with increasing rate contributed the highest mean proportion of precipitous blood pressure changes. It was also found that the mean proportion of precipitous blood pressure changes for unstable LSP with decreasing rate was higher than the other three LSP patterns (Figure 20.5).

## DISCUSSION

It is important to consider the autonomic neuroanatomical pathways that may be the basis for the LSP, since epileptogenic activity originating in the cortex could be transmitted to the hypothalamus and to the brain stem to alter autonomic neural control of blood pressure and cardiac rate and rhythm (Figure 20.6). The hypothalamus exerts control over the autonomic nervous system; the anterior and medial hypothalamus regulates parasympathetic function, and the posterior and lateral hypothalamus regulates sympathetic function. Direct projections exist from the hypothalamus to the preganglionic sympathetic neurons of the intermediolateral cell column and to the parasympathetic nuclei of the brain stem (Saper et al. 1976). The mammillotegmental tract connects the hypothalamus with the reticular formation, which contains multisynaptic descending pathways linking the hypothalamus with autonomic areas in the brain stem and spinal cord. The medullary reticular formation contains cardiovascular areas that can produce changes in heart rate and blood pressure. These areas produce their effects through reticulospinal connections to the intermediolateral cell column and through connections to preganglionic parasympathetic neurons (Willis and Grossman 1981). The intermediolateral cell column also receives input from the following regions of the medulla: A1 (norepinephrine-containing) neurons, C1 area (epinephrine-containing) neurons, raphe, and the nucleus tractus solitarius. The nucleus tractus solitarius receives afferent projections from the arterial baroreceptors. Aside from its medullary

input, the intermediolateral cell column receives projections from the A5 area, a group of norepinephrine-containing neurons that is located in the pons (Natelson 1985). The hypothalamus is also connected to the brain stem by the medial forebrain bundle, which projects to the midbrain reticular formation, providing another pathway for descending control over the autonomic nervous system. The medial forebrain bundle connects the hypothalamus with structures in the forebrain, such as septal area, anterior olfactory nucleus, and pyriform cortex. The medial forebrain bundle also contains fibers from the fornix and the orbitofrontal cortex. The orbitofrontal cortex projects to the thalamus and the amygdala (Korner 1979), which is connected to the hypothalamus by the stria terminalis and the ventral amygdalofugal pathway.

A close link between the hypothalamus and the limbic system exists through the Papez circuit. Papez (1937) postulated that information from the cortex travels by way of the cingulate gyrus to the hippocampus, which projects to the hypothalamus via the fornix. The mamillothalamic tract connects the mammillary bodies to the anterior nuclei of the thalamus. The circuit is completed by a pathway connecting the thalamus and the cingulate gyrus. Electrical stimulation of the hypothalamus or other structures in the Papez circuit results in autonomic responses. Autonomic responses also occur as a result of stimulation of other areas of the cortex. Wall and David (1951) described three cortical areas in monkeys in which blood pressure changes greater than 10–20 mm Hg could be produced with electrical stimulation. The first of these areas is the sensorimotor cortex; the descending pathway from this area is independent of the hypothalamus and closely related to the pyramidal tract. A direct corticospinal pathway that is independent of the hypothalamus was also described by Landau (1953). The second area is the orbitofrontal cortex; the pathway that begins in this area passes through the hypothalamus. The third of the areas described by Wall and David is the anterior temporal lobe; the pathway from this area of the cortex is partially dependent on the hypothalamus and partially direct to the tegmentum and pons. Although it

Motor cortex

Prefrontal cortex    Orbitofrontal cortex

Pyramidal tract

Pyriform cortex
Anterior olfactory nucleus
Septal area

Temporal lobe

MFB (Medial forebrain bundle)

?

Cingulate gyrus

Dorso medial    Thalamus
Anterior thalamic nuclei

Hippocampus

Mammillo thalamic tract

Fornix

?

Hypothalamus

MFB

Stria terminalis

Amygdala

Mammillo tegmental tract    MFB    Ventral amygdalo fugal pathway

Hypothalamo spinal tract

Reticular formation
Midbrain
Multi synaptic pathway    Pons    A5
Medulla
Cardiovascular areas

Baroreceptors

Reticulospinal/ reticulobulbar tracts    Other input from medulla[a]

Preganglionic neurons in spinal cord and brain stem

Preganglionic nerves

Autonomic ganglia

Postganglionic nerves

Heart and blood vessels

[a]Includes A1 neurona, raphe, nucleus tractus solitarius, and C1 area

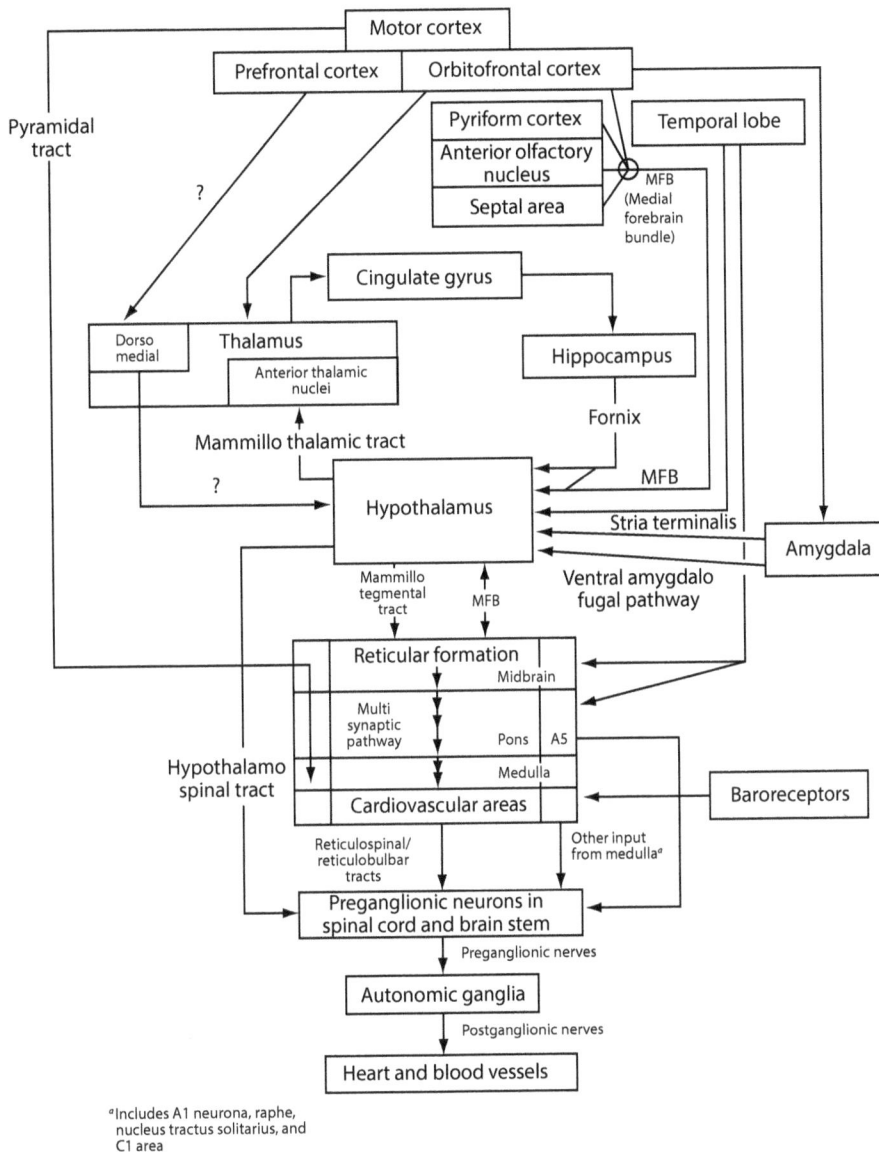

**FIGURE 20.6** Numerous neuroanatomical pathways exist by which epileptogenic activity may be transmitted to the autonomic nervous system, resulting in the lockstep phenomenon and associated autonomic changes.

has not been established that neocorticohypothalamic connections exist in man, the possibility has been raised that the dorsomedial nucleus of the thalamus, which connects with the prefrontal cortex, has projections to the hypothalamus (Breusch 1984), through which epileptogenic activity originating in the cortex could reach the hypothalamus and brain stem, resulting in discharge from the autonomic nervous system and phenomena such as blood pressure changes and cardiac arrhythmia. Electrical stimulation of the cerebral cortex in man and animals results in autonomic responses such as changes in blood pressure (Chapman et al. 1950; Hoff and Green 1936), changes in heart rate, and dilatation of the pupil (Hoff and Green 1936). Blood pressure changes have been evoked through stimulation of various regions of the cortex, including tips of temporal lobes (Chapman et al. 1950), motor cortex, premotor cortex, parietal cortex, and cingulate gyrus (Hoff and Green 1936). Furthermore, autonomic changes,

including alterations in blood pressure, have been associated with epileptogenic activity.

The precipitous blood pressure changes observed in our experiments were not consistent in terms of direction; there were a total of 46 increases and 48 decreases observed during the 60-minute periods monitored in each of the nine cats. Experiments involving electrical stimulation of the cortex have shown similar blood pressure changes in terms of direction. Wall and David (1951) and Delgado (1960) found both increases and decreases in blood pressure on stimulation of the cortex. Kaada et al. (1949) also elicited both increases and decreases in blood pressure with electrical stimulation of the cortex, as well as biphasic responses in which an increase in blood pressure was followed by a secondary decrease or a decrease in blood pressure was followed by a secondary increase. In our experiments, biphasic responses (defined for the purpose of this discussion as two precipitous blood pressure changes of opposite direction occurring within 10 seconds of each other) were seen nine times in four cats.

Hoff and Green (1936) demonstrated pressor and depressor points in the cortex, which are located 2–4 mm from each other. This observation may help to explain the inconsistency of the direction of precipitous blood pressure changes, the relationship of blood pressure changes to unstable LSP, and why the direction of blood pressure changes was not related to the direction of unstable LSP (increasing rate or decreasing rate). If, for example, predominantly pressor areas were being stimulated by epileptogenic activity and the frequency of the epileptogenic activity increased, the blood pressure might increase; if the frequency of the epileptogenic activity decreased, the blood pressure might decrease. If, however, predominantly depressor areas were stimulated by the epileptogenic activity, the blood pressure might decrease with increasing epileptogenic activity and increase with decreasing epileptogenic activity.

The question that remains is how the mean arterial blood pressure can decrease in the presence of an increased rate of postganglionic cardiac sympathetic discharge. In cats treated with ouabain, Lathers et al. (1977) demonstrated "nonuniformity" of postganglionic cardiac sympathetic discharge, i.e., some cardiac sympathetic branches showed increased activity, some showed decreased activity, and some branches showed no change in activity. This nonuniform discharge was associated with ouabain-induced arrhythmia (Lathers et al. 1977). Lathers and Schraeder (1982) found a similar nonuniform sympathetic discharge in cats treated with PTZ. If two or three branches of postganglionic cardiac sympathetic nerves exhibit this nonuniform discharge pattern, then the possibility exists that the discharge from the sympathetic nerves that innervate the blood vessels and control blood pressure may not be uniform. In this case, blood pressure could decrease, although discharge in some cardiac sympathetic branches was increased.

This discussion has concentrated mainly on epileptogenic activity originating in the cortex because one of the factors associated with SUD is the presence of structural lesions of the brain that are thought to cause seizures. In one study, autopsies of 60% of epileptic persons who died suddenly revealed structural lesions of the brain, including old contusions of the frontal and temporal lobes, brain tumors, cortical malformations, evidence of craniotomy, focal atrophy or hemiatrophy, Wernicke's encephalopathy, and cryptic vascular malformation (Leestma et al. 1984). In another study (Freytag and Ingraham 1964), 63% of cases of SUD associated with epilepsy were found to have structural brain lesions. However, epileptic persons without such lesions may also die suddenly; furthermore, autonomic symptoms occur in association with generalized epilepsy. It is thought that the thalamus and the midbrain reticular formation are involved in generalized epilepsy, perhaps as a site of origin for the seizure activity (Kiloh et al. 1980). The thalamus, being part of the Papez circuit and having connections to the cortex, is capable of transmitting epileptogenic activity to the hypothalamus, resulting in autonomic manifestations.

The reticular formation contains the multisynaptic pathways that connect the hypothalamus with the autonomic areas in the brain stem and spinal cord. Seizure activity occurring in the reticular formation could be transmitted to the autonomic areas of the brain stem and spinal cord by these pathways.

## SUMMARY

The results of this study show that autonomic changes, i.e., precipitous blood pressure changes, are associated with unstable LSP patterns. These findings indicate that the LSP (and its patterns) should be investigated further to determine its relationship to cardiac arrhythmias and epilepsy-related SUD. At least three mechanisms can be postulated through which LSP may be related to arrhythmia and SUD in persons with epilepsy. The first of these is excessive sympathetic stimulation of a heart that is already electrically unstable due to prior damage. It is the opinion of Jay and Leestma (1981) that this is the case; they describe pathological changes in the myocardium that several investigators have found in patients with epilepsy who died suddenly. The pathological changes are consistent with repeated high levels of catecholamines and resemble those produced in experimental animals by sympathetic stimulation. Jay and Leestma have suggested that this damage to the heart provides a locus where fatal arrhythmias can begin when the heart is again stimulated by sympathetic discharge. LSP may be the link between epileptogenic activity in the brain and sympathetic stimulation of the heart.

The second possible mechanism involves nonuniform discharge of postganglionic sympathetic nerve branches, which is associated with arrhythmias caused by administration of ouabain (Lathers et al. 1977). As mentioned earlier, Lathers and Schraeder (1982) found a similar nonuniform sympathetic discharge pattern in cats treated with PTZ. In the latter study, the nonuniform cardiac neural discharge was associated with epileptogenic activity and changes in the autonomic parameters of mean arterial blood pressure and cardiac rhythm. It was suggested that these changes may contribute to SUD.

The third mechanism is especially relevant to this study; precipitous blood pressure changes per se may be a factor in the development of arrhythmia in persons with epilepsy. In a study by Allen (1931), premature systolic arrhythmias followed increases in blood pressure induced by stimulation of the superior colliculus in rabbits. The arrhythmias were not observed when blood pressure was maintained at a constant level during stimulation of the superior colliculus; the conclusion was made that the arrhythmias could be attributed to the blood pressure changes. Evans and Gillis (1978) elicited blood pressure increases by stimulation of the hypothalamus and concluded that the arrhythmias that occurred after (not during) such stimulation were the result of a sudden surge of parasympathetic activity reflexly evoked by the increase in blood pressure.

A case reported by Kiok et al. (1986) describes a 23-year-old man who had sinus arrest lasting up to 9 seconds, as well as bradycardia of 40–50 bpm, during clinically observed seizures. The authors suggest that the parasympathetic nervous system may be involved in the production of some cases of arrhythmia in epileptic persons. Although the blood pressure remained stable during the seizures in this particular case, the autonomic manifestations suggest parasympathetic involvement. Interestingly, the patient described in the report was found by computed tomography to have right temporal lobe atrophy and had subtherapeutic blood levels of anticonvulsant drugs. According to Jay and Leestma (1981), structural abnormalities of the brain and subtherapeutic levels of anticonvulsants are two factors associated with epilepsy-related SUD.

The three mechanisms leading to arrhythmia and SUD that are outlined in this discussion are by no means mutually exclusive. It is quite possible that no single mechanism can explain all cases of SUD in epileptic persons. Perhaps some cases are caused by ventricular fibrillation related to a lower ventricular fibrillation threshold associated with increased cardiac sympathetic discharge, whereas other cases are caused by sinus arrest related to reflex parasympathetic discharge evoked by precipitous blood pressure changes (especially if there is some cardiac damage produced by prior sympathetic stimulation). The association of autonomic events with the LSP indicates that further investigation in this direction is warranted.

## ACKNOWLEDGMENTS

The authors gratefully acknowledge Dr. Adele Kaplan for statistical analyses and Carol Harwick, Darlene Spino, and Don Stauffer for typing the manuscript. Special thanks to Dr. Paul L. Schraeder for consultation. The research was funded by NIH grant BRSGRR-04518. A. Z. Stauffer received a 1986 Medical Student Research Fellowship from the Epilepsy Foundation of America.

## REFERENCES

Allen, WF. An experimentally produced premature systolic arrhythmia (pulsus bigeminus) in rabbits. *Am J Physiol* 1931;98:344–51.

Breusch SR. Anatomy of the human hypothalamus. In: Givens JR, ed. *The Hypothalamus*. Chicago, IL: Year Book Medical; 1984, p. 13.

Chapman WP, Livingston KE, Papper JL. Effect upon blood pressure of electrical stimulation of tips of temporal lobes in man. *J Neurophysiol* 1950;13:65–71.

Delgado JMR. Circulating effects of cortical stimulation. *Physiol Rev* 1960;40(54):146–71.

Evans DE, Gillis RA. Reflex mechanisms involved in cardiac arrhythmias induced by hypothalamic stimulation. *Am J Physiol* 1978;234(2):H199–209.

Freytag JR, Ingraham FD. 295 Medical autopsies in epileptics. *Arch Pathol* 1964;78:274–86.

Hoff EC, Green HG. Cardiovascular reactions induced by electrical stimulation of the cerebral cortex. *Am J Physiol* 1936;117:411–22.

Jay GW, Leestma JE. Sudden death in epilepsy. *Acta Neurol Scand* 1981;63 (Suppl 82):1–66.

Jun HW. Pharmacokinetic studies of pentylenetetrazol in dogs. *J Pharmacol Sci* 1976;65:1038–41.

Kaada BR, Pribram KH, Epstein JA. Respiratory and vascular responses in monkeys from temporal lobe pole, insula, orbital surface and cingulate gyrus. *J Neurophysiol* 1949;12:347–56.

Kiloh LG, McComas AJ, Osselton JW. *Clinical Electroencephalography*. London: Butterworths; 1980.

Kiok MC, Terrence CF, Fromm GH, Lavine S. Sinus arrest in epilepsy. *Neurology* 1986;36:115–6.

Korner PI. Central nervous control of autonomic cardiovascular function. In: Berne RM, Sperelaskis N, Geiger SR, eds. *Handbook of Physiology—The Cardiovascular System*, Vol. 1. Bethesda, MD: American Physiological Society; 1979, pp. 691–739.

Landau WM. Autonomic responses mediated via the corticospinal tract. *J Neurophysiol* 1953;16:299–311.

Lathers CM, Schraeder PL. Autonomic dysfunction in epilepsy: Characterization of autonomic cardiac neural discharge associated with pentylenetetrazol-induced epileptogenic activity. *Epilepsia* 1982;23:633–41.

Lathers CM, Roberts J, Kelliher GJ. Correlation of ouabain-induced arrhythmia and nonuniformity in the histamine-evoked discharge of cardiac sympathetic nerves. *J Pharmacol Exp Ther* 1977;203:461–19.

Lathers CM, Schraeder PL, Weiner FL. Synchronization of cardiac autonomic neural discharge with epileptogenic activity: The lockstep phenomenon. *Electroencephalogr Clin Neurophysiol* 1987;67:247–59.

Leestma JE, Kalelkar MB, Teas SS, Jay GW, Hughes JR. Sudden unexpected death associated with seizures: Analysis of 66 cases. *Epilepsia* 1984;25(1):84–8.

Natelson BH. Neurocardiology: An interdisciplinary area for the 80's. *Arch Neurol* 1985;42:178–84.

Papez JW. A proposed mechanism of emotion. *Arch Neurol Psychiatr* 1937;38:725–43.

Saper CB, Loewy AD, Swanson LW, Cowan WM. Direct hypothalamoautonomic connections. *Brain Res* 1976;117:305–12.

Schraeder PL, Lathers CM. Cardiac neural discharge and epileptogenic activity in the cat: An animal model for unexplained death. *Life Sci* 1983;32:1371–82.

Wall PD, David GD. Three cerebral cortical systems affecting autonomic function. *J Neurophysiol* 1951;14:507–17.

Willis WL, Grossman RG. *Medical Neurobiology*. St. Louis, MO: C. V. Mosby; 1981, p. 405.

Winer BJ. *Statistical Principles in Experimental Design*, 2nd ed. New York, NY: McGraw-Hill; 1971, p. 399.

# 21 Interspike Interval Histogram Characterization of Synchronized Cardiac Sympathetic Neural Discharge and Epileptogenic Activity in the Electrocorticogram of the Cat

*Daniel K. O'Rourke and Claire M. Lathers*

## CONTENTS

## INTRODUCTION

This is one of a series of articles (Lathers et al. 1987; Chapters 19 and 20, this book) attempting to characterize one potential mechanism in an animal model that may, in part, explain unexpected death in an epileptic patient. Because many of the mechanisms of death at the time of clinically observable seizures are known, our emphasis has been on determining one potential factor that may be a contributory mechanism behind unexplained interictal death.

Our model has used the anesthetized cat infused intravenously with pentylenetetrazol (PTZ). This chemical is known to produce seizures (Hahn 1960; Lathers et al. 1984). It is important to note that most epileptic patients who die unexpectedly are found on autopsy to have cortical lesions, which probably served as seizure foci during life (Leestma et al. 1984).

The lockstep phenomenon (LSP) theory may help explain sudden unexpected death in this population. It is defined by the occurrence of a one-to-one synchronization of the electrocorticogram (ECoG) discharge patterns with the discharge patterns of the peripheral autonomic nerves innervating the heart. An example of LSP is shown in Figure 21.1. We theorize that the LSP occurs when the oscillatory driver of the interictal cortical focus becomes linked to the oscillatory driver of the autonomic cardiac nerves. The actual cause of death is hypothesized to be dependent on the function of the neural discharge, which would then be driven at the rate of the interictal focus. Because these are autonomic nerves innervating the heart, the finely tuned electrical depolarization system of the heart could be disturbed. This autonomic dysfunction may directly produce cardiac arrhythmias. These and other theories are discussed and analyzed in terms of the science of chaos. Chaos is a concept in physics that is applicable in modeling these observed natural phenomena and aids in the interpretation of our data. Chaos identifies pattern and regularity in seemingly disorganized events (Winfree 1987). The science is most useful in predicting the activity of nonlinear, noncyclical functions, such as the plot of intervals between depolarizations in an electroencephalogram (EEG) showing LSP or in the plot of ventricular depolarizations in atrial fibrillation monitored by an electrocardiogram (ECG). The principles of chaos help to substantiate the association of LSP and sudden unexpected death in epilepsy (SUDEP).

Our goal in this series of papers is to demonstrate that LSP occurs and then to characterize LSP and its effects. This study demonstrated that, with the use of the interspike interval (ISI) technique, the discharges noted in the ECoG are correlated in several important ways with the simultaneous discharges occurring in two postganglionic sympathetic nerves monitored in the same cat.

## METHODS

The animal preparation used in this experiment has been described previously (Carnel et al. 1985; Lathers et al. 1977, 1984; and Chapter 19 of this book). Briefly, nine cats were intravenously anesthetized with 80 mg/kg $\alpha$-chloralose.

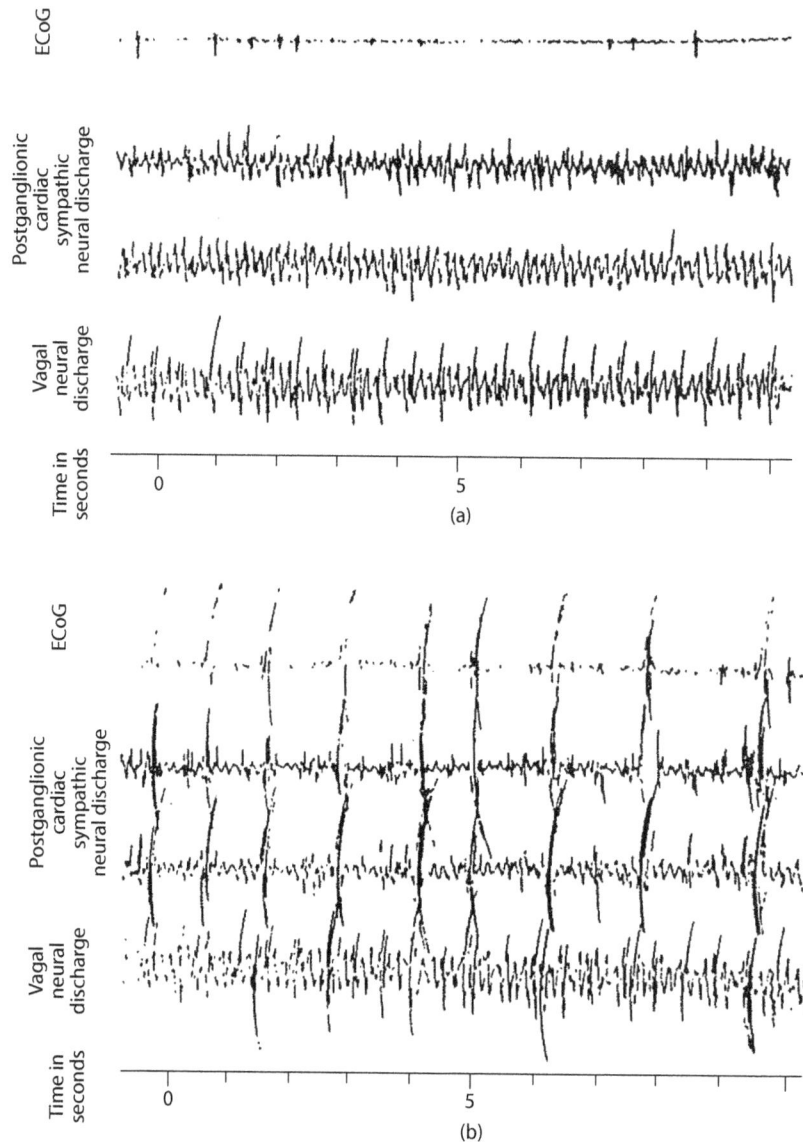

**FIGURE 21.1**   Electrocorticogram (ECoG) and two postganglionic cardiac sympathetic neural discharge patterns monitored simultaneously. (a) Pattern of neural discharges recorded during the control period, that is, the period just before the first dose of pentylenetetrazol administration. (b) Example of the lockstep phenomenon (LSP). ECoG neural burst discharge patterns are seen to be correlated one to one with those of both postganglionic cardiac sympathetic neural discharge patterns.

Gallamine 4 mg/kg (intravenous) was used to maintain paralysis. Leads were placed to monitor several postganglionic sympathetic nerves, the vagus nerve, the ECoG, and the ECG. A 20-mg/kg intravenous dose of phenobarbital administered over 10 minutes was followed by a 60-minute period of stabilization before the experiment was begun. PTZ was administered intravenously at 10, 20, 50, 100, 200, and 2000 mg/kg with a 10-minute interval between each dose. Differential amplitude discriminators were used to produce a better signal-to-noise ratio. The output from the differential amplitude discriminators was stored on magnetic tape and printed on a polygraph.

The data on the magnetic tapes were played back and fed into a Nuclear Chicago model 7100 Data Retrieval computer,

which analyzed the discharge patterns for the time between each depolarization (ISI). The tape was played from the time PTZ was first administered until the next dose was given. The summed ISIs were plotted as a histogram. An oscilloscope was used to monitor the patterns being displayed and to adjust the discriminator of the computer. A variable-pulse generator was used to standardize the discriminator and later to provide a standard peak on the ISI histogram. This was used to extrapolate the number of intervals in the unknown peaks by comparing the areas beneath the ISI histogram curve.

The ISI histograms were characterized by recording the number of peaks, height, mode, and least and greatest intervals. The area of the peak was approximated by assuming a triangle formed by the highest point (the mode) and the two baseline extremes. The area was then used to calculate the number of occurrences of that interval in seconds under the curve by comparing its number to the area of a known curve. Graphs of these data are illustrated in Figure 21.2. A one-way analysis of variance (ANOVA) was used for the calculation of modes of the intervals.

One cat was excluded from the computation of the statistical analysis because the ISIs showed no useful information. The signal-to-noise ratio was small enough that the discriminator on the computer could not be set to discern the interictal spikes from that of the background information. This appears to have been due to equipment failure of one of the second-stage amplifiers. All statistics were computed excluding this cat.

## RESULTS

Three characteristic time intervals seen on the ISI histograms are summarized in Table 21.1. Their average modes were approximately the same and their lengths were constant with

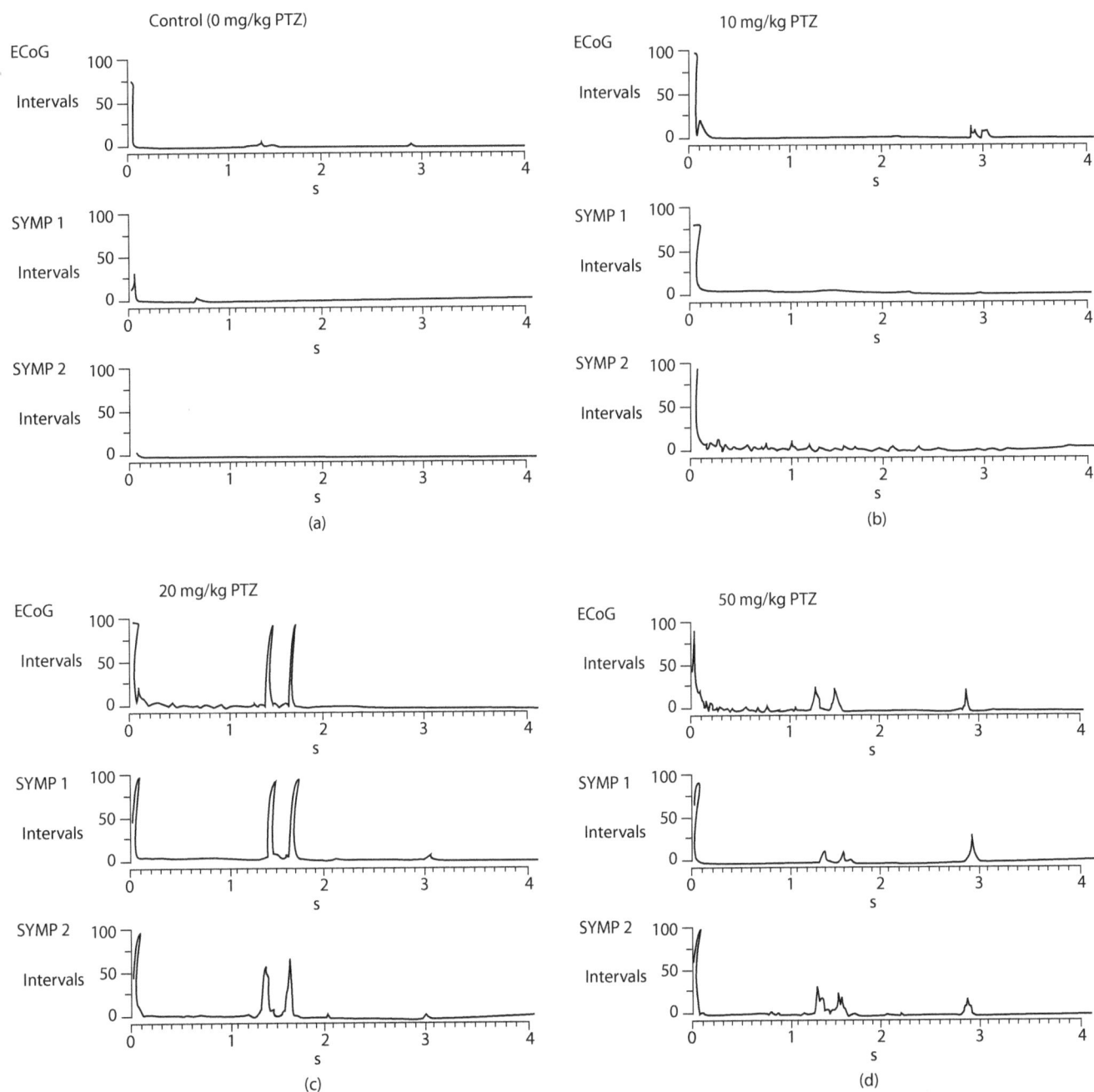

**FIGURE 21.2** (a–d) Ten-minute ISI histograms of electrocorticogram and two postganglionic sympathetics (SYMP) from representative cats.

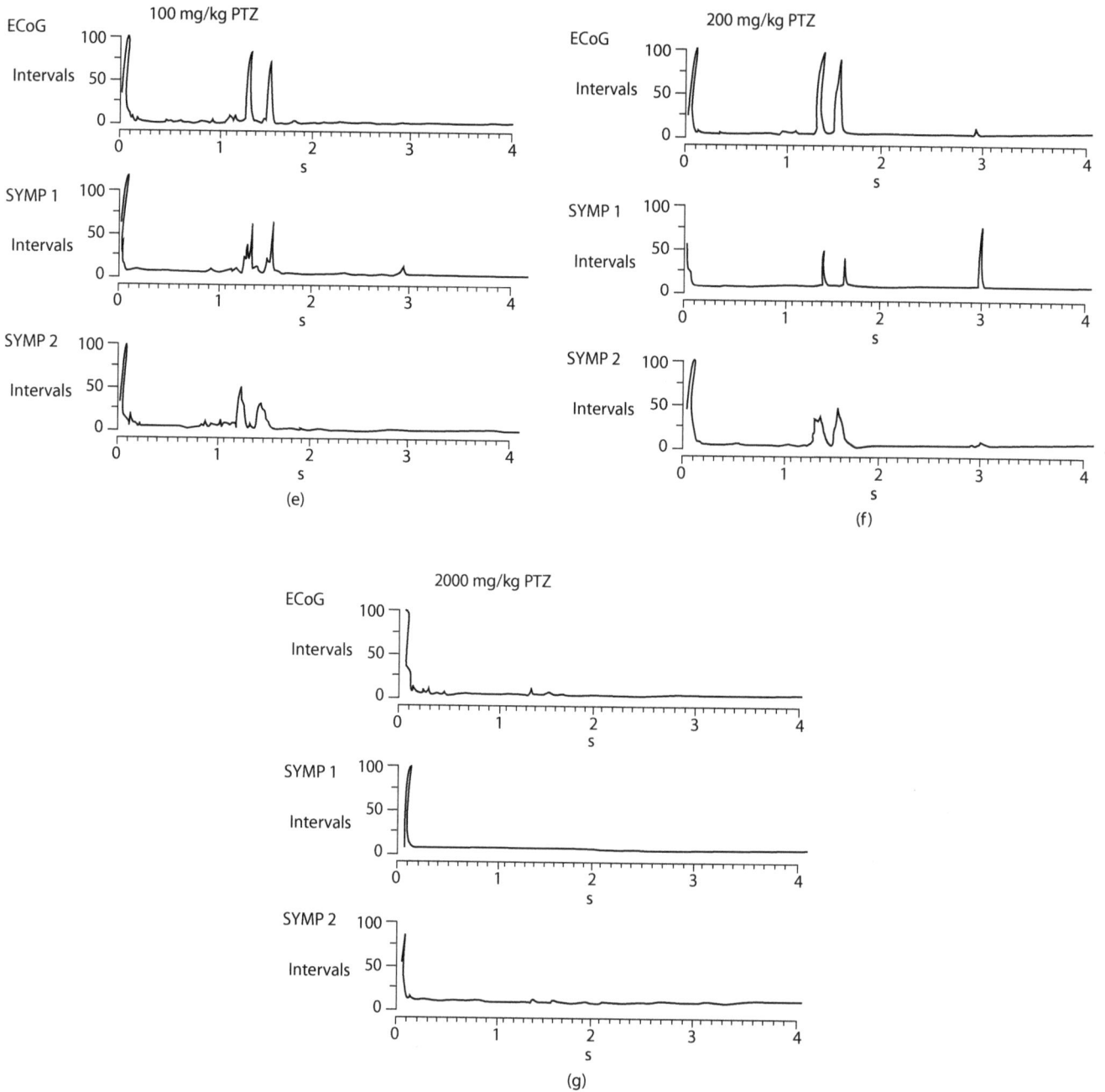

**FIGURE 21.2 (Continued)** (e–g) Ten-minute ISI histograms of electrocorticogram and two postganglionic sympathetics (SYMP) from representative cats.

**TABLE 21.1**

**Time Intervals for ECoG and Two Postganglionic Sympathetic Cardiac Neural Discharge Patterns**

| Peak | ECoG | Symp 1 | Symp 2 |
|------|------|--------|--------|
| 1 | 1.38 | 1.38 | 1.38 |
| 2 | 1.54 | 1.64 | 1.58 |
| 3 | 2.82 | 2.85 | 2.98 |
| *F* value for one-way ANOVA with two degrees of freedom | | | |
| | 1399[a] | 1755[a] | 177[a] |

[a] $p < .01$.

respect to the PTZ dose administered (see Figures 21.3 through 21.5).

The neural and ECoG discharge data produced in each experiment are shown in Figure 21.1. We analyzed these data using the techniques discussed earlier and produced the ISIs shown in Figure 21.2a through g. Note that as the dose of PTZ is increased, two characteristic peaks are seen. A third peak can be seen to occur at an interval of about 3 seconds. These peaks, which represent sums of intervals, were found to be statistically different with $p < .01$. In the control (Figure 21.2a) and at the lethal dose of 2000 mg/kg PTZ, no histogram peaks are seen because at these points the LSP does not occur. A peak at less than 0.1 second occurs on each of the histograms. This reflects the ictal activity that occurs

immediately after a dose of PTZ is given and represents the ISI histogram in ictus. The data from one cat are shown here for illustration, but eight cats were used in the computations and statistical analysis.

Figures 21.6 through 21.8 should be reviewed together. They were constructed by adding the total number of intervals that occurred at any of the three characteristic time intervals and plotting this against the dose of PTZ. These graphs show a rapid incline and then a plateau. In physiological terms, the LSP occurred at fairly characteristic time intervals, producing a similar number of intervals, independent of the dose of PTZ once the threshold dose was given. This is similar for the ECoG and for the two representative postganglionic sympathetic nerves.

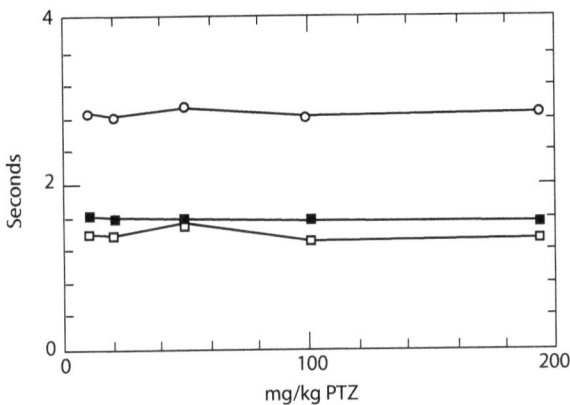

FIGURE 21.3 Mode of the interspike interval histogram in seconds for the three peaks seen on the ECoG versus pentylenetetrazol (PTZ) dose (eight cats included). This plot demonstrates the consistency of the interval length in seconds of the LSP. Average modes are 1.38 seconds (open square), 1.54 seconds (closed circle), and 2.82 seconds (open circle).

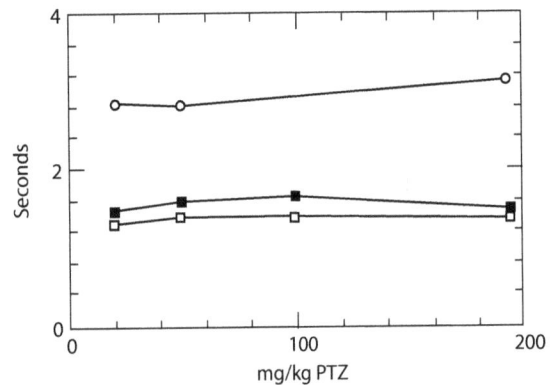

FIGURE 21.5 Mode of the interspike interval histogram in seconds for the three peaks seen on one postganglionic sympathetic nerve discharge pattern (#2) versus pentylenetetrazol (PTZ) dose (eight cats included). Average modes are 1.38 seconds (open square), 1.58 seconds (closed square), and 2.98 seconds (open circle) (compare with Figures 21.3 and 21.4).

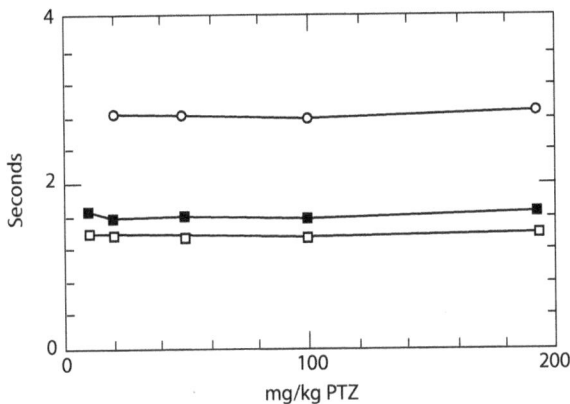

FIGURE 21.4 Mode of the interspike interval histogram in seconds for the three peaks seen on one postganglionic sympathetic nerve discharge pattern (#1) versus pentylenetetrazol (PTZ) dose (eight cats included). The average mode is very constant over all doses of PTZ. While the number of intervals changes with increasing PTZ dose, the length of the interval, as demonstrated here, does not change. Average modes are 1.38 seconds (open square), 1.64 seconds (closed circle), and 2.85 seconds (open circle).

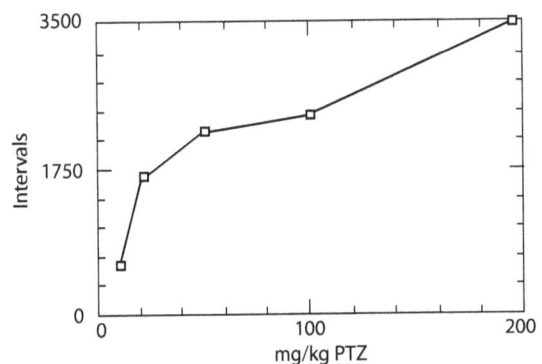

FIGURE 21.6 Summed interspike intervals (ISIs) for the electrocorticogram (ECoG) versus pentylenetetrazol (PTZ) dose (eight cats included). The total numbers of time intervals that produced the three characteristic peaks of the ECoG ISI were summed and plotted against the dose of PTZ administered. The number of intervals increases rapidly with increasing dose of PTZ until 50 mg/kg of PTZ is reached. There is a plateau period between 50 and 100 mg/kg of PTZ. The increase in the total number of intervals between 100 and 200 mg/kg of PTZ occurs only in the ECoG and represents no increase in the time spent in the LSP. Compare with Figures 21.7 and 21.8.

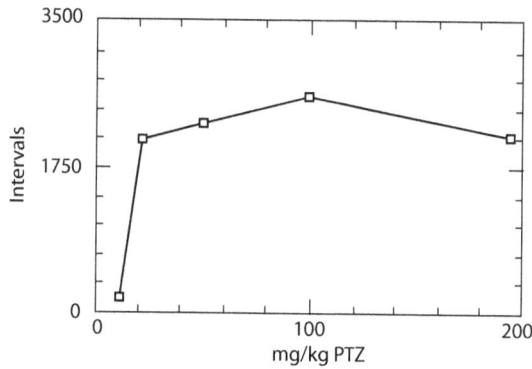

**FIGURE 21.7**  Summed interspike intervals for a postganglionic sympathetic nerve (#1) versus pentylenetetrazol (PTZ) dose (eight cats included). There is a sharp rise at low doses of PTZ and a plateau of PTZ doses greater than 50 mg/kg, which is probably the natural occurrence of this phenomenon.

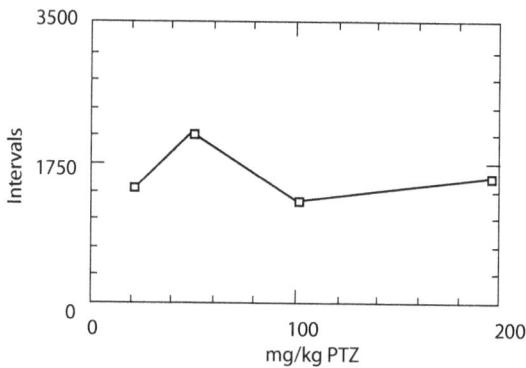

**FIGURE 21.8**  Summed interspike intervals for a postganglionic sympathetic nerve (#2) versus pentylenetetrazol (PTZ) dose (eight cats included). There is a sharp rise until 50 mg/kg of PTZ and then a dip to lower numbers of intervals with increasing doses of PTZ. Although the number of intervals is less than in Figures 21.6 and 21.7, the shape of the curve approximates that of the other postganglionic sympathetic cardiac nerve.

The number of intervals seen in each peak rose quickly with increasing PTZ dose and then reached a plateau. The implication is that the number of time intervals that constituted the three characteristic peaks of the ISI histogram rose until a certain plasma concentration was reached. Increasing the plasma concentration beyond this level did not increase the number of intervals at the three characteristic time intervals. The ECoG showed an increase in the number of intervals from 100 to 200 mg/kg PTZ. This was not associated with a concomitant rise in the number of intervals seen in either of the sympathetic nerves. There was, therefore, no further contribution to LSP for the increased number of intervals in this range.

Figures 21.9 through 21.11 are similar to Figures 21.6 through 21.8 except that the individual histograms from each ISI plot are shown separately, summed over eight cats. This plot was used to demonstrate that each of the individual peaks follows the general trend of rising sharply to 50 mg/kg and then leveling to a plateau. In other words, when the LSP

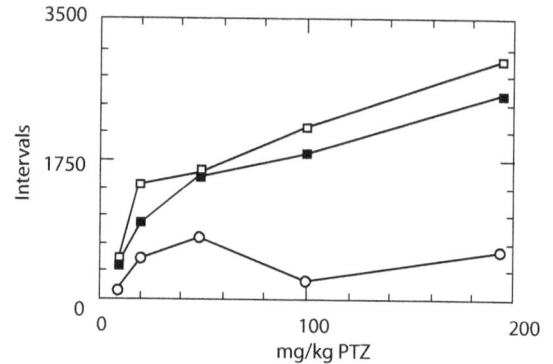

**FIGURE 21.9**  Summed interspike intervals (ISIs) for the three peaks seen on the electrocorticogram (ECoG) versus pentylenetetrazol (PTZ) dose (eight cats included). ECoG ISI number increases for each peak after the PTZ dose of 100 mg/kg PTZ. This trend is not repeated by the sympathetic nerves monitored. This increase represents intervals that do not appear to contribute to the LSP. Average modes are 1.38 seconds (open square), 1.54 seconds (closed square), and 2.82 seconds (open circle).

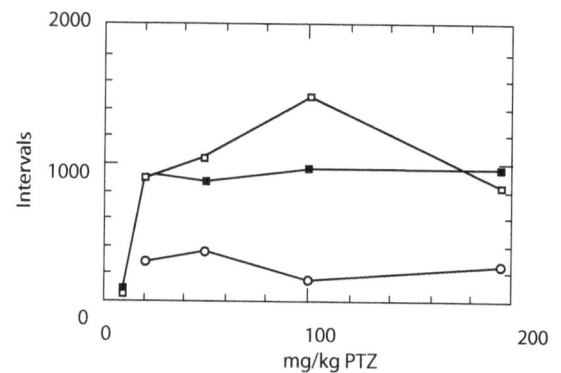

**FIGURE 21.10**  Summed interspike intervals (ISIs) for the three peaks seen from one postganglionic sympathetic nerve (#1) versus pentylenetetrazol (PTZ) dose (eight cats included). The plot with the 1.64-second average mode (closed square) curve represents what we surmise to be typical of the LSP, that is, there is a rapid increase in the number of intervals representing LSP beginning. A plateau thereafter signifies the maintenance of LSP. The other average modes are 1.38 seconds (open square) and 2.85 seconds (open circle).

occurred the number of intervals produced at each dose of PTZ remained fairly constant regardless of the dose of PTZ. Furthermore, it occurred at one of three characteristic time intervals. The LSP occurred at one of the two shorter time intervals more commonly than it did at the longer interval.

Figures 21.3 through 21.5 are plots of modes of time intervals in seconds versus the dose of PTZ administered. Note that the length of the time interval in seconds is very nearly constant. A series of straight, nonintersecting, and horizontal lines in this graph indicate that the modes of the ISI peaks are completely independent of PTZ dose. Note that the time interval with a mode at 3 seconds did not occur in every cat and at some doses of PTZ it did not occur at all, thus producing few data points.

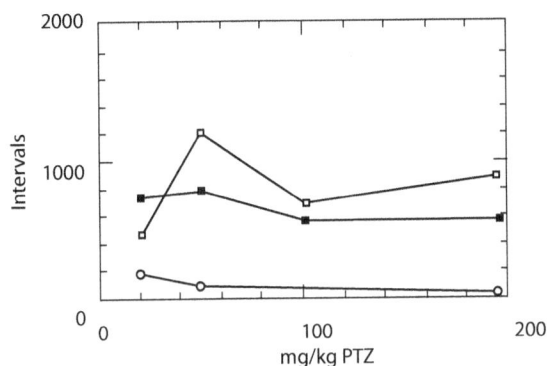

**FIGURE 21.11** Summed interspike intervals (ISIs) for the three peaks seen from one postganglionic sympathetic nerve (#2) versus pentylenetetrazol (PTZ) dose (eight cats included). Number of intervals increases with increasing PTZ dose until a critical value of PTZ is reached. The plots then begin to plateau. Average modes are 1.38 seconds (open square), 1.58 seconds (closed square), and 2.98 seconds (open circle). Compare this graph with Figures 21.9 and 21.10.

## DISCUSSION

Figure 21.12a is a representation of the anatomical location of the three oscillatory drivers of concern in LSP and cardiac arrhythmias: the cortex, cardiac medullary center, and sinoatrial (SA) node of the heart. In our experiment, the cardiac accelerator nerve was recorded to assess the partial output from the cardiac center in the medulla. The pathways involved in the brain between the cortex and the medullary centers were described by Stauffer et al. (Chapter 20, this book).

Figure 21.12b depicts schematically the normal association of the oscillatory drivers in the brain: the interictal activity in the cortex, cardiac medullary center in the medulla, and SA node of the heart. Note that springs have been used to represent the interaction between the centers. The centers influence each other, but the depolarizations are not synchronized one to one. In Figure 21.12c, a solid bar is used to depict the association between the interictal focus and the cardiac medullary center during LSP because there is a one-to-one association between the depolarizations of these two centers. In other words, the interictal discharge is driving the cardiac medullary center. A spring still depicts the connection between the medullary centers and the heart because the association is never one to one. When the first two drivers in the brain move in synchrony, their effect is translated to the SA node to produce a change in depolarization of the heart. A change in rate, rhythm, or aberration results.

The ISI histograms in this study show the dichotomy of LSP, that is, it is either on or off. The discharge pattern characteristic of LSP once present was not altered appreciably by increasing the dose of PTZ until the lethal dose was given. This is demonstrated in Figures 21.3 through 21.5. The intervals were shown to be distinct from one another by a one-way ANOVA with $p < .01$.

We suggest that the operative mechanism in the LSP may be that the cortex fires constantly, during both ictal and interictal

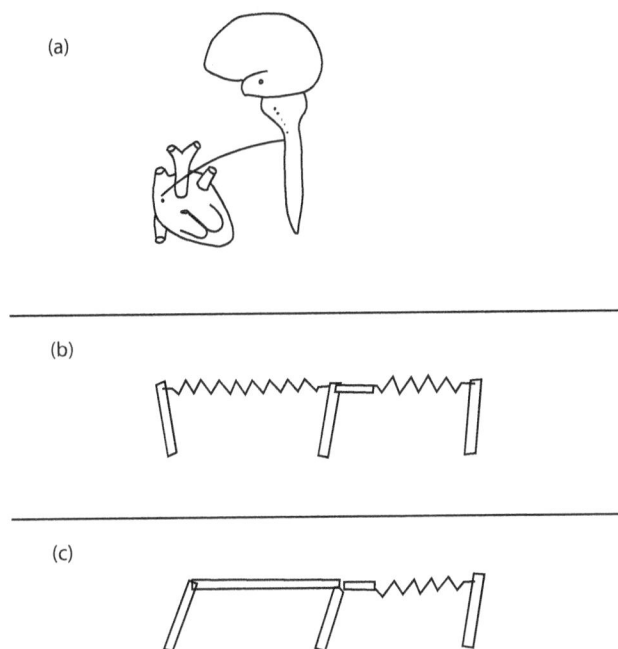

**FIGURE 21.12** A model for the interaction of the brain and heart in the LSP. (a) Brain-heart interaction resulting in LSP. (b) Springs represent interactions among interictal activity in the cortex, cardiac medullary center in the medulla and SA node of the heart. (c) Solid bar depicts the association between the interictalfocus and the cardiac medullary center during LSP. The spring depicts the connection between the medullary centers and the heart.

periods. In the ictal period, the interictal depolarizations overwhelm the nearby cells and thus the seizure discharges spread, becoming clinically noticeable. In the interictal period, the cells may continue to depolarize. If these cells fire with an electrical potential strong enough and at the proper frequency to overtake another group of cells, then the rate of depolarization of the latter group of cells will be driven to seizure activity that will serve as the pacemaker for the second group of cells. In this experiment, the second group of cells was the nucleus of the sympathetic nerves located in the cardiac centers of the medulla. These nerves innervate the heart and exhibit both chronotropic and inotropic effects; excessive stimulation will cause cardiac arrhythmias (Randall et al. 1978).

The spread of seizure activity to variable sites involves more than simply the intensity of the interictal discharge. Proximity to specialized tracts may also be of concern. During the ictal period, the intensity of the depolarization originating at the focus is strong enough to spread to areas of the brain that elicit clinically noticeable phenomena. In a generalized seizure, the spread is so extensive that the reticular activating system is involved and the patient loses consciousness. The former dichotomy proposed for the seizure focus—that is, it is intense enough either to cause a full-blown seizure or to be completely inoperative—seems incorrect. Interictal activity enables it to capture areas of the brain in close proximity by direct continuity and in distant areas by involvement of tracts that efficiently carry the impulses over long distances. The clinical expression of these dynamics is a link between the oscillatory drivers of the focus and those of, for instance, the medullary cardiac centers. Figure 21.12 diagrammatically shows our concept of the interaction among the cortex focus, medullary cardiac center, and heart. The SA node is a pacemaker that is influenced by the discharge of the parasympathetic and sympathetic autonomic nerves that innervate it; this neural connection between the medullary centers and the heart is represented by a spring. These centers have the ability to influence the activity of the SA node but not to directly drive it, just as a spring potentiates movement but does not directly drive it (Guyton 1981). In the normal state, the rate of firing of the SA node, and thus the rate of the heart, and the depolarizations of the nerves reaching the heart will not be correlated one to one because the heart has its own automatic pacemaker. However, it appears that with the development of interictal and ictal discharge and the occurrence of LSP cardiac arrhythmias may occur in an unpredictable manner. These arrhythmias may contribute to sudden death.

Many systems in nature are linked in a similar fashion to the proposed LSP link. The phenomenon is called entrainment or mode locking by physicists. Gleick (1987) used the example of the relationship of the Moon to the Earth to demonstrate this point. In the orbit of the Moon around the Earth, one lunar surface is always presented to the Earth. This is because the orbit of the Moon is locked to the rotation of the Earth. The rotation of the Earth and the orbit of the Moon are locked just as the oscillators of the epileptic focus and the medullary cardiac centers are locked one to one during the state of what we call the LSP, or what physicists call mode locking.

The occurrence of a very regular oscillator in the brain is theoretically dangerous, regardless of its mechanism of known effect. The science called chaos, which has arisen in the past few decades, is of great use in explaining the phenomenon of linked drivers. Ary Goldberger, a prominent physiologist and chaostician, has written: "Fractal processes associated with scaled, broad-band spectra are 'information-rich.' Periodic states, in contrast, reflect narrow-band spectra and are defined by monotonous repetitive sequences, depleted of information content" (Goldberger et al. 1985). The fractal processes of which he speaks, ubiquitous in biological systems including the brain, are those systems that convey different information, depending on how closely you look at them. A commonly used example is that of the *Mona Lisa*. At a great distance, the outside borders of its frame form a rectangle, and this is all that is conveyed to the observer. At an intermediate distance, the beauty of the woman may be appreciated. At a closer distance, the mastery of the artist can be known in terms of each brush stroke. Each of the observations is unique, but together they form the treasured masterpiece. The electrical depolarizations of the brain are an example of such a fractal process. The complexity of a fractal process may at times depreciate into a simple periodic process representing decay of the system and a dramatic change. The key message conveyed by the application of the science of chaos is that simple systems, such as

periodic ones, are easily perturbed and less able to return to the preperturbed state. Therefore, seeing a periodic rhythm in the brain, where there is normally rich complexity, implies a susceptibility to failure of the system, that is, death.

The ultimate cause of sudden unexpected death in this population is thought to be cardiac because at autopsy no obvious cause of death can be found. The only two possible causes are failure of one of the two major electrical systems of the body, the brain and the heart. If the brain fails to send out the impulses from respiratory centers, then respiratory failure will be the immediate cause of death. If the brain sends a message to the heart that causes it to enter a fatal arrhythmia, or if the heart enters an arrhythmia on its own, then once again sudden death will occur. It is probable that other associated factors play a role in the disturbance of the normal healthy state, such as a fixed lesion in the heart, which alone would not explain death and/or autonomic dysfunction, as has been published by several laboratories including ours (Stauffer et al., Chapter 20, this book; Van Buren 1958). Central respiratory failure and arrhythmia are the only obvious etiologies that would leave no signs at autopsy (Jay and Leestma 1981). Arrhythmia is much more likely, given the findings of this experiment. The perturbation of the electrical depolarization of the heart may have several mechanisms, any or several of which may be operational. Further investigation is necessary to sort out the causes. The difficulty in doing a study of this, however, may mandate empirical treatment. We must first have plausible mechanisms from which models can be built.

The specific mechanism of death in this population may be more complex than the sympathetic discharge rate, although even this theory has merit. An area of damage to the electrical stimulation system of the heart, that is, the His-Purkinje system, may be caused by continual stimulation of the β-receptors by the sympathetic nerves innervating these receptors; this stimulation might produce a fixed microscopic lesion, which alone would be harmless but sufficient to cause this portion of the myocardium to be less flexible in its response to other insults, for example, excessive sympathetic discharge. A second possibility concerns the arrangement of the receptors in the ventricle. β-Receptors in the ventricles are arranged in a pattern such that their highest density is in the apex with a gradually decreasing density near the base (Lathers et al. 1986). Downregulation of the β-receptors from continual sympathetic discharge might disturb this gradation, producing a potentially arrhythmic situation. A pattern of increased sympathetic depolarization could be the fatal step in a two-stage process.

A third possibility is that of a forbidden sequence of sympathetic depolarizations, that is, a pattern of depolarizations from the sympathetics, which can interrupt the regular electrical depolarization. Winfree (1987) has begun to characterize these processes in terms of chaos modeling of the heart. More work needs to be performed to identify which of these theories or combination of theories is active in the epileptic patient who dies of sudden unexpected death. Mathematical models like those developed for the heart by Jose Jalife and colleagues (Salata and Jalife 1985) will facilitate our understanding and provide a basis for continued investigation.

Our model for the demonstration of the interictal activity of LSP is, of course, only an approximation of the human with epilepsy. There are, however, the following important similarities. The focal lesions that have been demonstrated in the brains of patients who have died to interictal unexplained death have shown cortical lesions in as many as 60% of those patients autopsied (Leestma et al. 1984). Moreover, the cat has a more highly developed cortex than many other animals proposed for such models, for example, the rat, which makes the cat model more likely to represent human epilepsy. The inadequacies of any animal model clearly demonstrate why future research must be coupled with mathematical modeling to maintain good correlation and to add direction for future study.

The possibility exists that our model produces LSP in a way that does not simulate the natural phenomenon. First, epilepsy in our model was caused by the intravenous administration of a chemical, PTZ, which has access to parts of the brain in proportion to their perfusion with blood. Although many areas of the cortex are exposed to the drug, probably one area eventually becomes the pacemaker of interictal discharge activity.

The study used pretreatment with phenobarbital to dampen the epileptogenic activity of PTZ to allow a greater amount of time spent in interictal activity, that is, to prevent status epilepticus. This allowed us to maximize the time spent in the interictal period. Recall that our objective was to study the possible mechanism of interictal death, not ictal death. In a previous study (Lathers et al. 1987) that did not use phenobarbital, we showed that phenobarbital is not directly involved in the production of LSP.

The ISI technique is a novel way of analyzing LSP. It is a rapid method of analyzing the complex discharge patterns generated by a nerve and the brain. When computing an ISI, much information is lost; only an instantaneous picture is produced. It is rather like taking the first derivative of a function: the information obtained is valuable, but it is now only a useful trend of the original, more complex function. Therefore, the ISI will never serve as the sole measure of LSP but rather as a very useful indirect measure of the occurrence of LSP.

The computation of mean ISI and the calculation of the area from the ISI peaks were accomplished by approximating the patterns with a triangle. Several errors can be introduced in this operation. First, the area will almost always be underestimated; thus, it is more difficult to show statistical significance, making any results all the more valid. Second, the standard that was used to calculate the area-to-interval number was based on the area noted in the standard peak histograms, which were added to each ISI histogram. Because this area would also probably be underestimated, the calculated number of intervals would be greater than the actual number of intervals that created the histogram. We consider the actual difference to be negligible.

Sudden unexplained death in the epileptic patient may prove to have many causes, but it seems important to understand the possible mechanisms that have been discussed here and to contemplate their treatment. It seems practical to think that the administration of a pharmacological agent to an identified population at risk might be an effective means of prevention. To go about proving this, we must first have a valid animal model. Second, we must be able to quantitate very closely the degree of LSP occurring, enabling the comparison of various pharmacological agents in the prevention of LSP. The technique of using ISIs to examine the characteristic intervals is a rapid-assessment technique that could be used to analyze the effect of a pharmacological agent. Several authors have used the ISI to characterize discharge patterns, for example, the action of ouabain on autonomic nerves (Lathers et al. 1977).

The future application of this technique is intriguing. An ambulatory EEG monitor coupled with an ambulatory ECG monitor could be used to record the electrical events for 24 hours. Given that the characteristic intervals for LSP are identified, a statistical analysis of the EEG using the ISI technique could rapidly identify these characteristic intervals and pinpoint the precise time at which they occurred. Next, the ECG could be analyzed for aberrations. A statistical correlation would be sought for those times found to be suspect in the EEG with the aberrations noted in the ECG. This would eliminate the need for direct recording of the postganglionic cardiac stimulator nerve, as has been done in this experiment, because it is quite impractical in humans.

## SUMMARY

The association between epileptogenic activity in ECoG and aberrations in cardiac activity was investigated by further characterizing the LSP. The pattern of neuronal discharges from several postganglionic cardiac sympathetic branches with simultaneous recordings of the ECoG and the ECG monitored in nine anesthetized cats in which epileptogenic activity was induced with PTZ was analyzed based on time intervals between action potentials in the ECoG. A similar analysis was made of the time intervals between action potentials in the nerves innervating the heart.

Time intervals for both ECoG and cardiac sympathetic discharge were summed and plotted as ISI histograms using a data retrieval computer. The ISIs obtained for the ECoG and the cardiac accelerator nerve tracings were compared. Analysis and comparison of these ISIs demonstrated the occurrence of LSP. The intervals found to be most characteristic of the LSP when monitoring the ECoG were 1.38, 1.58, and 2.85 seconds. These intervals were found to be statistically different with $p < .01$.

The implications of our findings were discussed in terms of the science of chaos. The data suggest that the discharge patterns from the ECoG and the sympathetic nerves are synchronized. This aberrant discharge pattern may be associated with changes in the ECG, which may ultimately contribute to understanding the mechanism of sudden unexpected death in persons with epilepsy.

## REFERENCES

Carnel SB, Schraeder PL, Lathers CM. Effect of phenobarbital pretreatment on cardiac neural discharge and pentylenetetrazol-induced epileptic activity in the cat. *Pharmacology* 1985;30: 225–40.

Gleick J. *Chaos: Making a New Science.* New York, NY: Viking; 1987.

Goldberger AL, Bhargava V, West BJ. Nonlinear dynamics of the heart beat. *Physica* 1985;17D:207–14.

Guyton AC. Rhythmic excitation of the heart. In: Guyton AC, ed. *Textbook of Medical Physiology,* Philadelphia, PA: Saunders; 1981, pp. 165–175.

Hahn F. Analeptics. *Pharmacol Rev* 1960;12:447–530.

Jay G.W, Leestma JE. 1981. Sudden death in epilepsy. *Acta Neurol Scand* 1981;63(Suppl 82):1–66.

Lathers CM, Levin RM, Spivey WH. Regional distribution of myocardial receptors. *Eur J Pharmacol* 1986;130:111–7.

Lathers CM, Roberts J, Kelliher GJ. 1977. Correlation of ouabain-induced arrhythmia and nonuniformity in the histamine-evoked discharge of cardiac sympathetic nerves. *J Pharmacol Exp Ther* 1977;203:467–79.

Lathers CM, Schraeder PL, Carnel SB. Neural mechanisms in cardiac arrhythmias associated with epileptogenic activity: The effect of phenobarbital. *Life Sci* 1984;34:1919–36.

Lathers CM, Schraeder PL, Weiner FL. Synchronization of cardiac autonomic neural discharge with epileptogenic activity: The lockstep phenomenon. *Electroencephalogr Clin Neurophysiol* 1987;67: 247–59.

Leestma JE, Kalelkar MB, Teas SS, Jay GW, Hughes JR. 1984. Sudden unexpected death associated with seizures: Analysis of 66 cases. *Epilepsia* 25: 84–88.

Randall WC, Thomas JX, Euler DE, Rosanski GL. Cardiac dysrhythmias associated with autonomic nervous system imbalance in the conscious dog. In: Shwartz PJ, Brown AM, Malliani A, Zanchetti A, eds. *Perspectives in Cardiovascular Research vol. 2, Neural Mechanisms in Cardiac Arrhythmias.* New York, NY: Raven Press; 1978, 123–38.

Salata JJ, Jalife J. "Fade" of hyperpolarizing response to vagal stimulation at the sinoatrial and atrioventricular nodes of the rabbit heart. *Circ Res* 1985;56(5):718–27.

Van Buren JM. 1958. Some autonomic concomitants of ictal automatism. *Brain* 81: 505–28.

Winfree AT. 1987. *When Time Breaks Down: The Three-Dimensional Dynamics of Electrochemical Waves and Cardiac Arrhythmias.* Princeton, NJ: Princeton University Press.

# Section III

SUDEP Risk Mechanisms
Animal Models and Clinical Studies

# 22 Abnormal Brain Activity Triggers Long-Term Potentiation in Sympathetic Ganglia
## Implication for Sudden Death

*Karim Alkadhi and Karem Alzoubi*

## CONTENTS

Neural plasticity in the form of long-term potentiation (LTP) of synaptic transmission is known to occur in a variety of synapses including those of autonomic ganglia (Scott and Bennett 1993; Alkadhi et al. 1996). LTP of sympathetic ganglia (gLTP) is expressed in vitro following a brief period of high-frequency preganglionic nerve stimulation. Ganglionic LTP can also be produced in vivo by chronic psychosocial stress, which provides the repeated high-frequency presynaptic activity required for gLTP induction resulting in sustained elevation of sympathetic tone to cardiovascular system (Alkadhi and Alzoubi 2007). Ganglionic LTP in the rat sympathetic superior cervical ganglion is triggered by a serotonin receptor–dependent mechanism (Alkadhi et al. 2005a). The functional consequence of the chronic stress-induced expression of gLTP in sympathetic ganglia has been reported as marked elevation of blood pressure in various rat models including stress-induced hypertensive, spontaneously hypertensive (SHR), aged, and Zucker obese rats (Alkadhi et al. 2001; Alzoubi et al. 2008a,b; Alzoubi and Alkadhi 2009; Alzoubi et al. 2010). Expression of gLTP in sympathetic ganglia results in a significantly higher tonic sympathetic outflow to peripheral effector organs including the heart and blood vessels.

Chronic mental stress, which induces a sustained increase in brain efferent impulse outflow to sympathetic ganglia, provides repeated high-frequency presynaptic activity, which causes highly localized calcium ($Ca^{2+}$) influx into synaptic regions (Alkadhi et al. 2005a). This influx activates $Ca^{2+}$-dependent molecular messengers required for induction and expression of gLTP in sympathetic ganglia, which leads to a sustained increase in the sympathetic tone to the cardiovascular system. We have demonstrated that in vivo expression

of gLTP is fully responsible for the development of psychosocial stress-induced hypertension and accentuation of genetic forms of experimental hypertension (Alkadhi et al. 2005a; Alkadhi and Alzoubi 2011).

The expression of gLTP is believed to be the culmination of a cascade of molecular events, both in the postsynaptic and presynaptic regions, involving several enzymes, modulators, and second messengers. Although the function of gLTP is unclear, it may simply be that recurring activity invariably results in marked potentiation of synaptic transmission in any neural circuit. However, expression of LTP in autonomic ganglia as a result of hyperactivity of the central nervous system (CNS) can result in unwanted pathophysiological changes in the cardiovascular system.

In this chapter, we review possible conditions that cause an upsurge in brain activity that may induce in vivo expression of gLTP including CNS stimulants and certain brain disorders such as chronic stress, posttraumatic stress disorder (PTSD), and epilepsy.

## UNIQUE DEPENDENCE OF gLTP ON ENDOGENOUS SEROTONIN

Ganglionic LTP induction requires the presence of serotonin and $Ca^{2+}$. The requirement for certain patterns of stimulation for triggering the induction and expression of gLTP infers the involvement of an appropriate specific transmitter/modulator. The function of serotonin in the expression of gLTP has been recognized (Alkadhi et al. 2005a). Additionally, greater-than-usual amount of extracellular $Ca^{2+}$ must enter the cell to initiate intracellular steps in the cascade of events leading to enduring synaptic functional changes. Therefore, the receptor ion channel complexes required for the expression of LTP are largely $Ca^{2+}$ ionophores. It is known that the presence of $Ca^{2+}$ is critical for the release of neurotransmitters including serotonin, as well as for the activation of a number of intracellular $Ca^{2+}$-dependent signaling molecules essential for induction and maintenance of this long-lasting response. Indirect evidence indicates that $Ca^{2+}$ increases in the presynaptic nerve terminal during posttetanic potentiation and the initial few minutes of gLTP in autonomic ganglia (Briggs and McAfee 1988; Hogan et al. 1998). In rat superior cervical ganglion, decreasing extracellular $Ca^{2+}$ prevents the expression of gLTP (Briggs et al. 1985).

Induction and maintenance of gLTP involves activation of serotonin $5\text{-}HT_3$ receptors in addition to high-frequency stimulation (Alkadhi et al. 1996; Alkadhi et al. 2005a; Alkadhi and Alzoubi 2011). Repetitive stimulation and serotonin together are necessary but neither alone is sufficient for the expression of gLTP. Serotonin seems to be released from a source within the ganglion. The endogenous origin of serotonin is suggested by experiments in which pretreatment of isolated ganglia with the serotonin uptake inhibitor, fluoxetine (Prozac©, 10 μM), caused subsequent high-frequency stimulation to induce significantly larger gLTP magnitude than in untreated ganglia (Figure 22.1) (Alkadhi et al. 1996). Additionally, the contribution of endogenous serotonin is suggested by failure of high-frequency stimulation to express gLTP in ganglia excised from serotonin-depleted animals. In serotonin-depleted ganglia (from animals pretreated with 3 mg/kg reserpine, 24 hours prior to excision of ganglia), high-frequency stimulation did not produce gLTP. However, treatment of the same ganglia with serotonin or

the $5\text{-}HT_3$ receptor agonist, m-CPBG, followed by high-frequency stimulation readily resulted in full expression of gLTP (Alkadhi et al. 1996). Pretreatment of isolated ganglia with the $5\text{-}HT_3$ receptor antagonist bemesetron (MDL 72222) prevented the induction of gLTP. Additionally, superfusion of bemesetron on ganglia during the maintenance phase reversibly blocked gLTP (Figure 22.2) (Alkadhi et al. 1996). Therefore, there is compelling evidence indicating that activation of the $5\text{-}HT_3$ receptor by endogenous serotonin is required for both induction and maintenance of gLTP (Alkadhi et al. 1996).

The type 3 serotonin (5-HT3) receptor is the only ligand-gated ion channel receptor for serotonin in vertebrates. The 5-HT3 receptor is similar to the acetylcholine nicotinic (nACh) receptor (Lummis et al. 1990). These four-transmembrane domain receptors are associated with ion channels and are nonspecific for passing positively charged ions including sodium and potassium ions in addition to having relatively high permeability to $Ca^{2+}$ ions (Ronde and Nichols 1998). Two $5\text{-}HT_3$ receptor subtypes have been cloned: $5\text{-}HT_3A$ and $5\text{-}HT_3B$. Whereas $5\text{-}HT_3A$ is expressed in both central and peripheral neurons, the $5\text{-}HT_3B$ subtype is found only in autonomic neurons coexpressed with $5\text{-}HT_3A$. Although the exact function of 5-HT3 receptors in the expression of gLTP is not yet clear, it is possible that the activation of this receptor-channel complex allows a highly focused influx of $Ca^{2+}$ required for the activation of upstream enzymes including protein kinase C, calmodulin, and $Ca^{2+}$–calmodulin kinase II (CaMKII), whose levels were increased during the expression of gLTP (Alzoubi et al. 2004; Alzoubi et al. 2008b).

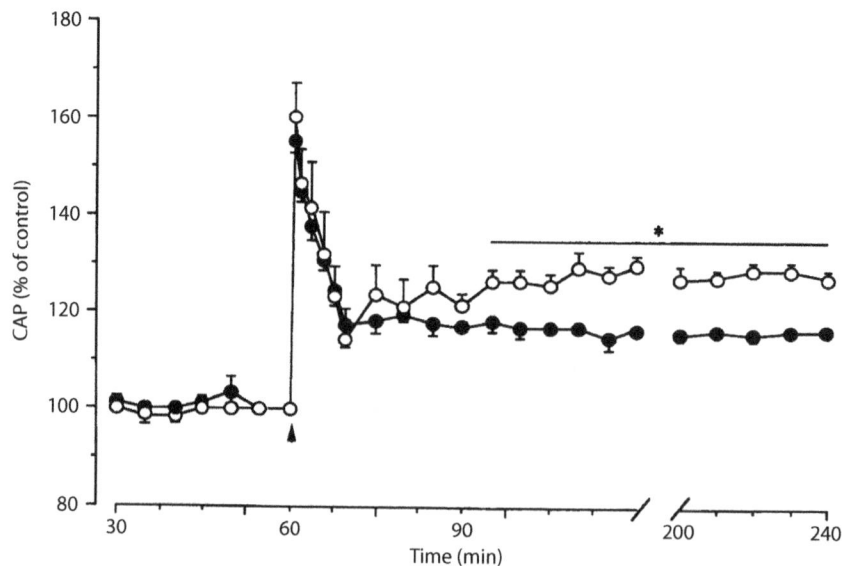

**FIGURE 22.1** Pretreatment of ganglia with the serotonin-specific transport inhibitor fluoxetine (Prozac) 30 minutes before high-frequency stimulation (arrowhead) significantly enhanced gLTP (○) but had no effect on posttetanic potentiation (response immediately after stimulation). Results from untreated ganglia (●) are also shown for comparison. The asterisk indicates significant difference (unpaired t-test) from corresponding points for untreated ganglia (n = 4/group). CAP = Compound Action Potential. (From Alkadhi, KA et al., *J Physiol*, 496(Pt 2), 479–89, 1996.)

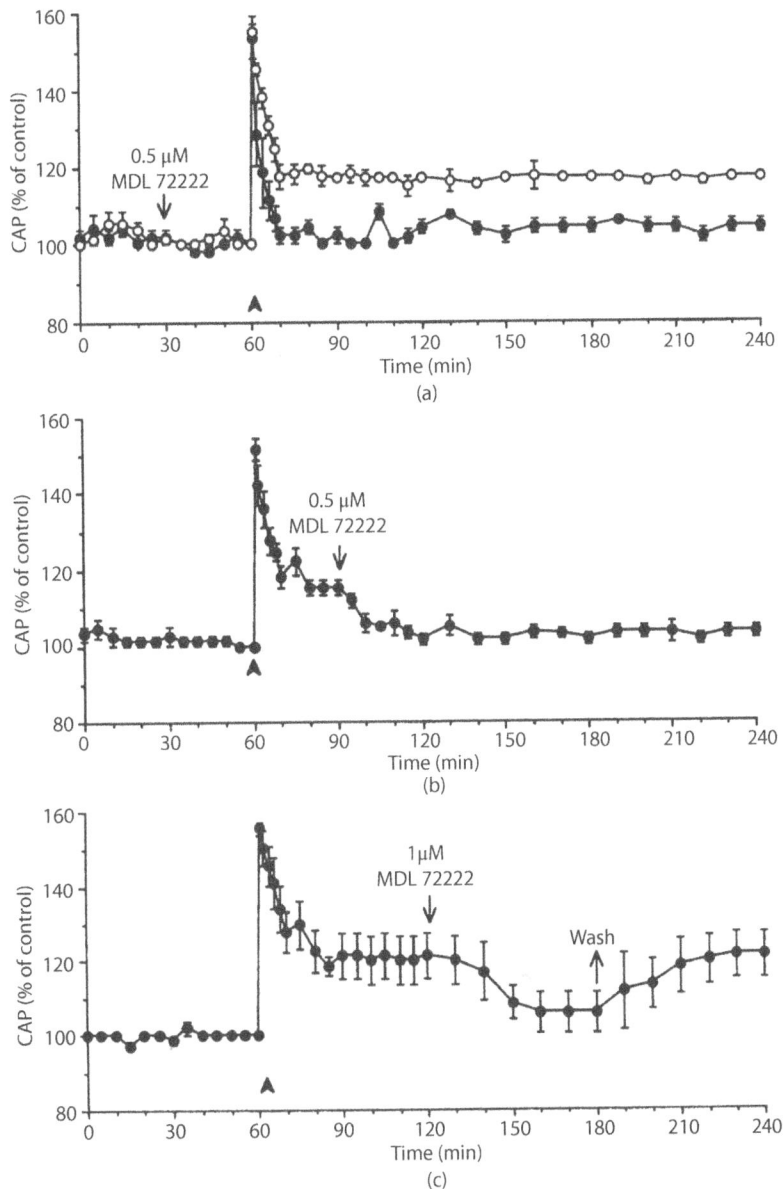

**FIGURE 22.2** Effects of 5-HT3 receptor antagonist MDL 72222 on induction and maintenance of gLTP. (a) MDL 72222 (●, 4 ganglia) superfused before high-frequency stimulation (at arrowhead) blocked the induction of gLTP. Results from untreated ganglia (○) are also shown for comparison. (b) MDL 72222, superfused 30 minutes ($n = 3$ ganglia) or 1 hour (c, 6 ganglia) after high-frequency stimulation, reversibly blocked the established gLTP. (From Alkadhi, KA et al., *J Physiol*, 496(Pt 2), 479–89, 1996.)

## POSSIBLE INDUCTION AND EXPRESSION OF gLTP BY BRAIN DISORDERS AND DRUGS

In vivo expression of gLTP in autonomic ganglia is expected to enhance tonic efferent impulses to neuroeffector organs such as the heart, blood vessels, and glands, which would negatively impact the normal functions of these organs. Increased activity of the sympathetic nervous system may be responsible for the development and/or aggravation of a variety of disorders including high blood pressure and cardiac arrhythmias.

Any mechanism that causes a continuous upsurge in impulse outflow to ganglia could provide the high-frequency presynaptic activity required for gLTP induction, which would result in a sustained elevation of sympathetic tone to the heart and blood vessels, leading to or contributing to cardiovascular disorder (Alkadhi et al. 2001; Gerges et al. 2002; Alkadhi et al. 2005a, b; Alkadhi and Alzoubi 2007; Alzoubi et al. 2008a, b). The expression of gLTP and its relation to cardiovascular disorders, such as hypertension and arrhythmias, are major risk factors for SUDEP. So far, evidence that links expression of gLTP with induction or aggravation of hypertension has been established only for chronic stress

(Alkadhi et al. 2001; Gerges et al. 2002; Alkadhi et al. 2005a, b; Alkadhi and Alzoubi 2007; Alzoubi et al. 2008a, b). In the following sections, we discuss various disorders and drugs that can be assumed to increase the risk of sudden death.

## CHRONIC PSYCHOSOCIAL STRESS

The role of chronic psychosocial stress in the expression of gLTP and the ensuing hypertension has been previously discussed at length (Alkadhi and Alzoubi 2011). Chronic stress is associated with the onset and aggravation of ischemic heart disease and is known to produce a greater rise in blood pressure in individuals with hypertension than in healthy subjects (Esler et al. 1977; Boone 1991; McEwen 1998). It is known that both genetic and stress-induced experimental hypertension involve a significant neural component that contributes to the development and maintenance of this disorder in humans (Mark 1996). Although stress-induced hypertension returns to normal within days of termination of the stress, lingering mild–moderate hypertension can result in cardiovascular diseases (Kannel et al. 1999) and cognitive impairment (Gerges et al. 2004; Aleisa et al. 2006). Enhanced impulse to the autonomic ganglia caused by psychosocial stress is also associated with sustained hypertension and increased risk of coronary heart disease (Siegrist 2001). There is compelling evidence for the role of enhanced influence of the sympathetic nervous system on cardiovascular function in young mildly hypertensive humans (Egan et al. 1987). Stress-induced sustained increase in central sympathetic outflow to ganglia seems to provide high-frequency presynaptic activity, which expresses gLTP in sympathetic ganglia leading to a sustained increase in sympathetic tone to blood vessels, causing hypertension (Alkadhi et al. 2005a; Alkadhi and Alzoubi 2007).

The function of the cardiovascular centers in the brain stem is greatly modulated by higher centers in the hippocampus, amygdala, and prefrontal cortex. This pathway is believed to have a profound effect on cardiovascular functions (Naftel and Hardy 1997). Stress perception involves participation of the frontal lobe, which alters cardiovascular function by influencing the autonomic regulatory systems (Szilagyi 1991). This has been demonstrated in psychosocially stressed pigs where the blockade of frontocortical brain stem pathways prevents the appearance of lethal arrhythmias (Skinner and Reed 1981). Interestingly, depression and anxiety are commonly associated with epilepsy (Selassie et al. 2014).

Our group conducted extensive study of the role of chronic psychosocial stress in the expression of gLTP, which leads to hypertension in rats. Psychosocially stressed animals developed reversible hypertension within 5 to 6 days of the initiation of stress (Alkadhi et al. 2005b). We found no significant difference between male and female rats in the magnitude of the chronic stress-induced increase in blood pressure or the number of stress days required to induce steady-state hypertension (Alkadhi et al. 2005b). One piece of evidence for the role of gLTP in the elevation of blood pressure by

stress comes from experiments in which pretreatment of rats with 5-HT3 receptor antagonists (e.g., Zofran, Navoban, Kytril etc.), which inhibit gLTP expression, prevents the development of hypertension (Alkadhi et al. 2005b). Further support for the expression of gLTP in vivo is provided by electrophysiological evidence obtained in sympathetic ganglia excised from stressed rat: (1) a shift of the input–output curve of stressed animals' ganglia to the left side of that of normotensive controls (Alkadhi et al. 2005b) suggests the expression of LTP (Johnston and Wu 1995). (2) The gLTP inhibitors (5HT3 receptor antagonists) block basal transmission in ganglia from stress-hypertensive animals but not in ganglia from normotensive controls, indicating the presence of gLTP in ganglia from hypertensive animals (Alkadhi et al. 2005b). (3) High-frequency stimulation that induces gLTP in normal ganglia has no effect on ganglia from stress-hypertensive animals indicating that in vivo expressed gLTP has prevented the effect of stimulation due to saturation, characteristic of LTP (Alkadhi et al. 2005b; Alzoubi et al. 2008b). (4) When two different types of stress, psychosocial stress and forced swim, are administered concurrently, they produce an increase in blood pressure equivalent to that produced by either stressor alone, which suggests that stress hypertension is due to a saturable mechanism and further supports the role of gLTP in stress-induced hypertension (Alkadhi et al. 2005b). (5) At the molecular level, experiments using Western blot analysis revealed augmented protein levels of gLTP-associated signaling molecules in ganglia isolated from stress-hypertensive animals equivalent to those in normal rat ganglia in which gLTP was expressed by high-frequency stimulation in vitro (Alzoubi et al. 2008b). These experiments provide ample evidence supporting the view that excessive activation of sympathetic ganglia leads to expression of gLTP with the consequence of dysregulation of the cardiovascular system.

## POSTTRAUMATIC STRESS DISORDER

PTSD is a debilitating and potentially chronic disorder characterized by significant morbidity. Many individuals with PTSD recover in the first few years after experiencing the traumatic event, but up to 40% remain chronically symptomatic (Kessler et al. 1995). This form of stress can result from exposure to severe traumatic events such as witnessing a severe injury or death, involvement in combat, natural disasters, or a life-threatening accident, most of which are commonly experienced more by men than women (Lasiuk and Hegadoren 2006). Neuroimaging has revealed three brain regions believed to be involved in the pathophysiology of PTSD: the amygdala, prefrontal cortex, and hippocampus (Brunello et al. 2001).

The amygdala is activated on exposure to a traumatic event, whereupon it sends increasing impulses to the frontal and prefrontal cortex, hypothalamus, hippocampus, as well as brain stem nuclei. An additional response to a traumatic event is activation of the hypothalamic-pituitary-adrenal (HPA) axis, which stimulates the release of corticotrophin releasing factor (CRF) from the hypothalamus. The CRF then stimulates the release of adrenocorticotrophin hormone from the pituitary, which in turn stimulates the release of cortisol from the adrenal glands. Cortisol serves as a negative feedback inhibition, terminating the HPA stress response (Yehuda et al. 1998). Under normal conditions, removal of the stressor returns adrenergic activity to normal homeostatic levels observed prior to the crisis.

PTSD is believed to be largely due to dysfunction of the HPA axis (Bhatnagar et al. 2006; de Kloet et al. 2006). Evidence indicates that although similar in some aspects to chronic stress, PTSD is unique in its pathology (Vieweg et al. 2006). Increased brain activity has been reported during the course of PTSD. For example, subjects with PTSD showed increased spontaneous activity in the amygdala, and a number of areas in the frontal cortex (Yan et al. 2013). Additionally, PTSD is associated with increased peripheral sympathetic activity exemplified by higher heart rate, and/or increased epinephrine/norepinephrine release (Morris and Rao 2013). It is yet to be investigated whether gLTP is being expressed in sympathetic ganglia during the course of PTSD and whether changes in cardiovascular measures, such as heart rate, are the results of already expressed gLTP in sympathetic ganglia of subjects/animals with PTSD.

## EPILEPSY

Epilepsy is a CNS disorder characterized by excessive and abnormal brain cortical nerve cell activity, which is transmitted to the periphery generally resulting in convulsive seizures. Seizures are often accompanied by intense activation of the sympathetic nervous system that can cause hypertension, diffuse myocyte damage, and increased susceptibility to ventricular arrhythmias (Ishiguro and Morgan 2001; Shimizu et al. 2008). The cardiovascular disturbances, with enhanced sympathetic activity, can persist even between seizures (Devinsky et al. 1994; Hilz et al. 2003; Pansani et al. 2010, 2011). Several centers in the brain have been implicated in the cardiopulmonary effect of seizures, including the hypothalamus and the medulla oblongata, specifically areas A1 and A5, nuclei of the nucleus tractus solitarius, and area postrema, among others (Colice 1985; Stauffer et al. 1987). These nuclei of the medulla are heavily involved in cardiovascular and respiratory regulation and receive input from the carotid sinus (Davison et al. 2012). Thus, excessive activity of these centers is transmitted down to autonomic ganglia and may result in the expression of synaptic plasticity in these ganglia. The expression of synaptic plasticity in the form of gLTP of sympathetic ganglia leads to enhanced sympathetic outflow to the cardiovascular system, resulting in hypertension and neurogenic cardiac arrhythmias. The fact that the major risk factors of SUDEP are linked to poorly controlled recurrent seizures suggests that most cases of SUDEP are seizure-related events (Surges et al. 2009).

## CHRONIC USE OF CNS STIMULANTS: IMPLICATION FOR SUDEP

### Nicotine

Nicotine, the active agent in tobacco products, is an agonist at nicotinic acetylcholine receptors in the CNS as well as in autonomic ganglia. Chronic use of nicotine is associated with increased neural cholinergic activity in the brain (Nguyen et al. 2004: Gozzi et al. 2006; Rose et al. 2007; Gloria et al. 2009; Beaver et al. 2011). Administration of nicotine in young rats resulted in epileptiform brain activity (Hralova et al. 2010). Moreover, nicotine increases peripheral sympathetic activity through direct activation of ganglionic nicotinic receptors (Kirpekar et al. 1980; Haass and Kubler 1997; Adamopoulos et al. 2008). Nicotine is known to induce the release of epinephrine into the bloodstream from the adrenal medulla (Hill and Wynder 1974; Grunberg et al. 1988). Thus, central as well as peripheral actions of nicotine cause stimulation of the cardiovascular system manifested as increase in heart rate and elevation of blood pressure (Hill and Wynder 1974). Therefore, the use of chronic tobacco products could lead to the expression of gLTP or at least the exacerbation of effects of already expressed gLTP in persons with epilepsy and thus increase the risk for SUDEP. Interestingly, persons with epilepsy are more likely to smoke (Ferguson et al. 2008).

### Caffeine

Caffeine is a methylxanthine that acts through competitive antagonism of the adenosine receptor. Its presence in various beverages, chocolate, and many prescription and over-the-counter drugs makes it the most widely consumed CNS stimulant. Neuroimaging studies revealed that caffeine increases attention and arousal by acting on various brain cortical regions (Koppelstaetter et al. 2008; Koppelstaetter et al. 2010; Park et al. 2014). Caffeine consumption has been associated with a number of human diseases; however, causal relationships have been difficult to substantiate. For example, earlier studies that showed an association between coffee consumption and coronary heart disease have been difficult to replicate. Contrary to common perception, the published literature revealed little evidence that caffeine in typical dosages increases the risk of cardiac infarction, sudden death, or arrhythmia. However, a relatively new source of caffeine is energy drinks, contain large amounts of caffeine. By self-report, up to 50% of teenagers and young adults consume energy drinks regularly (Seifert et al. 2011; de Kloet et al. 2006). Acute energy drink consumption may cause myocardial infarction due to platelet and endothelial dysfunction in healthy young adults (Worthley et al. 2010). Therefore, consumption of energy drinks in persons with epilepsy could increase the risk for SUDEP.

### Cocaine and Amphetamines

Although infrequent, the use of stimulants has been linked to sudden unexplained death in children and young people (Gould et al. 2009). Amphetamine exerts its CNS-stimulating effect mainly by altering catecholamine system in areas responsible for reward, such the brain mesocorticolimbic area (Mikkelsen et al. 1981; Bidwell et al. 2011; Miller 2011). Studies have shown that major catecholamines such as dopamine and norepinephrine are increased by amphetamine in a dose-dependent manner (Mikkelsen et al. 1981; Eiden and Weihe 2011; Miller 2011). Additionally, several studies have identified a cocaine- and amphetamine-regulated transcript "neuropeptide" at sympathetic ganglia and adrenal medulla. This neuropeptide seems to work as a neurotransmitter or neuromodulator involved in autonomic regulations (Dun et al. 2000; Babic and Ciriello 2004; Burman et al. 2004; Fenwick et al. 2006). The neuropeptide was shown to induce dose-dependent increases in mean arterial blood pressure and plasma noradrenaline in conscious rabbits (Matsumura et al. 2001) and to induce increases in mean arterial pressure and heart rate in anesthetized rats (Liu and Varner 1996; Scruggs et al. 2005).

Cocaine is an effective sympathomimetic agent that is associated with cardiovascular dysregulation including ventricular arrhythmia, systemic hypertension, acute myocardial infarction, and left ventricular hypertrophy. It acts, at least in part, by inhibiting monoamine reuptake in central and peripheral sympathetic nerve terminals in humans (Melon et al. 1997; Vongpatanasin et al. 1999; Lange and Hillis 2001). This increase in sympathetic nerve activity leads to the release of norepinephrine, peripheral vasoconstriction, increased mean arterial blood pressure, and prolonged inotropic and chronotropic responses of the heart (Matsuda et al. 1980; Mo et al. 1999; Vongpatanasin et al. 1999; Lange and Hillis 2001; Menon et al. 2007). It has been shown that these cardiovascular manifestations of cocaine are mainly mediated by stimulation of the peripheral sites of the sympathetic nervous system (Gillis et al. 1995). In contrast, studies in animal models show that cocaine reduces central and peripheral sympathetic activity (Gantenberg and Hageman 1991; Raczkowski et al. 1991; Abrahams et al. 1996; Hernandez et al. 1996; Abrahams and Varner 1998). Therefore, exposure of persons with epilepsy to CNS stimulants may increase the danger of SUDEP.

## CONSEQUENCE OF EXPRESSION OF gLTP

Moderately high-frequency electric stimulation of preganglionic nerves is known to express gLTP in the sympathetic and parasympathetic ganglia both in vivo and in vitro (Brown and McAfee 1982; Koyano et al. 1985; Briggs and McAfee 1988; Briggs et al. 1988; Alonso-deFlorida et al. 1991; Bachoo and Polosa 1992; Scott and Bennett 1993; Weinreich et al. 1995; Alkadhi et al. 1996; Alkadhi and Alzoubi 2011). Similarly, intense activation of the cardiovascular centers by certain chronic mental disorders or drugs may cause repeated high-frequency outflow of impulses from the brain, resulting in repetitive presynaptic activation of autonomic ganglia. Such activation has been shown in chronically stressed rats to evoke long-lasting gLTP, leading to neurogenic hypertension (Alzoubi et al. 2008a, b, 2010). Additionally, intense activation of the sympathetic nervous

system by any process can result in cardiac contractile dysfunction and ventricular arrhythmias (Ishiguro and Morgan 2001; Shimizu et al. 2008). This is best exemplified in epileptic seizures. A number of studies demonstrated that status epilepticus produces intense sympathetic activation in both patients and animal models (Sakamoto et al. 2008; Shimizu et al. 2008), leading to increased blood pressure and heart rate during seizures (Goodman et al. 1990; Johnston et al. 1997; Sakamoto et al. 2008). These findings suggest that prolonged seizures induce cardiac dysfunction and increase risk of lethal arrhythmias.

We hypothesize that gLTP expressed as a result of prolonged or recurrent seizures can be a major cause of SUDEP. A poorly understood complication, SUDEP is the most common cause of death directly related to epilepsy (Surges et al. 2009). Individuals with recurrent, poorly controlled chronic seizures are especially at high risk for SUDEP. SUDEP poses a considerable risk affecting up to 5000 patients a year in the United States alone (Bozorgi and Lhatoo 2013; Moghimi and Lhatoo 2013). The risk of sudden death in epileptic patients is 20 times more than that in the general population (Shorvon and Tomson 2011) and up to 90 times more frequent in epileptic children than in nonepileptic children (Donner 2011).

It has been suggested that SUDEP is caused by neurogenic cardiac arrhythmias and neurogenic pulmonary edema, which are often seen in autopsies of victims (Bateman et al. 2008; Lhatoo et al. 2010; Richerson and Buchanan 2011; Surges and Sander 2012; Cheshire 2013). Seizure-induced intense sympathetic discharge causes hypertension, diffuse myocyte damage, and increased susceptibility to ventricular arrhythmias (Ishiguro and Morgan 2001; Shimizu et al. 2008). The resulting increase in systemic vascular resistance subsequently leads to an increase in systemic blood pressure and a reduction in compliance of the left ventricle. These changes are followed by an increase in pulmonary capillary hydrostatic pressure due to constriction of pulmonary veins, resulting in intra-alveolar hemorrhage from damage to the alveolar wall and leakage of fluid into the interstitial and alveolar spaces characteristic of neurogenic pulmonary edema (Fontes et al. 2003; Kondo et al. 2004; Kandatsu et al. 2005; Leal Filho et al. 2005a, b). An indication that both cardiac arrhythmias and neurogenic pulmonary edema are associated with sympathetic ganglionic hyperactivity is suggested by the findings that ganglionic blockade prevented the development of these conditions (Healy and Guideri 1985; Sedy et al. 2007, 2009, 2011).

## SUMMARY AND CONCLUSION

Intense abnormal activity in the brain can cause marked stimulation of the sympathetic nervous system, which often induces the expression of gLTP in sympathetic ganglia leading to increased peripheral vascular resistance and abnormal cardiac rhythm. Abnormal activity in the brain can result from traumatic brain injuries, chronic mental stress, epilepsy, or chronic use of CNS stimulants. Although these disorders are known to cause marked hypertension and cardiac arrhythmias, their causative relationship to the expression of gLTP has not been studied except for chronic stress. Thus, it is essential to establish such connections to enhance therapeutic strategies for the prevention of dangerous consequences of these disorders such as SUDEP.

# REFERENCES

Abrahams TP, Varner KJ. Effects of cocaine on adrenal sympathetic nerve discharge in anesthetized rats. *Physiol Behav* 1998;63: 629–34.

Abrahams TP, Cuntapay M, Varner KJ. Sympathetic nerve responses elicited by cocaine in anesthetized and conscious rats. *Physiol Behav* 1996;59:109–15.

Adamopoulos D, van de Borne P, Argacha JF. New insights into the sympathetic, endothelial and coronary effects of nicotine. *Clin Exp Pharmacol Physiol* 2008;35:458–63.

Aleisa AM, Alzoubi KH, Gerges NZ, Alkadhi KA. Nicotine blocks stress-induced impairment of spatial memory and long-term potentiation of the hippocampal CA1 region. *Int J Neuropsychopharmacol* 2006;9:417–26.

Alkadhi K, Alzoubi K. Role of long-term potentiation of sympathetic ganglia (gLTP) in hypertension. *Clin Exp Hypertens* 2007;29:267–86.

Alkadhi K, Alzoubi K. Synaptic plasticity of autonomic ganglia: Role of chronic stress and implication in cardiovascular diseases and sudden death. Chapter 26 In: Lathers et al, eds. *Sudden death in epilepsy: Forensic and clinical issues*. Boca Raton, FL.: CRC Press/Taylor & Francis Group; 2011, pp. 395–425.

Alkadhi KA, Alzoubi KH, Aleisa AM. Plasticity of synaptic transmission in autonomic ganglia. *Prog Neurobiol* 2005a;75:83–108.

Alkadhi KA, Alzoubi KH, Aleisa AM, Tanner FL, Nimer AS. Psychosocial stress-induced hypertension results from in vivo expression of long-term potentiation in rat sympathetic ganglia. *Neurobiol Dis* 2005b;20:849–57.

Alkadhi KA, Salgado-Commissariat D, Hogan YH, Akpaudo SB. Induction and maintenance of ganglionic long-term potentiation require activation of 5-hydroxytryptamine (5-HT3) receptors. *J Physiol* 1996;496(Pt 2):479–89.

Alkadhi KA, Otoom SA, Tanner FL, Sockwell D, Hogan YH. Inhibition of ganglionic long-term potentiation decreases blood pressure in spontaneously hypertensive rats. *Exp Biol Med (Maywood)* 2001;226:1024–30.

Alonso-deFlorida F, Morales MA, Minzoni AA. Modulated long-term potentiation in the cat superior cervical ganglion in vivo. *Brain Res* 1991;544:203–10.

Alzoubi KH, Alkadhi KA. Calmodulin and guanylyl cyclase inhibitors block the in vivo expression of gLTP in sympathetic ganglia from chronically stressed rats. *Neurosci Res* 2009; 63:95–9.

Alzoubi KH, Aleisa AM, Alkadhi KA. Expression of gLTP in sympathetic ganglia of obese Zucker rats in vivo: Molecular evidence. *J Mol Neurosci* 2008a;35:297–06.

Alzoubi KH, Aleisa AM, Alkadhi KA. Expression of gLTP in sympathetic ganglia from stress-hypertensive rats: Molecular evidence. *J Mol Neurosci* 2008b;35:201–09.

Alzoubi KH, Aleisa AM, Alkadhi KA. In vivo expression of ganglionic long-term potentiation in superior cervical ganglia from hypertensive aged rats. *Neurobiol Aging* 2010;31:805–12.

Alzoubi KH, Bedawi AS, Aleisa AM, Alkadhi KA. Hypothyroidism impairs long-term potentiation in sympathetic ganglia: Electrophysiologic and molecular studies. *J Neurosci Res* 2004;78:393–402.

Babic T, Ciriello J. Medullary and spinal cord projections from cardiovascular responsive sites in the rostral ventromedial medulla. *J Comp Neurol* 2004;469:391–412.

Bachoo M, Polosa C. Preganglionic axons from the third thoracic spinal segment fail to induce long-term potentiation in the superior cervical ganglion of the cat. *Can J Physiol Pharmacol* 1992;70 (Suppl):S27–31.

Bateman LM, Li CS, Seyal M. Ictal hypoxemia in localization-related epilepsy: Analysis of incidence, severity and risk factors. *Brain* 2008;131:3239–45.

Beaver JD, Long CJ, Cole DM, Durcan MJ, Bannon LC, Mishra RG, Matthews PM. The effects of nicotine replacement on cognitive brain activity during smoking withdrawal studied with simultaneous fMRI/EEG. *Neuropsychopharmacology* 2011; 36:1792–800.

Bhatnagar S, Vining C, Iyer V, Kinni V.) Changes in hypothalamic–pituitary–adrenal function, body temperature, body weight and food intake with repeated social stress exposure in rats. *J Neuroendocrinol* 2006;18:13–24.

Bidwell LC, McClernon FJ, Kollins SH. Cognitive enhancers for the treatment of ADHD. *Pharmacol Biochem Behav* 2011;99: 262–74.

Boone JL. Stress and hypertension. *Prim Care* 1991;18:623–49.

Bozorgi A, Lhatoo SD. Seizures, cerebral shutdown, and SUDEP. *Epilepsy Curr* 2013;13:236–40.

Briggs CA, McAfee DA. Long-term potentiation at nicotinic synapses in the rat superior cervical ganglion. *J Physiol* 1988;404: 129–44.

Briggs CA, McAfee DA, McCaman RE. Long-term potentiation of synaptic acetylcholine release in the superior cervical ganglion of the rat. *J Physiol* 1985;363:181–90.

Briggs CA, McAfee DA, McCaman RE. Long-term regulation of synaptic acetylcholine release and nicotinic transmission: The role of cyclic AMP. *Br J Pharmacol* 1988;93:399–411.

Brown TH, McAfee DA. Long-term synaptic potentiation in the superior cervical ganglion. *Science* 1982;215:1411–3.

Brunello N, Davidson JR, Deahl M, Kessler RC, Mendlewicz J, Racagni G, Shalev AY, Zohar J. Posttraumatic stress disorder: Diagnosis and epidemiology, comorbidity and social consequences, biology and treatment. *Neuropsychobiology* 2001;43:150–62.

Burman KJ, Sartor DM, Verberne AJ, Llewellyn-Smith IJ. Cocaine-and amphetamine-regulated transcript in catecholamine and noncatecholamine presympathetic vasomotor neurons of rat rostral ventrolateral medulla. *J Comp Neurol* 2004;476:19–31.

Cheshire WP. Highlights in clinical autonomic neurosciences: Sudden unexpected death in epilepsy. *Auton Neurosci* 2013;179:5–8.

Colice GL. Neurogenic pulmonary edema. *Clin Chest Med* 1985;6: 473–89.

Davison DL, Terek M, Chawla LS. Neurogenic pulmonary edema. *Crit Care* 2012;16:212.

Devinsky O, Perrine K, Theodore WH. Interictal autonomic nervous system function in patients with epilepsy. *Epilepsia* 1994;35: 199–204.

de Kloet CS, Vermetten E, Geuze E, Kavelaars A, Heijnen CJ, Westenberg HG. Assessment of HPA-axis function in posttraumatic stress disorder: Pharmacological and non-pharmacological challenge tests, a review. *J Psychiatr Res* 2006;40:550–67.

Donner EJ. Explaining the unexplained; expecting the unexpected: Where are we with sudden unexpected death in epilepsy? *Epilepsy Curr* 2011;11:45–9.

Dun NJ, Dun SL, Kwok EH, Yang J, Chang J. Cocaine- and amphetamine-regulated transcript-immunoreactivity in the rat sympatho-adrenal axis. *Neurosci Lett* 2000;283:97–100.

Egan B, Panis R, Hinderliter A, Schork N, Julius S. Mechanism of increased alpha adrenergic vasoconstriction in human essential hypertension. *J Clin Invest* 1987;80:812–7.

Eiden LE, Weihe E. VMAT2: A dynamic regulator of brain monoaminergic neuronal function interacting with drugs of abuse. *Ann N Y Acad Sci* 2011;1216:86–98.

Esler M, Julius S, Zweifler A, Randall O, Harburg E, Gardiner H, DeQuattro V. Mild high-renin essential hypertension. Neurogenic human hypertension? *N Engl J Med* 1977; 296:405–11.

Fenwick NM, Martin CL, Llewellyn-Smith IJ. Immunoreactivity for cocaine- and amphetamine-regulated transcript in rat sympathetic preganglionic neurons projecting to sympathetic ganglia and the adrenal medulla. *J Comp Neurol* 2006;495:422–33.

Ferguson PL, Chiprich J, Smith G, Dong B, Wannamaker BB, Kobau R, Thurman DJ, Selassie AW. Prevalence of self-reported epilepsy, health care access, and health behaviors among adults in South Carolina. *Epilepsy & Behavior* 2008;13:529–34

Fontes RB, Aguiar PH, Zanetti MV, Andrade F, Mandel M, Teixeira MJ. Acute neurogenic pulmonary edema: Case reports and literature review. *J Neurosurg Anesthesiol* 2003;15:144–50.

Gantenberg NS, Hageman GR. Cocaine depresses cardiac sympathetic efferent activity in anesthetized dogs. *J Cardiovasc Pharmacol* 1991;17:434–9.

Gerges NZ, Aleisa AM, Alhaider AA, Alkadhi KA. Reduction of elevated arterial blood pressure in obese Zucker rats by inhibition of ganglionic long-term potentiation. *Neuropharmacology* 2002;43:1070–6.

Gerges NZ, Alzoubi KH, Park CR, Diamond DM, Alkadhi KA. Adverse effect of the combination of hypothyroidism and chronic psychosocial stress on hippocampus-dependent memory in rats. *Behav Brain Res* 2004;155:77–84.

Gillis RA, Hernandez YM, Erzouki HK, Raczkowski VF, Mandal AK, Kuhn FE, Dretchen KL. Sympathetic nervous system mediated cardiovascular effects of cocaine are primarily due to a peripheral site of action of the drug. *Drug Alcohol Depend* 1995;37:217–30.

Gloria R, Angelos L, Schaefer HS, Davis JM, Majeskie M, Richmond BS, Curtin JJ, Davidson RJ, Baker TB. An fMRI investigation of the impact of withdrawal on regional brain activity during nicotine anticipation. *Psychophysiology* 2009;46:681–93.

Goodman JH, Homan RW, Crawford IL. Kindled seizures elevate blood pressure and induce cardiac arrhythmias. *Epilepsia* 1990;31:489–95.

Gould MS, Walsh BT, Munfakh JL, Kleinman M, Duan N, Olfson M, Greenhill L, Cooper T. Sudden death and use of stimulant medications in youths. *Am J Psychiatry* 2009;166(9):992–1001.

Gozzi A, Schwarz A, Reese T, Bertani S, Crestan V, Bifone A. Region-specific effects of nicotine on brain activity: A pharmacological MRI study in the drug-naive rat. *Neuropsychopharmacology* 2006;31:1690–703.

Grunberg NE, Popp KA, Bowen DJ, Nespor SM, Winders SE, Eury SE. Effects of chronic nicotine administration on insulin, glucose, epinephrine, and norepinephrine. *Life Sci* 1988;42:161–70.

Haass M, Kubler W. Nicotine and sympathetic neurotransmission. *Cardiovasc Drugs Ther* 1997;10:657–65.

Healy C, Guideri G. DOCA-salt induced myocardial sensitization to ventricular fibrillation by isoprenaline in rats. Role of the autonomic nervous system. *J Auton Pharmacol* 1985;5: 271–8.

Hernandez YM, Raczkowski VF, Dretchen KL, Gillis RA. Cocaine inhibits sympathetic neural activity by acting in the central nervous system and at the sympathetic ganglion. *J Pharmacol Exp Ther* 1996;277:1114–21.

Hill P, Wynder EL. Smoking and cardiovascular disease. Effect of nicotine on the serum epinephrine and corticoids. *Am Heart J* 1974;87:491–96.

Hilz MJ, Platsch G, Druschky K, Pauli E, Kuwert T, Stefan H, Neundorfer B, Druschky A. Outcome of epilepsy surgery correlates with sympathetic modulation and neuroimaging of the heart. *J Neurol Sci* 2003;216:153–62.

Hogan YH, Hawkins R, Alkadhi KA. Adenosine A1 receptor activation inhibits LTP in sympathetic ganglia. *Brain Res* 1998;807: 19–28.

Hralova M, Maresova D, Riljak V. Effect of the single-dose of nicotine-administration on the brain bioelectrical activity and on behaviour in immature 12-day-old rats. *Prague Med Rep* 2010;111:182–90.

Ishiguro Y, Morgan JP. Effect of endogenous catecholamine on myocardial stunning in a simulated ischemia model. *Fundam Clin Pharmacol* 2001;15:111–6.

Johnston D, Wu S. Cellular neurophysiology of learning and memory. In: Johnston D and Wu S, eds. *Foundations of Cellular Neurophysiology*. Cambridge, MA: MIT press; 1995, pp. 441–75.

Johnston SC, Siedenberg R, Min JK, Jerome EH, Laxer KD. Central apnea and acute cardiac ischemia in a sheep model of epileptic sudden death. *Ann Neurol* 1997;42:588–94.

Kandatsu N, Nan YS, Feng GG, Nishiwaki K, Hirokawa M, Ishikawa K, Komatsu T, Yokochi T, Shimada Y, Ishikawa N. Opposing effects of isoflurane and sevoflurane on neurogenic pulmonary edema development in an animal model. *Anesthesiology* 2005;102:1182–9.

Kannel WB, Peter WF, Wilson MD. Cardiovascular risk factors and hypertension. In: Izzo JL, Black HR, eds. *Hypertension primer: The Essentials of High Blood Pressure*. Philadelphia, PA: Lippincot Williams & Wilkens; 1999, pp. 199–200.

Kessler RC, Sonnega A, Bromet E, Hughes M, Nelson CB. Posttraumatic stress disorder in the National Comorbidity Survey. *Arch Gen Psychiatry* 1995;52:1048–60.

Kirpekar SM, Garcia AG, Prat JC. Action of nicotine on sympathetic nerve terminals. *J Pharmacol Exp Ther* 1980;213:133–8.

Kondo H, Feng GG, Nishiwaki K, Shimada Y, Hirokawa M, Komatsu T, Yokochi T, Ishikawa N. A role for L-glutamate ionotropic receptors in the development of rat neurogenic pulmonary edema. *Eur J Pharmacol* 2004;499:257–63.

Koppelstaetter F, Poeppel TD, Siedentopf CM, Ischebeck A, Kolbitsch C, Mottaghy FM, Felber SR, Jaschke WR, Krause BJ. Caffeine and cognition in functional magnetic resonance imaging. *J Alzheimers Dis* 2010;20(Suppl 1):S71–84.

Koppelstaetter F, Poeppel TD, Siedentopf CM, Ischebeck A, Verius M, Haala I, Mottaghy FM et al. Does caffeine modulate verbal working memory processes? An fMRI study. *Neuroimage* 2008;39:492–9.

Koyano K, Kuba K, Minota S. Long-term potentiation of transmitter release induced by repetitive presynaptic activities in bull-frog sympathetic ganglia. *J Physiol* 1985;359:219–33.

Lange RA, Hillis LD. Cardiovascular complications of cocaine use. *N Engl J Med* 2001;345:351–8.

Lasiuk GC, Hegadoren KM. Posttraumatic stress disorder part II: Development of the construct within the North American psychiatric taxonomy. *Perspect Psychiatr Care* 2006;42: 72–81.

Leal Filho MB, Morandin RC, de Almeida AR, Cambiucci EC, Borges G, Gontijo JA, Metze K. Importance of anesthesia for the genesis of neurogenic pulmonary edema in spinal cord injury. *Neurosci Lett* 2005a;373:165–70.

Leal Filho MB, Morandin RC, de Almeida AR, Cambiucci EC, Metze K, Borges G, Gontijo JA. Hemodynamic parameters and neurogenic pulmonary edema following spinal cord injury: An experimental model. *Arq Neuropsiquiatr* 2005b;63:990–6.

Lhatoo SD, Faulkner HJ, Dembny K, Trippick K, Johnson C, Bird JM. An electroclinical case-control study of sudden unexpected death in epilepsy. *Ann Neurol* 2010;68:787–96.

Liu W, Varner KJ. Characterization of the sympathetic nerve responses to amphetamine: Role of central alpha 2-adrenergic receptors. *J Cardiovasc Pharmacol* 1996;28:712–22.

Lummis SC, Kilpatrick GJ, Martin IL. Characterization of 5-HT3 receptors in intact N1E-115 neuroblastoma cells. *Eur J Pharmacol* 1990;189(2–3):223–7.

Mark AL. The sympathetic nervous system in hypertension: A potential long-term regulator of arterial pressure. *J Hypertens* 1996;(Suppl 14):S159–65.

Matsuda Y, Masuda Y, Blattberg B, Levy MN. The effects of cocaine, chlorpheniramine and tripelennamine on the cardiac responses to sympathetic nerve stimulation. *Eur J Pharmacol* 1980;63:25–33.

Matsumura K, Tsuchihashi T, Abe I. Central human cocaine- and amphetamine-regulated transcript peptide 55-102 increases arterial pressure in conscious rabbits. *Hypertension* 2001;38:1096–100.

McEwen BS. Protective and damaging effects of stress mediators. *N Engl J Med* 1998;338:171–9.

Melon PG, Boyd CJ, McVey S, Mangner TJ, Wieland DM, Schwaiger M. Effects of active chronic cocaine use on cardiac sympathetic neuronal function assessed by carbon-11-hydroxyephedrine. *J Nucl Med* 1997;38:451–6.

Menon DV, Wang Z, Fadel PJ, Arbique D, Leonard D, Li JL, Victor RG, Vongpatanasin W. Central sympatholysis as a novel countermeasure for cocaine-induced sympathetic activation and vasoconstriction in humans. *J Am Coll Cardiol* 2007;50:626–33.

Mikkelsen E, Lake CR, Brown GL, Ziegler MG, Ebert MH. The hyperactive child syndrome: Peripheral sympathetic nervous system function and the effect of d-amphetamine. *Psychiatry Res* 1981;4:157–69.

Miller GM. The emerging role of trace amine-associated receptor 1 in the functional regulation of monoamine transporters and dopaminergic activity. *J Neurochem* 2011;116:164–76.

Mo W, Arruda JA, Dunea G, Singh AK. Cocaine-induced hypertension: Role of the peripheral sympathetic system. *Pharmacol Res* 1999;40:139–45.

Moghimi N, Lhatoo SD. Sudden unexpected death in epilepsy or voodoo heart: Analysis of heart/brain connections. *Curr Cardiol Rep* 2013;15:424.

Morris MC, Rao U. Psychobiology of PTSD in the acute aftermath of trauma: Integrating research on coping, HPA function and sympathetic nervous system activity. *Asian J Psychiatr* 2013;6:3–21.

Naftel JP, Hardy SG. Visceral motor pathways. In: Haines, DE, ed. *Fundamental Neuroscience.* New York, NY: Churchill-Livingstone; 1997, pp. 417–429.

Nguyen HN, Rasmussen BA, Perry DC. Binding and functional activity of nicotinic cholinergic receptors in selected rat brain regions are increased following long-term but not short-term nicotine treatment. *J Neurochem* 2004;90:40–9.

Pansani AP, Colugnati DB, Sonoda EY, Arida RM, Cravo SL, Schoorlemmer GH, Cavalheiro EA, Scorza FA. Tachycardias and sudden unexpected death in epilepsy: A gold rush by an experimental route. *Epilepsy Behav* 2010;19:546–7.

Pansani AP, Colugnati DB, Schoorlemmer GH, Sonoda EY, Cavalheiro EA, Arida RM, Scorza FA, Cravo SL. Repeated amygdala-kindled seizures induce ictal rebound tachycardia in rats. *Epilepsy Behav* 2011;22:442–9.

Park CA, Kang CK, Son YD, Choi EJ, Kim SH, Oh ST, Kim YB, Park CW, Cho ZH. The effects of caffeine ingestion on cortical areas: Functional imaging study. *Magn Reson Imaging* 2014;32:366–71.

Raczkowski VF, Hernandez YM, Erzouki HK, Abrahams TP, Mandal AK, Hamosh P, Friedman E, Quest JA, Dretchen KL, Gillis RA. Cocaine acts in the central nervous system to inhibit sympathetic neural activity. *J Pharmacol Exp Ther* 1991;257:511–9.

Richerson GB, Buchanan GF. The serotonin axis: Shared mechanisms in seizures, depression, and SUDEP. *Epilepsia* 2011;52(Suppl 1):28–38.

Ronde P, Nichols RA. High calcium permeability of serotonin 5-HT3 receptors on presynaptic nerve terminals from rat striatum. *J Neurochem* 1998;70:1094–103.

Rose JE, Behm FM, Salley AN, Bates JE, Coleman RE, Hawk TC, Turkington TG. Regional brain activity correlates of nicotine dependence. *Neuropsychopharmacology* 2007;32:2441–52.

Sakamoto K, Saito T, Orman R, Koizumi K, Lazar J, Salciccioli L, Stewart M. Autonomic consequences of kainic acid-induced limbic cortical seizures in rats: Peripheral autonomic nerve activity, acute cardiovascular changes, and death. *Epilepsia* 2008;49:982–96.

Scott TR, Bennett MR. The effect of ions and second messengers on long-term potentiation of chemical transmission in avian ciliary ganglia. *Br J Pharmacol* 1993;110:461–9.

Scruggs P, Lai CC, Scruggs JE, Dun NJ. Cocaine- and amphetamine-regulated transcript peptide potentiates spinal glutamatergic sympathoexcitation in anesthetized rats. *Regul Pept* 2005;127: 79–85.

Sedy J, Kunes J, Zicha J. Neurogenic pulmonary edema induced by spinal cord injury in spontaneously hypertensive and Dahl salt hypertensive rats. *Physiol Res* 2011;60:975–9.

Sedy J, Urdzikova L, Likavcanova K, Hejcl A, Burian M, Jendelova P, Zicha J, Kunes J, Sykova E. Low concentration of isoflurane promotes the development of neurogenic pulmonary edema in spinal cord injured rats. *J Neurotrauma* 2007;24:1487–1501.

Sedy J, Zicha J, Kunes J, Hejcl A, Sykova E. The role of nitric oxide in the development of neurogenic pulmonary edema in spinal cord-injured rats: The effect of preventive interventions. *Am J Physiol Regul Integr Comp Physiol* 2009;297:R1111–7.

Seifert SM, Schaechter JL, Hershorin ER, Lipshultz SE. Health effects of energy drinks on children, adolescents, and young adults. *Pediatrics* 2011;127:511–28.

Selassie AW, Wilson DA, Martz GU, Smith GG, Wagner JL, Wannamaker BB. Epilepsy beyond seizure: A population-based study of comorbidities. *Epilepsy Res* 2014;108:305—15.

Shimizu M, Kagawa A, Takano T, Masai H, Miwa Y. Neurogenic stunned myocardium associated with status epileptics and postictal catecholamine surge. *Intern Med* 2008;47:269–73.

Shorvon S, Tomson T. Sudden unexpected death in epilepsy. *Lancet* 2011;378:2028–38.

Siegrist J. [Psychosocial factors influencing development and course of coronary heart disease]. *Herz* 2001;26:316–25.

Skinner JE, Reed JC. Blockade of frontocortical-brain stem pathway prevents ventricular fibrillation of ischemic heart. *Am J Physiol* 1981;240:H156–63.

Stauffer AZ, Dodd-O J, Lathers CM. The relationship of the lock-step phenomenon and precipitous changes in mean arterial blood pressure. *Electroencephalogr Clin Neurophysiol* 1989 72(4):340–345.

Surges R, Sander JW. Sudden unexpected death in epilepsy: Mechanisms, prevalence, and prevention. *Curr Opin Neurol* 2012;25:201–7.

Surges R, Thijs RD, Tan HL, Sander JW. Sudden unexpected death in epilepsy: Risk factors and potential pathomechanisms. *Nat Rev Neurol* 2009;5(9):492–504.

Szilagyi JE. Psychosocial stress elevates blood pressure via an opioid dependent mechanism in normotensive rats. *Clin Exp Hypertens A* 1991;13:1383–94.

Vieweg WV, Julius DA, Fernandez A, Beatty-Brooks M, Hettema JM, Pandurangi AK. Posttraumatic stress disorder: Clinical features, pathophysiology, and treatment. *Am J Med* 2006;119: 383–90.

Vongpatanasin W, Mansour Y, Chavoshan B, Arbique D, Victor RG. Cocaine stimulates the human cardiovascular system via a central mechanism of action. *Circulation* 1999;100:497–502.

Weinreich D, Undem BJ, Taylor G, Barry MF. Antigen-induced long-term potentiation of nicotinic synaptic transmission in the superior cervical ganglion of the guinea pig. *J Neurophysiol* 1995;73:2004–16.

Worthley MI, Prabhu A, De Sciscio P, Schultz C, Sanders P, Willoughby SR. Detrimental effects of energy drink consumption on platelet and endothelial function. *Am J Med* 2010; 123(2):184–7.

Yan X, Brown AD, Lazar M, Cressman VL, Henn-Haase C, Neylan TC, Shalev A et al. Spontaneous brain activity in combat related PTSD. *Neurosci Lett* 2013;547:1–5.

Yehuda R, McFarlane AC, Shalev AY. Predicting the development of posttraumatic stress disorder from the acute response to a traumatic event. *Biol Psychiatry* 1998;44:1305–13.

# 23 $\beta_1$-Adrenergic Blockade Prevents Cardiac Dysfunction and Increased Susceptibility to Experimental Arrhythmias Following Status Epilepticus in Rats

*Steven L. Bealer, Cameron S. Metcalf, and Jason G. Little*

## CONTENTS

## INTRODUCTION

The precise mechanisms of sudden unexplained death in epilepsy (SUDEP), and mortality during and following status epilepticus (SE), have not been completely determined. However, a number of studies indicate that cardiac ventricular abnormalities and arrhythmias produce sudden cardiac death and may contribute to seizure-related mortality (Painter et al. 1993; Walton 1993; Boggs et al. 1998; Lathers and Schraeder 2002; Nei et al. 2004; Leung et al. 2006). The mechanisms of seizure-induced arrhythmogenic changes in the heart have not been defined. However, a number of studies support the proposal that sympathetic nervous system (SymNS) activation during seizures contributes to the cardiac effects and dysfunction that culminate in potentially lethal arrhythmias.

It is well documented that SE is associated with intense SymNS activation in humans (Walton 1993; Shimizu et al. 2008) and in animals (Kreisman et al. 1993; Kanter et al. 1996; Sakamoto et al. 2008). Furthermore, isolated epileptic seizures are also accompanied by SymNS activation (Simon et al. 1984; Di Gennaro et al. 2004; Mayer et al. 2004; Rugg-Gunn et al. 2004; Ryvlin et al. 2006). These findings are consistent with the proposed role of SymNS activation in generating seizure-associated arrhythmias.

SymNS activation can significantly increase the risk of lethal cardiac arrhythmias and sudden death when acting on cardiac tissue with anatomical damage and/or electrical dysfunction (Anderson 2003; Dorian 2005; Hohnloser 2005). Seizure activity can result in cardiac structural damage that may provide an anatomical substrate for arrhythmias. For example, as described in our accompanying chapter in this book (Chapter 24) and previously published data (Metcalf et al. 2009b; Bealer et al. 2010),

we observed seizure-related cardiac injury, as indicated by increased plasma cardiac troponin I (cTnI) concentrations and diffuse TUNEL staining in cardiac tissue following SE. In addition, several reports show that epileptic seizures can induce cardiac myocyte damage, also evaluated by postictal increases in plasma cTnI concentration (Brobbey and Ravakhah 2004; Stollberger and Finsterer 2004a; Parvulescu-Codrea et al. 2006). Consequently, both SE and isolated seizures are associated with structural damage, which promote arrhythmias in response to SymNS activation.

In addition to, or as a result of, anatomical damage to cardiac myocytes during seizures, there are changes in cardiac function that increase susceptibility to arrhythmias. For example, SE often produces chronic cardiac electrical abnormalities and left ventricular pump dysfunction (Boggs et al. 1993; Manno et al. 2005; Legriel et al. 2008) that promote arrhythmias for an extended period following seizure activity. Furthermore, self-limited seizures are also associated with arrhythmogenic changes in cardiac electrical activity, including lengthening and/or shortening of the QT interval (Brotherstone et al. 2009; Kandler et al. 2005; Surges et al. 2010b).

Taken together, these data are consistent with the hypothesis that seizures can produce anatomical, functional, and electrical abnormalities that increase susceptibility to lethal cardiac arrhythmias in response to ictal SymNS activation. However, the role of increased SymNS activity during seizures in the development of cardiac damage and electrocardiographic dysfunction that increase susceptibility to arrhythmias has not been completely elucidated. This chapter describes studies that evaluate the contribution of cardiac SymNS activity during seizures on arrhythmogenic changes in the heart.

## CARDIAC EFFECTS OF SYMPATHETIC NERVOUS SYSTEM ACTIVATION DURING SEIZURES

### EFFECTS OF β-ADRENERGIC BLOCKADE ON SEIZURE-INDUCED CARDIAC DAMAGE

We examined the effects of $\beta_1$-adrenergic blockade during SE on cardiac myocyte damage. SE was induced in rats by administration of lithium and pilocarpine using previously described procedures (Kulkarni and George 1995; Glien et al. 2001). Seizures were terminated with valproic acid following 90 minutes of continuous stage 4 to 5 activity. We previously demonstrated that 90 minutes of SE in this model results in chronic cardiac and autonomic dysfunction (Metcalf et al. 2009a). Control rats underwent similar procedures but were not administered pilocarpine. Separate groups of animals undergoing SE or control procedures were administered either the $\beta_1$-adrenergic antagonist atenolol (AT) (1 mg/kg) or vehicle prior to the initiation of seizure activity and at 30- to 45-minute intervals during seizures. Furthermore, additional atenolol was given to appropriate animals when heart rate exceeded preseizure values by 10 bpm. This protocol and dose of AT administration was selected because it completely inhibits seizure-related tachycardia in rats (Bealer et al. 2010; Little and Bealer 2012).

To evaluate seizure-induced myocyte damage, the plasma concentration of cTnI, a sensitive and specific blood-borne indicator of myocardial damage in humans (Antman 2002; Sarko and Pollack 2002) and experimental animals (O'Brien et al. 2006; Kurata et al. 2007), was measured in arterial plasma. Blood was obtained at 60 minutes following the onset of SE and at an identical time in control animals.

SE induced damage to cardiac myocytes within 60 minutes of the initiation of seizure activity in vehicle-treated rats, as denoted by the significant increase in plasma concentration of cTnI (Figure 23.1). However, SE animals that received atenolol before and during seizures (SE+AT) had plasma cTnI concentrations that were comparable to control and control+atenolol rats. These data demonstrate that SE-related cardiac damage was prevented by systemic $\beta_1$-adrenergic receptor blockade. These findings suggest that inhibition of the seizure-related tachycardia by $\beta_1$-adrenergic receptor blockade during SE protected the cardiomyocytes from seizure-induced damage.

### $\beta_1$-ADRENERGIC BLOCKADE PREVENTS DETRIMENTAL EFFECTS OF SE ON LEFT VENTRICULAR FUNCTION

These experiments were designed to determine if SE diminished cardiac function at 24 hours following seizures. In these studies, we used a model of self-sustaining limbic SE induced by stimulation of the amygdala (Nissinen et al. 2000). SE was terminated with valproic acid following 90 minutes of seizure activity. Animals were treated with either vehicle or atenolol using the aforementioned procedures.

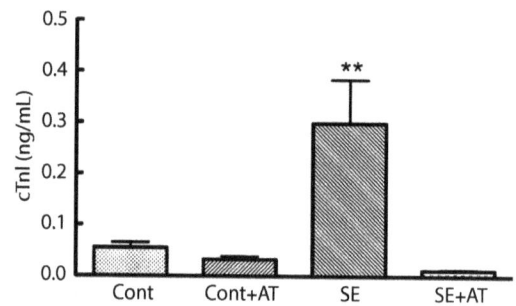

**FIGURE 23.1** Concentrations of plasma cardiac troponin I (cTnI) at 60 minutes following the onset of seizures in animals treated with vehicle (status epilepticus [SE]) or atenolol (SE+AT) and at comparable times in control rats given vehicle (Cont) or atenolol (Cont+AT). $^{**}p < .01$ compared to all other groups. (From Bealer, SL et al., *Epilepsy Res*, 91, 66–73, 2010. With permission.)

These groups were compared to control animals that did not experience seizures. At 24 hours after SE or control treatments, cardiac output and left ventricular pressures were measured in anesthetized animals. From these values, the first derivatives of the maximum and minimum left ventricular pressure changes over time ($dP/dt$ max and min), which are estimates of ventricular contractility and relaxation, were calculated.

Figure 23.2 shows that ventricular contractility and relaxation are diminished at 24 hours following SE. The decrease in ventricular contractility resulted in a significant reduction in cardiac output. Furthermore, the detrimental effects on cardiac output and contractility were prevented by $\beta_1$-adrenergic receptor blockade. However, seizure-induced reduction in ventricular relaxation was not altered by atenolol administration.

These data show that diminished left ventricular function following SE, which may contribute to lethal arrhythmias, results from $\beta_1$-adrenergic receptor stimulation during seizures.

### EFFECT OF $\beta_1$-ADRENERGIC RECEPTOR BLOCKADE ON QT-INTERVAL PROLONGATION

To determine the effects of SE-related $\beta_1$-adrenergic receptor activation on cardiac electrical activity, we evaluated electrocardiographic recordings from rats following recovery from SE, which was induced with lithium-pilocarpine injections and terminated after 90 minutes by the administration of valproic acid (Metcalf et al. 2009a). Animals were treated with either vehicle or atenolol prior to and during SE as described earlier. Electrocardiogram recordings were obtained from anesthetized animals at 10–12 days following SE and were evaluated for heart rate and QT interval corrected for heart rate (QTc). We found that this 10- to 12-day period allows animals to recover from the acute, debilitating effects of pilocarpine-induced SE and regain normal patterns of food

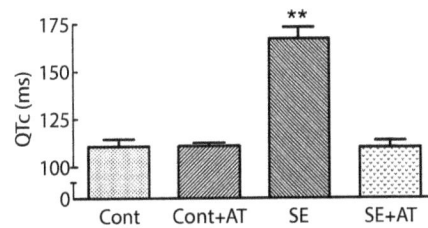

**FIGURE 23.3** QTc interval at 12–14 days following status epilepticus (SE) or control procedures (Cont) in animals treated with vehicle (SE) or atenolol (SE+AT) prior to seizures. $^{**}p < .01$ compared to all other groups. (From Bealer, SL et al., *Epilepsy Res*, 91, 66–73, 2010. With permission.)

## β₁-ADRENERGIC RECEPTORS MEDIATE SEIZURE-RELATED SUSCEPTIBILITY TO ARRHYTHMIAS

Seizures can induce cardiac damage and alter myocyte electrical processes that increase susceptibility to lethal ventricular arrhythmias. Indeed, we have shown that both SE (Metcalf et al. 2009b) and repeated self-limiting seizures that are characteristic of epilepsy (Bealer and Little 2013) increase susceptibility to experimentally induced arrhythmias in rat models. We evaluated the contribution of β₁-adrenergic receptor activation during SE on susceptibility to experimentally induced arrhythmias at 2 weeks following SE induced by lithium-pilocarpine in animals treated with atenolol or vehicle as described earlier. Susceptibility to arrhythmias was determined by measuring the latency to premature ventricular contractions, ventricular tachycardia, and ventricular fibrillation induced by intravenous administration of the arrhythmogenic agent aconitine (Grippo et al. 2004; Shu et al. 2004).

As previously demonstrated (Metcalf et al. 2009b), SE increased susceptibility to all aconitine-induced arrhythmias, as indicated by the decreased latency between the initiation of infusion and the appearance of the arrhythmias (Figure 23.4). However, the onsets of these arrhythmias in SE rats treated with atenolol before and during SE were similar to those observed in untreated control animals and in control rats treated with atenolol (Figure 23.4). These data demonstrate that β₁-adrenergic blockade during SE prevents increased susceptibility to experimentally induced arrhythmias following SE activity.

## DISCUSSION

These data demonstrate that β₁-adrenergic receptor blockade during SE prevents cardiomyocyte damage, diminished cardiac performance, and chronic electrical dysfunctions that are associated with increased susceptibility to lethal arrhythmias. Specifically, increased plasma concentrations of cTnI, acute decreases in cardiac output and ventricular contractility, and chronic QTc prolongation during and following SE were prevented by β₁-adrenergic blockade during the seizure. Furthermore, prevention of these cardiac effects protected

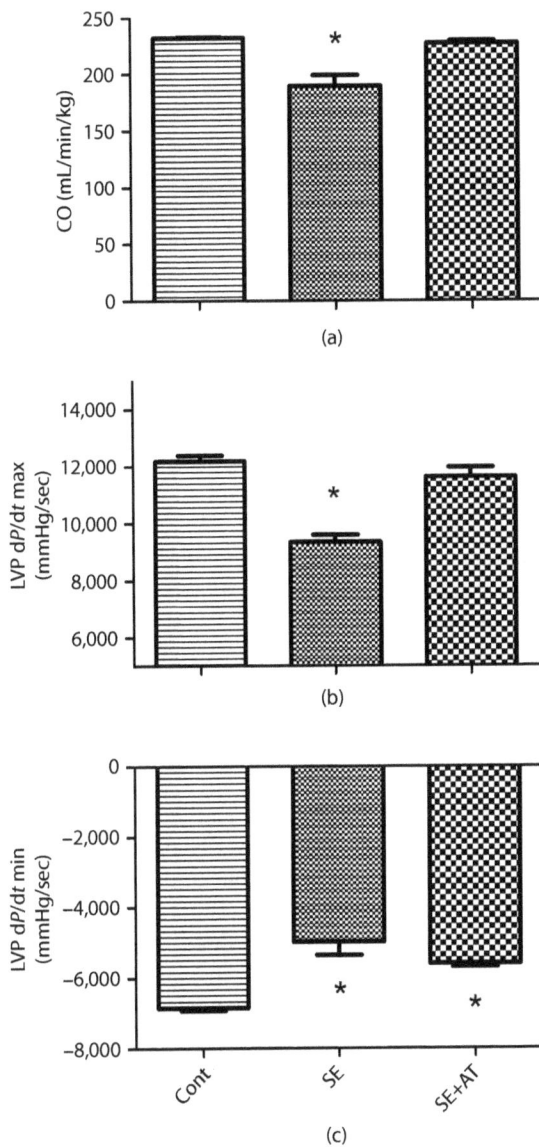

**FIGURE 23.2** Cardiac output, (a) left ventricular pressure (LVP) max (b) and LVP min (c) 24 hours following treatment in status epilepticus (SE) rats given vehicle (SE) or atenolol (SE+AT), and control animals (Cont). $^{*}p < .05$ compared to Cont and SE+AT. (From Little, JG and SL Bealer, *Epilepsy Res*, 99, 233–9, 2012. With permission.)

and water ingestion, but they still exhibit arrhythmogenic cardiac effects (Metcalf et al. 2009b; Bealer et al. 2010). QTc prolongation is a well-recognized indicator of risk for sudden cardiac death (Darbar et al. 1996; Chugh et al. 2009).

SE caused a chronic increase in QTc interval (Figure 23.3) compared to control rats given either vehicle or atenolol. Furthermore, lengthening of the QTc interval by SE was prevented by atenolol (1 mg/kg) administration. These data demonstrate that β₁-adrenergic blockade prevents arrhythmogenic changes in cardiac repolarization induced by SE and suggest that ictal SymNS activation induces cardiac electrical dysfunction that increases susceptibility to lethal arrhythmias.

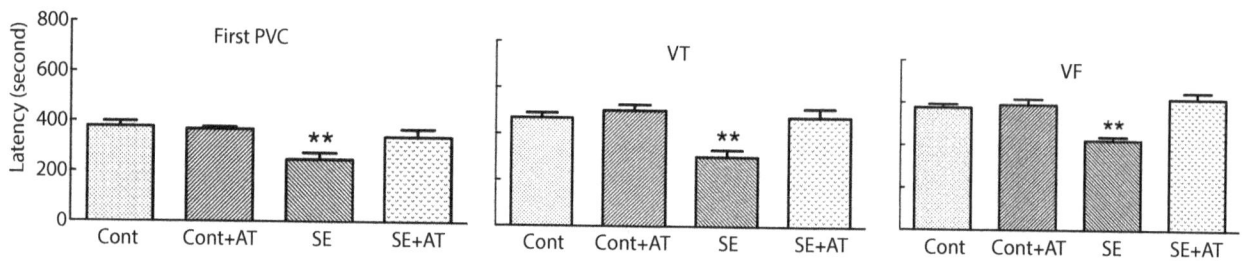

**FIGURE 23.4** Latency to first premature ventricular contraction (PVC), ventricular tachycardia (VT), and ventricular fibrillation (VF) in animals undergoing SE and treated with vehicle (SE) or atenolol (SE+AT) compared to similarly treated control rats (Cont; Cont+AT). **$p < .01$ compared to all other groups. (From Bealer, SL et al., *Epilepsy Res*, 91, 66–73, 2010. With permission.)

animals from increased susceptibility to experimentally induced arrhythmias.

Previous studies demonstrate that central actions of β-adrenergic blocking agents can reduce seizure activity (Lathers et al. 1989; Luchowska et al. 2002; Nakamura et al. 2008) and inhibit the associated cardiac arrhythmias (Lathers et al. 1989). However, the effect of selective, peripheral blockade of β$_1$-adrenergic receptors on arrhythmogenic effects of seizures was not known. Atenolol was selected for our studies because it is a peripherally acting β$_1$-adrenergic antagonist that does not cross the blood–brain barrier and has no effects on seizure intensity or threshold (De Sarro et al. 2002; Luchowska et al. 2002). Consistent with these reports, the treatment protocol used in our studies did not alter seizure duration or intensity, or evoked central nervous system damage (Bealer et al. 2010; Little and Bealer 2012). Taken together, these data indicate that the cardioprotective effects of peripheral β$_1$-adrenergic blockade were due to diminished stimulation of β$_1$-receptors in the heart, and not to a nonspecific decrease in seizure intensity, in contrast to the cardioprotection following the administration of central β-adrenergic antagonists that may be due to reduced seizure intensity and/or reduced ictal SymNS activation.

A number of previous studies demonstrated that SE produces intense activation of the SymNS both in patients and in animal models (Sakamoto et al. 2008; Shimizu et al. 2008), increasing both heart rate and blood pressure during seizures (Goodman et al. 1990; Johnston et al. 1997; Sakamoto et al. 2008). In patients, SE induces a reversible decrement in cardiac function (Legriel et al. 2008) and increased risk of lethal arrhythmias for a period following seizure activity (Gao et al. 1995; Sato et al. 1999). Data from the studies discussed in this chapter are consistent with the proposal that the cardiac dysfunction and increased risk of lethal arrhythmias observed following SE are due to intense cardiac stimulation by the SymNS during the period of SE. The arrhythmogenic responses produced by SE include cardiomyocyte damage and QT-interval prolongation, likely due to the downregulation of cardiac Kv4.2 potassium channels (Bealer et al. 2010). As both of these effects are prevented by β$_1$-adrenergic receptor blockade, it seems probable that ictal activation of the SymNS mediates these cardiac effects. This interpretation is consistent with the proposal that ischemia resulting from intense positive inotropic and chronotropic tachycardia

in response to catecholamine stimulation produces myocyte damage and results in detrimental effects on cardiac function (Bolli 1990), such as decreased cardiac output and left ventricular contractility (Goodman et al. 1990; Johnston et al. 1997; Sakamoto et al. 2008; Metcalf et al. 2009b).

These studies investigated cardiac effects of the protracted seizures characteristic of SE. However, epilepsy is characterized by multiple much shorter, self-limiting seizures. The role of SymNS activity and β$_1$-adrenergic receptor blockade in cardiac dysfunction and SUDEP is currently unknown. However, similar to SE, isolated epileptic seizures are associated with SymNS activation (Simon et al. 1984) and characterized by tachycardia and increased blood pressure (Di Gennaro et al. 2004; Mayer et al. 2004; Rugg-Gunn et al. 2004; Ryvlin et al. 2006). Furthermore, such seizures can produce myocyte damage (Brobbey and Ravakhah 2004; Stollberger and Finsterer 2004a; Parvulescu-Codrea et al. 2006) and arrhythmogenic changes in repolarization (Kandler et al. 2005; Brotherstone et al. 2009; Surges et al. 2010b). In addition, we found that repeated, self-limiting seizures in kindled rats produce QT-interval prolongation and increased susceptibility to arrhythmias, similar to cardiac dysfunction observed following SE (Bealer and Little 2013). Therefore, both ictal activation of the SymNS and cardiac dysfunction in association with self-limited seizures typical of epilepsy are similar to those described in SE, suggesting that similar mechanisms mediate cardiac related SUDEP. Indeed, it has recently been suggested that risk for lethal arrhythmias in SUDEP is due to progressive cardiac damage sustained by excessive catecholaminergic stimulation during repeated seizures (P-Codrea Tigaran et al. 2005) and that the catecholamine surge during seizures is related, and may be causative, to SUDEP (Stollberger and Finsterer 2004b; P-Codrea Tigaran et al. 2005; Shimizu et al. 2008).

These studies examined the effects of β$_1$-adrenergic blockade on the cardiac effects of stage 4 to 5 seizures during SE. As described in our accompanying chapter (Chapter 24), we observed similar changes in QT interval and susceptibility to experimental arrhythmias following administration of multiple isolated seizures in kindled rats. However, both SE and the isolated seizures in kindled animals examined in these studies were stage 4 to 5 on the Racine scale. Although not yet studied, it is likely that less severe seizure intensity would produce more moderate cardiac effects. Consequently, we would anticipate that patients most at risk for SUDEP routinely experience more severe seizures.

In summary, both SE and isolated epileptic seizures are associated with intense activation of the SymNS. The resulting stimulation of cardiac β₁-adrenergic receptors produces chronotropic and inotropic effects that may induce cardiac ischemia and result in cardiomyocyte damage and cardiac electrical abnormalities that increase the risk of sudden cardiac death. In support of this proposal, studies reported in this chapter demonstrate that blockade of peripheral β₁-adrenergic receptors during SE prevents cardiomyocyte damage, diminished cardiac performance, and QT-interval prolongation. However, the role of the SymNS and β₁-adrenergic receptor stimulation in cardiac dysfunction following the repeated, self-limited seizures characteristic of epilepsy has not been examined.

Many of the cardiac effects characteristic of SE have been reported in patients with epilepsy during seizures (Brotherstone et al. 2009), as well as in the immediate post-ictal (Kandler et al. 2005; Surges et al. 2010a) and interictal (Ramadan et al. 2013) periods. As a result, it has been proposed that the repeated seizures in patients with epilepsy may cause cumulative, progressive cardiac damage that could possibly culminate in cardiac related SUDEP. Although not yet directly tested, we propose that the cardiac effects of repeated, self-limiting seizures are due to ictal SymNS activation and thus could be attenuated or prevented by β₁-adrenergic receptor blockade. Indeed, any drug that attenuates seizure-associated tachycardia may be cardioprotective. Taken together, these data indicate that patients with epilepsy who are at increased risk of SUDEP may benefit from cardioprotective agents shown to diminish the incidence of lethal arrhythmias in other pathological conditions. Specifically, routine administration of β₁-adrenergic antagonists and electrocardiographic evaluation of cardiac function may reduce the incidence of lethal arrhythmias and detrimental cardiac adaptations associated with both SE and epilepsy.

# REFERENCES

Anderson KP. Sympathetic nervous system activity and ventricular tachycardias: Recent advances. *Ann Noninvasive Electrocardiol* 2003;8:75–89.

Antman EM. Decision making with cardiac troponin tests. *New England J Med* 2002;346:2079–82.

Bealer SL, Little JG. Seizures following hippocampal kindling induce QT interval prolongation and increased susceptibility to arrhythmias in rats. *Epilepsy Res* 2013;105:216–9.

Bealer SL, Little JG, Metcalf CS, Brewster AL, Anderson AE. Autonomic and cellular mechanisms mediating detrimental cardiac effects of status epilepticus. *Epilepsy Res* 2010;91:66–73.

Boggs JG, Painter JA, DeLorenzo RJ. Analysis of electrocardiographic changes in status epilepticus. *Epilepsy Res* 1993;14:87–94.

Boggs JG, Marmarou A, Agnew JP, Morton LD, Towne AR, Waterhouse EJ, Pellock JM, DeLorenzo RJ. Hemodynamic monitoring prior to and at the time of death in status epilepticus. *Epilepsy Res* 1998;31:199–209.

Bolli R. Mechanisms of myocardial "stunning." *Circulation* 1990;82:173–738.

Brobbey A, Ravakhah K. Elevated serum cardiac troponin I level in a patent after a grand mal seizure and with no evidence of cardiac disease. *Am J Med Sci* 2004;328:189–91.

Brotherstone R, Blackhall B, McLellan A. Lengthening of corrected QT during epileptic seizures. *Epilepsia* 2009;51:221–32.

Chugh SS, Reiner K, Singh T, Uy-Evanado A, Socoteanu C, Peters D, Mariani R, Gunson K, Jui J. Determinants of prolonged QT interval and their contribution to sudden death risk in coronary artery disease: The Oregon sudden unexpected death study. *Circulation* 2009;119:663–70.

Darbar D, Luck J, Davidson N, Pringle T, Main G, McNeill G, Struthers AD. Sensitivity and specificity of QTc dispersion for identification of risk of cardiac death in patients with peripheral vascular disease. *BMJ* 1996;312:874–8.

De Sarro G, Di Paola ED, Ferreri G, De Sarro A, Fischcher W. Influence of some beta-adrenoceptor antagonists on the anticonvulsant protency of antiepileptic drugs against audiogenic seizures in DBA/2 mice. *Eur J Pharmacol* 2002;442:205–13.

Di Gennaro G, Quarato PP, Sebastiano F, Esposito V, Onorati P, Grammaldo LG, Meldolesi GN et al. Ictal heart rate increase precedes EEG discharge in drug-resistant mesial temporal lobe seizures. *Clin Neurophysiol* 2004;115:1169–77.

Dorian P. Antiarrhythmic action of B-blockers: Potential mechanisms. *J Cardiovasc Pharmacol Therapeut* 2005;10(Suppl 1): S15–22.

Gao WD, Atar D, Backx PH, Marban E. Relationoship between intracellular calcium and contractile force in stunned myocardium. Direct evidence for decreased myofilament Ca2+ responsiveness and altered diastolic function in intact ventricular muscle. *Circ Res* 1995;76:1036–48.

Glien M, Brandt B, Potschke P, Voigt H, Ebert U, Loscher W. Repeated low dose treatment of rats with pilocarpine: Low mortality but high proportion of rats developing epilepsy. *Epilepsy Res* 2001;46:111–9.

Goodman JH, Homan RW, Crawford IL. Kindled seizures elevate blood pressure and induce cardiac arrhythmias. *Epilepsia* 1990;31:489–95.

Grippo AJ, Santos CM, Johnson RF, Beltz TG, Martins JB, Felder RB, Johnson AK. Increased susceptibility to ventricular arrhythmias in a rodent model of experimental depression. *Am J Physiol* 2004;286:H619–26.

Hohnloser SH. Ventricular arrhythmias: Antiadrenergic therapy for the patient with coronary artery disease. *J Cardiovasc Pharmacol Therapeut* 2005;10(Suppl 1):S23–31.

Johnston SC, DSiedenberg R, Min JK, Jerome EH, Laxer KD. Central apnea and acute cardiac ischemia in a sheep model of epileptic sudden death. *Ann Neurol* 1997;42:588–94.

Kandler L, Fiedler A, Scheer K, Wild F, Frick U, Schneider P. Early post-convulsive prolongation of QT time in children. *Acta Paediatr* 2005;94:1243–7.

Kanter RK, Strauss JA, Sauro MD. Comparison of neurons in rat medulla oblongata with fos immunoreactivity evoked by seizures, chemoreceptor, or baroreceptor stimulation. *Neurosci* 1996;73:807–16.

Kreisman NR, Gauthier-Lewis ML, Conklin SG, Voss NF, Barbee RW. Cardiac output and regioinal hemodynamics during recurrent seizures in rats. *Brain Res* 1993;626:295–302.

Kulkarni SK, George B. Lithium-pilocarpine neurotoxicity: A potential model of status epilepticus. *Methods Find Exp Clin Pharamacol* 1995;17:551–67.

Kurata M, Iidaka T, Sasayama Y, Fukushima T, Sakimura M, Shirai N. Correlation among clinicopathological parameters of myocardial damage in rats treated with isoproterenol. *Exp Anim* 2007;56:57–62.

Lathers CM, Schraeder PL. Clinical pharmacology: Drugs as a benefit and/or risk in sudden unexpected death in epilepsy? *J Clin Pharmacol* 2002;42:123–6.

Lathers CM, Stauffer AZ, Tumer N, Kraras CM, Goldman BD. Anticonvulsant and antiarrhythmic actions of the beta blocking agent timolol. *Epilepsy Res* 1989;4:42–54.

Legriel S, Bruneel F, Dalle L, Apere-de-Vecchi C, Georges JL, Abbosh N, Hernry-Lagarrigue M et al. Recurrent Takotsubo cardiomyopathy triggered by convulsive status epilepticus. *Neurocrit Care* 2008;9:118–21.

Leung H, Kwan P, Elger CE. Finding the missing link between ictal bradyarrhythmia, ictal asystole, and sudden unexpected death in epilepsy. *Epilepsy Behav* 2006;9:19–30.

Little JG, Bealer SL. B-adrenergic blockade prevents cardiac dysfunction following status epilepticus in rats. *Epilepsy Res* 2012;99:233–9.

Luchowska E, Luchowska P, Wielosz M, Kleinrok Z, Czuczwar SJ, Urbanska EM. Propranolol and metopropolol enhance the anticonvulsant action of valproate and diazepam against maximal electroshock. *Pharmacol Biochem Behav* 2002; 71:223–31.

Manno EM, Pfeifer EA, Cascino GD, Noe KH, Wijdicks EFM. Cardiac pathology in status epilepticus. *Ann Neurol* 2005; 58:954–7.

Mayer H, Benninger F, Urak L, Plattner B, Geldner J, Feucht M. EKG abnormalities in children and adolsecence with symptomatic temporal lobe epilepsy. *Neurology* 2004;63:324–8.

Metcalf CS, Radwanski PB, Bealer SL. Status epileticus produces chronic alterations in cardiac sympathovagal balance. *Epilepsia* 2009a;50:747–54.

Metcalf CS, Poelzing S, Little JG, Bealer SL. Status epilepticus induces cardiac myofilament damage and increased susceptibility to arrhythmias in rat. *Am J Physiol* 2009b;297:H2120–7.

Nakamura T, Oda Y, Takahashi R, Tanaka K, Hase I, Asada A. Propranolol increases the threshold for lidocaine-induced convulsions in awake rats: A direct effect on the brain. *Anesth Analg* 2008;106:1450–5.

Nei M, Ho RT, Abou-Khalil BW, Drislane FW, Liporace J, Romeo A, Sperling MR. EEG and ECG in sudden unexplained death in epilepsy. *Epilepsia* 2004;45:338–45.

Nissinen JT, Halonen T, Kolvisto E, Pitkanen A. A new model of chronic temporal lobe epilepsy induced by electrical stimulation of the amygdala in rat. *Epilepsy Res* 2000;38:177–205.

O'Brien PJ, Smith DEC, Knechtel TJ, Marchak MA, Pruimboom-Brees I, Brees DJ, Spratt DP et al. Cardiac troponin I is a sensitive, specific biomarker of cardiac injury in laboratory animals. *Lab Anim* 2006;40:153–71.

P-Codrea Tigaran S, Dalager-Pedersen S, Baandrup U, Dam M, Vesterby-Charles A. Sudden unexpected death in epilepsy: Is death by seizures a cardiac event? *Am J Forensic Med Pathol* 2005;26:99–105.

Painter JA, Shiel FO, DeLorenzo RJ. Cardiac pathology findings in status epilepticus. *Epilepsia* 1993;34(Suppl 6):30.

Parvulescu-Codrea S, Britton JW, Bruce CJ, Cascino GD, Jaffe AS. Elevations of troponin in patients with epileptic seizures? What do they mean? *Clin Cardiol* 2006;29:325–6.

Ramadan M, El-Shahat N, Omar A, Gomaa M, Belal T, Sakr S, Abu-Hegazy M, Hakim H, Selim H, Omar S. Interictal electrocardiographic and echocardiographic changes in patients with generalized tonic-clonic seizures. *Int Heart J* 2013;54:171–5.

Rugg-Gunn FJ, Simister RJ, Squirrell M, Holdbright DR, Duncan JS. Cardiac arrhythmias in focal epilepsy: A prospective long-term study. *Lancet* 2004;364:2212–9.

Ryvlin P, Montavont A, Kahane P. Sudden unexplained death in epilepsy: From mechanisms to prevention. *Curr Opin Neurol* 2006;19:194–9.

Sakamoto K, Saito T, Orman R, Koizumi K, Lazar J, Salciccioli L, Stewart M. Autonomic consequences of kainic acid-induced limbic cortical seizures in rats: Peripheral autonomic nerve activity, acute cardiovascular changes, and death. Epilepsia 2008;49:982–96.

Sarko J, Pollack CV. Cardiac troponins. *J Emerg Med* 2002;23:57–65.

Sato K, Masuda T, Izumi T. Subarachnoid hemorrhage and myocardial damage: Clinical and experimental studies. *Jpn Heart J* 1999;40:683–701.

Shimizu M, Kagawa A, Takano T, Masai H, Miwa Y. Neurogenic stunned myocardium associated with status epilepticus and postictal catecholamine surge. *Intern Med* 2008;47:269–73.

Shu H, Yi-Ming W, Xu LP, Miao CY, Su DF. Increased susceptibility of ventricular arrhythmias to aconitine in anaesthetized rats in attributed to the inhibition of baroreflex. *Clin Exp Pharmacol Physiol* 2004;31;249–53.

Simon RP, Aminoff MJ, Benowitz NL. Changes in plasma catecholamines after tonic-clonic seizures. *Neurology* 1984;34:255–7.

Stollberger C, Finsterer J. Cardiac troponin levels following monitored seizures. Neurology 2004a;62:1453.

Stollberger C, Finsterer J. Cardiorespiratory findings in sudden unexplained/unexpected death in epilepsy (SUDEP). *Epilepsy Res* 2004b;59:51–60.

Surges R, Scott CA, Walker MC. Enhanced QT shortening and persistent tachycardia after generalized siezures. *Neurology* 2010a;74:421–6.

Surges R, Taggart P, Sander JW, Walker MC. Too long or too short? New insights into abnormal cardiac repolarization in people with chronic epilepsy and its potential role in sudden unexpected death. *Epilepsia* 2010b;51:738–44.

Walton NY. Systemic effects of generalized convulsive status epilepticus. *Epilepsia* 1993;34(Suppl 1):S54–8.

# 24 Cardiac Myocyte Damage, Electrocardiographic Dysfunction, and Ion Channel Remodeling in Rodent Models of Seizure Disorders

*Steven L. Bealer, Cameron S. Metcalf, Steven Poelzing,
Jason G. Little, Amy Brewster, and Anne Anderson*

## CONTENTS

## CARDIAC MORTALITY IN SEIZURE DISORDERS

Seizure disorders can increase cardiac morbidity and mortality. Both status epilepticus (SE), a single seizure or single series of rapidly recurring seizures lasting more than 30 minutes (Shorvon 1994; Logroscino et al. 2005), and the much shorter, but chronically recurring seizures of epilepsy increase the risk of sudden cardiac death (Lathers and Schraeder 2002; So 2008; Devinsky 2011). Death in individuals with epilepsy can occur suddenly and without explanation, known as sudden unexpected death in epilepsy (SUDEP) (Lathers and Schraeder 2002; So 2008; Devinsky 2011). Although the mechanisms of seizure-related mortality are not fully understood, lethal arrhythmias appear to contribute to death during and following SE (Walton 1993; Boggs et al. 1998), and to SUDEP (Lathers and Schraeder 2002; Nei et al. 2004; Ryvlin et al. 2006).

## PREDISPOSING FACTORS FOR VENTRICULAR ARRHYTHMIAS

Sudden cardiac death can result from physiological facilitators acting on myocyte substrates that trigger lethal arrhythmias (Campbell 1991; Willich et al. 1993). Cardiac substrates for arrhythmias can be anatomical, functional, and/or electrophysiological abnormalities of cardiomyocytes (Campbell 1991; Willich et al. 1993). For example, damaged myocardium or altered cardiac electrical activity, such as QT interval prolongation, can serve as substrates for triggered, life-threatening arrhythmias and sudden cardiac death (Kloner and Jennings 2001; Fallavollita et al. 2005; Pizzuto et al. 2006). Although earlier studies

indicate that seizure activity may cause myocyte damage (Woodruff et al. 2003; Brobbey and Ravakhah 2004; Stollberger and Finsterer 2004; Parvulescu-Codrea et al. 2006) and cardiac electrical dysfunction, including QT interval prolongation (Brotherstone et al. 2009; Surges et al. 2010; Isik et al. 2011; Seyal et al. 2011) in patients, the contributions of seizures to generation of arrhythmogenic substrates have not been fully elucidated. This chapter describes our studies using animal models of SE and epilepsy to evaluate the effects of seizures on cardiac myocyte damage and cardiac electrical activity.

### SEIZURE-INDUCED ARRHYTHMOGENIC SUBSTRATES

#### Myocyte Damage Following Status Epilepticus

Several studies have indicated that epileptic seizures can increase plasma concentrations of troponin I levels (Woodruff et al. 2003; Brobbey and Ravakhah 2004; Stollberger and Finsterer 2004; Parvulescu-Codrea et al. 2006,), indicative of cardiac myocyte damage. We have extended this area of investigation by combining analysis of plasma concentrations of troponin I with histological staining of cardiac tissue from animals following 60 minutes of SE induced by treatment with pilocarpine. Plasma troponin I concentrations are significantly elevated within 60 minutes of cardiac injury in rats (York et al. 2007).

Arterial blood was obtained from animals following 60 minutes of continuous seizure activity and analyzed for cardiac troponin I concentration. Furthermore, to determine if SE produced gross anatomical damage to cardiac myocytes, we stained cardiac tissue for hematoxylin-eosin

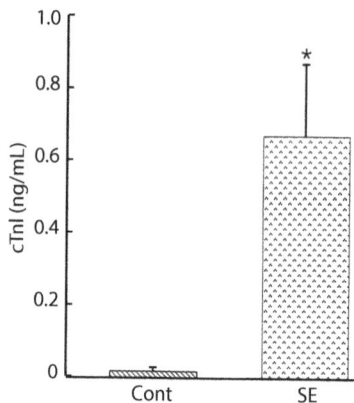

**FIGURE 24.1** Plasma troponin I concentrations in control (Cont) rats and animals following 60 minutes of status epilepticus (SE). $^*p < .01$ compared to Cont. (Reprinted from Metcalf, CS et al., *Am J Physiol*, 297, H2120–7, 2009. With permission.)

(H&E) and terminal deoxynucleotidyl transferase-mediated dUTP-biotin nick end labeling (TUNEL) in hearts taken from animals following 90 minutes of seizure activity. Hearts were classified as H&E and/or TUNEL positive if any image exhibited positive staining. Hearts with no observable H&E or TUNEL positive in any image were classified as negative.

Figure 24.1 demonstrates that plasma troponin I concentration is significantly elevated in rats following 60 minutes of SE, suggestive of damage to cardiac myocytes. Analyses of H&E staining in transversely sliced tissue from the anterior left ventricular subepicardium showed that contraction band necrosis, deposition of fibrotic tissue, and other gross structural changes (positive H&E stain) were not observed in any image section obtained from control or SE animals (Figure 24.2a). In distinction, positive TUNEL staining was present in both control rats and SE animals (Figure 24.2b). Although images from control animals were predominantly TUNEL negative, sections obtained from two of nine control rats showed some TUNEL-positive staining. However, the number of hearts from SE rats demonstrating TUNEL-positive staining was significantly higher than control animals (Figure 24.2c). It is important to note that TUNEL-positive staining in post-ictal rats ranged from diffuse and localized in small regions of the myocardium (Figure 24.2b, center) to strong TUNEL staining distributed more widely throughout the section (Figure 24.2b, right).

These anatomical results are consistent with increased troponin I concentrations and demonstrate that SE can cause subtle myocyte damage that may increase susceptibility to life-threatening arrhythmias, with little or no gross anatomical or structural cardiac damage.

## QT Interval Prolongation and Susceptibility to Arrhythmias in Kindled Rats

We previously demonstrated that the protracted seizures of SE result in arrhythmogenic alterations in cardiac function, including QT interval prolongation and increased

susceptibility to experimentally induced arrhythmias (Metcalf et al. 2009; Bealer et al. 2010). We extended these studies to determine effects of self-limiting seizures in rats following hippocampal kindling, a model of human epilepsy, on electrocardiographic activity and susceptibility to experimental arrhythmias.

Rats underwent rapid hippocampal kindling using previously described techniques (Lothman et.al. 1985; Lothman and Williamson 1993). After kindling, some kindled rats were administered six to eight stage 4 to 5 (Racine scale) motor seizures (K-MS) on Monday, Wednesday, and Friday for 2 consecutive weeks. A separate group of animals underwent kindling but were not given subsequent seizures (K-Cont). A final group of animals received all surgical procedures but did not undergo kindling or seizures (Cont). At 4–6 days following the final day of seizure administration (K-MS) or the control period (K-Cont; Cont), all animals were prepared for evaluation of electrocardiograms. In addition, to determine susceptibility to experimentally induced cardiac arrhythmias, the latencies to premature ventricular contraction (PVC), ventricular tachycardia, and ventricular fibrillation during continuous intravenous infusion of the arrhythmogenic agent, aconitine, were measured.

K-MS rats had a total of 35–48 seizures. Figure 24.3 shows QT intervals adjusted for heart rate (QTc) measured in Cont, K-Cont, and K-MS animals. K-MS rats demonstrated significant QTc interval prolongation compared to both Cont and K-Cont animals.

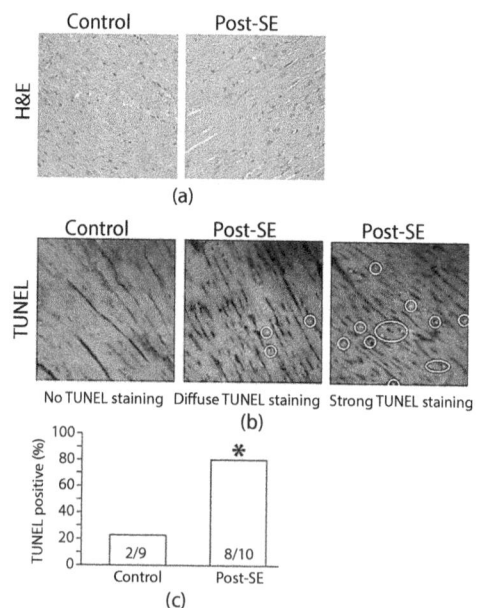

**FIGURE 24.2** Representative images of (a) H&E- and (b) TUNEL-stained myocardial sections from control and status epilepticus (SE) animals. Panel C represents summary data of percentage of animals demonstrating positive TUNEL staining. $^*p < .05$ compared to control. (Reprinted from Metcalf, CS et al., *Am J Physiol*, 297, H2120–7, 2009. With permission.)

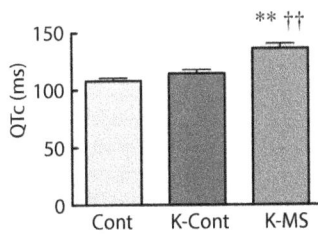

**FIGURE 24.3** Adjusted QT interval in control (Cont) animals and kindled rats given no seizures (K-Cont) or administered seizures (K-MS). **,†† $p < .01$ re: Cont, K-Cont. (Reprinted from Bealer, SL and Little JG, *Epilepsy Res*, 105, 216–219, 2013. With permission.)

Figure 24.4 illustrates the latencies between the initiation of aconitine infusion and the first primary ventricular contraction, ventricular tachycardia, and ventricular fibrillation. All three arrhythmias occurred significantly sooner in K-MS rats than in Cont or K-Cont animals. These data indicate that repeated seizures in kindled animals cause significant QT interval prolongation, which is associated with increased susceptibility to cardiac arrhythmias.

## Cardiac Channel Remodeling Following Status Epilepticus

The cardiac mechanisms responsible for the seizure-related changes in QT interval that we observed in animal models of seizure disorders are unknown. One potential contributing mechanism is seizure-induced cardiomyocyte ion channel remodeling. In the heart, Kv4.x channels are critical for repolarization of myocytes (Birnbaum et al. 2004). Decreased expression of these channels is reported in several cardiomyopathies characterized by an increased risk of sudden cardiac death, including myocardial infarction (Kaprielian et al. 1999), ventricular hypertrophy (Kassiri et al. 2002), and diabetes (Xu et al. 1996). Earlier studies demonstrated that Kv4.2 channels are decreased in neuronal tissue following SE (Birnbaum et al. 2004; Lugo et al. 2008; Su et al. 2008). In addition, we have previously shown that Kv4.2 knockout mice have a decrease in seizure threshold and experience sudden unexplained death following chemoconvulsant stimulation (Barnwell et al. 2009). However, changes in Kv4.x channels in cardiac tissue following SE had not been investigated. Thus, we proposed that one candidate mechanism underlying the arrhythmogenic electrical activity and

increased susceptibility to arrhythmias following SE is cardiac ion channel remodeling, specifically Kv4.x channel downregulation.

The protein levels of cardiac Kv4.2 and Kv4.3 channels were evaluated in hearts obtained from Cont rats and animals subjected to 90 minutes of SE, 1 week and 2 weeks following treatment. The optical densities of immunoreactive bands following Western blotting for Kv4.2 and Kv4.3 protein levels, normalized to GapDH levels, were evaluated. Figure 24.5 shows Western blot analyses of Kv4.2 and Kv4.3 potassium channels in cardiac tissue 1 week and 2 weeks following SE or control procedures. Protein levels for Kv4.2 channels were significantly decreased by more than 60% both 1 week and 2 weeks following SE, compared to control animals. In contrast, protein levels for Kv4.3 channels are unchanged following seizures. Thus, we conclude that ion channel remodeling of Kv4.2 potassium channels in cardiomyocytes results from seizure activity and may account for arrhythmogenic changes in repolarization that contribute to sudden death in seizure disorders.

These findings confirm and extend earlier reports that seizure activity can result in the generation of well-accepted cardiac substrates for lethal arrhythmias. Specifically, cardiac myocyte damage and electrocardiographic dysfunction are present in animal models of seizure activity. Furthermore, these data indicate that the mechanism of QT interval prolongation is downregulation of Kv4.2 potassium channels in these models of seizure disorders. In conclusion, these cardiac responses to seizures can provide the cardiac substrates promoting arrhythmias.

## ICTAL FACILITATORS OF ARRHYTHMIAS

### Ictal Sympathetic Nervous System Activation

It is well recognized that increased sympathetic nervous system (SymNS) activity, particularly acting on abnormal cardiac tissue, significantly increases the risk of lethal ventricular arrhythmias and sudden death (Anderson 2003; Dorian 2005; Hohnloser 2005). Numerous reports have demonstrated that seizure activity is associated with intense SymNS activation during SE in humans (Shimizu et al. 2008; Walton 1993) and animals (Kreisman et al. 1993; Kanter et al. 1996; Sakamoto et al. 2008). Similar to the seizure activity of SE, the self-limiting seizures of epilepsy also produce SymNS activation (Simon et al. 1984; Di Gennaro

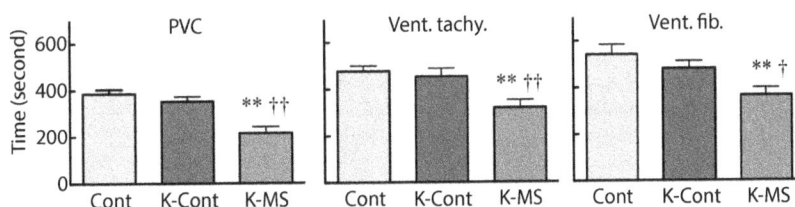

**FIGURE 24.4** Latency to aconitine-induced premature ventricular contraction (PVC), ventricular tachycardia (Vent. tachy.), and ventricular fibrillation (Vent. fib.) in control (Cont), kindled control (K-Cont), and kindled animals administered motor seizures (K-MS). **,†† $p < .01$ re: Cont, K-Cont; † $p < .05$ re: K-Cont. (Reprinted from Bealer, SL and Little, JG, *Epilepsy Res*, 105, 216–219, 2013. With permission.)

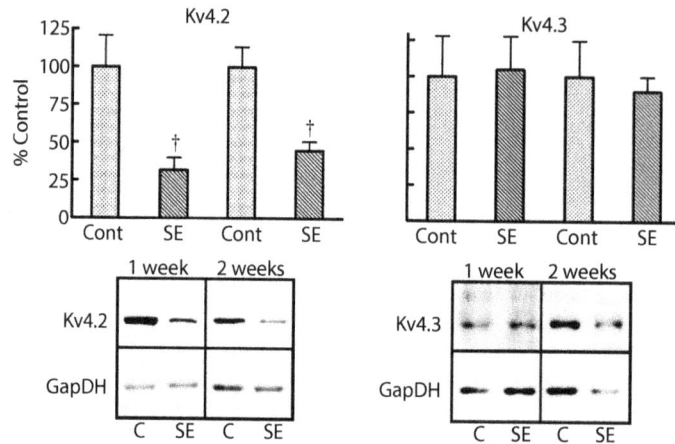

**FIGURE 24.5** Western blot analyses of Kv4.2 and Kv4.3 potassium channel proteins in cardiac tissue obtained 1 week or 2 weeks following seizure status epilepticus (SE) or control (Cont) procedures. $^\dagger p < .01$ re: Cont. (Reprinted from Bealer, SL et al., *Epilepsy Res*, 91, 66–73, 2010. With permission.)

et al. 2004; Mayer et al. 2004; Rugg-Gunn et al. 2004; Ryvlin et al. 2006). These reports are consistent with the proposal that seizures of SE and epilepsy induce SymNS activation, which may act on damaged or dysfunctional cardiac tissue to initiate a lethal arrhythmia and could produce death following SE or SUDEP.

## Ictal Hypoxemia

In addition to increased SymNS activity, seizures are associated with respiratory distress due to peripheral pulmonary effects and decreased central respiratory drive (Johnston et al. 1997; Langan et al. 2000; Tomson et al. 2008; Bateman et al. 2010). Impaired respiration results in hypoxemia, i.e., decreased plasma $O_2$ saturation ($SaO_2$), which reduces $O_2$ delivery to the heart and thus enhances cardiac hypoxia, a facilitator of arrhythmias. In one study of monitored patients during presurgical workups, clinically significant falls in $SaO_2$ occurred in one-third of patients during seizures (Bateman et al. 2008), and some patients exhibited severe hypoxemia with $SaO_2$ falling below 60% (Seyal et al. 2010). Furthermore, arrhythmogenic changes in cardiac function, characterized by QT interval prolongation, were significantly more likely to occur during seizures associated with decreased $SaO_2$ than during seizures with no oxygen desaturation (Seyal et al. 2011). Finally, there is a positive association between duration of oxygen desaturation, QT interval prolongation, and death (Seyal et al. 2011). These data suggest that respiratory depression, associated ictal hypoxemia, and the resulting arrhythmogenic changes in cardiac repolarization (QT prolongation) contribute to SUDEP. We propose that in addition to SymNS activation ictal hypoxemia acts as a facilitator on cardiac substrates to promote cardiac arrhythmias.

## SUMMARY

These studies have demonstrated that seizure activity results in cardiac tissue damage and electrocardiographic abnormalities, which can serve as substrates for potentially lethal,

triggered cardiac arrhythmias. Furthermore, seizure-induced electrocardiographic dysfunction, i.e., QT interval prolongation, represents a ventricular repolarization abnormality resulting from decreased expression of cardiac Kv4.x potassium channels. Finally, generation of these arrhythmogenic cardiac substrates increases susceptibility to cardiac arrhythmias.

Based on these studies utilizing animal models of seizure activity (Metcalf et al. 2009; Bealer et al. 2010; Little and Bealer 2012) and reports from the clinical literature, we propose the model for development of cardiac dysfunction and arrhythmias resulting in SE-related mortality and SUDEP that is presented in Figure 24.6. Specifically, we hypothesize that during SE the continuous exposure to the arrhythmogenic facilitators SymNS activation and hypoxemia induces a progressively severe repolarization abnormality and myocyte damage over the duration of the continuous seizure (pathway 2, Figure 24.6). The increasingly severe cardiac dysfunction and damage eventually becomes sufficient to induce a lethal, triggered arrhythmia in response to facilitator presence either during or following seizure activity (pathway 1, Figure 24.6). The proposed critical role of SymNS activation is supported by studies described in our accompanying chapter (Chapter 23), which demonstrate that seizure-related cardiac dysfunction is prevented by $\beta_1$-adrenergic blockade.

Similarly, we hypothesize that SUDEP events involving cardiac arrhythmias in patients with epilepsy also result from activation of pathway 1, Figure 24.6. However, in human epilepsy we propose that the cardiac substrates (repolarization

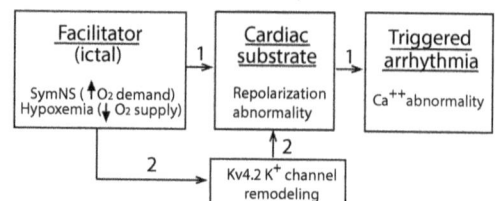

**FIGURE 24.6** Proposed model for generation of seizure-associated cardiac arrhythmias.

abnormality and myocyte damage) develop and become progressively more severe in response to repeated exposure to ictal SymNS activation and hypoxemia occurring during each of the multiple, self-limiting seizures (pathway 2, Figure 24.6). As the cumulative effects of repeated seizures in epilepsy increase the severity of substrate dysfunction, the interaction with the ictal facilitators develops the capacity to induce triggered arrhythmias (pathway 1, Figure 24.6), resulting in SUDEP.

## REFERENCES

Anderson KP. Sympathetic nervous system activity and ventricular tachycardias: Recent advances. *Ann Noninvasive Electrocardiol* 2003;8:75–89.

Barnwell LF, Lugo JN, Lee WL, Willis SE, Gertz SE, Hrachovy RA, Anderson AE. Kv4.2 knockout mice demonstrate increased susceptibility to convulsant stimulation. *Epilepsia* 2009;50:1741–51.

Bateman LM, Li C-S, Seyal M. Ictal hypoxemia in localization-related epilspsy: Analysis of incidence, severity and risk factors. *Brain* 2008;131:3239–45.

Bateman LM, Spitz M, Seyal M. Ictal hypoventilation contributes to cardiac arrhythmia and SUDEP: Report on two deaths in video-EEG-monitored patients. *Epilepsia* 2010;51:916–20.

Bealer SL, Little JG, Metcalf CS, Brewster AL, Anderson AE. Autonomic and cellular mechanisms mediating detrimental cardiac effects of status epilepticus. *Epilepsy Res* 2010;91:66–73.

Bealer SL, Little JG. Seizures following hippocampal kindling induce QT interval prolongation and increased susceptibility to arrhythmias in rats. *Epilepsy Res* 2013;105:216–219.

Birnbaum SG, Varga AW, Yuan L-L, Anderson AE, Sweatt JD, Schraeder LA. Structure and function of the Kv4-family of transient potassium channels. *Physiol Rev* 2004;84:803–33.

Boggs JG, Marmarou A, Agnew JP, Morton LD, Towne AR, Waterhouse EJ, Pellock JM, DeLorenzo RJ. Hemodynamic monitoring prior to and at the time of death in status epilepticus. *Epilepsy Res* 1998;31:199–209.

Brobbey A, Ravakhah K. Elevated serum cardiac troponin I level in a patent after a grand mal seizure and with no evidence of cardiac disease. *Am J Med Sci* 2004;328:189–91.

Brotherstone R, Blackhall B, McLellan A. Lengthening of corrected QT during epileptic seizures. *Epilepsia* 2009;51:221–32.

Campbell RW. Predisposing factors for ventricular arrhythmias. *J Cardiovasc Pharmacol* 1991;17:S9–12.

Devinsky O. Sudden, unexpected death in epilepsy. *N Engl J Med* 2011;365:1801–11.

Di Gennaro G, Quarato PP, Sebastiano F, Esposito V, Onorati P, Grammaldo LG, Meldolesi GN et al. Ictal heart rate increase precedes EEG discharge in drug-resistant mesial temporal lobe seizures. *Clin Neurophysiol* 2004;115:1169–77.

Dorian P. Antiarrhythmic action of B-blockers: Potential mechanisms. *J Cardiovasc Pharmacol Therapeut* 2005;10(Suppl 1): S15–22.

Fallavollita JA, Riegel BJ, Suzuki G, Valeti U, Canty JM, Jr. Mechanism of sudden cardiac death in pigs with viable chronically dysfunctional myocardium and ischemic cardiomyopathy. *Am J Physiol* 2005;289:H2688–96.

Hohnloser SH. Ventricular arrhythmias: Antiadrenergic therapy for the patient with coronary artery disease. *J Cardiovasc Pharmacol Therapeut* 2005; 10(Suppl 1): S23–31.

Isik U, Akyabakan C, Tokel K, Ozek MM. Ictal electrocradiographic changes in children presenting wiht seizures. *Pediatr Int* 2011;54: 27–31.

Johnston SC, DSiedenberg R, Min JK, Jerome EH, Laxer KD. Central apnea and acute cardiac ischemia in a sheep model of epileptic sudden death. *Ann Neurol* 1997;42:588–94.

Kanter RK, Strauss JA, Sauro MD. Comparison of neurons in rat medulla oblongata with fos immunoreactivity evoked by seizures, chemoreceptor, or baroreceptor stimulation. *Neurosci* 1996;73:807–16.

Kaprielian R, Wickenden AD, Kassiri Z, Parker TG, Liu PP, Backx PH. Relationship between $K^+$ channel down-regulation and $[Ca^{2+}]i$ in rat ventricular myocytes following myocardial infarction. *J Physiol* 1999;517:229–45.

Kassiri Z, Zobel C, Nguyen TT, Molkentin JD, Backx PH. Reduction of I (to) causes hypertrophy in neonatal rat ventricular myocytes. *Circ Res* 2002;90:578–85.

Kloner RA, Jennings DB. Consequences of brief ischemia: Stunning, predonditioning, and their clinical implications. *Circulation* 2001;104:158–67.

Kreisman NR, Gauthier-Lewis ML, Conklin SG, Voss NF, Barbee RW. Cardiac output and regioinal hemodynamics during recurrent seizures in rats. *Brain Res* 1993;626:295–302.

Langan Y, Nashef L, Sander JW. Sudden unexpected death in epilepsy: A series of witnessed deaths. *J Neurol Neurosurg Psychiatry* 2000;68:211–3.

Lathers CM, Schraeder PL. Clinical pharmacology: Drugs as a benefit and/or risk in sudden unexpected death in epilepsy? *J Clin Pharmacol* 2002;42:123–6.

Little JG, Bealer SL. B-adrenergic blockade prevents cardiac dysfunction following status epilepticus in rats. *Epilepsy Res* 2012;99:233–9.

Logroscino G, Hesdorffer DC, Cascino G, Hauser WA, Coeytaux A, Glalobardes B, Morabia A, Jallon P. Mortality after a first episode of status epilepticus in the United States and Europe. *Epilepsia* 2005;46:46–8.

Lothman EW, Hatlelid JM, Zorumski CF, Conry JA, Moon PF, Perlin JB. Kindling with rapidly recurring hippocampal seizures. *Brain Res* 1985;360:83–91.

Lothman EW, Williamson JM. Rapid kindling with recurrent hippocampal seizures. *Epilepsy Res* 1993;14:209–20.

Lugo JN, Barnwell LF, Ren Y, Lee WL, Johnston LD, Kim R, Hrachovy RA, Sweatt JD, Andersen AE. Altered phosphorlyation and localization of the A-type channel, Kv4.2 in status epilepticus. *J Neurochem* 2008;106:1929–40.

Mayer H, Benninger F, Urak L, Plattner B, Geldner J, Feucht M. EKG abnormalities in children and adolsecence with symptomatic temporal lobe epilepsy. *Neurology* 2004;63:324–8.

Metcalf CS, Poelzing S, Little JG, Bealer SL. Status epilepticus induces cardiac myofilament damage and increased susceptibility to arrhythmias in rat. *Am J Physiol* 2009;297:H2120–7.

Nei M, Ho RT, Abou-Khalil BW, Drislane FW, Liporace J, Romeo A, Sperling MR. EEG and ECG in sudden unexplained death in epilepsy. *Epilepsia* 2004;45:338–45.

Parvulescu-Codrea S, Britton JW, Bruce CJ, Cascino GD, Jaffe AS. Elevations of troponin in patients with epileptic seizures? What do they mean? *Clin Cardiol* 2006;29:325–6.

Pizzuto MF, Valverde AM, Heavey BM, Banas MD, Michelakis N, Suzuki G, Fallavollita JA, Canty JM, Jr. Brief sympathetic activation precedes the development of ventricular tachycardia and ventricular fibrillation in hibernating myocardium. *J Electrocardiol* 2006;39:S140–5.

Rugg-Gunn FJ, Simister RJ, Squirrell M, Holdbright DR, Duncan JS. Cardiac arrhythmias in focal epilepsy: A prospective long-term study. *Lancet* 2004;364:2212–9.

Ryvlin P, Montavont A, Kahane P. Sudden unexplained death in epilepsy: From mechanisms to prevention. *Curr Opin Neurol* 2006;19:194–9.

Sakamoto K, Saito T, Orman R, Koizumi K, Lazar J, Salciccioli L, Stewart M. Autonomic consequences of kainic acid-induced limbic cortical seizures in rats: Peripheral autonomic nerve activity, acute cardiovascular changes, and death. *Epilepsia* 2008;49:982–96.

Seyal M, Bateman LM, Albertson TE, Lin TC, Li CS. Respiratory changes with seizures in localization-related epilepsy: Analysis of periictal hypercapnia and ariflow patterns. *Epilepsia* 2010;51:1359–64.

Seyal M, Pascual F, Lee C-YM, Li C-S, Bateman LM. Seizure-related cardiac repolarization abnormalities are associated with ictal hypoxemia. *Epilepsia* 2011;52:2105–11.

Shimizu M, Kagawa A, Takano T, Masai H, Miwa Y. Neurogenic stunned myocardium associated with status epilepticus and postictal catecholamine surge. *Intern Med* 2008;47: 269–73.

Shorvon S. *Status Epilepticus: Its Clinical Features and Treatment in Children and Adults.* Cambridge, UK: Cambridge University Press; 1994.

Simon RP, Aminoff MJ, Benowitz NL. Changes in plasma catecholamines after tonic-clonic seizures. *Neurology* 1984;34:255–7.

So E. What is known about the mechanim underlying SUDEP? *Epilepsia* 2008;49(Suppl 9):93–98.

Stollberger C, Finsterer J. Cardiac troponin levels following monitored seizures. *Neurology* 2004;62:1453.

Su T, Cong WD, Long YS, Luo AH, Sun WW, Deng WY, Liao WP. Altered expression of voltage-gated potassium channel 4.2 and voltage-gated potassium channel 4-interacting protein, and changes in intracellular calcium levels following lithium-pilocarpine-indcued status epilepticus. *Neuroscience* 2008;157:566–76.

Surges R, Adjei P, Kallis C, Erhuero J, Scott CA, Bell GS, Sander JW, Walker MC. Pathologic cardiac repolarization in pharmacoresistanct epilepsy and its potential role in sudden unexpected death in epilepsy: A case-control study. *Epilepsia* 2010;51:233–42.

Tomson T, Nashef L, Ryvlin P. Sudden unexpected death in epilepsy: Current knowledge and future directions. *Lancet Neurol* 2008;7:1021–31.

Walton NY. Systemic effects of generalized convulsive status epilepticus. *Epilepsia* 1993;34(Suppl 1):S54–8.

Willich SN, Maclure M, Mittleman M, Arntz H-R, Muller JE. Sudden cardiac death-Support for a role of triggering in causation. *Circulation* 1993;87:1442–50.

Woodruff BK, Britton JW, Tigaran S, Cascino GD, Burritt MF, McConnell JP, Ravkilde J et al. Cardiac troponin levels following monitored epiletic seizures. *Neurology* 2003;60:1690–2.

Xu Z, Patel KP, Rozanski GJ. Metabolic basis of decreased outward K = current in ventricular myocytes from diabetic rats. *Am J Physiol* 1996;271:H2190–6.

York M, Scudamore C, Brady S, Chen C, Wilson S, Curtis M, Evans G et al. Characterization of troponin responses in isoproterenol-induced cardiac injury in the Hanover Wistar rat. *Toxicol Pathol* 2007;35:606–17.

# 25 A Rat Model for Exploring the Contributions of Ventricular Arrhythmias to Sudden Death in Epilepsy

*Isaac Naggar and Mark Stewart*

## CONTENTS

Seizures can weakly or profoundly impact autonomic nervous system (ANS) function. Seizure spread from limbic or neocortical regions through various subcortical structures including hypothalamus and medullary centers impacts sympathetic and parasympathetic divisions to cause diverse systemic effects, including pupillary constriction or dilation, salivation, piloerection, diaphoresis, changes in cardiac rhythm, derangements of peristalsis, and urinary incontinence (Van Buren 1958; Baumgartner et al. 2001; Devinsky 2004). Significant autonomic effects of seizures more commonly occur in association with generalized tonic-clonic seizures or partial seizures originating in the temporal lobe (Opherk et al. 2002; Leutmezer et al. 2003; Devinsky 2004) than in association with absence seizures or focal seizures that minimally impact limbic or insular cortices. The severity of some autonomic effects of seizures makes seizure-induced autonomic derangements and the resulting consequences popular candidates for consideration as contributing to or causing sudden unexpected death in epilepsy (SUDEP) (Lathers et al. 2008; Sakamoto et al. 2008; Devinsky 2011; Stewart 2011; Surges and Sander 2012; Tolstykh and Cavazos 2013).

Multiple studies have sought to define the extent to which the autonomic consequences of seizures alter cardiac rhythm (e.g., Nei et al. 2000; Opherk et al. 2002; Rugg-Gunn et al. 2004). Seizures that produce sinus arrhythmias provoke tachycardia in up to 99% of cases (Schuele 2009), with heart rate (HR) increases to 120–150 bpm (Nei et al. 2004; Rugg-Gunn et al. 2004; Sevcencu and Struijk 2010). Episodes of ictalbradycardia to an HR of 20–40 bpm have been reported (Sevcencu and Struijk 2010). Other changes to cardiac rhythm have been noted during seizures, including premature atrial and ventricular contractions (Nei et al. 2000) and ST-segment changes indicating cardiac ischemia (Tigaran 2002; Tigaran et al. 2003).

Ictalbradycardia has been recognized since the early 1900s (Finny 1906; Russell 1908) and ictalasystole has been observed in a significant number of patients with refractory focal epilepsy (Rugg-Gunn et al. 2004). Asystole in patients with epilepsy is thought to be induced by vagal overactivity (Schuele et al. 2008), as has been demonstrated in animal models (see section "Final Remarks"). Some cases have been treated with implantable pacemakers (Rugg-Gunn et al. 2004; Stokes et al. 2012).

Ictalasystole is a severe cardiac outcome of seizures that has been documented in human and animal research and is thought to be an important clue toward a mechanistic explanation of SUDEP (Schuele 2009; So 2008). Interestingly, animal studies that demonstrate severe bradycardia have also shown that these bradyarrhythmias are capable of reducing cardiac output and cerebral perfusion, which terminates the underlying seizure and thus permits a return to normal sinus rhythm (Sakamoto et al. 2008; Hotta et al. 2010; Stewart 2011). In patients with epilepsy, a similar sequence of cerebral hypoperfusion due to ictalasystole terminating the seizure has also been suggested (Moseley et al. 2011; Schuele et al. 2010).

Seizures produce significant respiratory changes in addition to their cardiac effects. Ictal apnea has long been recognized (Blum 2009), and it results in oxygen desaturation during seizures (Bateman et al. 2008; Seyal et al. 2010). Brainstem serotonergic respiratory circuits may be involved in ictal hypoxemia (see Chapter 26), as patients taking selective serotonin reuptake inhibitors (SSRIs) experienced better oxygen saturation during seizures compared to those patients with epilepsy not on SSRIs (Bateman et al. 2010). The protective action of SSRIs or specific serotonergic agonists has been studied extensively in mice (Faingold et al. 2010, 2011). Earlier studies in sheep established the importance of ictal hypoxemia in seizure-induced death: ictal hypoventilation led to severe bradycardia and death (Johnston et al. 1995, 1997). Similar findings have been demonstrated in rats

(Sakamoto et al. 2008; Stewart 2011), mice (Faingold et al. 2010; Uteshev et al. 2010), and cats (Lathers and Schraeder 1982; Schraeder and Lathers 1983).

## CHRONIC AUTONOMIC AND CARDIAC CHANGES FROM SEIZURES

A challenging problem has been determining whether and defining to what extent seizures have a cumulative and lasting impact on autonomic or cardiac function. Patients with temporal lobe epilepsy exhibit reduced baroreflex sensitivity as compared to controls (Dutsch et al. 2006). A meta-analysis of heart rate variability (HRV) studies in epilepsy concluded that vagal tone is lower in epilepsy patients than in controls (Lotufo et al. 2012). In addition, an HRV study of patients at high risk for SUDEP revealed an inverse correlation between vagal tone by HRV and risk of SUDEP (DeGiorgio et al. 2010).

A growing body of evidence indicates changes in cardiac repolarization during seizures, as QT interval prolongation (Tavernor et al. 1996; Seyal et al. 2010) and ST segment changes (Tigaran et al. 1997; Nei et al. 2000; Tigaran et al. 2003) have been noted to occur during seizures. Cardiac repolarization abnormalities during seizures, in addition, may be related to ictal hypoxemia (Bateman et al. 2008; Seyal et al. 2011). Increased QT interval length and increased QT dispersion also have been noted during interictal EKG recordings from epileptic patients as compared to controls (Akalin et al. 2003; Neufeld et al. 2009; Dogan et al. 2010; Surges et al. 2010; Ramadan et al. 2013). QT interval prolongation and increased QT dispersion may be associated with increased risk for ventricular arrhythmias (e.g., Day et al. 1990; Schouten et al. 1991), but this association and the value of QT interval measurements for predicting risk remain controversial (e.g., Malik and Batchvarov 2000, Food and Drug Administration, HHS 2005). These repolarization findings suggest that beta-adrenergic blocking agents, a drug class used for the treatment of long QT syndrome, may be useful for cardiogenic SUDEP prevention by addressing the repolarization derangements. Beta-blockade has also been suggested as a preventive treatment for patients to combat possible consequences of tachycardia during seizures (Opherk et al. 2002), a finding shown much earlier in animals in which beta-blockade had both antiarrhythmic and anticonvulsant effects (Lathers et al. 1989).

Animal studies support the concept of altered interictal autonomic tone leading to persistent cardiac abnormalities. In rats, 2 weeks after lithium/pilocarpine-induced status epilepticus (SE), it was found that a period of SE could cause increased sympathetic tone, as determined by the evaluation of basal HR (HR due to resting autonomic inputs) and intrinsic HR (HR in the absence of all autonomic inputs; i.e., after combined atenolol and atropine administration) (Metcalf et al. 2009b). This evaluation pointed clearly to a shift in sympathovagal balance toward relatively increased sympathetic influence. Decreased cardiac contractility in these rats could be prevented in this model by administering atenolol with the convulsant (Little

and Bealer 2012), implying sympathetically-mediated long-term cardiac effects of seizures. In the same model, it was found that in the period soon after SE, QT intervals were increased and the rats required a lower dose of aconitine, an arrhythmogenic drug, to induce ventricular fibrillation (VF) than did controls (Metcalf et al. 2009a).

Human autopsy studies have focused on presumed cases of SUDEP (Schuele 2009). Gross and microscopic cardiac changes have been noted in these cases. In one study, heart, lung, and liver weights were greater in SUDEP cases than calculated expected values (Leestma et al. 1989). Increased interstitial and perivascular fibrosis have also been identified in SUDEP cases (Falconer and Rajs 1976; Natelson et al. 1998), along with greater cardiac fibrosis as compared to controls (CodreaTigaran et al. 2005). However, it should be noted that not all postmortem SUDEP studies agree with these findings (Opeskin et al. 2000). Contradictory findings may be due in part to the fact that SUDEP is a diagnosis of exclusion; actual cases are difficult to confirm (Nashef et al. 2012), and there may be other noncardiogenic causes of SUDEP.

The specific nature of the chronic cardiac derangement that may occur in patients with epilepsy as demonstrated in autopsy studies has been explored in animal models. Rats have been observed to develop myofilament damage in the period after lithium/pilocarpine-induced SE (Metcalf et al. 2009a) and cardiac hypertrophy 2 weeks later (Walton et al. 1995). However, cardiac hypertrophy has not been noted in an echocardiographic study of patients with epilepsy (Ramadan et al. 2013).

The examples of cardiac fibrosis and hypertrophy, increased QT interval lengths and dispersion, evidence for increased sympathetic tone and decreased parasympathetic tone, and the commonly acknowledged observations of ictal tachycardia all raise the question of whether VF may be a cause of SUDEP (e.g., Lotufo et al. 2012). Generally, decreased vagal protection increases the risk for VF (Thayer et al. 2010). To date, four cases of VF arising from seizures (Dasheiff and Dickinson 1986; Swallow et al. 2002; Espinosa et al. 2009; Ferlisi et al. 2013), plus one case of VF in relation to seizure-induced takotsubo cardiomyopathy (Cunnington et al. 2012) have been documented. In addition, epilepsy has been recently shown to be a risk factor for sudden cardiac arrest ending in ventricular fibrillation (Bardai et al. 2012). Originally shown in a minority subset of cats receiving pentylenetetrazol as a convulsant (Carnel et al. 1985), VF is a likely outcome in mice with a mutation in the potassium channel KCNQ1 resulting in an epileptic phenotype, abnormalities in cardiac repolarization, and high risk for ventricular fibrillation (Goldman et al. 2009). Our work with rats speaks directly to this question and is summarized in the next three sections.

## USE OF KAINIC ACID AND URETHANE TO EXPLORE CARDIAC PHYSIOLOGY OF SEIZURES

We have developed and used a rat preparation to explore seizure spread and systemic consequences of limbic seizures (Saito et al. 2006; Sakamoto et al. 2008; Hotta et al. 2009; Stewart 2011). The combination of urethane anesthesia and the convulsant kainic acid permits invasive and noninvasive monitoring of sympathetic nerve activity and systemic function during seizure activity that is difficult or impossible to accomplish with other preparations. Because seizures are confined to limbic cortex in this model, animals can be studied in the absence of paralytic agents, permitting examination of seizure spread into autonomic and respiratory centers. Animals anesthetized with urethane remain stable for hours, and the drug is suitable for cardiovascular study (Maggi and Meli 1986). A limitation of the model, however, is that kainic acid-induced seizures occur in an otherwise normal brain and the patterns of seizure origin, spread, and resulting systemic consequences may differ from those occurring in epileptic animals. Subsets of measures can be obtained in unanesthetized preparations using telemetry for some signals as an example, but the special advantage of the urethane/kainate preparation is the array of invasive measures that can be simultaneously made during seizure activity.

Kainic acid can also be used to produce spontaneous seizures in animals (Sperk 1994; Dudek et al. 2006) and, therefore, is one of the best models of epilepsy in rats. Rats that have been made epileptic by this method exhibit cell death in their hippocampal and parahippocampal regions, a condition very similar to hippocampal sclerosis seen in many patients with temporal lobe epilepsy (Dudek et al. 2006; Sperk 1994). In addition, hippocampal sclerosis has been posited to play a role in increasing the autonomic changes in epilepsy (Koseoglu et al. 2009), making it a suitable model for studying cardiac and autonomic changes that accompany chronic seizures.

## CAN AUTONOMIC ACTIVITY INITIATE VENTRICULAR FIBRILLATION?

With direct recordings, we have shown significant increases in sympathetic nerve activity (including cervical sympathetic ganglion, cardiac sympathetic nerves, renal sympathetic nerve, and splanchnic nerve) during seizures (Sakamoto et al. 2008; Hotta et al. 2009). In an otherwise healthy heart, or perhaps more likely in a heart that has experienced numerous seizures, this increased sympathetic activity may trigger a severe tachyarrhythmia. Experimentally, various cardiac arrhythmias have been produced with direct or indirect sympathetic stimulation in dog (Han and Moe 1964; Hockman et al. 1966; Armour et al. 1972) and cat (Lathers et al. 1977, 1978). Sympathomimetic amines and sympathetic stimulation also cause a decrease in the electrical stimulus current necessary to produce VF in dog hearts (Han et al. 1964). Conversely, blocking sympathetic innervation has been shown to be protective against ventricular tachyarrhythmias. In a coronary ligation model of myocardial infarction-related arrhythmias, dogs that underwent stellectomy required a greater current to produce VF than control animals (Kliks et al. 1975; Schwartz et al. 1984). This concept is the basis for a large body of evidence showing that blocking beta-adrenergic input specifically to the heart reduces sudden cardiac death after myocardial infarction (MI) (Hjalmarson 1997).

The most common cause of VF in humans is regional cardiac ischemia in the setting of myocardial infarction. However, global hypoxemia has been implicated in some conditions to produce arrhythmias (e.g., obstructive apnea) (Fava et al. 2011). Although VF does not typically occur due to severe blood loss or asphyxia alone (Surawicz 1964), hypoxemia may aid in VF induction. Conversely, greater oxygen availability can be cardioprotective against VF. Chardack et al. (1964) observed following coronary ligation in dogs, that placing the dogs in hyperbaric oxygen chambers increased survival and decreased VF occurrence.

In rats, we explored the autonomic and oxygen status necessary to initiate ventricular fibrillation. We used combinations of vagotomyto induce severe parasympathetic nerve decreases that could be manipulated with stimulation of the distal nerve, systemic isoproterenol to produce levels of sympathetic activation, and hypoxemia of various degrees and time course to define the conditions necessary to evoke VF (Naggar et al. 2012). It was possible to initiate VF by manipulating these parameters. VF required high sympathetic drive accompanied by minor or no vagal activity within a specific "window" of oxygen saturation.

In manipulating parasympathetic and sympathetic activity as well as systemic oxygen status, we detected a narrow window within this parameter set that permitted spontaneous ventricular fibrillation (Naggar et al. 2012). Spontaneous entry into VF could result from the combination of severe decreases in parasympathetic tone (experimentally produced by bilateral vagal transection), severe increases in sympathetic tone (experimentally produced by isoproterenol infusions that could exceed doses necessary for maximal HR), and a decreased oxygen saturation that was neither too abrupt nor too severe (Figure 25.1). Oxygen saturations that were less significant under the same autonomic conditions often led to premature ventricular contractions and tachycardia, whereas more severe desaturations resulted in severe bradyarrhythmias and eventually death. In animals with intact, unaltered spontaneous vagal activity, VF never occurred. However, in one animal during strong vagus nerve stimulation (VNS) with a train of pulses at 50 Hz, a manipulation we have used to produce asystole (see "Final Remarks" section), the period of asystole contributed to cardiac ischemia. During the stimulus train, we observed a spontaneous run of ventricular tachycardia. We concluded that it is difficult, but not impossible, to provoke VF in a normal heart by autonomic overactivation, with or without concomitant hypoxemia. In fact, we found that VNS could actually cardiovert VF to normal sinus rhythm by bringing about cardiac standstill, and this effect occurred via the cholinergic action of the vagus nerve (Naggar et al. 2012).

Other investigators have shown that vagal input to the heart is proarrhythmic in diseases such as Brugada syndrome, where increased vagal activity can cause VF (Kasanuki et al. 1997; Antzelevitch 2006; Kaufman 2009), and long QT3 syndrome, where increased vagal activity leads to irregular bradyarrhythmias and eventually death (Kaufman 2009).

One of the physiologic features of the autonomic/hypoxia-driven VF was sudden and marked dilation of the left

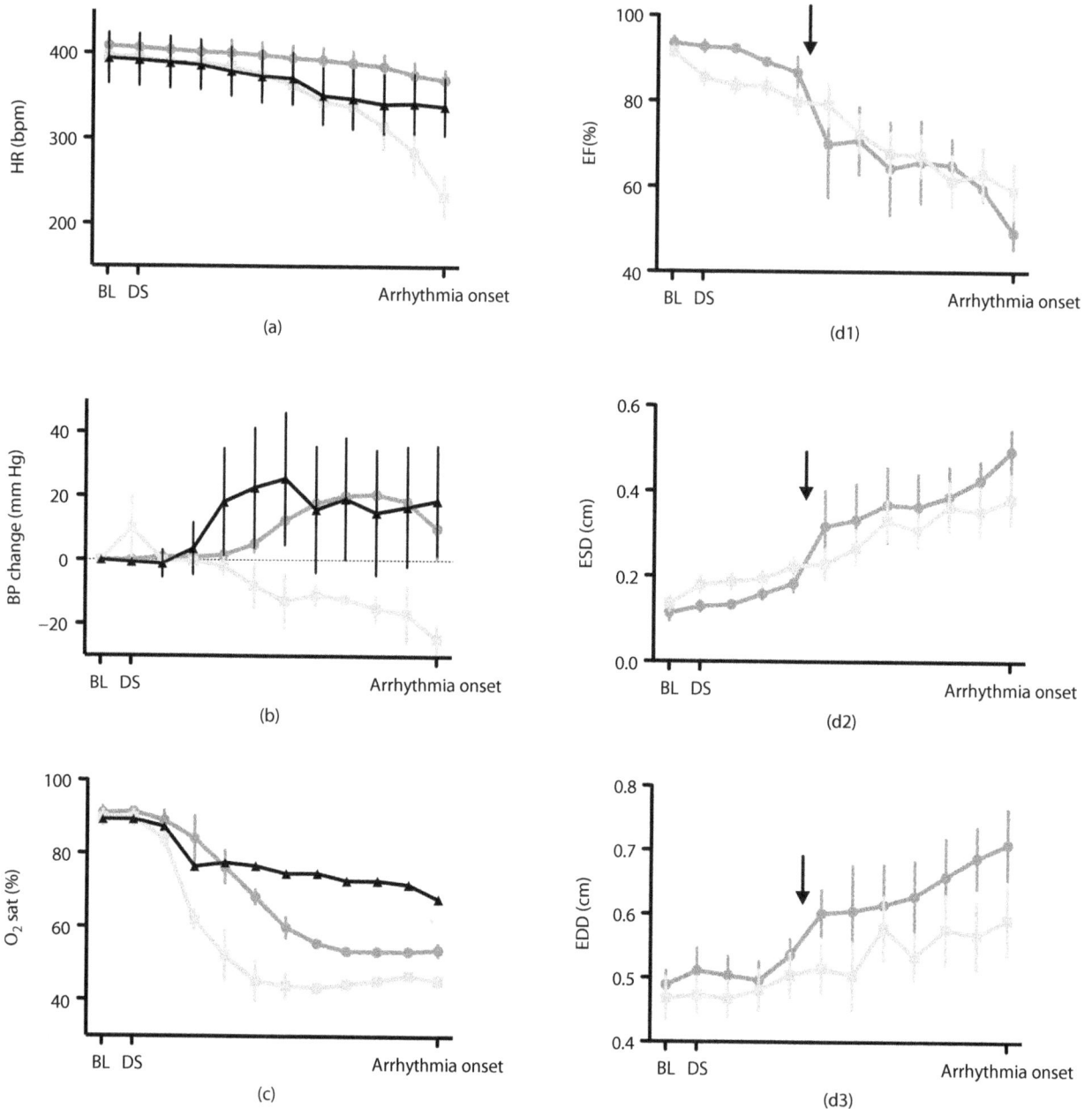

**FIGURE 25.1** Changes in systemic and cardiac variables in the time before arrhythmia onset in a rat model used to explore conditions necessary to trigger ventricular fibrillation. Changes in HR over time after the switch to an abnormally large ventilatory dead space (DS) by connecting a fixed length and diameter segment of tubing to the endotracheal tube are shown in (a). This was preceded immediately by a baseline (BL) measurement. HR was measured for overlapping groups of animals entering VF (dark gray), non-sinus bradycardia (light gray), and sinus bradycardia (black). Measurements were made over normalized time, i.e., at time intervals relative to the dead space placement and arrhythmia onset (VF, sinus/non-sinus bradycardia). The interval between dead space change and arrhythmia onset was generally about 1–3 minutes in duration. (b) Shows the change in BP over the same time scale, where the BP in the non-sinus bradycardia group decreases significantly compared to the other two groups ($p = .004$ at last time point). (c) Shows oxygen saturation at this time scale, and a measurement from one animal with sinus bradycardia is shown for reference. (d1–d3) show echocardiographic measurements of end-systolic diameter (ESD), end-diastolic diameter (EDD), and ejection fraction (EF) along the same time scale as (a)–(c). No appreciable differences could be seen between VF and non-sinus bradycardia, except for a shift in EF in the VF group (black arrow). This was observed as a change in systolic function, as can be seen in the drastic shift in ESD (D2). While the shifts are suggestive, the data do not show statistical significance. (Adapted from Naggar, I et al., *J Physiol Sci*, 2012, 62(6), 479–92, 2012.)

ventricular (LV) wall. This finding is consistent with a prior porcine study showing that an increase in end-diastolic length of the ischemic cardiac region following coronary occlusion was associated with a higher likelihood of developing VF. This response held true for animals given nitroglycerin or no drug; i.e., it was independent of whether or not the myocardium was stretched (Barrabes et al. 2002). Dilation and hypoperfusion of a given area of myocardium was important for induction of

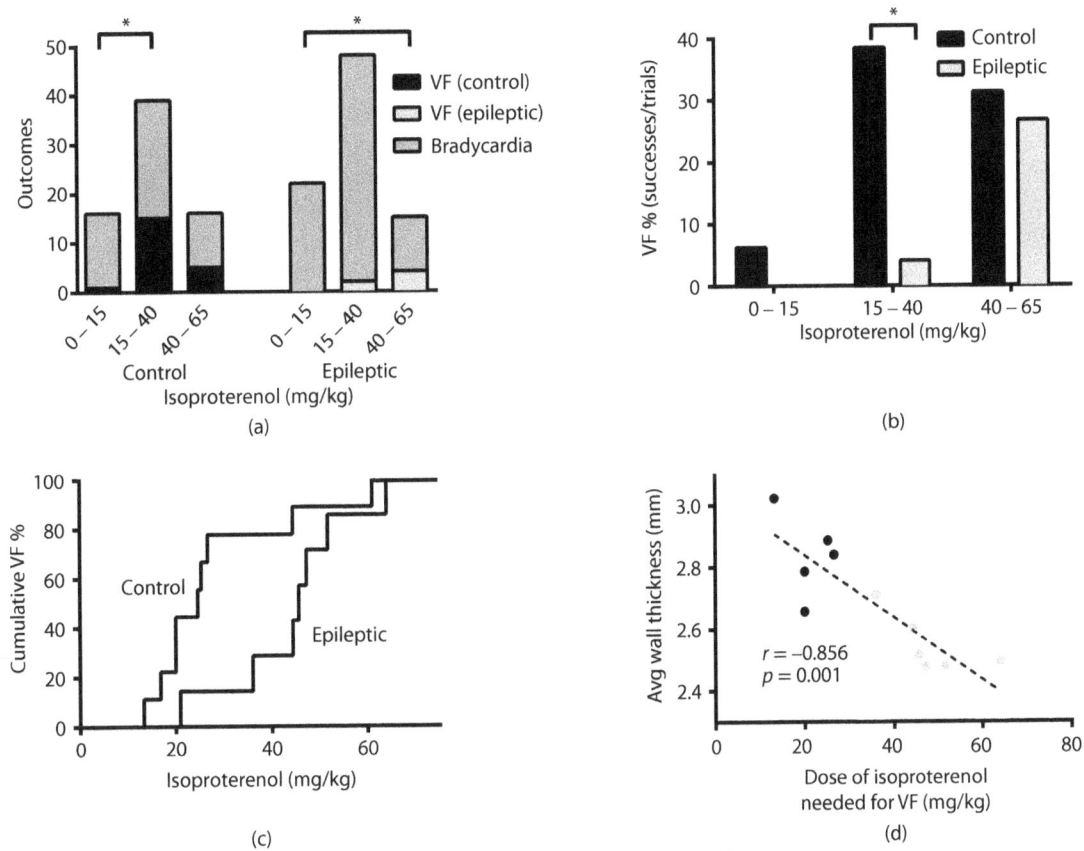

**FIGURE 25.2** Decreased VF susceptibility in epileptic rats. Counts of total outcomes of trials of hypoxemia across isoproterenol dosage are shown for control (black) and epileptic (light gray) rats in (a), and the percent success rate at achieving VF in these outcomes is shown in (b). Bradycardia as an outcome is shown in dark gray for both groups in (a). Panel (c) shows an empirical cumulative probability density function plot of incidence of VF over isoproterenol dose using all animals with isoproterenol doses >65 mg/kg (control $N = 10$, epileptic $N = 7$). A strong correlation between the isoproterenol dose necessary for VF and left ventricular average wall thickness is shown in (d). Control rats showing VF (black) and epileptic rats showing VF (light gray). (Adapted from Naggar, I et al., *Epilepsy Res*, 108(1), 44–56, 2014a.)

VF in our experiments. In our study, the end-diastolic diameter (EDD) was increased in animals entering either VF or severe bradycardia compared to baseline. Taken together with the systolic dysfunction in rats ultimately entering VF (Figure 25.1d), it appears that sudden mechanical dysfunction may contribute to provoking ventricular arrhythmias such as VF.

Autonomic derangements may contribute to SUDEP (DeGiorgio et al. 2010), and they are certainly common during seizures (Opherk et al. 2002; Sakamoto et al. 2008). A combination of these autonomic derangements with global cardiac hypoxia can produce VF. The conditions are very specific, however, so that the types of autonomic derangements occurring during seizures, which include activation of both parasympathetic and sympathetic divisions, even with hypoxemia, are unlikely to precipitate VF (Sakamoto et al. 2008; Stewart 2011). Indeed, vagal activity, even a minor amount, is cardioprotective against VF (e.g., Naggar et al. 2012). Seizures cause increases in activity in both branches of the ANS (Sakamoto et al. 2008; Hotta et al. 2009). Put another way, the autonomic derangements caused by seizures are such that VF is an unlikely outcome. Interestingly, one of the reported cases of VF in an epileptic patient occurred after the patient received both atropine and adrenaline (Swallow

et al. 2002) on a background of pulmonary edema and asystole, conditions that closely resemble those in our rat experiments. On the basis of our animal data, VF triggered by seizure activity is an extremely unlikely cause of SUDEP.

## DO PERSISTENT AUTONOMIC AND CARDIAC CHANGES INCREASE SUSCEPTIBILITY TO VF?

As discussed in the previous section, the impact of autonomic activity and hypoxemia on otherwise healthy hearts may differ from the impact on diseased hearts, and seizures may damage the heart. To examine these observations further, we studied the relations between seizures and autonomic and cardiac derangements in a chronic seizure model (Naggar et al. 2014a). A single exposure to kainic acid (10–12 mg/kg ip) induced a period of SE that was terminated in some animals at 1 hour with pentobarbital (25–50 mg/kg ip). After approximately 2 to 4 weeks, animals displayed spontaneous seizure activity in this well-established model of epilepsy. In addition to producing a chronic seizure condition, epileptic rats displayed a number of long-term cardiac effects, including (1) decreased vagal tone and increased sympathetic tone, (2) increased QT dispersion, and (3) eccentric cardiac hypertrophy without significant cardiac fibrosis. Of these three findings, decreased vagal tone correlated with cardiac hypertrophy.

Epileptic rats displayed severe systolic dysfunction the day after acute seizures, but animals with long-standing chronic seizures were actually less susceptible to autonomic/hypoxemia-driven VF than were nonepileptic animals tested under the same conditions, and their decreased susceptibility was correlated with their average cardiac wall thickness (Figure 25.2).

The findings of eccentric hypertrophy and decreased susceptibility to VF were surprising. The mechanism of this hypertrophy is unclear, although it may arise from constant increased sympathetic input to the heart or from the cardiac myofilament damage that occurs after severe seizures (Metcalf et al. 2009). However, it is likely that the hypertrophy arises mainly from altered autonomic tone, as an inverse correlation was found between SDNN, the standard deviation of all normal R-R intervals, and heart weights (Naggar et al. 2014). The finding of eccentric hypertrophy may suggest that rats experience a tachycardia-induced dilated cardiomyopathy, in which there was marked chamber dilation, although without hypertrophy, as described previously in other animal models (Shinbane et al. 1997).

In general, it appears that autonomic changes are related to significant, persistent cardiac alterations that accompany epilepsy. Others have shown that beta-blockade during the period of SE in rats prevents a decrease in LV contractility, QT-interval prolongation, and hypertension in the period after SE (Little and Bealer 2012). These findings, coupled with the correlation of autonomic tone with increased cardiac mass in our experiments, suggest that: (1) uninhibited sympathetic tone produces substantial cardiac changes in epilepsy, (2) cardiac damage decreases systolic function, which increases sympathetic tone to compensate, or (3) cardiac structural and autonomic changes occur in parallel from seizures.

Prior studies of severe seizures in otherwise normal animals have shown that VF can occur from seizures in a minority of cases, as 1 of 5 sheep was observed to develop VF during unanesthetized bicuculline-induced seizures (Johnston et al. 1995). In a study in anesthetized cats with PTZ-induced seizures, 2 of 9 died from VF while the others died in asystole (Schraeder and Lathers 1983). In spite of the sustained, although not clearly cumulative, cardiac derangements in patients and animals with epilepsy, our rat data suggest that the narrow window for VF described earlier is even narrower in the presence of these cardiac alterations. In other words, the epileptic rats had significantly lower VF susceptibility. The finding of lower VF susceptibility in epileptic rats has implications for SUDEP. These data suggest that VF arising from autonomic/hypoxemia is even less likely to be a cause of SUDEP. Ictalbradycardia and asystole, which are thought to be more dangerous than ictal tachycardia (Opherk et al. 2002) and have been shown to account for death in a rat model (Stewart 2011) may be a more likely mechanism for death.

Several potential explanations exist linking decreased wall thickness to VF susceptibility in our VF model. Perhaps decreased wall thickness and increased heart size produce a greater surface area over which cardiac electrical activity must be conducted, reducing the likelihood of reentrant arrhythmias and VF. Alternatively, it is well known that tonically increased sympathetic tone down-regulates beta-adrenergic receptor density (Bristow et al. 1982; Fowler et al. 1986). A decreased beta-receptor density induced by sympathetic overdrive may lead to a blunted ischemic response to isoproterenol or sympathetic nervous system activation. Conversely, beta-receptor antagonists are known to increase beta-adrenergic receptor density (e.g., Lathers et al. 1986; Lathers et al.1988; Lathers and Levin 2011 for an epilepsy-relevant review). Decreased average wall thickness, in this sense, may have been an indirect measure of the extent of beta-receptor density changes, since increased heart rate may have provoked eccentric hypertrophy. If this explanation is true, it suggests that the use of beta-blockers in patients with epilepsy is not protective against seizure-induced tachyarrhythmias, including VF (Opherk et al. 2002); rather, the cardiac changes that result from repeated seizures may actually be protective against VF. Finally, the mechanism of protection may be that recurrent seizures produce a conditioning response by incurring multiple repeated episodes of ischemia, as one model with fluorothyl ether-induced SE has demonstrated hypoxic-preconditioning prior to cerebral artery occlusion in rats (Towfighi et al. 1999; Giorgi et al. 2005).

It should be noted that the decreased VF susceptibility does not contradict our finding of increased QT dispersion, as QT dispersion is a measure of abnormalities in ventricular repolarization (Day et al. 1990; Schouten et al. 1991), and is not a marker of overall arrhythmogenicity. Others have found increased susceptibility to VF by aconitine infusion in the period following SE or kindling in rats (Metcalf et al. 2009a; Bealer and Little 2013). The change in VF susceptibility was found to accompany decreased vagal tone and increased sympathetic tone (Metcalf et al. 2009b), QT interval prolongation (Bealer and Little 2013), and cardiac myofilament damage (Metcalf et al. 2009a). A major difference between our findings and these reports is that aconitine may have advantages inducing arrhythmias in an enlarged heart because of its capacity to activate essentially every cardiac cell, whereas the suggested mechanisms for protection in our model would all contribute to prevention of autonomic/hypoxic causes of ventricular arrhythmias. Measures of wall thickness findings are certainly worthwhile to follow clinically, especially among patients with epilepsy over time and may serve as a specific marker for cardiac risk within this group.

## FINAL REMARKS

In earlier discussions of SUDEP mechanisms based on our animal experiments, we made the point that while severe autonomic derangements induced by seizure activity can produce extreme cardiac arrhythmias, the most severe arrhythmias reduce cardiac output and brain blood flow, stopping the seizure. We suggested that asphyxiation as a result of airway obstruction is a pathophysiological occurrence during some seizures that can sustain autonomic derangements that are qualitatively identical to derangements of ANS function caused directly by seizure activity, and these asphyxiation-induced ANS derangements can persist (depending on the obstruction) even after a seizure ended, resulting in death (e.g., Stewart 2011). Clearly, ventricular fibrillation is a cardiac condition that can be seizure-induced, but would be inescapable even if the seizure terminated. The much more likely occurrence of ventricular tachycardia during seizures has contributed to the general attitude that a tachyarrhythmia rather than a bradyarrhythmia is more likely to be the terminal event.

Among the bradyarrhythmias, cardiac asystole is an established and dangerous consequence of seizures. Cardiac asystole appears to be a vagally mediated phenomenon, as the atrioventricular block noted during ictalasytole (Altenmuller et al. 2004) resembles the atrioventricular block that occurs as a complication of VNS (Ali et al. 2004) and the atrioventricular block noted during VNS in pigs (Naggar et al. 2014b) (Figure 25.3). Just as the normal sinus rhythm returns after the vagal stimulation ends, we believe that a seizure-induced vagal storm ends when the cardiac output drops sufficiently to reduce brain blood flow (Hotta et al. 2010).

Based on the data from our model to this point, we believe that SUDEP risk is entirely an issue of the specific physiological parameter set associated with any single seizure (and this can vary from seizure to seizure within an individual). We believe that the increased risk in patients whose seizures are poorly controlled relates only to the number of seizures that might put them at risk, rather than a cumulative cardiac or autonomic pathology. From our data, and those of others, reviewed in this chapter, it is clear that seizure-induced cardiac damage is possibly cumulative, but our data indicate that such cardiac damage does not appear to contribute to sudden death as expected. Rather, the cardiac changes associated with epilepsy may actually lower the risk for ventricular fibrillation, as we illustrated with several explanations for mechanism.

We are certainly aware that our conclusions regarding VF as a cause of SUDEP are controversial because some cases of seizure-induced VF have been reported and there is a pervasive view that tachycardia and arrhythmias during seizures predict VF in cardiovascular disease. Further, markers such as decreased heart rate variability or repolarization derangements (discussed in the previous section see also Strzelczyk et al. 2011) in patients with epilepsy are also suggestive that the risk for VF is elevated. In this chapter, we reviewed evidence for the likelihood of VF as a cause of SUDEP in a rat model that actually shows similar changes in HRV and cardiac repolarization to those reported in patients with epilepsy. A major point of this review is to summarize data that, notwithstanding the presence of these clinical markers and clinical reports of increased VF risk in patients with epilepsy, the observed result in our rat model is decreased susceptibility to ventricular fibrillation. Although we do not suggest that the full set of mechanisms for SUDEP has been established or that antiarrhythmic therapies are never indicated in patients with epilepsy, our data in rats indicate that seizure-induced VF is physiologically unlikely as a consequence of seizure-driven conditions. Certainly, this is true in our rat model, and we believe the findings are suggestive and relevant for patients with epilepsy.

Although rat is an animal in which VF is typically non-sustained because of its small critical mass, at variance with larger mammalian hearts including that of humans, our work focused on entry into in VF, not its duration. Furthermore, at least one clinical report of VF arising from a seizure appears to confirm the relevance of our model (Swallow et al. 2002), as VF arose only once the patient entered the necessary physiologic state we studied, i.e., with adrenaline and atropine on a background of pulmonary edema. More data in larger mammalian species in which cardiac electrophysiology and autonomic innervation more closely resemble the human heart may provide further details of the linkage of physiological variables to terminal arrhythmias.

In addition, we would hypothesize that the probability of seizure-induced VF in patients is inversely proportional to the duration of disease, i.e., the probability of VF in association with any given seizure in the life of a patient is highest with the first seizure. Much more data will be necessary to test this hypothesis, including the expansion of animal work where mechanisms can be explored with detailed monitoring and controlled manipulation of the physiology. We believe that the evidence from our rat model regarding entry into VF

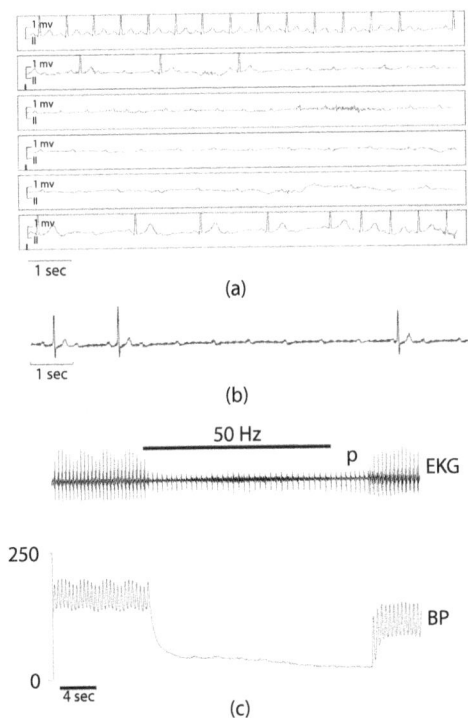

**FIGURE 25.3** Seizures and vagus nerve stimulation produce complete heart block and asystole. Panel (a) (Altenmuller et al. 2004) shows complete heart block and asystole from the period during a focal left temporal seizure. Vagus nerve stimulation in a patient with epilepsy produces the same, as in (b) (Iriarte et al. 2009). Our study in pigs and sheep produced complete heart block and asystole upon vagus nerve stimulation as well (c). (From Naggar, I. et al., *Auton Neurosci*, 183, 12–22, 2014b.)

and risk associated with chronic disease strongly suggests that VF cannot be the main cause of SUDEP, despite clinical case reports (reviewed in the section "Chronic Autonomic and Cardiac Changes from Seizures") and markers of VF risk in patients with epilepsy (Verrier and Schachter, Chapter 14 in this book).

Physical and functional cardiac changes may serve as useful biomarkers for SUDEP risk and clearly deserve further study, especially in larger animals (e.g., epileptic dogs) and patients, keeping in mind that our animal data point in the opposite direction of what some may expect—i.e., the cardiac changes we observed were apparently protective against fatal tachyarrhythmias.

## REFERENCES

Akalin F, Tirtir A, Yilmaz Y. Increased QT dispersion in epileptic children. *Acta Paediatr* 2003;92(8):916–20.

Ali II, Pirzada NA, Kanjwal Y, Wannamaker B, Medhkour A, Koltz MT, Vaughn BV. Complete heart block with ventricular asystole during left vagus nerve stimulation for epilepsy. *Epilepsy Behav* 2004;5(5):768–71.

Altenmuller DM, Zehender M, Schulze-Bonhage A. High-grade atrioventricular block triggered by spontaneous and stimulation-induced epileptic activity in the left temporal lobe. *Epilepsia* 2004;45(12):1640–4.

Antzelevitch C. Brugada syndrome. *Pacing Clin Electrophysiol* 2006; 29(10):1130–59.

Armour JA, Hageman GR, Randall WC. Arrhythmias induced by local cardiac nerve stimulation. *Am J Physiol* 1972;223(5):1068–75.

Bardai A, Lamberts RJ, Blom MT, Spanjaart AM, Berdowski J, van der Staal SR, Brouwer HJ, Koster RW, Sander JW, Thijs RD, Tan HL. Epilepsy is a risk factor for sudden cardiac arrest in the general population. *PLoS One* 2012;7(8):e42749.

Barrabes JA, Garcia-Dorado D, Padilla F, Agullo L, Trobo L, Carballo J, Soler-Soler J. Ventricular fibrillation during acute coronary occlusion is related to the dilation of the ischemic region. *Basic Res Cardiol* 2002;97(6):445–51.

Bateman LM, Li CS, Lin TC, Seyal M. Serotonin reuptake inhibitors are associated with reduced severity of ictal hypoxemia in medically refractory partial epilepsy. *Epilepsia* 2010;51(10):2211–4.

Bateman LM, Li CS, Seyal M. Ictal hypoxemia in localization-related epilepsy: Analysis of incidence, severity and risk factors. *Brain* 2008;131(Pt 12):3239–45.

Baumgartner C, Lurger S, Leutmezer F. Autonomic symptoms during epileptic seizures. *Epileptic Disord* 2001;3(3):103–16.

Bealer SL, Little JG. Seizures following hippocampal kindling induce QT interval prolongation and increased susceptibility to arrhythmias in rats. *Epilepsy Res* 2013;105 (1–2):216–9.

Blum AS. Respiratory physiology of seizures. *J Clin Neurophysiol* 2009;26(5):309–15.

Bristow MR, Ginsburg R, Minobe W, Cubicciotti RS, Sageman WS, Lurie K, Billingham ME, Harrison DC, Stinson EB. Decreased catecholamine sensitivity and beta-adrenergic-receptor density in failing human hearts. *N Engl J Med* 1982;307(4):205–11.

Carnel SB, Schraeder PL, Lathers CM. Effect of phenobarbital pretreatment on cardiac neural discharge and pentylenetetrazol-induced epileptogenic activity in the cat. *Pharmacology* 1985;30(4):225–40.

Chardack WM, Gage AA, Federico AJ, Cusick JK, Matsumoto PJ, Lanphier EH. Reduction by hyperbaric oxygenation of the mortality from ventricular fibrillation following coronary artery ligation. *Circ Res* 1964;15:497–502.

Codrea Tigaran S, Dalager-Pedersen S, Baandrup U, Dam M, Vesterby-Charles A. Sudden unexpected death in epilepsy: Is death by seizures a cardiac disease? *Am J Forensic Med Pathol* 2005;26(2):99–105.

Cunnington C, Garg S, Balachandran KP. Seizure-associated takotsubo cardiomyopathy presenting with unheralded ventricular fibrillation. *Int J Cardiol* 2012;162 (1):e21–3.

Dasheiff RM, Dickinson LJ. Sudden unexpected death of epileptic patient due to cardiac arrhythmia after seizure. *Arch Neurol* 1986;43(2):194–6.

Day CP, McComb JM, Campbell RW. QT dispersion: An indication of arrhythmia risk in patients with long QT intervals. *Br Heart J* 1990;63(6):342–4.

DeGiorgio CM, Miller P, Meymandi S, Chin A, Epps J, Gordon S, Gornbein J, Harper RM. RMSSD, a measure of vagus-mediated heart rate variability, is associated with risk factors for SUDEP: The SUDEP-7 Inventory. *Epilepsy Behav* 2010;19(1):78–81.

Devinsky O. Effects of Seizures on Autonomic and Cardiovascular Function. *Epilepsy Curr* 2004;4(2):43–6.

Devinsky O. Sudden, unexpected death in epilepsy. *N Engl J Med* 2011;365(19):1801–11.

Dogan EA, Dogan U, Yildiz GU, Akilli H, Genc E, Genc BO, Gok H. Evaluation of cardiac repolarization indices in well-controlled partial epilepsy: 12-Lead ECG findings. *Epilepsy Res* 2010;90(1–2):157–63.

Dudek FE, Clark S, Williams PA, Grabenstatter HL. Kainate-induced status epilepticus: A chronic model of acquired epilepsy. In: Pitkänen A, Schwartzkroin PA, Moshé SL, eds. *Models of Seizures and Epilepsy*. Oxford, UK: Elsevier Academic; 2006, Chapter 34, pp. 415–32.

Dutsch M, Hilz MJ, Devinsky O. Impaired baroreflex function in temporal lobe epilepsy. *J Neurol* 2006;253(10):1300–8.

Espinosa PS, Lee JW, Tedrow UB, Bromfield EB, Dworetzky BA. Sudden unexpected near death in epilepsy: Malignant arrhythmia from a partial seizure. *Neurology* 2009;72(19):1702,3 .

Faingold C., Randall M, Tupal S. DBA/1 mice exhibit chronic susceptibility to audiogenic seizures followed by sudden death associated with respiratory arrest. *Epilepsy Behav* 2010;17(4):436–40.

Faingold CL, Tupal S, Randall M. Prevention of seizure-induced sudden death in a chronic SUDEP model by semichronic administration of a selective serotonin reuptake inhibitor. *Epilepsy Behav* 2011;22(2):186–90.

Falconer B, Rajs J. Post-mortem findings of cardiac lesions in epileptics: A preliminary report. *Forensic Sci* 1976;8(1):63–71.

Fava C, Montagnana M, Favaloro EJ, Guidi GC, Lippi G. Obstructive sleep apnea syndrome and cardiovascular diseases. *Semin Thromb Hemost* 2011;37(3):280–97.

Ferlisi M, Tomei R, Carletti M, Moretto G, Zanoni T. Seizure induced ventricular fibrillation: A case of near-SUDEP. *Seizure* 2013;22 (3):249–51.

Finny JM. Bradycardia, with arrhythmia and epileptiform seizures. *Br Med J* 1906;1:967–71.

Food and Drug Administration, HHS. International Conference on Harmonisation; guidance on E14 Clinical Evaluation of QT/QTc Interval Prolongation and Proarrhythmic Potential for Non-Antiarrhythmic Drugs; availability. Notice. *Fed Regist* 2005;70(202):61134–5.

Fowler MB, Laser JA, Hopkins GL, Minobe W, Bristow MR. Assessment of the beta-adrenergic receptor pathway in the intact failing human heart: Progressive receptor down-regulation and subsensitivity to agonist response. *Circulation* 1986;74(6):1290–302.

Giorgi FS, Malhotra S, Hasson H, Veliskova J, Rosenbaum DM, Moshe SL. Effects of status epilepticus early in life on susceptibility to ischemic injury in adulthood. *Epilepsia* 2005;46 (4):490-8.

Goldman AM, Glasscock E, Yoo J, Chen TT, Klassen TL, Noebels JL. Arrhythmia in Heart and Brain: KCNQ1 Mutations Link Epilepsy and Sudden Unexplained Death. *Sci Transl Med* 2009;1:98–106.

Han J, Garciadejalon P, Moe GK. Adrenergic Effects on Ventricular Vulnerability. *Circ Res* 1964;14:516–24.

Han J, Moe GK. Nonuniform Recovery of Excitability in Ventricular Muscle. *Circ Res* 1964;14:44–60.

Hjalmarson A. Effects of beta blockade on sudden cardiac death during acute myocardial infarction and the postinfarction period. *Am J Cardiol* 1997;80(9B):35J–9.

Hockman CH, Mauck HP Jr., Hoff EC. ECG changes resulting from cerebral stimulation. II. A spectrum of ventricular arrhythmias of sympathetic origin. *Am Heart J* 1966;71(5):695–700.

Hotta H, Koizumi K, Stewart M. Cardiac sympathetic nerve activity during kainic acid-induced limbic cortical seizures in rats. *Epilepsia* 2009;50(4):923–7.

Hotta H, Watanabe N, Orman R, Stewart M. Efferent and afferent vagal actions on cortical blood flow and kainic acid-induced seizure activity in urethane anesthetized rats. *Auton Neurosci* 2010;156(1–2):144–8.

Iriarte J, Urrestarazu E, Alegre M, Macias A, Gomez A, Amaro P, Artieda J, Viteri C. Late-onset periodic asystolia during vagus nerve stimulation. *Epilepsia* 2009;50(4):928–32.

Johnston SC, Horn JK, Valente J, Simon RP. The role of hypoventilation in a sheep model of epileptic sudden death. *Ann Neurol* 1995;37(4):531–7.

Johnston SC, Siedenberg R, Min JK, Jerome EH, Laxer KD. Central apnea and acute cardiac ischemia in a sheep model of epileptic sudden death. *Ann Neurol* 1997;42(4):588–94.

Kasanuki H, Ohnishi S, Ohtuka M, Matsuda N, Nirei T, Isogai R, Shoda M, Toyoshima Y, Hosoda S. Idiopathic ventricular fibrillation induced with vagal activity in patients without obvious heart disease. *Circulation* 1997;95(9):2277–85.

Kaufman ES. Mechanisms and clinical management of inherited channelopathies: Long QT syndrome, Brugada syndrome, catecholaminergic polymorphic ventricular tachycardia, and short QT syndrome. *Heart Rhythm* 2009;6(8 Suppl):S51–5.

Kliks BR, Burgess MJ, Abildskov JA. Influence of sympathetic tone on ventricular fibrillation threshold during experimental coronary occlusion. *Am J Cardiol* 1975;36(1):45–9.

Koseoglu E, Kucuk S, Arman F, Ersoy AO. Factors that affect interictal cardiovascular autonomic dysfunction in temporal lobe epilepsy: Role of hippocampal sclerosis. *Epilepsy Behav* 2009;16(4):617–21.

Lathers CM, Kelliher GJ, Roberts J, Beasley AB. Nonuniform cardiac sympathetic nerve discharge: Mechanism for coronary occlusion and digitalis-induced arrhythmia. *Circulation* 1978;57(6):1058–65.

Lathers CM, Levin RM. Animal model for sudden cardiac death. Sympathetic and myocardial beta-receptor densities. In: LathersCM, SchraederPL, Bungo MW, Leetsma JE, eds. *Sudden Death in Epilepsy: Forensic and Clinical Issues.* Boca Raton, FL: Taylor & Francis Group; 2011, pp. 539–49.

Lathers CM, Roberts J, Kelliher GJ. Correlation of ouabain-induced arrhythmia and nonuniformity in the histamine-evoked discharge of cardiac sympathetic nerves. *J Pharmacol Exp Ther* 1977;203(2):467–79.

Lathers CM, Schraeder PL. Autonomic dysfunction in epilepsy: Characterization of autonomic cardiac neural discharge associated with pentylenetetrazol-induced epileptogenic activity. *Epilepsia* 1982;23(6):633–47.

Lathers CM, Schraeder PL, Bungo MW. The mystery of sudden death: Mechanisms for risks. *Epilepsy Behav* 2008;12 (1):3–24.

Lathers CM, Spivey WH, Levin RM. The effect of chronic timolol in an animal model for myocardial infarction. *J Clin Pharmacol* 1988;28(8):736–45.

Lathers C, Spivey WH, Suter LE, Lerner JP, Tumer N, Levin RM. The effect of acute and chronic administration of timolol on cardiac sympathetic neural discharge, arrhythmia, and beta adrenergic receptor density associated with coronary occlusion in the cat. *Life Sci* 1986;39(22):2121–41.

Lathers CM, Stauffer AZ, Tumer N, Kraras CM, Goldman BD. Anticonvulsant and antiarrhythmic actions of the beta blocking agent timolol. *Epilepsy Res* 1989;4(1):42–54.

Leestma JE, Walczak T, Hughes JR, Kalelkar MB, Teas SS. A prospective study on sudden unexpected death in epilepsy. *Ann Neurol* 1989;26(2):195–203.

Leutmezer F, Schernthaner C, Lurger S, Potzelberger K, Baumgartner C. Electrocardiographic changes at the onset of epileptic seizures. *Epilepsia* 2003;44(3):348–54.

Little JG, Bealer SL. beta adrenergic blockade prevents cardiac dysfunction following status epilepticus in rats. *Epilepsy Res* 2012;99(3):233–9.

Lotufo PA, Valiengo L, Bensenor IM, Brunoni AR. A systematic review and meta-analysis of heart rate variability in epilepsy and antiepileptic drugs. *Epilepsia* 2012;53(2):272–82.

Maggi CA, Meli A. Suitability of urethane anesthesia for physiopharmacological investigations in various systems. Part 2: Cardiovascular system. *Experientia* 1986;42(3):292–7.

Malik M, Batchvarov VN. Measurement, interpretation and clinical potential of QT dispersion. *J Am Coll Cardiol* 2000; 36(6):1749–66.

Metcalf CS, Poelzing S, Little JG, Bealer SL. Status epilepticus induces cardiac myofilament damage and increased susceptibility to arrhythmias in rats. *Am J Physiol Heart Circ Physiol* 2009a;297(6):H2120–7.

Metcalf CS, Radwanski PB, Bealer SL. Status epilepticus produces chronic alterations in cardiac sympathovagal balance. *Epilepsia* 2009b;50(4):747–54.

Moseley BD, Ghearing GR, Benarroch EE, Britton JW. Early seizure termination in ictal asystole. *Epilepsy Res* 2011;97(1–2): 220–4.

Naggar I, Lazar J, Kamran H, Orman R, Stewart M. Relation of autonomic and cardiac abnormalities to ventricular fibrillation in a rat model of epilepsy. *Epilepsy Res* 2014a;108(1):44–56.

Naggar I, Nakase K, Lazar J, Salciccioli L, Selesnick I, Stewart M. Vagal control of cardiac electrical activity and wall motion during ventricular fibrillation in large animals. *Auton Neurosci* 2014b;183:12–22.

Naggar I, Uchida S, Kamran H, Lazar J, Stewart M. Autonomic boundary conditions for ventricular fibrillation and their implications for a novel defibrillation technique. *J Physiol Sci* 2012;62(6):479–92.

Nashef L, So EL, Ryvlin P, Tomson T. Unifying the definitions of sudden unexpected death in epilepsy. *Epilepsia* 2012; 53(2): 227–33.

Natelson BH, Suarez RV, Terrence CF, Turizo R. Patients with epilepsy who die suddenly have cardiac disease. *Arch Neurol* 1998;55(6):857–60.

Nei M, Ho RT, Abou-Khalil BW, Drislane FW, Liporace J, Romeo A, Sperling MR. EEG and ECG in sudden unexplained death in epilepsy. *Epilepsia* 2004;45(4):338–45.

Nei M, Ho RT, Sperling MR. EKG abnormalities during partial seizures in refractory epilepsy. *Epilepsia* 2000;41(5):542–8.

Neufeld G, Lazar JM, Chari G, Kamran H, Akajagbor E, Salciccioli L, Kassotis J, Stewart M. Cardiac repolarization indices in epilepsy patients. *Cardiology* 2009;114(4):255–60.

Opeskin K, Thomas A, Berkovic SF. Does cardiac conduction pathology contribute to sudden unexpected death in epilepsy? *Epilepsy Res* 2000;40(1):17–24.

Opherk C, Coromilas J, Hirsch LJ. Heart rate and EKG changes in 102 seizures: Analysis of influencing factors. *Epilepsy Res* 2002;52(2):117–27.

Ramadan MM, El-Shahat N, Omar AA, Gomaa M, Belal T, Sakr SA, Abu-Hegazy M, Hakim H, Selim AH, Omar SA. 2013. Interictal electrocardiographic and echocardiographic changes in patients with generalized tonic-clonic seizures. *Int Heart J* 2013;54(3):171–5.

Rugg-Gunn FJ, Simister RJ, Squirrell M, Holdright DR, Duncan JS. Cardiac arrhythmias in focal epilepsy: A prospective long-term study. *Lancet* 2004;364(9452):2212–9.

Russell AE. The pathology of epilepsy. *Proc R Soc Med* 1908;1(Med Sect):72–118.

Saito T, Sakamoto K, Koizumi K, Stewart M. Repeatable focal seizure suppression: A rat preparation to study consequences of seizure activity based on urethane anesthesia and reversible carotid artery occlusion. *J Neurosci Methods* 2006; 155(2):241–50.

Sakamoto K, Saito T, Orman R, Koizumi K, Lazar J, Salciccioli L, Stewart M. Autonomic consequences of kainic acid-induced limbic cortical seizures in rats: Peripheral autonomic nerve activity, acute cardiovascular changes, and death. *Epilepsia* 2008;49(6):982–96.

Schouten EG, Dekker JM, Meppelink P, Kok FJ, Vandenbroucke JP, Pool J. QT interval prolongation predicts cardiovascular mortality in an apparently healthy population. *Circulation* 1991;84(4):1516–23.

Schraeder PL, Lathers CM. Cardiac neural discharge and epileptogenic activity in the cat: An animal model for unexplained death. *Life Sci* 1983;32(12):1371–82.

Schuele SU. Effects of seizures on cardiac function. *J Clin Neurophysiol* 2009;26(5):302–8.

Schuele SU, Bermeo AC, Alexopoulos AV, Burgess RC. Anoxia-ischemia: A mechanism of seizure termination in ictal asystole. *Epilepsia* 2010;51(1):170–3.

Schuele SU, Bermeo AC, Locatelli E, Burgess RC, Luders HO. Ictal asystole: A benign condition? *Epilepsia* 2008;49(1):168–71.

Schwartz PJ, Billman GE, Stone HL. Autonomic mechanisms in ventricular fibrillation induced by myocardial ischemia during exercise in dogs with healed myocardial infarction. An experimental preparation for sudden cardiac death. *Circulation* 1984;69(4):790–800.

Sevcencu C, Struijk JJ. Autonomic alterations and cardiac changes in epilepsy. *Epilepsia* 2010;51(5):725–37.

Seyal, Bateman LM, Albertson TE, Lin TC, and Li, CS. Respiratory changes with seizures in localization-related epilepsy: Analysis of periictal hypercapnia and airflow patterns. *Epilepsia* 2010;51(8):1359–64.

Shinbane JS, Wood MA, Jensen DN, Ellenbogen KA, Fitzpatrick AP, Scheinman MM. Tachycardia-induced cardiomyopathy: A review of animal models and clinical studies. *J Am Coll Cardiol* 1997;29(4):709–15.

So EL. What is known about the mechanisms underlying SUDEP? *Epilepsia* 2008;49(Suppl 9):93–8.

Sperk G. Kainic acid seizures in the rat. *Prog Neurobiol* 1994; 42(1):1–32.

Stewart M. The urethane/kainate seizure model as a tool to explore physiology and death associated with seizures. In: Lathers CM, Schraeder PL, Bungo MW, Leetsma JE, eds. *Sudden Death in Epilepsy: Forensic and Clinical Issues.* Boca Raton, FL: Taylor & Francis; 2011, 627–44.

Stokes MB, Palmer S, Moneghetti KJ, Mariani JA, Wilson AM. Asystole following complex partial seizures. *Heart Lung Circ* 2012.

Strzelczyk A, Adjei P, Scott CA, Bauer S, Rosenow F, Walker MC, Surges R. Postictal increase in T-wave alternans after generalized tonic-clonic seizures. *Epilepsia* 2011;52(11):2112–7.

Surawicz, Borys. Methods of Production of Ventricular Fibrillation. In: Surawicz B, Pellegrino ED, eds. *Sudden Cardiac Death.* New York: Grune & Stratton;1964, pp. 64–76.

Surges R, Sander JW. Sudden unexpected death in epilepsy: Mechanisms, prevalence, and prevention. *Curr Opin Neurol* 2012;25(2):201–7.

Surges R, Taggart P, Sander JW, Walker MC. Too long or too short? New insights into abnormal cardiac repolarization in people with chronic epilepsy and its potential role in sudden unexpected death. *Epilepsia* 2010;51(5):738–44.

Swallow RA, Hillier CE, Smith PE. Sudden unexplained death inepilepsy (SUDEP) following previous seizure-related pulmonary oedema: Case report and review of possible preventative treatment. *Seizure* 2002;11(7):446–8.

Tavernor SJ, Brown SW, Tavernor RM, and Gifford C. Electrocardiograph QT lengthening associated with epileptiform EEG discharges—a role in sudden unexplained death in epilepsy? *Seizure* 1996;5(1):79–83.

Thayer JF, Yamamoto SS, Brosschot JF. The relationship of autonomic imbalance, heart rate variability and cardiovascular disease risk factors. *Int J Cardiol* 2010;141(2):122–31.

Tigaran S, Rasmussen V, Dam M, Pedersen S, Hogenhaven H, Friberg B. ECG changes in epilepsy patients. *Acta Neurol Scand* 1997;96(2):72–75.

Tigaran S, Molgaard H, McClelland R, Dam M, Jaffe AS. Evidence of cardiac ischemia during seizures in drug refractory epilepsy patients. *Neurology* 2003;60(3):492–5.

Tolstykh GP, Cavazos JE. Potential mechanisms of sudden unexpected death in epilepsy. *Epilepsy Behav* 2013;26(3):410–4.

Towfighi J, Housman C, Mauger D, Vannucci RC. Effect of seizures on cerebral hypoxic-ischemic lesions in immature rats. *Brain Res Dev Brain Res* 1999;113(1–2):83–95.

Uteshev VV, Tupal S, Mhaskar Y, Faingold CL. Abnormal serotonin receptor expression in DBA/2 mice associated with susceptibility to sudden death due to respiratory arrest. *Epilepsy Res* 2010;88(2–3):183–8.

Van Buren JM. Some autonomic concomitants of ictal automatism; a study of temporal lobe attacks. *Brain* 1958; 81(4):505–28.

Walton NY, Rubinstein BK, Treiman DM. Cardiac hypertrophy secondary to status epilepticus in the rat. *Epilepsy Res* 1995;20(2):121–4.

# 26 Neurotransmitters Implicated in Control of Sudden Unexpected Death in Epilepsy in Animal Models

*Carl L. Faingold, Marc Randall, Xiaoyan Long, Victor V. Uteshev,*
*Srinivasa P. Kommajosyula, and Srinivasan Tupal*

## CONTENTS

Sudden unexpected death in epilepsy (SUDEP) is a rare but devastating outcome, and respiratory dysfunction following generalized convulsive seizure is the most common sequence of events observed in SUDEP cases that have been witnessed. Several neurotransmitters are known to be released during generalized seizures, observations that have led to the investigation of potential neurotransmitter involvement in SUDEP in seizure models. These models include dilute brown non-Agouti (DBA)/1 and DBA/2 mice that exhibit generalized convulsive seizures in response to high-intensity acoustic stimuli, called audiogenic seizures, which provoke seizure-induced respiratory arrest in a large percentage of DBA mice. By contrast, other seizure models that exhibit audiogenic seizures, such as genetically epilepsy-prone rats (GEPR-9s), rarely exhibit seizure-induced death.

As detailed further below, respiration is governed by neuronal networks in the brainstem, which are modulated by several neurotransmitters. These transmitters include serotonin (5-hydroxytryptamine, 5-HT), which enhances respiration, and adenosine and other neurotransmitters, which depress respiration. The levels of several of these same neurotransmitters are also known to rise during seizures and contribute to the postictal depression that follows generalized convulsive seizures. Our studies indicate that certain

drugs that enhance the activation of 5-HT receptors, including selective serotonin reuptake inhibitors (SSRIs), significantly reduce seizure-induced respiratory arrest incidence in DBA/1 and DBA/2 mice at doses that do not block seizures. Although the susceptibility of DBA/1 and DBA/2 mice to seizure-induced respiratory arrest can be blocked with SSRIs, particularly fluoxetine, the effectiveness and selectivity for seizure-induced respiratory arrest suppression of several SSRIs varies considerably among the different agents, with one agent, paroxetine, being minimally effective. By contrast, a 5-HT receptor antagonist will induce SUDEP in the DBA mice that exhibit tonic audiogenic seizures without seizure-induced respiratory arrest. Expression of specific 5-HT receptor subtype proteins within the neuronal network that controls respiration in the rostral ventrolateral medulla (RVLM) of DBA mice is significantly altered with important variations between DBA/1 and DBA/2 mice as compared to seizure-resistant mice.

Levels of another neurotransmitter, adenosine, are highly elevated in the brain during and following seizures in animals and in patients with epilepsy. Since adenosine exerts a major depressant effect on the brainstem neuronal network that controls normal respiration, the postictal increases of this neurotransmitter may contribute to the induction of SUDEP.

Agents that alter the actions of adenosine exert significant effects on seizure-induced respiratory arrest in DBA mice and in GEPR-9s. Preseizure treatment of these animals with adenosine itself or metabolism blockers of adenosine induces significant changes in respiration and incidence of seizure-induced respiratory arrest. Respiratory depression, as indicated by significant decreases in blood oxygen saturation and increases in autoresuscitation efforts and a significant increase in the incidence of death were observed following seizures in GEPR-9s treated with adenosine metabolism blockers. DBA/2 mice that exhibited audiogenic seizures but did not initially exhibit seizure-induced respiratory arrest also exhibited a significant increase in the incidence of seizure-induced respiratory arrest after adenosine metabolism blockers or adenosine administration. In contrast, preseizure treatment with an adenosine antagonist, caffeine, significantly reduced seizure-induced respiratory arrest in DBA/2 mice that exhibited it.

The present findings indicate that GEPR-9s may be able to model seizure-induced respiratory dysfunction, which can lead to death when adenosine metabolism is blocked. These findings also indicate that seizure-induced respiratory arrest, leading to death in both models, can be induced by blocking adenosine breakdown, and an adenosine antagonist can block seizure-induced respiratory arrest in DBA/2 mice. Alcohol drinking and withdrawal are factors predisposing to human SUDEP, and alcohol withdrawal in GEPR-9s will also cause them to exhibit respiratory dysfunction and seizure-related death. Taken together, the data on 5-HT and adenosine suggest that preventative measures for SUDEP should explore the use of a combination of agents that reduce the effect of adenosine as well as agents that enhance the action of serotonin.

This chapter describes the role of neurotransmitters in controlling normal respiratory function and the effects of seizures on respiration, and synthesizes this information with insights from animal models concerning neurotransmitters involved in respiration that are implicated in the development and control of seizure-related sudden unexpected death, culminating in suggestions for translating these findings to the clinic.

## RESPIRATORY MALFUNCTION AS A CAUSE OF SUDEP

SUDEP is a devastating consequence of epilepsy and has long been recognized as an important concern in both adult and pediatric epilepsy patients, particularly those who experience generalized convulsive seizures (Langan et al. 2000, 2005; Donner et al. 2001; So 2006, 2008; Donner 2011; Duncan and Brodie 2011; Tomson et al. 2008; Asadi-Pooya and Sperling 2009; Shorvon and Tomson 2011; Schuele et al. 2011; Devinsky 2011; Nashef et al. 1995, 2012; Ryvlin et al. 2013).

The most common behavioral pattern, which is observed in >80% of cases of SUDEP prior to death, was syndromes that involved a generalized convulsive seizure, particularly tonic–clonic seizures (Opeskin and Berkovic 2003; Tomson et al. 2008; Ryvlin et al. 2013). Diminished respiratory function, irregular cardiac rhythm, and postictal electroencephalogram (EEG) suppression, also called cerebral shutdown, are commonly seen in patients and animals in association with generalized convulsive seizure (Schraeder and Lathers 1989; Nashef et al. 1996; Langan et al. 2000; So et al. 2000; Ryvlin et al. 2006, 2013; Bateman et al. 2008, 2010; Lathers et al. 2008; Seyal et al. 2010; Surges and Sander 2012; Moseley et al. 2012; Auerbach et al. 2013; Pavlova et al. 2013).

Respiratory dysfunction is a major proposed cause for SUDEP, since in witnessed cases of human SUDEP, respiratory difficulties were observed prior to death in a majority of cases (Langan et al. 2000; Lear-Kaul et al. 2005; Bateman et al. 2010; Kalume 2013; Seyal et al. 2012; Ryvlin et al. 2013). For example, case reports on human SUDEP indicated that death occurred in the postictal period following generalized seizures primarily resulting from respiratory dysfunction leading to cardiac dysfunction (Lear-Kaul et al. 2005; Seyal et al. 2010; Sowers et al. 2013). SUDEP and near-SUDEP cases have been observed in epilepsy monitoring units in the ongoing Mortality in Epilepsy Monitoring Unit Study, and a major percentage of these cases exhibited respiratory difficulties (Ryvlin et al. 2006, 2013). Significantly compromised respiratory function was found in most observed seizures, and patients exhibiting generalized convulsive seizure showed ~50% decline in respiration in epilepsy monitoring units (Bateman et al. 2008; Seyal et al. 2012; Nadkarni et al. 2012).

Thus, the preponderance of clinical observations suggests an important role of respiratory difficulties during and after generalized convulsive seizures, and respiratory arrest in observed cases of SUDEP and near-SUDEP. Hypoxia-inducible factor (HIF)$_1$-alpha is involved in critical aspects of cell survival in response to hypoxia, and postmortem data from patients with epilepsy have indicated high HIF$_1$-alpha labeling scores in SUDEP cases, supporting a role of hypoxia in these cases (Feast et al. 2012).

Cardiac and brain mechanisms for SUDEP have also been proposed, and these system failures may also be related to respiratory dysfunction due to dysregulation of brainstem mechanisms (Lhatoo et al. 2010; Freitas et al. 2013). The heightened levels of a number of neurotransmitters and neuromodulators resulting from generalized seizures can contribute both to cessation of seizures and to the postictal depression that follows these seizures in humans and animal models (Fisher and Schachter 2000; Lado and Moshe 2008).

## DBA/2 MICE: ACUTELY SUSCEPTIBLE SUDEP MODEL

DBA/2 mice have been used as a model of SUDEP (Venit et al. 2004; Tupal and Faingold 2006) and DBA/1 mice as a chronically susceptible SUDEP model (Faingold et al. 2010a, b). DBA mice are genetically susceptible to generalized convulsive seizures evoked by acoustic stimulation, audiogenic seizures, which result in sudden death due to seizure-induced respiratory arrest, but this strain of mice has only a relatively short period of consistent susceptibility to sudden death. Exposure to intense acoustic stimulation induces generalized convulsive audiogenic seizures, which is very common in rodents, including DBA mice and GEPR-9s, due to genetic factors. Audiogenic seizures can also be induced in previously normal rodents with several types of treatments (Faingold 2002; Faingold et al. 2014).

DBA/2 mice exposed to intense broadband acoustic stimuli from an electrical bell exhibit generalized convulsive, audiogenic seizures consisting of wild running (100% incidence), generalized clonus (100%), and tonic seizures, culminating in tonic hind limb extension (85%). During the postictal period, ~75% of DBA/2 mice exhibit sudden death (Willott and Henry 1976; Seyfried and Glaser 1985; Tupal and Faingold 2006; Uteshev et al. 2010). That death was due to seizure-induced respiratory arrest can be concluded because in a large proportion of DBA/2 mice, sudden death can be prevented if respiration is supported promptly (Tupal and Faingold 2006; Uteshev et al. 2010). A minority, ~25%, of DBA/2 mice exhibit audiogenic seizures but not seizure-induced respiratory arrest (Tupal and Faingold 2006). The response to audiogenic seizures in each DBA/2 mouse shows a stable pattern of seizure behaviors, including seizure-induced respiratory arrest, at postnatal days 21–25, but susceptibility to seizure-induced respiratory arrest declines subsequently due, in part, to loss of hearing (Collins 1972; Turner and Willott 1998; Tupal and Faingold 2006). After postnatal day 25, the incidence of seizure-induced respiratory arrest begins to decline, reaching zero by postnatal day 35 (Tupal and Faingold 2006). Cessation of respiration and subsequent anoxia are likely to be the initial lethality-inducing events, since sudden death can be prevented in >90% of DBA/2 mice that are given prompt respiratory support (Tupal and Faingold 2006). Increasing oxygen supply in the vicinity of DBA/2 mice also increases survival rates (Venit et al. 2004). During seizure-induced respiratory arrest in a DBA/2 mouse when the animal is not breathing, the electrocardiogram is detectable for 4–6 minutes with frequent dysrhythmias before cessation of the electrocardiogram, indicating that cardiac function remains temporarily after seizure-induced respiratory arrest (Faingold et al. 2010b).

## DBA/1 MICE: CHRONICALLY SUSCEPTIBLE MODEL OF SUDEP

Susceptibility to seizure-induced respiratory arrest in DBA/2 mice lasts for ~7 days, allowing these mice to serve only as an acutely susceptible model of SUDEP. However, a closely related mouse strain, DBA/1 mice, exhibits susceptibility to seizure-induced respiratory arrest that lasts much longer (Faingold et al. 2010b, 2011, 2013), allowing evaluation of semichronic drug treatments for seizure-induced respiratory arrest prevention, such as would be administered to patients. With a repetitive protocol of seizure induction once daily for 3–4 consecutive days prior to postnatal day 30, DBA/1 mice exhibit an incidence of seizure-induced respiratory arrest of 80%–100% of animals. The seizure-induced respiratory arrest in DBA/1 mice is fatal unless prompt respiratory support is given, as described above for DBA/2 mice. The incidence of respiratory arrest resulting from the first seizure is ~33%, but the incidence rises to ~100% with 3 to 4 seizures in DBA/1

mice (Faingold et al. 2010a, b). The initial incidences in different shipments of DBA/1 mice varied in subsequent studies.

During seizure-induced respiratory arrest in DBA/1 mice, when the animal is not breathing, the electrocardiogram remains consistently detectable for ~4 to 6 minutes with fluctuating heart rates and abnormal rhythms that alternate irregularly prior to complete cessation (Faingold et al. 2010a) in a manner similar to that seen in DBA/2 mice, as noted above. The onset of arrhythmic electrocardiographic patterns begins at a mean of ~15 seconds after the onset of respiratory arrest. DBA/1 mice that begin daily testing at postnatal day 24 to 30 remain consistently susceptible to seizure-induced respiratory arrest for at least as long as postnatal day 80, which is a significantly greater duration of susceptibility as compared to DBA/2 mice, and which allows these mice to serve as a chronically susceptible SUDEP model. Female DBA/1 mice also exhibit a high degree of susceptibility to seizure-induced respiratory arrest when seizure testing begins at postnatal day 24 to 30, similar to males. However, if initial seizure testing is delayed to >7 weeks of age, DBA/1 mice of both sexes exhibit significant reductions of seizure-induced respiratory arrest susceptibility as compared to mice tested initially at postnatal days 24 to 30 (Figure 26.1) (Faingold and Randall 2013). Although a small percentage (<10%) of DBA/1 mice die despite resuscitation efforts, a somewhat larger percentage (~15%) died spontaneously over a 3 month period in recent preliminary studies, which suggests that the mice are also experiencing unwitnessed spontaneous seizures that result in death, which may be analogous to the unwitnessed deaths that are common in human SUDEP. The lack of spontaneous seizures had been a source of concern about the DBA mouse models meeting the criteria for SUDEP (Massey et al. 2014).

## MODULATION OF RESPIRATION BY SEROTONIN

Since respiratory malfunction is the key precipitating event in the seizure-induced death in DBA mice and is common in observed SUDEP cases, the brain mechanisms responsible for control of respiration may help to explain the susceptibility to SUDEP. The central respiratory network encompasses the RVLM, including the nucleus of the solitary tract, the pre-Bötzinger complex of the brainstem, as well as the midbrain periaqueductal gray as critical network hubs (Bonham et al. 2006; Kubin et al. 2006; Potts 2006; Subramanian 2013; Subramanian and Holstege 2013; Bautista et al. 2014). Intrinsic pacemaker currents in neurons in the pre-Bötzinger complex are modulated by several neurotransmitters, including serotonin (5-HT) and adenosine as well as other neurotransmitters (Chen and Bonham 1998; Kline et al. 2002; Pena and Ramirez 2002; Ramirez and Viemari 2005; Bonham et al. 2006; Brisson-Thoby and Greer 2008; Smith et al. 2013).

Endogenous 5-HT is one of the major brain neurotransmitters and is involved in generating and transmitting normal respiratory rhythm in the brainstem respiratory network (Al-Zubaidy et al. 1996; Wong-Riley and Liu 2005; Ramirez

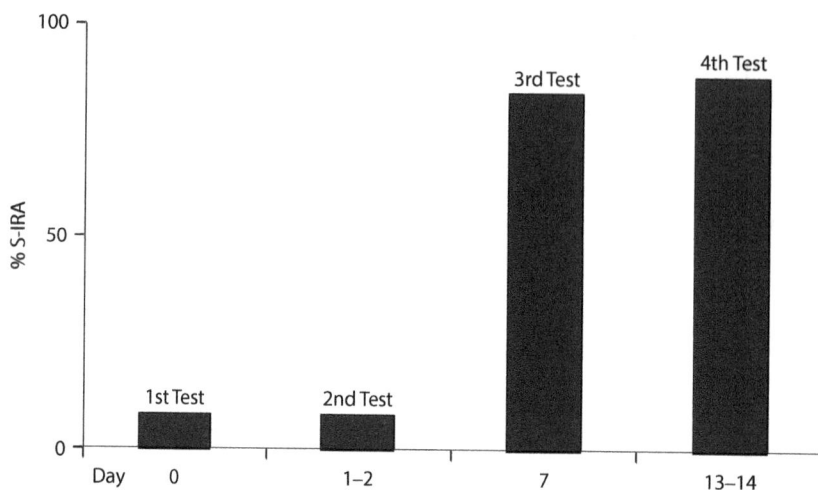

**FIGURE 26.1** The age of first seizure testing of dilute brown non-Agouti (DBA)/1 mice influenced the percentage of mice that exhibited audiogenic seizures (AGS) followed by respiratory arrest. The percentage of DBA/1 mice that exhibited seizure-induced respiratory arrest (S-IRA) was examined in 60 male and female mice in which initial daily testing was delayed. The incidence of S-IRA in DBA/1 mice when the first test was delayed to >7 weeks (postnatal day [PND] 53–73) (day 0) was reduced. These DBA/1 mice initially showed an 8% incidence of S-IRA, which is a significantly reduced degree of S-IRA susceptibility ($p < .05$, Mann–Whitney $U$ test), compared to mice that began testing on PND 24–30. This significantly reduced incidence of S-IRA was also seen when the mice were tested 1–2 days later. However, when the DBA/1 mice were tested at 7 and 13 to 14 days later, they exhibited a much higher incidence of S-IRA, reaching 88% at 13 to 14 days, a result that was not significantly different from that seen in the DBA/1 mice tested initially at PND 24 to 30 days. (From Faingold, CL and Randall, M, *Epilepsy Behav*, 28, 78–82, 2013. With permission.)

et al. 2012; Smith et al. 2013; Feldman et al. 2013). Specific subtypes of 5-HT receptors are thought to be selectively relevant to control of respiration and to epilepsy (Carley and Radulovacki 1999; Richter et al. 2003; Toczek et al. 2003). Pharmacological, electrophysiological, and immunohisto-chemical studies indicate that expression of at least 7 of the 5-HT receptor subtypes occur in the brainstem (Raul 2003; Jordan 2005). Of those subtypes, the subfamily of $5\text{-HT}_2$ receptors (i.e., $5\text{-HT}_{2A}$, $5\text{-HT}_{2B}$, and $5\text{-HT}_{2C}$) is especially relevant to epilepsy and seizures, as discussed below. Although all three $5\text{-HT}_2$ receptors act via activation of Gq/11 receptors coupled to phospholipase C, their net effects are not identical, and stimulation of $5\text{-HT}_2$ receptors could produce either excitation or inhibition. In the brainstem, and specifically in the nucleus of the solitary tract, activation of $5\text{-HT}_{2C}$ is usually inhibitory (Jordan 2005). By contrast, activation of $5\text{-HT}_{2A}$ and $5\text{-HT}_{2B}$ receptors exhibited predominantly excitatory effects (Jordan 2005). Consistent with this mechanism, the absence of $5\text{-HT}_{2C}$ receptors in transgenic mice is associated with audiogenic seizure susceptibility that can result in death (Applegate and Tecott 1998).

As discussed above, endogenous activation of 5-HT receptors is required for the generation of the respiratory rhythm. Therefore, enhanced activation of 5-HT receptors following generalized convulsive seizure may be effective in preventing seizure-induced respiratory arrest. Activation of 5-HT receptors, particularly $5\text{-HT}_4$ receptors (Manzke et al. 2003; Meyer et al. 2006), effectively controls respiratory disturbances, and activation of 5-HT pathways may be an important approach to treatment of life-threatening respiratory disorders in patients (Richter et al. 2003). Blockade of $5\text{-HT}_1$ and $5\text{-HT}_2$ receptors by the 5-HT antagonist, methysergide,

decreased respiratory frequency in vivo and in vitro (Bodineau et al. 2004). A selective serotonin reuptake inhibitor, paroxetine, significantly increased respiratory rates in rodents (Olsson et al. 2004).

## MODULATION OF SEIZURES BY SEROTONIN

5-HT is also implicated in control of seizures. Anticonvulsant effects both in humans and in rat epilepsy models are seen with drugs that enhance the action of 5-HT. A rat model of generalized epilepsy that is susceptible to audiogenic seizures exhibits an extensive loss of 5-HT throughout the brain (Welsh et al. 2002; Merrill et al. 2003). SSRIs, such as fluoxetine, exert anticonvulsant effects in several seizure models, and diminished 5-HT neurotransmission is seen in genetic epilepsy models (Browning et al. 1997; Applegate and Tecott 1998; Hernandez et al. 2002). Reduced $5\text{-HT}_{1A}$ receptor binding has been observed in certain forms of human epilepsy (Merlet et al. 2004; Meschaks et al. 2005). $5\text{-HT}_{2C}$ receptor knockout mice exhibit susceptibility to audiogenic seizures, and these animals exhibit respiratory arrest if the seizure pattern includes tonic hind limb extension, indicative of a very severe convulsion (Heisler et al. 1998). Differences have been observed in 5-HT effects on seizures that vary with receptor subtype and seizure model (Gharedaghi et al. 2014).

## SEROTONIN MODULATES SUDEP SUSCEPTIBILITY IN DBA MICE

The SSRI fluoxetine (Prozac) is known to elevate synaptic 5-HT levels (Malagie et al. 1995). Administration of this agent (15–25 mg/kg, intraperitoneally [i.p.]) significantly reduced seizure-induced respiratory arrest in DBA/2 mice (Tupal and Faingold 2006). This finding is consistent with previous studies indicating that SSRIs, including fluoxetine, exert anticonvulsant effects except in toxic doses (Dailey and Naritoku 1996; Specchio et al. 2004; Merrill et al. 2005; Hamid and Kanner 2013). Susceptibility to seizure-induced respiratory arrest returned in DBA/2 mice by 72 hours after drug administration ceased, a finding that is consistent with the half-life of this agent (Holladay et al. 1998). Suppression of respiratory arrest in this SUDEP model occurred following fluoxetine administration in DBA/2 mice in doses that did not reduce seizure severity, indicating that the effect on respiratory arrest was not dependent on an anticonvulsant effect. The onset of the respiratory arrest suppression by fluoxetine began at 30 minutes, consistent with the time course of significant elevations in 5-HT levels in several rodent brain areas (Malagie et al. 1995). These findings support the importance of enhancing 5-HT neurotransmission in prevention of respiratory arrest in this SUDEP model.

The major clinical use for fluoxetine is to treat depression, and this agent and similar SSRIs are commonly used to treat patients with epilepsy who have comorbid depression (LaFrance et al. 2008). However, the suppressive effect on seizure-induced respiratory arrest in DBA/2 mice occurs much earlier than the several weeks of treatment often required for remission of depression clinically (Tupal and Faingold 2006). The time course of the effect of fluoxetine in DBA/2 mice is consistent with the half-life of this agent in mice (Holladay et al. 1998) and with the onset of the therapeutic effects of antidepressants, such as fluoxetine, in treating certain human sleep disorders, which also does not require weeks of treatment (Nishino and Mignot 1997). The onset of the antidepressant effect in humans is currently thought to be delayed because the increase in 5-HT levels results in neuroplastic brain changes, which take time to develop (Racagni and Popoli 2008).

Systemic administration of a 5-HT$_{1A}$ partial agonist buspirone (10 mg/kg i.p.) significantly reduced the incidence of SUDEP but only to 50%. This agent did not reduce the incidence of seizure-induced respiratory arrest in DBA/2 mice any further despite doubling the dose, a finding that is in keeping with its incomplete effect on 5-HT receptors. These findings further support the importance of enhancing 5-HT neurotransmission in prevention of respiratory arrest in this SUDEP model. These data suggest that these novel serotonergic agonists, which enhance 5-HT neurotransmission more selectively, may potentially be useful in patients for prevention of SUDEP.

As noted above, ~25% of DBA/2 mice exhibited audiogenic seizures but not seizure-induced respiratory arrest (Tupal and Faingold 2006). Cyproheptadine, a nonselective 5-HT receptor antagonist (1 or 2 mg/kg, i.p.), was administered to DBA/2 mice that exhibited tonic extension during audiogenic seizures but not seizure-induced respiratory arrest. Significant increases in the incidence of seizure-induced respiratory arrest were observed (Tupal and Faingold 2006). Audiogenic seizures without seizure-induced respiratory arrests were again observed 24 hours after cyproheptadine

treatment in these DBA/2 mice. These findings further support the importance of 5-HT neurotransmission in control of respiratory arrest in this SUDEP model. These data suggest that the use of agents that block 5-HT neurotransmission may be problematic in patients with epilepsy.

Fluoxetine (45–70 mg/kg, i.p.) also induced significant reductions in seizure-induced respiratory arrest in DBA/1 mice, requiring the highest dose for complete suppression. Notably, these doses are considerably higher than those required in the DBA/2 mice. Semichronic, 5-day, fluoxetine administration (20 mg/kg, i.p., once daily) to DBA/1 mice also significantly reduced seizure-induced respiratory arrest by day 5. The suppression of seizure-induced respiratory arrest was reversible 2–4 days after termination of the chronic treatment (Faingold et al. 2011). These findings further support the importance of enhancing 5-HT neurotransmission in prevention of respiratory arrest in this SUDEP model.

Several other SSRIs are currently available. The effects of sertraline on seizure-induced respiratory arrest were also evaluated in the DBA/1 mice (Figure 26.2). Significant reductions in the incidence of seizure-induced respiratory arrest were seen following sertraline (40–75 mg/kg) administration, and seizure-induced respiratory arrest was completely blocked at 75 mg/kg. At the 40- and 50-mg/kg doses of sertraline, the DBA/1 mice all continued to exhibit audiogenic seizures, but the incidence of the tonic component of seizures was significantly reduced. Susceptibility to seizure-induced respiratory arrest returned at 24 to 48 hours after sertraline administration in most DBA/1 mice. These data indicate that this SSRI is also effective in blocking seizure-induced respiratory arrest induced by generalized convulsive seizures in DBA/1 mice without blocking audiogenic seizure susceptibility (Faingold and Randall 2013).

These results suggested that the SSRIs as a group may be effective in blocking seizure-induced respiratory arrest in DBA/1 mice. Therefore, two other clinically used SSRIs, namely, fluvoxamine and paroxetine and the serotonin–norepinephrine reuptake inhibitor venlafaxine, were evaluated to determine if these agents were also effective in blocking seizure-induced respiratory arrest. Fluvoxamine administration significantly reduced seizure-induced respiratory arrest at 60 to 80 mg/kg 30 minutes after administration of this SSRI. Even at the highest dose tested, the mice remained susceptible to audiogenic seizures. However, the incidence of the tonic phase of the seizure was also significantly reduced by fluvoxamine at each of the effective doses. Susceptibility to seizure-induced respiratory arrest was again observed at 24 hours after fluvoxamine administration. However, paroxetine at doses up to 120 mg/kg did not exert significant effects on any seizure-related behavior in DBA/1 mice at 30 minutes after administration. At 2 hours, a significant reduction ($p < .05$) in seizure-induced respiratory arrest began to be observed with the 120 mg/kg dose (Faingold et al. 2014). A delayed effect of paroxetine was seen at 24 hours (Figure 26.3), and 100 and 120 mg/kg doses induced significant reductions of seizure-induced respiratory arrest and tonic seizures, although the degree of the effect was

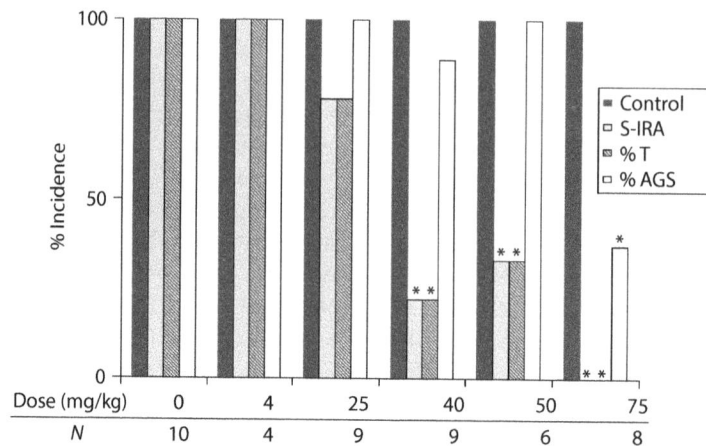

**FIGURE 26.2** Effect on DBA/1 mice on administration of the selective serotonin reuptake inhibitor (SSRI) sertraline on the incidence of audiogenic S-IRA. Dark bars indicate the incidence of S-IRA in DBA/1 mice before the drug or vehicle (dimethyl sulfoxide, 10% in saline, intraperitoneally [i.p.]) injection, and gray bars indicate the incidence of AGS at 30 minutes after sertraline (4–75 mg/kg, i.p.) or vehicle (0.1 mL/g body weight mg/kg) administration. Hatched bars indicate the incidence of tonic hind limb convulsion (T), and open bars indicate the incidence of AGS. Sertraline in doses of 40, 50, or 75 mg/kg significantly reduced the incidence of S-IRA compared to 24 hours before treatment. Note: All of the mice remained susceptible to AGS, but the incidence of tonic hind limb convulsions was significantly reduced at the 40–75 mg/kg doses. Susceptibility to S-IRA returned at 24–48 hours. Those DBA/1 mice that did not return to susceptibility to S-IRA after sertraline exhibited health problems and were euthanized. *Significantly different from vehicle control, $p < .05$; Wilcoxon signed ranks test. $N$ is the number of animals given each dose. (From Faingold, CL and Randall, M, *Epilepsy Behav*, 28, 78–82, 2013. With permission.)

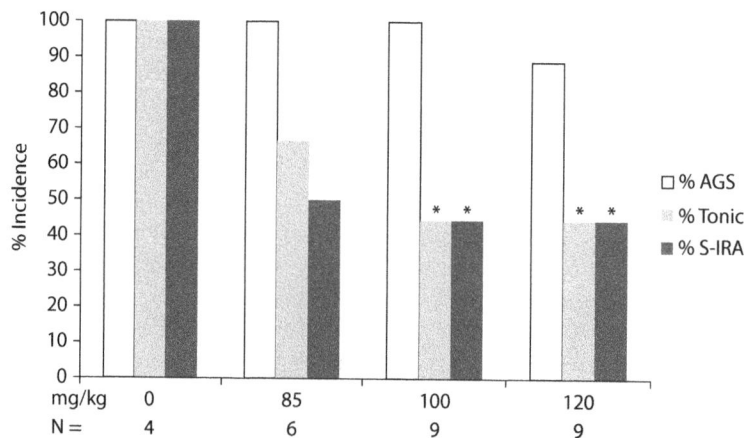

**FIGURE 26.3** Paroxetine effects on audiogenic S-IRA in DBA/1 mice. Paroxetine is an SSRI that exerted only a partial blockade of S-IRA without blocking AGS, which were delayed in onset, requiring 24 hours for the maximal effect to be seen. Open bars indicate incidence of AGS. Gray bars indicate incidence of tonic hind limb convulsions (Tonic), and black bars indicate the incidence of S-IRA. The dose required to reduce S-IRA was near toxic levels. *$p < .05$; Wilcoxon signed rank test; $N$ = number of mice given each dose; 0 mg/kg = vehicle control.

only slightly >50%. This observation contrasts with the degree of prevention seen with fluvoxamine, which reached 100% effectiveness at the highest dose. Paroxetine was also administered to DBA/1 mice in a semichronic paradigm, 20–50 mg/kg daily for 5 days. No significant reduction of seizure behaviors was induced when tested on day 5, and higher doses were toxic. The differences between the effectiveness of SSRIs may be due to additional actions of some of these agents, excluding paroxetine, on sigma-1 receptors (Sugimoto et al. 2012). Venlafaxine exhibited a U-shaped dose–effect relationship wherein only intermediate doses of this agent significantly reduced seizure-induced respiratory arrest, which may be due to its dual effect on serotonin and norepinephrine uptake (Faingold et al. 2014).

We also examined the effects of the 5-HT$_{2B/2C}$ agonist m-chlorophenylpiperazine (mCPP) to test the generality of serotonergic effects on DBA mice. In DBA/2 mice, mCPP pretreatment (5 or 10 [but not 2] mg/kg, i.p.) significantly reduced the incidence of seizure-induced respiratory arrest without blocking seizure susceptibility. However, in DBA/1 mice, mCPP in doses up to 40 mg/kg was ineffective in blocking seizure-induced respiratory arrest, and 60 mg/kg was toxic. The cause of this strain difference was perplexing (Faingold et al. 2011) and led to the evaluation of 5-HT receptor subtype expression in the two strains of DBA mice, as discussed below. The effects of a selective 5-HT$_7$ agonist AS-19 (10–60 mg/kg) on audiogenic seizures in DBA/1 mice indicated that this agent was also not effective in blocking any seizure-related behavior, including seizure-induced respiratory arrest, in DBA/1 mice (Faingold et al. 2014). In higher doses, AS-19 was toxic and even proconvulsant, since spontaneous seizures not triggered by the acoustic stimulus were seen. The 5-HT$_7$ agonist was evaluated because 5-HT$_7$ receptors are involved in control of respiration by the spinal cord (Liu et al. 2009), suggesting that these receptors may not be critical in the therapeutic effects of elevating 5-HT on seizure-induced respiratory arrest in DBA/1 mice. These data indicate that 5-HT in DBA/1 mice also modulates seizure-induced respiratory arrest susceptibility, but that not all drugs that increase the activation of 5-HT receptors are effective.

The incidence of seizure-induced respiratory arrest at 30 minutes after administration of the nonselective 5-HT antagonist, cyproheptadine, was also evaluated. A drug-induced increase in the incidence of seizure-induced respiratory arrest in DBA/1 mice was observed. Thus, 2 mg/kg (but not higher doses) of cyproheptadine induced a significant increase in seizure-induced respiratory arrest incidence when given prior to the first audiogenic seizure test in DBA/1 mice at age 31–38 days (Faingold et al. 2014). This observation parallels the findings with the same 5-HT antagonist in DBA/2 mice (Tupal and Faingold 2006).

## SEROTONIN RECEPTOR PROTEIN ABNORMALITIES IN DBA MICE

The apparent deficit in serotonergic activation in DBA mice, which are susceptible to seizure-induced respiratory arrest, may be related to altered expression of specific subtypes of 5-HT receptors in respiratory centers of the brainstem. Specific receptor subtypes in the brainstem have been previously observed, and 5-HT neurotransmission is important to brainstem respiratory networks as well as seizure networks, as noted above (Brennan et al. 1997; Applegate and Tecott 1998; Feldman, et al. 2003; Di Giovanni et al. 2006; Benarroch 2007; Hodges and Richerson 2008; Doi and Ramirez 2008; Hodges et al. 2008). The expression of 5-HT receptor proteins in the medial–caudal brainstem of DBA/2 and DBA/1 mice was evaluated and compared to C57BL/6J mice, which are genetically related to DBA mice but do not exhibit susceptibility to audiogenic seizure or seizure-induced respiratory arrest, as indicated by Western blots (Uteshev et al. 2010; Faingold et al. 2011). In DBA/1 mice, 5-HT$_{2C}$ and 5-HT$_{3B}$ receptor expression was significantly reduced, a pattern similar to that seen in DBA/2 mice. However, 5-HT$_{2B}$ receptor expression was also reduced in DBA/1 mice, in contrast with the 5-HT$_{2B}$ receptor elevation seen in DBA/2 mice. This difference may explain the differential effects of the 5-HT$_{2B/2C}$ agonist mCPP in these SUDEP models, as described earlier.

## MODULATION OF RESPIRATION BY ADENOSINE

As noted above, adenosine is another major brain neurotransmitter involved in generating and transmitting respiratory rhythm (Vandam et al. 2008; Del Negro 2011; Zwicker et al.

2011), and this substance has also been implicated in SUDEP mechanisms in animals (Shen et al. 2010; Fukuda et al. 2012). Adenosine is a purine that is a transmitter or cotransmitter in many peripheral and central nervous system (CNS) sites in the nervous system including neurons and glia (Burnstock 2013). Adenosine in the brain exerts its action by activating multiple G-protein-coupled receptors including A1, A2$_A$, A2$_B$, and A3 receptor subtypes. A1 and A3 receptors inhibit, whereas A2$_A$ and A2$_B$ receptors stimulate production of the second messenger, cyclic adenosine monoamine phosphate. A1 and A2$_A$ receptors are activated by nanomolar concentrations of adenosine, whereas A2$_B$ and A3 receptors become activated only when adenosine levels rise into the micromolar range during inflammation, hypoxia, ischemia, or seizures (Paul et al. 2011).

Adenosine in the brain acts as a neuromodulator. It mediates inhibition of neuronal activity in many signaling pathways, producing sedation and anticonvulsant and protective actions by acting on adenosine A1 receptors on neurons and glia. Imaging in the human brain has shown that the distribution of the major subtype A1 is highest in the striatum and thalamus, moderate in the cerebral cortices and pons, and low in the cerebellum (Fukumitsu et al. 2005). Normal increases in adenosine levels are associated with induction of sleep (Brown et al. 2012), which is of interest because nocturnal seizures have been associated with a higher risk of SUDEP (Lamberts et al. 2012). Tissue samples from patients with epilepsy and animal models show extensive changes in A1 receptor density and binding (Paul et al. 2011). Adenosine is released from pre- and postsynaptic neurons and from glial cells, and the concentration of extracellular adenosine normally ranges from 25 to 250 nanomolar. During ischemia, hypoxia, or seizures, these values may rise 3- to 10-fold (Lopes et al. 2011). Many of the inhibitory actions of adenosine at synapses are due to inhibition of Ca$^{2+}$-dependent excitatory neurotransmitter release presynaptically and are mediated by G-protein-coupled receptors that lead to inhibition of voltage-dependent calcium channels.

The four adenosine receptors that have been identified are related to seven transmembrane-domain G-protein-coupled receptors that have been cloned in a variety of species, including man, and all are present in the nervous system. The A1 receptor is widely expressed and mediates most of the inhibitory effects of adenosine in the brain, whereas the A2$_A$ and A3 receptors are present in a lower density and may have more restricted and localized actions; the A2$_A$ receptors are particularly abundant in the basal ganglia and are predominantly excitatory. The A3 receptor is found mostly in peripheral tissues, and its density in the brain is low except in hippocampus and cerebellum. The affinity of this subtype for adenosine is considerably lower than the A1 and A2$_A$ and the A3 receptor may play a role only when adenosine levels are elevated, such as during and following seizures (Lopes et al. 2011).

The central control of respiration involves complex network interactions among neurons distributed throughout the brain, and the network that generates respiratory rhythm is composed of micronetworks within larger networks to generate distinct rhythms and patterns that characterize breathing (Feldman and Del Negro 2006). As noted above, the pre-Bötzinger complex in the RVLM plays a critical role in generating the respiratory rhythm and contains subnetworks with specific synaptic and intrinsic membrane properties that control the different types of respiratory rhythmic activities, such as eupneic, sigh, and gasping activities (Bautista et al. 2014). The pre-Bötzinger complex is part of a larger network that receives important inputs from the pons and retrotrapezoid nucleus/parafacial nucleus (Garcia et al. 2011). The neurons in the RVLM that control respiration are inhibited by adenosine, which acts at A1 receptors to inhibit respiration, and this depression of central mechanisms of respiration is long-lasting (Del Negro 2011).

A key human finding implicating the importance of adenosine in the potential prevention of SUDEP is the role of adenosine antagonists in treating apnea of prematurity (Kumral et al. 2012), which is characterized by an unstable respiratory rhythm due to immaturity of the respiratory network. Ventilatory responses to hypoxia and hypercarbia in the neonate are impaired, and inhibitory reflexes are exaggerated, leading to the development of apnea. A nonselective adenosine antagonist, caffeine, is the primary pharmacological treatment for neonatal apnea and is thought to work via blockade of adenosine receptors A1 and A2, although blockade of $A2_A$ receptors may also play an important role (Mathew 2011).

## MODULATION OF SEIZURES BY ADENOSINE

Extracellular levels of adenosine in the brain are determined primarily by the adenosine cycle, involving adenosine triphosphate (ATP) release and degradation of ATP into adenosine, reuptake of adenosine via nucleoside transporters, and phosphorylation by adenosine kinase (ADK), which occur in astrocytes (Boison 2012). Overexpression of astroglial ADK leads to adenosine deficiency and increased neuronal excitability and has been observed in astrogliosis and in rodent and human forms of epilepsy (Boison 2012). These ADK changes result in changes in the level of extracellular adenosine, which exerts its CNS effects by activation of pre- and postsynaptic adenosine $A_1$ receptors.

An ADK hypothesis of epileptogenesis has been proposed, which suggests that adenosine dysfunction in epilepsy is biphasic, with an acute surge of adenosine triggered by injury contributing to the development of astrogliosis associated with overexpression of ADK, which can then trigger spontaneous seizures (Boison 2012). Adenosine levels in the brain are known to rise precipitously to micromolar levels in human and animal forms of seizures during postictal depression and thereby activate all subtypes of adenosine receptors (During and Spencer 1992; Berman et al. 2000; Pedata et al. 2001). A significant increase in adenosine levels in the blood was observed in DBA/1 mice after seizures as compared to DBA/1 mice that were not subjected to a seizure (Figure 26.4). Adenosine has been proposed to act as an endogenous anticonvulsant mechanism (During and Spencer 1992; Shen

et al. 2010; Boison 2012). However, the respiratory depressant effect of adenosine may make an important contribution to the respiratory dysfunction commonly seen during seizures in patients with epilepsy (Bateman et al. 2008). Adenosine agonists acting at the A1 receptor prolong postictal depression and adenosine antagonists shorten it (Kostopoulos et al. 1989; Angelatou et al. 1991). Significant increases of hippocampal levels of adenosine and its metabolites, hypoxanthine and inosine, were observed with seizures induced by several different convulsant drugs (Berman et al. 2000). Dialysis probes implanted in the hippocampus of patients with epilepsy detected 6- to 31-fold increases of extracellular adenosine during seizure activity (During and Spencer 1992) (Figure 26.5).

Adenosine exerts an anticonvulsant action primarily by acting on inhibitory A1 receptors that control excessive neuronal activity, and mice lacking A1 receptors are more susceptible to seizures, exhibit spontaneous seizures, and develop lethal status epilepticus (Fedele et al. 2006; Lopes et al. 2011). Electrical kindling seizures result in decreased extracellular adenosine levels and reduced A1 receptor activation, which may contribute importantly to seizure generation (Rebola et al. 2003; Dulla et al. 2005). Adenosine receptor density changes in human and animal models of epilepsy, depending on the duration of the treatment as well as on the convulsant drug used. Thus, increases in A1 receptors are observed following acute or chronic induction of seizures (Pagonopoulou et al. 2006). Seizure-induced release of adenosine regulates synaptic activity via A1, $A2_A$, $A2_B$, and A3 receptors (Boison and Stewart 2009). Activation of A1 receptors inhibits network excitability, limits the extension of seizures, and mediates seizure arrest (Etherington and Frenguelli 2004; Fedele et al. 2006; Li et al. 2007).

Seizures in the nonepileptic brain are thought to be prevented, in part, by a sustained anticonvulsant effect of endogenous adenosine (Dunwiddie and Masino 2001; Fredholm et al. 2001; Pagonopoulou et al. 2006). Under normal conditions, adenosine concentrations are kept in the normal range by phosphorylation via ADK into 5′-adenosine monophosphate and deamination into inosine by adenosine deaminase (Boison 2012). During prolonged seizures or traumatic brain injury, a surge of adenosine to micromolar levels occurs that far exceeds the affinity of A1 receptors. Thus, any combination of prolonged or excessive seizure activity with impaired adenosine clearance is likely to result in overactivation of adenosine receptors (Shen et al. 2010).

These data led to the development of an animal model for SUDEP that involves administration of inhibitors of adenosine deaminase and ADK prior to induction of seizures with kainic acid. Both the controls and the adenosine metabolism blocked animals exhibited seizures, but seizures in control animals were less severe and none of these animals died. Animals treated with the adenosine metabolism inhibitors exhibited more severe seizures and died within 20 minutes. The nonselective adenosine receptor antagonist, caffeine, prevented the deaths in these mice, and the authors suggested that the action of this agent may have been primarily on $A2_A$ receptors (Shen et al. 2010).

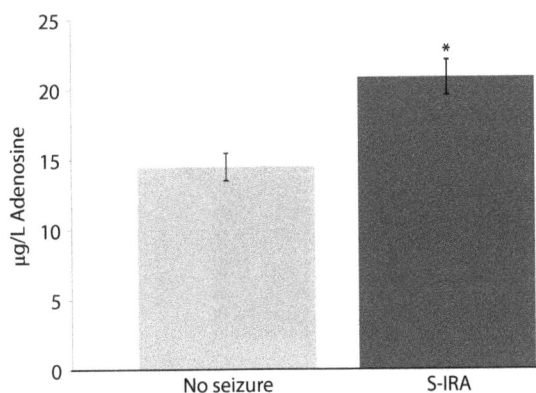

**FIGURE 26.4** Adenosine blood levels in DBA/1 mice. DBA/1 mice ($N = 7$ each) were sacrificed either immediately after seizure during S-IRA or sacrificed without audiogenic seizure. The blood was immediately frozen until analysis was performed by mass spectrometry. The results indicated that a significantly greater level of adenosine was seen in mice with S-IRA than in mice without seizure. $*p < .005$, $t$ test.

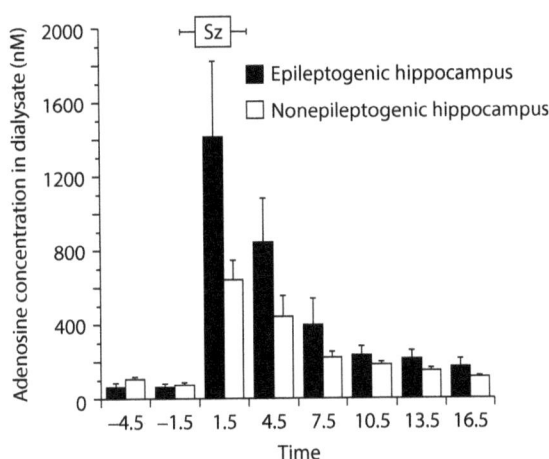

**FIGURE 26.5** Bilateral hippocampal extracellular fluid adenosine levels during complex partial seizures. Data represent the means $\pm$ SEM of adenosine levels in hippocampal dialysates collected at 3-minute intervals during four secondary generalized seizures in four patients. The box with Sz represents the seizures (mean $\pm$ SEM); standard errors show the imprecision in determining time of onset and the range of seizure duration. Adenosine is increased above basal levels ($-4.5$ and $-1.5$ minute samples) during the 1.5-minute interval and in all subsequent samples. Adenosine levels are significantly higher in the epileptogenic hippocampus during the seizure at 1.5 minutes compared with the contralateral hippocampus ($p < .05$, two-way analysis of variance with repeated measures and paired $t$ test). (Modified from During, MJ and Spencer, DD, *Ann Neurol*, 32, 618–24, 1992. With permission.)

## ADENOSINE MODULATES SUDEP SUSCEPTIBILITY IN DBA MICE

Recent data from our laboratory indicate that adenosine may also play a role in susceptibility to seizure-induced respiratory arrest in DBA/2 mice. As noted above, although ~75% of DBA/2 mice exhibited seizure-induced respiratory arrest, the remainder exhibited seizures without seizure-induced respiratory arrest. We examined whether agents that modify adenosine action would alter seizure-induced respiration changes and incidence of seizure-induced death in DBA/2 mice. This investigation involved administering adenosine or 5-iodotubericidin (5-ITU), an ADK inhibitor (Shen et al. 2010), or an adenosine antagonist, caffeine. DBA/2 mice that did not initially exhibit seizure-induced respiratory arrest showed a significant incidence of seizure-induced respiratory arrest at 30 minutes after 5-ITU or certain doses of

adenosine (Figure 26.6). Thus, adenosine (2 mg/kg) significantly increased the incidence of seizure-induced respiratory arrest in DBA/2 mice that did not exhibit it prior to drug, but higher adenosine doses produced a paradoxical effect, reducing the incidence of seizures in DBA/2 mice, so that audiogenic seizures were no longer consistently evoked. This anticonvulsant effect has also been seen in kindled seizures in rats and spontaneous seizures in mice (Boison 2013). Likewise, certain doses (~0.5 mg/kg) of the nonselective adenosine antagonist caffeine significantly reduced the incidence of seizure-induced respiratory arrest in DBA/2 mice that had exhibited it previously (Figure 26.7). However, neither higher nor lower doses of caffeine induced significant changes. This result may be related to the biphasic effects of adenosine, since at higher doses the proconvulsant effect of caffeine may predominate. Recent preliminary studies indicate that a selective $A2_A$ antagonist was also effective in

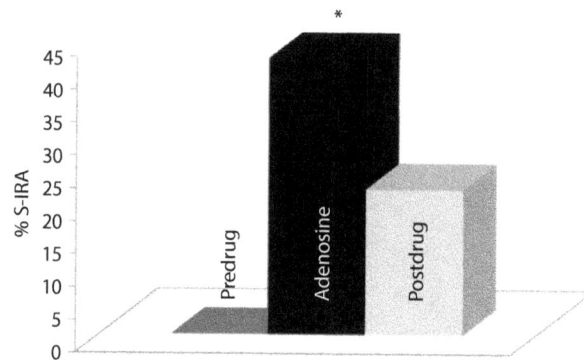

**FIGURE 26.6**  Adenosine effects on audiogenic S-IRA. Administration of a nonselective adenosine receptor agonist, adenosine (2 mg/kg, i.p.), at 30 minute prior to seizure significantly increased the incidence of susceptibility to S-IRA in DBA/2 mice that were susceptible to AGS but did not initially exhibit S-IRA compared to saline control. A number of these mice returned to not being S-IRA susceptible at 24 hours postdrug. Higher doses produced a paradoxical effect, since administration of 4 mg/kg and higher doses (not shown) actually reduced the incidence of seizures so that S-IRA could not be evaluated. $N = 14$ mice. $*p < 0.05$ (Wilcoxon signed rank test).

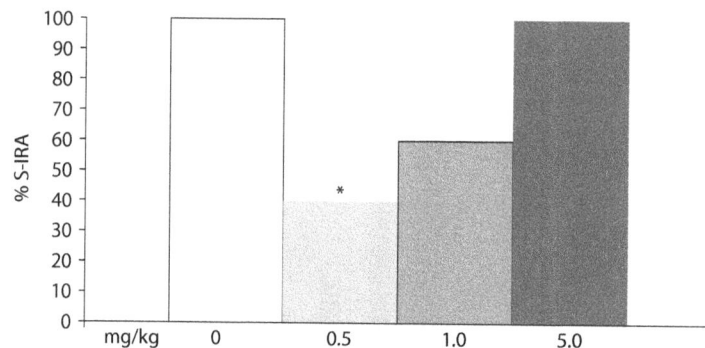

**FIGURE 26.7**  Caffeine effects in DBA/2 mice. The nonselective adenosine antagonist, caffeine, significantly decreased S-IRA in DBA/2 mice at 30 minutes after administration. However, this effect was observed only at a relatively low dose (0.5 mg/kg). Slightly lower and slightly higher doses induced nonsignificant effects. Higher and lower doses were totally ineffective. $*p < .05$; Mann–Whitney $U$ test; N = 5.

blocking seizure-induced respiratory arrest in DBA/2 mice, but a selective A1 antagonist was ineffective.

Since human SUDEP is relatively uncommon, we also examined the effects of blocking adenosine metabolism in another seizure model induced by auditory stimulation, the GEPR-9s, which rarely die from their seizures. We examined the effects on respiration and seizure-related deaths of administration of 5-ITU, the ADK inhibitor, and erythro-9-(2-hydroxy-3-nonyl)-adenine (EHNA), an adenosine deaminase inhibitor (Shen et al. 2010). Blood oxygen saturation (SpO$_2$%) in GEPR-9s was measured using a pulse oximetry sensor. Audiogenic seizures were induced at 30 minutes after drug administration and following seizures there was a significant decrease in SpO$_2$% in GEPR-9s after EHNA/5-ITU treatment. A significant increase in the incidence of death was also observed in these GEPR-9s at 1 to 24 hours after treatment but not in untreated GEPR-9s. These findings indicate that if adenosine metabolism is blocked, GEPR-9s may be able to model seizure-induced respiratory dysfunction, which can lead to death. These results also indicate that audiogenic seizures, which lead to death in both models, can be induced by blocking adenosine breakdown, and that an adenosine antagonist can block seizure-induced respiratory arrest in

DBA/2 mice (Faingold et al. 2013). However, the biphasic effects of the nonselective adenosine agonist and antagonist greatly complicate evaluation of the potential usefulness of these agents, and more selective adenosinergic agents need to be evaluated for their effects on seizure-induced respiratory arrest. Further work will be needed to determine if these biphasic effects can be dissected out using selective agonists and antagonists for adenosine receptor subtypes.

## NEURONAL NETWORK INTERACTIONS THAT MEDIATE SUDEP

The neuronal network in the brain that mediates audiogenic seizures in DBA mice has been proposed to involve a positive interaction between the network that mediates normal hearing (Brozoski and Bauer 2014) and the normal brainstem locomotion network (Jordan and Sławinska 2014), which interact to produce the sound-induced seizures (Faingold et al. 2014) (Figure 26.8). These seizures involve a subsequent negative interaction of this seizure network with the normal respiratory network (Bautista et al. 2014), which has been proposed to induce respiratory arrest that leads to cardiac failure and cerebral shutdown, resulting in sudden death (Faingold and

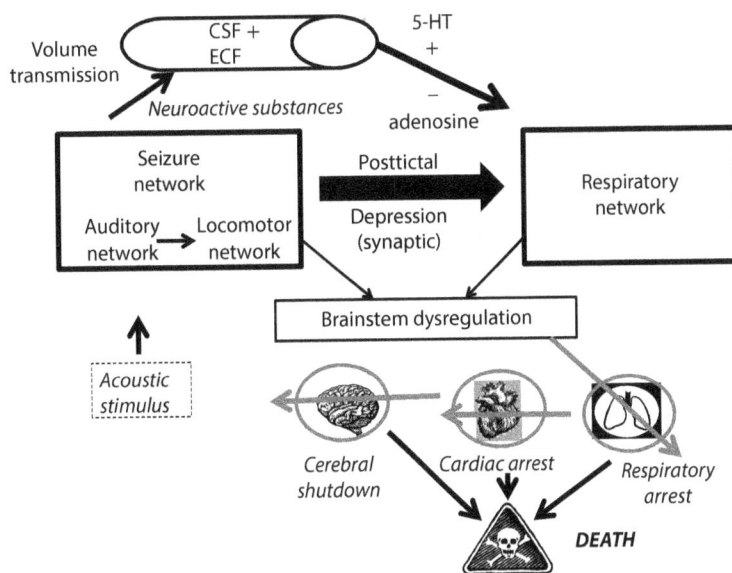

**FIGURE 26.8** Diagram of network interactions leading to seizure-induced death in DBA mouse models of human sudden unexpected death in epilepsy (SUDEP). AGS are induced by a high-intensity acoustic stimulus in the DBA mouse SUDEP models. These mice exhibit AGS, leading to death due to respiratory arrest as a result of seizure-induced brainstem dysregulation. The network that mediates AGS involves an additive interaction of the normal auditory network with the normal brainstem locomotor network. The seizure network interacts with the respiratory network in a negative fashion by synaptic and volume transmission. Volume transmission is mediated by the cerebrospinal fluid (CSF) and extracellular fluid (ECF), which carry neuroactive substances to the brainstem respiratory network. These neuroactive substances include agents that enhance respiration, such as 5-hydroxytryptamine (5-HT), and agents that depress respiration, including adenosine. If the negative influences, including physical restraints such as loose bed clothes (in human SUDEP) predominate, then respiratory arrest occurs, which leads to cardiac arrest, cerebral shutdown, and death. SUDEP in DBA mice can be prevented by enhancing 5-HT neurotransmission or by blocking the action of adenosine.

Tupal 2014). This seizure-related dysregulation of the brainstem involves the network interaction between the seizure network and the respiratory network, which may be mediated by anatomical and physiological interactions involving synaptic transmission. This network interaction may also involve volume transmission of neuroactive substances via diffusion through the cerebrospinal and extracellular fluids (Agnati et al. 2014), including the competing stimulatory effects of 5-HT and inhibitory effects on respiration of adenosine, respectively, discussed above (Figure 26.8) (Faingold and Tupal 2014).

## ALCOHOL AND SUDEP

It is well known that individuals who imbibe ethyl alcohol in excess can undergo ethanol withdrawal (ETX) seizures (McKeon et al. 2008; Manasco et al. 2012). In patients with a predisposition to epilepsy, intake of ethanol can cause their latent epilepsy to be expressed, and patients with epilepsy can experience worsened symptoms if they imbibe ethanol. These observations have led to the recommendation that patients with epilepsy avoid ethanol (Hauser et al. 1988; Brathen et al. 1999; Leach et al. 2012). There is also evidence suggesting that ethanol intake can increase the risk of SUDEP (McGugan 1999; Scorza et al. 2009; Hesdorffer and Tomson 2013). Therefore, we performed preliminary studies in the epilepsy model described above, GEPR-9s, which exhibit audiogenic seizures but rarely die as a result

of their seizures. Following a four-day Machrowicz binge ethanol paradigm (Faingold 2008; Feng and Faingold 2008) and subjected to the audiogenic seizure-inducing stimulus during ETX, they exhibited more intense and longer duration seizures and nearly 30% of them died. Immediately after seizure, these rats exhibited considerable respiratory dysfunction, with a significantly greater duration of gasping and agonal breathing, which are autoresuscitation mechanisms, than seen after seizures normally in GEPR-9s. Initial data suggest that seizure-induced death could be prevented with early respiratory support. This is based on the observations that in this animal model that normally does not exhibit seizure-induced death, ETX can result in seizure-related deaths with evidence of a respiratory causation. This may be relevant to human SUDEP, and further work on this model appears to be warranted.

## CONCLUSIONS AND FUTURE DIRECTIONS

Previous literature and the recent findings enumerated above indicate that neurotransmitters, including 5-HT and adenosine, which are known to be released during generalized seizures, play key roles in postictal depression (Fisher and Schachter 2000; Lado and Moshe 2008). These endogenous substances are also known to exert significant effects on normal respiration, particularly in the brainstem neuronal network that mediates central control of respiration. Since depression of respiration is strongly implicated as a major causation of human SUDEP, drugs that modify the action of these endogenous substances have the potential to alter SUDEP susceptibility. This idea has been tested in animal models of SUDEP in DBA mice. These mice continue to be useful models of human SUDEP because they exhibit seizure-induced respiratory arrest. Agents that alter the action of the neurotransmitters 5-HT and adenosine exert major effects on susceptibility of these mice to seizure-induced respiratory arrest, leading to cardiac arrhythmias and death. DBA/2 mice are acutely susceptible to seizure-induced respiratory arrest, but this susceptibility is relatively brief, ~1 week, after which they lose consistent susceptibility at ~1 month of age, due to hearing loss. DBA/1 mice are chronically susceptible to seizure-induced respiratory arrest, and consistent susceptibility can last for over 2–3 months in many mice. However, most DBA/1 mice require 3–4 consecutive daily seizures at postnatal day 24–30 before the majority of these animals, ~70%–100%, exhibit susceptibility to seizure-induced respiratory arrest. If the testing is not begun until after ~7 weeks of age, susceptibility to seizure-induced respiratory arrest may initially be very low and may require several seizures to establish consistent susceptibility. In both DBA mouse strains, the generalized convulsive seizures are induced with intense acoustic stimuli (audiogenic seizures). However, a rat model of audiogenic seizures, the GEPR-9s, rarely exhibits death associated with audiogenic seizures under normal conditions unless the action of adenosine is blocked or if the rats are subjected to ETX.

In addition to respiratory dysfunction, cardiovascular dysfunction and cerebral shutdown associated with postictal EEG suppression are the major phenomena associated with human SUDEP, and the latter events may also be related to respiratory dysfunction. Attribution of these phenomena to seizure-induced brainstem dysregulation is based on the critical role that the brainstem structures play in control of respiration, cardiac function, and consciousness (Brown et al. 2012; Garcia et al. 2013; Feldman et al. 2013), and in generalized seizures (Faingold 2012). Generalized seizures are known to result in the release of several neuroactive substances, including 5-HT and adenosine, and drugs that affect the action of 5-HT and adenosine affect susceptibility to seizure-induced respiratory arrest in DBA mice. Thus, certain agents that enhance the action of 5-HT, including several (but not all) SSRIs, prevent seizure-induced respiratory arrest without blocking seizures in both DBA/2 and DBA/1 mice. However, significant differences between the different clinically used SSRIs are seen in terms of effectiveness and selective effects on seizure-induced respiratory arrest. Thus, fluoxetine is the most effective and selective, whereas paroxetine is minimally effective and only in near-toxic doses.

Administration of a $5\text{-HT}_{2B/2C}$ agonist significantly reduced seizure-induced respiratory arrest incidence in DBA/2 mice, but this relatively selective agonist was ineffective in blocking seizure-induced respiratory arrest in DBA/1 mice. The 5-HT receptor subtype expression differs significantly from normal and from each other for the $5\text{-HT}_{2B}$ subunit in the two strains of DBA mice. A selective $5\text{-HT}_7$ agonist was also not effective in DBA/1 mice (Faingold et al. 2014). It is not known whether these differences are relevant to human SUDEP, although SSRI treatment was associated with a reduced degree of peri-ictal respiratory depression in one group of patients in a retrospective study (Bateman et al. 2010). The ability of one of the selective 5-HT agonists to suppress seizure-induced respiratory arrest in the DBA/2 mice suggests that selective agonists may be potentially useful for SUDEP prevention. However, further exploration of other selective agonists in both models is needed to provide guidance on this issue.

Since many patients with epilepsy are treated for comorbid depression with SSRIs, a thorough examination of existing case information as well as a prospective evaluation of patients undergoing seizures, particularly in epilepsy monitoring units, may provide data on the potential usefulness of agents that enhance the activity of 5-HT neurotransmission in the prevention of SUDEP in patients.

It would also be useful to know if DBA mice display differences in levels of 5-HT, the enzymes that mediate 5-HT synthesis or metabolism, or altered 5-HT uptake mechanisms. The finding that a nonselective 5-HT antagonist increased SUDEP susceptibility in DBA/2 and DBA/1 mice (Tupal and Faingold 2006; Faingold et al. 2014 submitted) also suggests that these agents, which are also used clinically for allergies and migraine headaches, should be avoided in patients who display the clinical characteristics associated with higher risk for SUDEP susceptibility.

Altering the effects of adenosine may also be a potential approach to understanding and preventing SUDEP, as suggested by Boison and colleagues (Shen et al. 2010). Adenosine levels in the brain are known to rise during seizures in animals and man, and adenosine is also known for its CNS depressant effects, including respiratory depression. In DBA/2 mice and in the GEPR-9s that were previously not susceptible to seizure-induced respiratory arrest, increasing adenosine receptor activation by blocking its metabolic breakdown increases seizure-induced respiratory depression and causes both species to exhibit an elevated incidence of susceptibility to death, requiring resuscitative intervention (Faingold et al. 2013). A nonselective adenosine antagonist also blocks seizure-induced respiratory arrest in DBA/2 mice. Future work will need to determine if subtype-selective adenosine receptor antagonists exert more selective effects on seizure-induced respiratory arrest. The biphasic action of adenosine seen in current studies makes further investigations more complicated, and the relative importance of adenosine receptor subtypes in these actions needs to be further evaluated. However, the agents' capacity to potentiate adenosine effects and increase the incidence of seizure-induced death in rodents that did not previously exhibit it by blocking the breakdown of adenosine, described above, does suggest the relative importance of this neurotransmitter in SUDEP mechanisms.

A number of other neurotransmitters/neuromodulators are also released during seizures, and several of them, including neurosteroids and endorphins, also exert significant effects on respiration. The role of these agents in seizure-induced respiratory arrest in these SUDEP models requires extensive further investigation.

## ACKNOWLEDGMENTS

We wish to thank Manish Raisinghani, Yashanad Mhaskar, and Kristin Plath for their parts in the experiments from our laboratory; Gayle Stauffer for her manuscript assistance; and Citizens United for Research in Epilepsy (CURE) Collaborative Grant and the CURE Christopher Donalty Grant award and the Epilepsy Foundation for funding our work on SUDEP.

## REFERENCES

Agnati LF, Genedani S, Spano P, Guidolin D, KjellFuxe K. Volume transmission and the Russian-doll organization of brain cell networks: Aspects of their integrative actions. In: Faingold C, Blumenfeld H, eds. *Neuronal Networks in Brain Function, CNS Disorders, and Therapeutics*. San Diego, CA: Academic Press/Elsevier; 2014, pp. 103–19.

Al-Zubaidy ZA, Erickson RL, Greer JJ. Serotonergic and noradrenergic effects on respiratory neural discharge in the medullary slice preparation of neonatal rats. *Pflugers Arch* 1996;431:942–9.

Angelatou F, Pagonopoulou O, Kostopoulos G. Changes in seizure latency correlate with alterations in A1 adenosine receptor binding during daily repeated pentylentetrazol-induced convulsions in different mouse brain areas. *Neurosci Lett* 1991;132(2):203–6.

Applegate CD, Tecott LH. Global increases in seizure susceptibility in mice lacking 5-HT2C receptors: A behavioral analysis. *Exp Neurol* 1998;154(2):522–30.

Asadi-Pooya AA, Sperling MR. Clinical features of sudden unexpected death in epilepsy. *J Clin Neurophysiol* 2009;26(5):297–301.

Auerbach DS, Jones J, Clawson BC, Offord J, Lenk GM, Ogiwara I, Yamakawa K, Meisler MH, Parent JM, Isom LL. Altered cardiac electrophysiology and SUDEP in a model of Dravet syndrome. *PLoSOne* 2013;8(10):e77843.

Bateman LM, Li CS, Seyal M. Ictal hypoxemia in localization-related epilepsy: Analysis of incidence, severity and risk factors. *Brain* 2008;131(Pt 12):3239–45.

Bateman LM, Spitz M, Seyal M. Ictal hypoventilation contributes to cardiac arrhythmia and SUDEP: Report on two deaths in video-EEG-monitored patients. *Epilepsia* 2010;51(5):916–20.

Bautista TG, Pitts Pilowsky PM, Morris KF. The brainstem respiratory network. In: Faingold CL, Blumenfeld H, eds. *Neuronal Networks in Brain Function, CNS Disorders, and Therapeutics*. San Diego, CA: Academic Press/Elsevier; 2014, pp. 235–45.

Benarroch EE. Brain stem respiratory control: Substrates of respiratory failure of multiple system atrophy. *MovDisord* 2007;22(2):155–61.

Berman RF, Fredholm BB, Aden U, O'Connor WT. Evidence for increased dorsal hippocampal adenosine release and metabolism during pharmacologically induced seizures in rats. *Brain Res* 2000;872(1–2):44–53.

Bodineau L, Cayetanot F, Marlot D, Collin T, Gros F, Frugiere A. Endogenous 5-HT (1/2) systems and the newborn rat respiratory control. A comparative in vivo and in vitro study. *Respir Physiol Neurobiol* 2004;141: 47–57.

Boison D. Adenosine dysfunction in epilepsy. *Glia* 2012;60(8): 1234–43.

Boison D. Role of adenosine in status epilepticus: A potential new target? *Epilepsia* 2013;54(Suppl 6):20–2.

Boison D, Stewart KA. Therapeutic epilepsy research: From pharmacological rationale to focal adenosine augmentation. *Biochem Pharmacol* 2009;78:1428–37.

Bonham AC, Chen CY, Sekizawa S, Joad JP. Plasticity in the nucleus tractus solitarius and its influence on lung and airway reflexes. *J Appl Physiol* 2006;101:322–7.

Brathen G, Brodtkorb E, Helde G, Sand T, Bovim G. The diversity of seizures related to alcohol use. A study of consecutive patients. *Eur J Neurol* 1999;6(6):697–703.

Brennan TJ, Seeley WW, Kilgard M, Schreiner CE, Tecott LH. Sound-induced seizures in serotonin 5-HT2c receptor mutant mice. *Nat Genet* 1997;16:387–90.

Brisson-Thoby M, Greer JJ. Anatomical and functional development of the pre-Bötzinger complex in prenatal rodents. *J Appl Physiol* 2008;104(4):1213–9.

Brown RE, Basheer R, McKenna JT, Strecker RE, McCarley RW. Control of sleep and wakefulness. *Physiol Rev* 2012;92(3):1087–187.

Browning RA, Wood AV, Merrill MA, Dailey JW, Jobe PC. Enhancement of the anticonvulsant effect of fluoxetine following blockade of 5-HT1A receptors. *Eur J Pharmacol* 1997;336(1):1–6.

Brozoski TJ, Bauer CA. Auditory neuronal networks and chronic tinnitus. In: Faingold C, Blumenfeld H, eds. *Neuronal Networks in Brain Function, CNS Disorders, and Therapeutics*. San Diego, CA: Academic Press/Elsevier; 2014, pp. 261–75.

Burnstock G. Introduction to purinergic signalling in the brain. *Adv Exp Med Biol* 2013;986:1–12.

Carley DW, Radulovacki M. Role of peripheral serotonin in the regulation of central sleep apneas in rats. *Chest* 1999;115:1397–401.

Chen CY, Bonham AC. Non-NMDA and NMDA receptors transmit area postrema input to aortic baroreceptor neurons in NTS. *Am J Physiol* 1998;275:H1695–706.

Collins RL. Audiogenic seizures. In: Purpura DP, Penry JK, Tower DB, Woodbury DM, Walter RD, eds. *Experimental Models of Epilepsy A Manual for the Laboratory Worker*. New York, NY: Raven Press; 1972, pp. 347–72.

Dailey JW, Naritoku DK. Antidepressants and seizures: Clinical anecdotes overshadow neuroscience. *Biochem Pharmacol* 1996;52:1323–9.

Del Negro CA. Disparate purinergic modulation of respiration in rats and mice. *J Physiol* 2011;589(Pt 18):4409–10.

Devinsky O. Sudden, unexpected death in epilepsy. *N Engl J Med* 2011;365(19):1801–11.

Di Giovanni G, Di Matteo V, Pierucci M, Benigno A, Esposito E. Central serotonin 2C receptor: From physiology to pathology. *Curr Top Med Chem* 2006;6(18):1909–25.

Doi A, Ramirez JM. Neuromodulation and the orchestration of the respiratory rhythm. *Respir Physiol Neurobiol* 2008;164(1–2):96–104.

Donner EJ. Explaining the unexplained; expecting the unexpected: Where are we with sudden unexpected death in epilepsy? *Epilepsy Curr* 2011;11(2):45–9.

Donner EJ, Smith CR, Snead OC III. Sudden unexplained death in children with epilepsy. *Neurology* 2001;57(3): 430–4.

Dulla CG, Dobelis P, Pearson T, Frenguelli BG, Staley KJ, Masino SA. Adenosine and ATP link P-CO$_2$ to cortical excitability via pH. *Neuron* 2005;48:1011–23.

Duncan S, Brodie MJ. Sudden unexpected death in epilepsy. *Epilepsy Behav* 2011;21(4):344–51.

Dunwiddie TV, Masino SA. The role and regulation of adenosine in the central nervous system. *Annu Rev Neurosci* 2001;24:31–55.

During MJ, Spencer DD. Adenosine: A potential mediator of seizure arrest and postictal refractoriness. *Ann Neurol* 1992;32(5):618–24.

Etherington LA, Frenguelli BG. Endogenous adenosine modulates epileptiform activity in rat hippocampus in a receptor sub-type-dependent manner. *Eur J Neurosci* 2004;19:2539–50.

Faingold CL. Role of GABA abnormalities in the inferior colliculus pathophysiology: Audiogenic seizures. *Hear Res* 2002;168:223–37.

Faingold CL. The Majchrowicz binge alcohol protocol: An intubation technique to study alcohol dependence in rats. *Curr Protoc Neurosci* 2008; Chapter 9: Unit 9.28.

Faingold CL. Brainstem networks: Reticulo-cortical synchronization in generalized convulsive seizures. In: Noebels JL, Avoli M, Rogawski MA, Olsen RW, Delgado-Escueta AV, eds. *Jasper's Basic Mechanisms of the Epilepsies*. 4th ed. New York, NY: Oxford University Press; 2012, pp. 257–71.

Faingold CL, Kommajosyula SP, Long X, Plath K, Randall M. Serotonin and sudden death: Differential effects of serotonergic drugs on seizure-induced respiratory arrest in DBA/1 mice. *Epilepsy Behav* 2014;37:198–203.

Faingold C, Raisinghani M, N'Gouemo P. Neuronal networks in epilepsy: Comparative audiogenic seizure networks. In: Faingold C, Blumenfeld H, eds. *Neuronal Networks in Brain Function, CNS Disorders, and Therapeutics*. San Diego, CA: Academic Press/Elsevier; 2014, pp. 349–73.

Faingold CL, Randall M. Effects of age, sex, and sertraline administration on seizure-induced respiratory arrest in the DBA/1 mouse model of sudden unexpected death in epilepsy (SUDEP). *Epilepsy Behav* 2013;28(1):78–82.

Faingold CL, Randall M, Kommajosyula SP. Role of adenosine in seizure-induced death in DBA/2 mice and genetically epilepsy-prone rats (GEPRs): Potential relevance to SUDEP. *Amer Epil Soc Abs* 2013;3.038.

Faingold CL, Randall M, Mhaskar Y, Uteshev VV. Differences in serotonin receptor expression in the brainstem may explain the differential ability of a serotonin agonist to block seizure-induced sudden death in DBA/2 vs. DBA/1 mice. *Brain Res* 2011;1418:104–10.

Faingold CL, Randall M, Tupal S. DBA/1 mice exhibit chronic susceptibility to audiogenic seizures followed by sudden death associated with respiratory arrest. *Epilepsy Behav* 2010a;17(4):436–40.

Faingold CL, Tupal S. Neuronal network interactions in the startle reflex, learning mechanisms, and CNS disorders, including sudden unexpected death in epilepsy. In: Faingold C, Blumenfeld H, eds. *Neuronal Networks in Brain Function, CNS Disorders, and Therapeutics*. San Diego, CA: Academic Press/Elsevier; 2014, pp. 407–18.

Faingold CL, Tupal S, Mhaskar Y, Uteshev VV. DBA mice as models of sudden unexpected death in epilepsy. In: Lathers CM, Schraeder PL, Bungo MW, Leestma JE, eds. *Sudden Death in Epilepsy: Forensic and Clinical Issues*. Boca Raton, FL: CRC Press; 2010b, pp. 659–76.

Faingold CL, Tupal S, Randall M. Prevention of seizure-induced sudden death in a chronic SUDEP model by semichronic administration of a selective serotonin reuptake inhibitor. *Epilepsy Behav* 2011;22(2):186–90.

Feast A, Martinian L, Liu J, Catarino CB, Thom M, Sisodiya SM. Investigation of hypoxia-inducible factor-1alpha in hippocampal sclerosis: A postmortem study. *Epilepsia* 2012;53(8):1349–59.

Fedele DE, Li T, Lan JQ, Fredholm BB, Boison D. Adenosine A1 receptors are crucial in keeping an epileptic focus localized. *Exp Neurol* 2006;200:184–90.

Feldman JL, Del Negro CA. Looking for inspiration: New perspectives on respiratory rhythm. *Nat Rev Neurosci* 2006;7(3):232–42.

Feldman JL, Del Negro CA, Gray PA. Understanding the rhythm of breathing: So near, yet so far. *Annu Rev Physiol* 2013;75:423–52.

Feldman JL, Mitchell GS, Nattie EE. Breathing: Rhythmicity, plasticity, chemosensitivity. *Annu Rev Neurosci* 2003;26:239–66.

Feng HJ, Faingold CL. The effects of chronic ethanol administration on amygdala neuronal firing and ethanol withdrawal seizures. *Neuropharmacology* 2008;55(5):648–53.

Fisher RS, Schachter SC. The postictal state: A neglected entity in the management of epilepsy. *Epilepsy Behav* 2000;1(1):52–9.

Fredholm BB, Ijzerman AP, Jacobson KA, Klotz KN, Linden J. International union of pharmacology. XXV. Nomenclature and classification of adenosine receptors. *Pharmacol Rev* 2001;53:527–52.

Freitas J, Kaur G, Fernandez GB, Tatsuoka C, Kaffashi F, Loparo KA, Rao S, et al. Age-specific periictal electro clinical features of generalized tonic-clonic seizures and potential risk of sudden unexpected death in epilepsy (SUDEP). *Epilepsy Behav* 2013;29(2):289–94.

Fukuda M, Suzuki Y, Hino H, Ishii E. Over-activation of adenosine A (2A) receptors and sudden unexpected death in epilepsy. *Epilepsy Behav* 2012;23(3):387–8.

Fukumitsu N, Ishii K, Kimura Y, Oda K, Sasaki T, Mori Y, Ishiwata K. Adenosine A1 receptor mapping of the human brain by PET with 8-dicyclopropylmethyl-1-11C-methyl-3-propylxanthine. *J Nucl Med* 2005;46(1):32–7.

Garcia AJ III, Koschnitzky JE, Dashevskiy T, Ramirez JM. Cardiorespiratory coupling in health and disease. *Autonom Neurosci* 2013;175(1–2):26–37.

Garcia AJ III, Zanella S, Koch H, Doi A, Ramirez JM. Chapter 3—Networks within networks: The neuronal control of breathing. *Prog Brain Res* 2011;188:31–50.

Gharedaghi MH, Seyedabadi M, Ghia JE, Dehpour AR, Rahimian R. The role of different serotonin receptor subtypes in seizure susceptibility. *Exp Brain Res* 2014;232(2):347–67.

Hamid H, Kanner AM. Should antidepressant drugs of the selective serotonin reuptake inhibitor family be tested as antiepileptic drugs? *Epilepsy Behav* 2013;26(3):261–5.

Hauser WA, Ng SKC, Brust JCM. Alcohol, seizures and epilepsy. *Epilepsia* 1988;29(Suppl 2):S66–78.

Heisler LK, Chu HM, Tecott LH. Epilepsy and obesity in serotonin 5-HT2C receptor mutant mice. *Ann N Y Acad Sci* 1998;861:74–8.

Hernandez EJ, Williams PA, Dudek FE. Effects of fluoxetine and TFMPP on spontaneous seizures in rats with pilocarpine-induced epilepsy. *Epilepsia* 2002;43:1337–45.

Hesdorffer DC, Tomson T. Sudden unexpected death in epilepsy. Potential role of antiepileptic drugs. *CNS Drugs* 2013;27(2):113–9.

Hodges MR, Richerson GB. Contributions of 5-HT neurons to respiratory control: Neuromodulatory and trophic effects. *Respir Physiol Neurobiol* 2008; 164(1–2):222–32.

Hodges MR, Tattersall GJ, Harris MB, McEvoy SD, Richerson DN, Deneris ES, Johnson RL, Chen ZF, Richerson GB. Defects in breathing and thermoregulation in mice with near-complete absence of central serotonin neurons. *J Neurosci* 2008;28(10):2495–505.

Holladay JW, Dewey MJ, Yoo SD. Pharmacokinetics and antidepressant activity of fluoxetine in transgenic mice with elevated serum alpha-1-acid glycoprotein levels. *Drug Metab Dispos* 1998;26(1):20–4.

Jordan D. Vagal control of the heart: Central serotonergic (5-HT) mechanisms *Exp Physiol* 2005;90:175–81.

Jordan LM, Sławinska U. The brain and spinal cord networks controlling locomotion. In: Faingold CL, Blumenfeld H, eds. *Neuronal Networks in Brain Function, CNS Disorders, and Therapeutics.* San Diego, CA: Academic Press/Elsevier; 2014, pp. 215–33.

Kalume F. Sudden unexpected death in Dravet syndrome: Respiratory and other physiological dysfunctions. *Respir Physiol Neurobiol* 2013;189(2):324–8.

Kline DD, Takacs KN, Ficker E, Kunze DL. Dopamine modulates synaptic transmission in the nucleus of the solitary tract. *J Neurophysiol* 2002;88:2736–44.

Kostopoulos G, Drapeau C, Avoli M, Olivier A, Villemeure JG. Endogenous adenosine can reduce epileptiform activity in the human epileptogenic cortex maintained in vitro. *Neurosci Lett* 1989;106(1–2):119–24.

Kubin L, Alheid GF, Zuperku EJ, McCrimmon DR. Central pathways of pulmonary and lower airway vagal afferents. *J Appl Physiol* 2006;101:618–27.

Kumral A, Tuzun F, Yesilirmak DC, Duman N, Ozkan H. Genetic basis of apnoea of prematurity and caffeine treatment response: Role of adenosine receptor polymorphisms: Genetic basis of apnoea of prematurity. *Acta Paediatr* 2012;101 (7):e299–303.

Lado FA, Moshe SL. How do seizures stop? *Epilepsia* 2008; 49(10):1651–64.

LaFrance WC Jr., Kanner AM, Hermann B. Psychiatric comorbidities in epilepsy. *Int Rev Neurobiol* 2008;83:347–83.

Lamberts RJ, Thijs RD, Laffan A, Langan Y, Sander JW. Sudden unexpected death in epilepsy: People with nocturnal seizures may be at highest risk. *Epilepsia* 2012;53(2):253–7.

Langan Y, Nashef L, Sander JW. Sudden unexpected death in epilepsy: A series of witnessed deaths. *J Neurol Neurosurg Psychiatry* 2000;68(2):211–3.

Langan Y, Nashef L, Sander JW. Case-control study of SUDEP. *Neurology* 2005;64(7):1131–3.

Lathers CM, Schraeder PL, Bungo MW. The mystery of sudden death: Mechanisms for risks. *Epilepsy Behav* 2008;12(1):3–24.

Leach JP, Mohanraj R, Borland W. Alcohol and drugs in epilepsy: Pathophysiology, presentation, possibilities, and prevention. *Epilepsia* 2012;53(Suppl 4):48–57.

Lear-Kaul KC, Coughlin L, Dobersen MJ. Sudden unexpected death in epilepsy: A retrospective study. *Am J Forensic Med Pathol* 2005;26:11–7.

Lhatoo SD, Faulkner HJ, Dembny K, Trippick K, Johnson C, Bird JM. An electroclinical case-control study of sudden unexpected death in epilepsy. *Ann Neurol* 2010;68(6):787–96.

Li T, Steinbeck JA, Lusardi T, Koch P, Lan JQ, Wilz A, Segschneider M, Simon RP, Brüstle O, Boison D. Suppression of kindling epileptogenesis by adenosine releasing stem cell-derived brain implants. *Brain* 2007;130:1276–88.

Liu J, Akay T, Hedlund PB, Pearson KG, Jordan LM. Spinal 5-HT7 receptors are critical for alternating activity during locomotion: In vitro neonatal and in vivo adult studies using 5-HT7 receptor knockout mice. *J Neurophysiol* 2009;102(1):337–48.

Lopes LV, Sebastiao AM, Ribeiro JA. Adenosine and related drugs in brain diseases: Present and future in clinical trials. *Curr Top Med Chem* 2011;11(8):1087–101.

Malagie I, Trillat AC, Jacquot C, Gardier AM. Effects of acute fluoxetine on extracellular serotonin levels in the raphe: An in vivo microdialysis study. *Eur J Pharmacol* 1995;286:213–7.

Manasco A, Chang S, Larriviere J, Hamm LL, Glass M. Alcohol withdrawal. *South Med J* 2012;105(11):607–12.

Manzke T, Guenther U, Ponimaskin EG, Haller M, Dutschmann M, Schwarzacher S, Richter DW. 5-HT4(a) receptors avert opioid-induced breathing depression without loss of analgesia. *Science* 2003;301:226–9.

Massey CA, Sowers LP, Dlouhy BJ, Richerson GB. Mechanisms of sudden unexpected death in epilepsy: The pathway to prevention. *Nat Rev Neurol* 2014;10(5):271–82.

Mathew OP. Apnea of prematurity: Pathogenesis and management strategies. *J Perinatol* 2011;31(5):302–10.

McGugan EA. Sudden unexpected deaths in epileptics—A literature review. *Scott Med J* 1999;44(5):1379.

McKeon A, Frye MA, Delanty N. The alcohol withdrawal syndrome. *J Neurol Neurosurg Psychiatry* 2008;79(8):854–62.

Merlet I, Ostrowsky K, Costes N, Ryvlin P, Isnard J, Faillenot I, Lavenne F, Dufournel D, Le BD, Mauguiere F. 5-HT1A receptor binding and intracerebral activity in temporal lobe epilepsy: An [18F]MPPF-PET study. *Brain* 2004;127:900–13.

Merrill MA, Clough RW, Jobe PC, Browning RA. Role of the superior colliculus and the intercollicular nucleus in the brainstem seizure circuitry of the genetically epilepsy-prone rat. *Epilepsia* 2003;44:305–14.

Merrill MA, Clough RW, Jobe PC, Browning RA. Brainstem seizure severity regulates forebrain seizure expression in the audiogenic kindling model. *Epilepsia* 2005;46:1380–8.

Meschaks A, Lindstrom P, Halldin C, Farde L, Savic I. Regional reductions in serotonin 1A receptor binding in juvenile myoclonic epilepsy. *Arch Neurol* 2005;62:946–50.

Meyer LC, Fuller A, Mitchell D. Zacopride and 8-OH-DPAT reverse opioid-induced respiratory depression and hypoxia but not catatonic immobilization in goats. *Am J Physiol Regul Integr Comp Physiol* 2006;290:R405–13.

Moseley BD, Britton JW, Nelson C, Lee RW, So E. Periictal cerebral tissue hypoxemia: A potential marker of SUDEP risk. *Epilepsia* 2012;53(12):e208–11.

Nadkarni MA, Friedman D, Devinsky O. Central apnea at complex partial seizure onset. *Seizure* 2012;21(7):555–8.

Nashef L, Fish DR, Garner S, Sander JW, Shorvon SD. Sudden death in epilepsy: A study of incidence in a young cohort with epilepsy and learning difficulty. *Epilepsia* 1995;36:1187–94.

Nashef L, So EL, Ryvlin P, Tomson T. Unifying the definitions of sudden unexpected death in epilepsy. *Epilepsia* 2012;53(2):227–33.

Nashef L, Walker F, Allen P, Sander JW, Shorvon SD. Fish DR. Apnoea and bradycardia during epileptic seizures: Relation to sudden death in epilepsy. *J Neurol Neurosurg Psychiatry* 1996;60(3):297–300.

Nishino S, Mignot E. Pharmacological aspects of human and canine narcolepsy. *Prog Neurobiol* 1997;52:27–78.

Olsson M, Annerbrink K, Hedner J, Eriksson E. Intracerebroventricular administration of the angiotensin II receptor antagonist saralasin reduces respiratory rate and tidal volume variability in freely moving Wistar rats. *Psychoneuroendocrinology* 2004;29(1):107–12.

Opeskin K, Berkovic SF. Risk factors for sudden unexpected death in epilepsy: A controlled prospective study based on coroners cases. *Seizure* 2003;12:456–64.

Pagonopoulou O, Efthimiadou A, Asimakopoulos B, Nikolettos NK. Modulatory role of adenosine and its receptors in epilepsy: Possible therapeutic approaches. *Neurosci Res* 2006;56(1):14–20.

Paul S, Elsinga PH, Ishiwata K, Dierckx RA, van Waarde A. Adenosine A (1) receptors in the central nervous system: Their functions in health and disease, and possible elucidation by PET imaging. *Curr Med Chem* 2011;18(31):4820–35.

Pavlova M, Singh K, Abdennadher M, Katz ES, Dworetzky BA, White DP, Llewellyn N, Kothare SV. Comparison of cardiorespiratory and EEG abnormalities with seizures in adults and children. *Epilepsy Behav* 2013;29(3):537–41.

Pedata F, Corsi C, Melani A, Bordoni F, Latini S. Adenosine extracellular brain concentrations and role of A2A receptors in ischemia. *Ann N Y Acad Sci* 2001;939:74–84.

Pena F, Ramirez JM. Endogenous activation of serotonin-2A receptors is required for respiratory rhythm generation in vitro. *J Neurosci* 2002;22:11055–64.

Potts JT. Inhibitory neurotransmission in the nucleus tractus solitarii: Implications for baroreflex resetting during exercise. *Exp Physiol* 2006;91(1):59–72.

Racagni G, Popoli M. Cellular and molecular mechanisms in the long-term action of antidepressants. *Dialogues Clin Neurosci* 2008;10(4):385–400.

Ramirez JM, Doi A, Garcia AJ III, Elsen FP, Koch H, Wei AD. The cellular building blocks of breathing. *Compr Physiol* 2012;2(4):2683–731.

Ramirez JM, Viemari JC. Determinants of inspiratory activity. *Respir Physiol Neurobiol* 2005;147(2–3):145–57.

Raul L. Serotonin 2 receptors in the nucleus tractus solitarius: Characterization and role in the baroreceptor reflex arc. *Cell Mol Neurobiol* 2003;23(4–5):709–26.

Rebola N, Coelho JE, Costenla AR, Lopes LV, Parada A, Oliveira CR, Soares-da-Silva P, de Mendonca A, Cunha RA. Decrease of adenosine A₁ receptor density and of adenosine neuromodulation in the hippocampus of kindled rats. *Eur J Neurosci* 2003;18(4):820–8.

Richter DW, Manzke T, Wilken B, Ponimaskin E. Serotonin receptors: Guardians of stable breathing. *Trends Mol Med* 2003;9(12):542–8.

Ryvlin P, Montavont A, Kahane P. Sudden unexpected death in epilepsy: From mechanisms to prevention. *Curr Opin Neurol* 2006;19:194–9.

Ryvlin P, Nashef L, Lhatoo SD, Bateman LM, Bird J, Bleasel A, Boon P, et al. Incidence and mechanisms of cardiorespiratory arrests in epilepsy monitoring units (MORTEMUS): A retrospective study. *Lancet Neurol* 2013;12(10):966–77.

Schraeder PL, Lathers CM. Paroxysmal autonomic dysfunction, epileptogenic activity and sudden death. *Epilepsy Res* 1989;3:55–62.

Schuele SU, Afshari M, Afshari ZS, Macken MP, Asconape J, Wolfe L, Gerard EE. Ictal central apnea as a predictor for sudden unexpected death in epilepsy. *Epilepsy Behav* 2011;22(2):401–3.

Scorza CA, Cysneiros RM, Arida RM, Terra VC, Machado HR, de Almeida AC, Cavalheiro EA, Scorza FA. Alcohol consumption and sudden unexpected death in epilepsy: Experimental approach. *Arq Neuropsiquiatr* 2009;67(4):1003–6.

Seyal M, Bateman LM, Albertson TE, Lin TC, Li CS. Respiratory changes with seizures in localization-related epilepsy: Analysis of periictal hypercapnia and airflow patterns. *Epilepsia* 2010;51(8):1359–64.

Seyal M, Hardin KA, Bateman LM. Postictal generalized EEG suppression is linked to seizure-associated respiratory dysfunction but not postictal apnea. *Epilepsia* 2012;53(5):825–31.

Seyfried TN, Glaser GH. A review of mouse mutants as genetic models of epilepsy. *Epilepsia* 1985;26:143–50.

Shen HY, Li T, Boison D. A novel mouse model for sudden unexpected death in epilepsy (SUDEP): Role of impaired adenosine clearance. *Epilepsia* 2010;51(3):465–8.

Shorvon S, Tomson T. Sudden unexpected death in epilepsy. *Lancet* 2011;378(9808):2028–38.

Smith JC, Abdala AP, Borgmann A, Rybak IA, Paton JF. Brainstem respiratory networks: Building blocks and microcircuits. *Trends Neurosci* 2013;36(3):152–62.

So EL. Demystifying sudden unexplained death in epilepsy—are we close? *Epilepsia* 2006;47(Suppl 1):87–92.

So EL. What is known about the mechanisms underlying SUDEP? *Epilepsia* 2008;49(Suppl 9):93–8.

So EL, Sam MC, Lagerlund TL. Postictal central apnea as a cause of SUDEP: Evidence from near-SUDEP incident. *Epilepsia* 2000;41:1494–7.

Sowers LP, Massey CA, Gehlbach BK, Granner MA, Richerson GB. Sudden unexpected death in epilepsy: Fatal post-ictal respiratory and arousal mechanisms. *Respir Physiol Neurobiol* 2013;189(2):315–23.

Specchio LM, Iudice A, Specchio N, La NA, Spinelli A, Galli R, Rocchi R, Ulivelli M, de TM, Pizzanelli C, Murri L. Citalopram as treatment of depression in patients with epilepsy. *Clin Neuropharmacol* 2004;27:133–6.

Subramanian HH. Descending control of the respiratory neuronal network by the midbrain periaqueductal grey in the rat in vivo. *J Physiol* 2013;591(Pt 1):109–122.

Subramanian HH, Holstege G. Stimulation of the midbrain peri aqueductal gray modulates preinspiratory neurons in the ventrolateral medulla in the rat in vivo. *J Comp Neurol* 2013;521(13):3083–98.

Sugimoto Y, Tagawa N, Kobayashi Y, Mitsui-Saito K, Hotta Y, Yamada J. Involvement of the sigma-1 receptor in the antidepressant-like effects of fluvoxamine in the forced swimming test in comparison with the effects elicited by paroxetine. *Eur J Pharmacol* 2012;696(1–3):96–100.

Surges R, Sander JW. Sudden unexpected death in epilepsy: Mechanisms, prevalence, and prevention. *Curr Opin Neurol* 2012;25(2):201–7.

Toczek MT, Carson RE, Lang L, Ma Y, Spanaki MV, Der MG, Fazilat S, et al. PET imaging of 5-HT1A receptor binding in patients with temporal lobe epilepsy. *Neurology* 2003;60(5):749–56.

Tomson T, Nashef L, Ryvlin P. Sudden unexpected death in epilepsy: Current knowledge and future directions. *Lancet Neurol* 2008;7(11):1021–31.

Tupal S, Faingold CL. Evidence supporting a role of serotonin in modulation of sudden death induced by seizures in DBA/2 mice. *Epilepsia* 2006;47(1):21–6.

Turner JG, Willott JF. Exposure to an augmented acoustic environment alters auditory function in hearing-impaired DBA/2J mice. *Hear Res* 1998;118(1–2):101–13.

Uteshev VV, Tupal S, Mhaskar Y, Faingold CL. Abnormal serotonin receptor expression in DBA/2 mice associated with susceptibility to sudden death due to respiratory arrest. *Epilepsy Res* 2010;88(2–3):1838.

Vandam RJ, Shields EJ, Kelty JD. Rhythm generation by the pre-Bötzinger complex in medullary slice and island preparations: Effects of adenosine A (1) receptor activation. *BMC Neurosci* 2008;9:95.

Venit EL, Shepard BD, Seyfried TN. Oxygenation prevents sudden death in seizure-prone mice. *Epilepsia* 2004;45:993–6.

Welsh JP, Placantonakis DG, Warsetsky SI, Marquez RG, Bernstein L, Aicher SA. The serotonin hypothesis of myoclonus from the perspective of neuronal rhythmicity. *Adv Neurol* 2002;89:307–29.

Willott JF, Henry KR. Roles of anoxia and noise-induced hearing loss in the postictal refractory period for audiogenic seizures in mice. *J Comp Physiol Psychol* 1976;90:373–81.

Wong-Riley MT, Liu Q. Neurochemical development of brain stem nuclei involved in the control of respiration. *Respir Physiol Neurobiol* 2005;149:83–98.

Zwicker JD, Rajani V, Hahn LB, Funk GD. Purinergic modulation of pre Bötzinger complex inspiratory rhythm in rodents: The interaction between ATP and adenosine. *J Physiol* 2011;589(Pt 18):4583–600.

# 27 Omega-3 Fatty Acids and Sudden Unexpected Death in Epilepsy
## A Translational Approach

*Fulvio A. Scorza, Esper A. Cavalheiro, Antonio-Carlos G. de Almeida,*
*Carla A. Scorza, Mariana B. Nejm, and Roberta M. Cysneiros*

## CONTENTS

People with epilepsy are more likely to die prematurely than those without epilepsy, and the most common epilepsy-related cause of death is sudden unexpected death in epilepsy (SUDEP) (Surges et al. 2009). Information concerning risk factors for SUDEP is conflicting, but potential risk factors include young age of epilepsy onset, frequency of generalized tonic-clonic seizures (GTCSs), nocturnal seizures, uncontrolled seizures, seizure type, longer duration of epilepsy, number of antiepileptic drugs used, symptomatic etiology of epilepsy, male gender, alcohol abuse, and winter temperatures. Additionally, the cause of SUDEP is still unknown; however, the most commonly suggested mechanisms are cardiac or respiratory abnormalities during and between seizures.

This review first provides an overview of the epidemiology, risk factors, and etiology of SUDEP and then focuses on possible preventative measures, in particular n-3 fatty acids (omega-3 FAs). Some but not all animal and clinical studies have shown that omega-3 FAs could have direct cardiac benefits and may be useful in the prevention and treatment of epilepsy and, hence, possibly in the prevention of SUDEP.

## SUDDEN UNEXPECTED DEATH IN EPILEPSY: GENERAL APPROACH

Epilepsy is one of the most common serious brain disorders; it knows no age, racial or social class, or geographic or national boundaries (de Boer et al. 2008). Often, epilepsy is seen as a benign condition in which affected individuals only have seizures. Unfortunately, the story is not as simple as it seems. People with epilepsy have a 2.6-fold increased risk of premature death compared with the general population (Neligan et al. 2011; Surges et al. 2012). SUDEP is responsible for 7.5%–17% of all deaths in people with epilepsy and has an incidence among adults between 1:500 and 1:1000 patient-years (Ficker et al. 1998; Schuele et al. 2007). SUDEP is defined as sudden, unexpected, witnessed or unwitnessed, nontraumatic, and nondrowning deaths in patients with epilepsy, with or without evidence of a seizure and excluding documented status epilepticus, in which postmortem examination does not reveal a toxicological or anatomical cause of death (Nashef 1997). The main risk factors currently recognized in the literature include the presence or number of GTCSs, nocturnal seizures, young age at epilepsy onset, longer duration of epilepsy, dementia, absence of cerebrovascular disease, asthma, male gender, symptomatic etiology of epilepsy, and alcohol abuse (Hesdorffer and Tomson 2013).

Many predisposing and initiating factors may coexist and contribute to SUDEP, but the mechanisms are poorly understood (Terra et al. 2013). Suggested mechanisms predisposing to SUDEP include autonomic dysregulation, i.e., respiratory and cardiovascular abnormalities during and after seizures (Nei et al. 2010; Hesdorffer and Tomson 2013). Taking cardiovascular dysfunctions into consideration, relevant putative mechanisms involved in SUDEP are fatal cardiac arrhythmias due to myocardial ischemia, electrolyte disturbances, arrhythmogenic drugs, or transmission of the epileptic activity via the autonomic nervous system to the heart (Nei et al. 2004; Stollberger and Finsterer 2004; Surges et al. 2009).

## POSSIBLE CARDIAC ABNORMALITIES RELATED TO SUDDEN UNEXPECTED DEATH IN EPILEPSY

A better understanding of the mechanisms of SUDEP is essential. The causes of death in SUDEP are currently unknown; however, clues for cardiogenic SUDEP may be present in postmortem examinations of the heart as well as demonstrations of ictal and interictal cardiovascular dysfunction (Schuele et al 2007; Stollberger and Finsterer 2004).

Postmortem examinations: Postmortem examination of the hearts of SUDEP victims has revealed increased weight and dilatation (Stollberger and Finsterer 2004; Colugnati et al. 2005; Bell and Sander 2006). Moreover, pathological alterations have included fibrosis of the walls of small coronary arteries, atrophy of cardiomyocytes, myofibrillar degeneration, edema of the conductive tissue, and morphological abnormalities of the cardiac conduction system (Stollberger and Finsterer 2004; Colugnati et al. 2005; Bell and Sander 2006). Most likely, these abnormalities are the consequence of repeated hypoxemia and/or associated with the sympathetically mediated release of catecholamines during seizures (Stollberger and Finsterer 2004; Colugnati et al. 2005; Lathers et al. 2008).

Ictal period: Many studies evaluated the frequency and character of potentially fatal ictal cardiac rhythms (Stollberger and Finsterer 2004; Ryvlin et al. 2006; Lathers et al. 2008), including the demonstration of ictal arrhythmias (Ryvlin et al. 2006). Thus, in 1996 Nashef and colleagues noninvasively recorded ictal cardiorespiratory variables in patients with epilepsy. They found an increase in heart rate in 91% of 41 seizures monitored and a transient bradycardia in five seizures (four patients). Furthermore, Nei and colleagues (Nei et al. 2000) evaluated the electrocardiographic alterations in 51 seizures in 43 patients with drug-resistant epilepsy and found that 70% of patients had either electrocardiographic abnormalities (16%) or tachycardia (30%) or both (23%) during the ictal and/or postictal periods. These authors suggest that these changes may be relevant to the pathophysiology of SUDEP. More compelling published evidence for potentially fatal ictal cardiac arrhythmias is needed.

Interictal period: Investigations of cardiac rhythms during the interictal period have included those by Drake and coworkers (Drake et al. 1993), who reviewed resting electrocardiograms (ECGs) in 75 patients with epilepsy and compared ventricular rate, PR interval, QRS duration, and QT interval corrected for heart rate ($QT_C$) with ECGs recorded in healthy age-matched controls. Patients with epilepsy had a faster heart rate and a longer QT duration than controls. Heart rate and QT duration, however, were not outside the normal range. In 2003, Tigaran and colleagues investigated whether patients with drug refractory epilepsy have cardiovascular abnormalities that might be related to sudden death. In their study, 23 subjects underwent comprehensive cardiovascular evaluations (ECG, Holter monitoring, echocardiography, ergometric exercise test, and myocardial scintigraphy and, if abnormalities were found, coronary angiography) before and during video-electroencephalogram monitoring. They found ST-segment depression in 40% of the patients that was associated with a higher maximum heart rate during seizures, suggesting that cardiac ischemia may occur in these patients (Tigaran et al. 2003).

Recently, Ramadan and collaborators investigated possible interictal electrocardiographic abnormalities in patients with GTCSs and looked for evidence of structural heart changes with echocardiography and compared the findings with healthy controls. They demonstrated that patients with epilepsy may be predisposed to disturbances of autonomic functions with subsequent cardiac arrhythmias due to the effects of recurrent seizures on cardiac microstructure (Ramadan et al. 2013). Although interictal changes in heart rate variability have been demonstrated in patients with epilepsy, their contribution to SUDEP remains to be determined.

## OMEGA-3 FATTY ACIDS, EPILEPSY, AND SUDDEN UNEXPECTED DEATH IN EPILEPSY

Based on the available information of possible cardiac causes of SUDEP, the role of omega-3 FAs in the diet as a potential agent to reduce the risk of SUDEP is of great interest, from the perspective of reducing both seizure frequency and severity and direct cardiac effects.

Potential anticonvulsant effects: Studies of epilepsy and omega-3 FAs are promising. In 1994, Spirer and colleagues (Spirer et al. 1994) speculated that dietary supplementation with omega-3 FAs may prevent febrile seizures in susceptible children. At the same time, Yehuda and colleagues (Yehuda et al. 1994) demonstrated that a mixture of nonesterified α-linolenic acid and linoleic acid with a ratio of 1:4 (SR-3) reduced the number and duration of seizures in four animal models of epilepsy. Using a cortical stimulation seizure model in rats, Voskuyil and others (Voskuyl et al. 1998) showed a moderate anticonvulsant effect with a long duration from omega-3 FAs. Furthermore, omega-3 FAs applied extracellularly have been shown to raise the stimulatory thresholds of CA1 neurons in hippocampal slices (Xiao and Li 1999).

In a series of studies, a research group led by Scorza demonstrated that chronic treatment with omega-3 FAs promoted positive plastic changes and neuroprotection in the hippocampus in epileptic rats (Ferrari et al. 2008; Cysneiros et al. 2010). Similarly, Taha and coworkers (Taha et al. 2009) demonstrated that linoleic and α-linolenic polyunsaturated fatty acids in a 4:1 ratio increased resistance to pentylenetetrazol-induced seizures. More recently, Musto and colleagues (Musto et al. 2011) studied the effect of docosahexaenoic acid (DHA) or its derived lipid mediator, neuroprotectin D1 (NPD1), in evoked seizures using a rapid kindling model of temporal lobe epilepsy and showed that DHA or direct injection of NPD1 into the third ventricle resulted in attenuation of kindling progression and hippocampal hyperexcitability.

Daily intake of a moderate amount of omega-3 FAs was shown to be effective in a case of drug-resistant canine epilepsy (Scorza et al. 2009). Unfortunately, the results of clinical studies in patients with drug-resistant epilepsy have been mixed at best. In an open label study of five subjects, Schlanger and colleagues (Schlanger et al. 2002) reported that high-dose omega-3 FA supplements (5 g/day in a special spread containing 65% omega-3 FAs) added to the daily breakfast diet for 6 months reduced seizure frequency and severity. After this promising exploratory study, three small randomized trials of high-dose omega-3 FAs (at doses ranging from 1.7 to 2.2 g/day) failed to demonstrate a convincing anticonvulsant effect (DeGiorgio and Miller 2008). In 2005, Yuen et al. performed the first double-blind, randomized controlled trial of omega-3 FAs in patients with drug-resistant epilepsy. Fifty-seven patients were randomized to 1.7 g of eicosapentaenoic acid (EPA) and DHA or placebo for 12 weeks (Yuen et al. 2005). Seizure frequency was reduced over the first 6 weeks of treatment in the omega-3 FAs–supplemented group, but this effect was not sustained over the final 6 weeks of the 12-week treatment period (Yuen et al. 2005). The authors believe that the loss of effect following the initial 6 weeks may have been the result of the dose used, treatment duration, and sample sizes (Yuen et al. 2005). Similarly, Bromfield and others (Bromfield et al. 2008) studied even higher doses of omega-3 FA (2.2 g/day of EPA and DHA) and found no benefit compared to placebo in reducing seizures. In fact, none of the 12 subjects on omega-3 FAs had a >50% reduction in seizures (Bromfield et al. 2008). Recently, Yuen and coworkers (Yuen et al. 2012) conducted a nonrandomized, open assessment of EPA (1000 mg/day, the lowest total dose of omega-3 FAs reported to date), in 10 patients with drug-refractory focal seizures. Six patients had fewer seizures during the supplementation period compared with baseline and one person had markedly reduced seizure severity, suggesting, despite the small number of participants and open nature of the study, a possible weak effect of EPA on seizures (Yuen et al. 2012). Given the trends in this open label trial, it is possible that low doses of omega-3 FAs may be better than higher doses, as the trials with higher doses have been negative to date. Further studies are needed to determine the optimum dose of omega-3 FAs to be used in individuals with epilepsy (Taha et al. 2010).

Potential cardiac benefits: The beneficial effects of omega-3 FAs in the cardiovascular system have been described since the last century. It was demonstrated that the low prevalence of cardiac diseases in Eskimos might be due to their high dietary ingestion of omega-3 FAs (Dyerberg and Bang 1979). Over the years, studies have confirmed the positive cardiac effects of omega-3 FAs. Fish consumption (one or two times per week) has been associated with a 50% reduction of sudden cardiac death (Albert et al. 1998; Siscovick et al. 2003). In the GISSI-Prevenzione trial, which enrolled 11,324 subjects presenting with a first myocardial infarction, a dosage of 850 mg/day of omega-3 FAs was associated with a significant reduction of fatal cardiovascular complications (30%) as well as sudden death (45%), compared to control subjects, suggesting an antiarrhythmic role for omega-3 FAs (Marchioli 1999; Marchioli et al. 2002).

On the whole, current data provide strong concordant evidence that omega-3 FAs reduce the risk of ventricular arrhythmia, atrial fibrillation, and sudden cardiac death (Mozaffarian and Wu 2011; Rix et al. 2013). Research gaps still persist, and further studies are needed to accurately assess the relative importance of different physiological and molecular mechanisms, precise dose responses of physiological and clinical effects, and optimal duration of treatment (Mozaffarian and Wu 2011; Rix et al. 2013).

In relation to SUDEP and considering that omega-3 FAs may improve vascular and cardiac hemodynamics, triglycerides, autonomic control, inflammation, thrombosis, and arrhythmia and reduce the risk of cardiac death (Calder 2004; Mozaffarian and Wu 2011), Yuen and Sander (2004) hypothesized that omega-3 FAs supplementation in people with refractory epilepsy may not only reduce seizures but also reduce cardiac arrhythmias and hence SUDEP. Following this reasoning, DeGiorgio and colleagues conducted a pilot, randomized, double-blind, and two-period crossover clinical trial of high-dose omega-3 FAs in 11 subjects with refractory seizures (DeGiorgio et al. 2008). The study provided very preliminary evidence of possible beneficial effects of omega-3 FAs on cardiac risk factors and heart rate variability in people with epilepsy, although, as mentioned earlier, there was no evidence of a reduction in seizure frequency.

Scorza and colleagues (Scorza et al. 2008) hypothesized that omega-3 FAs may play a role in preventing SUDEP and pointed out the need for further study in animal models. Accordingly, in an interesting study reported by Taha and collaborators (Taha et al. 2008), FAT-1 mice, which produce high levels of omega-3 FAs, had numerically higher survival rates after exposure to pentylenetetrazol (80% of FAT-1 mice survived, vs. only 44% of wild-type mice). Though this difference did not achieve statistical significance, it may provide an insight into a possible protective effect of omega-3 FAs on SUDEP risk (Taha et al. 2008). Quite interesting, Lopes and colleagues (Lopes et al. 2013) recently demonstrated that chronic supplementation with omega-3 FAs restored the heart rate of epileptic rats toward control values, suggesting a potential preventive effect of omega-3 FAs against SUDEP. Of note, a recent meta-analysis of omega-3 FAs has caused a reappraisal of the effects of omega-3 FAs in cardiac disease (Rizos et al. 2012) because the findings are at odds with large well-executed randomized trials after myocardial infarction demonstrating significant reduction in mortality with omega-3 FAs.

Overall, given the inconsistencies in laboratory-based studies and the even greater absence of demonstrated efficacy in clinical trials in epilepsy to date, physicians lack the data they require to recommend omega-3 FAs for people with seizure disorders. However, in light of the strong experimental laboratory data, we believe that further research into the potential protective effects of omega-3 FAs in epilepsy and SUDEP is warranted.

## CONCLUSION AND FUTURE RECOMMENDATIONS

Given the strong experimental animal data and some promising results in clinical trials in epilepsy, as well as the well-documented cardiac benefits of omega-3 FAs, we believe that there is a potential role for this dietary component to reduce the risk of SUDEP. Further laboratory-based and clinical studies in patients with epilepsy are warranted to examine different omega-3 FAs preparations, different doses, longer treatment durations, and larger sample sizes.

Although results to date have been inconsistent, we should not forget the famous words of the physicist Albert Einstein: "If we knew what it was we were doing, it would not be called research, would it?"

## ACKNOWLEDGMENTS

This chapter is supported by grants from FAPESP (Fundação de Amparo à Pesquisa do Estado de São Paulo), CNPq (Conselho Nacional de Desenvolvimento Científico e Tecnológico), FAPESP/CNPq/MCT (Instituto Nacional de Neurociência Translacional), FAPESP/FAPEMIG, and PRONEX FAPESP.

## REFERENCES

Albert CM, Hennekens CH, O'Donnell CJ, Ajani UA, Carey VJ, Willett WC, Ruskin JN, Manson JE. Fish consumption and risk of sudden cardiac death. *JAMA* 1998;279:23–8.

Bell GS, Sander JW. Sudden unexpected death in epilepsy. Risk factors, possible mechanisms and prevention: A reappraisal. *Acta Neurol Taiwan* 2006;15:72–83.

Bromfield E, Dworetzky B, Hurwitz S, Eluri Z, Lane L, Replansky S, Mostofsky D. A randomized trial of polyunsaturated fatty acids for refractory epilepsy. *Epilepsy Behav* 2008;12:187–90.

Calder PC. n-3 Fatty acids and cardiovascular disease: Evidence explained and mechanisms explored. *Clin Sci* 2004;107:1–11.

Calder PC, Yaqoob P. Understanding omega-3 polyunsaturated fatty acids. *Postgrad Med* 2009;121:148–57.

Colugnati DB, Gomes PA, Arida RM, de Albuquerque M, Cysneiros RM, Cavalheiro EA, Scorza FA. Analysis of cardiac parameters in animals with epilepsy: Possible cause of sudden death? *Arq Neuropsiquiatr* 2005;63:1035–41.

Cysneiros RM, Arida RM, Terra VC, Sonoda EY, Cavalheiro EA, Scorza FA. To sushi or not to sushi: Can people with epilepsy have sushi from time to time? *Epilepsy Behav* 2009;16:565–6.

Cysneiros RM, Ferrari D, Arida RM, Terra VC, de Almeida AC, Cavalheiro EA, Scorza FA. Qualitative analysis of hippocampal plastic changes in rats with epilepsy supplemented with oral omega-3 fatty acids. *Epilepsy Behav* 2010;17: 33–8.

de Boer HM, Mula M, Sander JW. The global burden and stigma of epilepsy. *Epilepsy Behav* 2008;12:540–6.

DeGiorgio CM, Miller P. n-3 Fatty acids (eicosapentanoic and docosahexanoic acids) in epilepsy and for the prevention of sudden unexpected death in epilepsy. *Epilepsy Behav* 2008;13:712–3.

DeGiorgio CM, Miller P, Meymandi S, Gornbein JA. n-3 Fatty acids (fish oil) for epilepsy, cardiac risk factors, and risk of SUDEP: Clues from a pilot, double-blind, exploratory study. *Epilepsy Behav* 2008;13:681–4.

Drake ME, Reider CR, Kay A. Electrocardiography in epilepsy patients without cardiac symptoms. *Seizure* 1993;2:63–5.

Dyerberg J, Bang HO. Haemostatic function and platelet polyunsaturated fatty acids in Eskimos. *Lancet* 1979;2:433–5.

Ferrari D, Cysneiros RM, Scorza CA, Arida RM, Cavalheiro EA, de Almeida AC, Scorza FA. Neuroprotective activity of omega-3 fatty acids against epilepsy-induced hippocampal damage: Quantification with immunohistochemical for calcium-binding proteins. *Epilepsy Behav* 2008;13:36–42.

Ficker DM, So EL, Shen WK, Annegers JF, O'Brien PC, Cascino GD, Belau PG. Population-based study of the incidence of sudden unexplained death in epilepsy. *Neurology* 1998;51:1270–4.

Hesdorffer DC, Tomson T. Sudden unexpected death in epilepsy: Potential role of antiepileptic drugs. *CNS Drugs* 2013;27:113–9.

Jeejeebhoy KN. Benefits and risks of a fish diet—Should we be eating more or less? *Nat Clin Pract Gastroenterol Hepatol* 2008;5:178–9.

Lathers CM, Schraeder PL, Bungo MW. The mystery of sudden death: Mechanisms for risks. *Epilepsy Behav* 2008;12:3–24.

Lopes MD, Colugnati DB, Lopes AC, Scorza CA, Cavalheiro EA, Cysneiros RM, Scorza FA. Omega-3 fatty acid supplementation reduces resting heart rate of rats with epilepsy. *Epilepsy Behav* 2013;27:504–6.

Marchioli R. Results of GISSI Prevenzione: Diet, drugs, and cardiovascular risk. Researchers of GISSI Prevenzione. *Cardiologia* 1999;44:745–6.

Marchioli R, Barzi F, Bomba E, Chieffo C, Di Gregorio D, Di Mascio R, Franzosi MG, Geraci E, Levantesi G, Maggioni AP, Mantini L, Marfisi RM, Mastrogiuseppe G, Mininni N, Nicolosi GL, Santini M, Schweiger C, Tavazzi L, Tognoni G, Tucci C, Valagussa F, GISSI-Prevenzione Investigators. Early protection against sudden death by n-3 polyunsaturated fatty acids after myocardial infarction: Time-course analysis of the results of the Gruppo Italiano per lo Studio della Sopravvivenza nell'Infarto Miocardico (GISSI)-Prevenzione. *Circulation* 2002;105:1897–903.

Mozaffarian D, Wu JH. Omega-3 fatty acids and cardiovascular disease: Effects on risk factors, molecular pathways, and clinical events. *J Am Coll Cardiol* 2011;58:2047–67.

Musto AE, Gjorstrup P, Bazan NG. The omega-3 fatty acid-derived neuroprotectin D1 limits hippocampal hyperexcitability and seizure susceptibility in kindling epileptogenesis. *Epilepsia* 2011;52:1601–8.

Nashef L. Sudden unexpected death in epilepsy: Terminology and definitions. *Epilepsia* 1997;38:S6–8.

Nashef L, Walker F, Allen P, Sander JW, Shorvon SD, Fish DR. Apnoea and bradycardia during epileptic seizures: Relation to sudden death in epilepsy. *J Neurol Neurosurg Psychiatry* 1996;60:297–300.

Nei M, Hays R. Sudden unexpected death in epilepsy. *Curr Neurol Neurosci Rep* 2010;10:319–26.

Nei M, Ho RT, Abou-Khalil BW, Drislane FW, Liporace J, Romeo A, Sperling MR. EEG and ECG in sudden unexplained death in epilepsy. *Epilepsia* 2004;45:338–45.

Nei M, Ho RT, Sperling MR. EKG abnormalities during partial seizures in refractory epilepsy. *Epilepsia* 2000;41:542–8.

Neligan A, Bell GS, Johnson AL, Goodridge DM, Shorvon SD, Sander JW. The long-term risk of premature mortality in people with epilepsy. *Brain* 2011;134:388–95.

Ramadan M, El-Shahat N, A Omar A, Gomaa M, Belal T, A Sakr S, Abu-Hegazy M, Hakim H, A Selim H, A Omar S. Interictal electrocardiographic and echocardiographic changes in patients with generalized tonic-clonic seizures. *Int Heart J* 2013;54:171–5.

Rix TA, Christensen JH, Schmidt EB. Omega-3 fatty acids and cardiac arrhythmias. *Curr Opin Clin Nutr Metab Care* 2013;16:168–73.

Rizos EC, Ntzani EE, Bika E, Kostapanos MS, Elisaf MS. Association between omega-3 fatty acid supplementation and risk of major cardiovascular disease events: A systematic review and meta-analysis. *JAMA* 2012;308:1024–33.

Ryvlin P, Montavont A, Kahane P. Sudden unexpected death in epilepsy: From mechanisms to prevention. *Curr Opin Neurol* 2006;19:194–9.

Schlanger S, Shinitzky M, Yam D. Diet enriched with omega-3 fatty acids alleviates convulsion symptoms in epilepsy patients. *Epilepsia* 2002;43:103–4.

Schuele SU, Widdess-Walsh P, Bermeo A, Lüders HO. Sudden unexplained death in epilepsy: The role of the heart. *Cleve Clin J Med* 2007;74:S121–7.

Scorza FA, Cavalheiro EA, Arida RM, Terra VC, Scorza CA, Ribeiro MO, Cysneiros RM. Positive impact of omega-3 fatty acid supplementation in a dog with drug-resistant epilepsy: A case study. *Epilepsy Behav* 2009;15:527–28.

Scorza FA, Cysneiros RM, Arida RM, Terra-Bustamante VC, de Albuquerque M, Cavalheiro EA. The other side of the coin: Beneficiary effect of omega-3 fatty acids in sudden unexpected death in epilepsy. *Epilepsy Behav* 2008;13:279–83.

Siscovick DS, Lemaitre RN, Mozaffarian D. The fish story: A diet-heart hypothesis with clinical implications: n-3 Polyunsaturated fatty acids, myocardial vulnerability, and sudden death. *Circulation* 2003;107:2632–4.

Spirer Z, Koren L, Finkelstein A, Jurgenson U. Prevention of febrile seizures by dietary supplementation with n-3 polyunsaturated fatty acids. *Med Hypotheses* 1994;43:43–5.

Stollberger C, Finsterer J. Cardiorespiratory findings in sudden unexplained/unexpected death in epilepsy (SUDEP). *Epilepsy Res* 2004;59:51–60.

Surges R, Thijs RD, Tan HL, Sander JW. Sudden unexpected death in epilepsy: Risk factors and potential pathomechanisms. *Nat Rev Neurol* 2009;5:492–504.

Surges R, Taggart P, Sander JW, Walker MC. Too long or too short? New insights into abnormal cardiac repolarization in people with chronic epilepsy and its potential role in sudden unexpected death. *Epilepsia* 2010;51:738–44.

Surges R, Sander JW. Sudden unexpected death in epilepsy: Mechanisms, prevalence, and prevention. *Curr Opin Neurol* 2012;25:201–7.

Taha AY, Burnham WM, Auvin S. Polyunsaturated fatty acids and epilepsy. *Epilepsia* 2010;51:1348–58.

Taha AY, Filo E, Ma DW, McIntyre Burnham W. Dose-dependent anticonvulsant effects of linoleic and alpha-linolenic polyunsaturated fatty acids on pentylenetetrazol induced seizures in rats. *Epilepsia* 2009;50:72–82.

Taha AY, Huot PS, Reza-López S, Prayitno NR, Kang JX, Burnham WM, Ma DW. Seizure resistance in fat-1 transgenic mice endogenously synthesizing high levels of omega-3 polyunsaturated fatty acids. *J Neurochem* 2008;105:380–8.

Terra VC, Cysneiros RM, Cavalheiro EA, Scorza FA. Sudden unexpected death in epilepsy: From the lab to the clinic setting. *Epilepsy Behav* 2013;26:415–20.

Tigaran S, Molgaard H, McClelland R, Dam M, Jaffe AS. Evidence of cardiac ischemia during seizures in drug refractory epilepsy patients. *Neurology* 2003;60:492–5.

Unknown. Fish: Friend or foe? In addition to heart-healthy omega-3 fats, seafood can carry mercury and other toxins. For most people, the benefits of eating fish far outweigh the risks. *Harv Heart Lett* 2007;17:4–6

Voskuyl RA, Vreugdenhil M, Kang JX, Leaf A. Anticonvulsant effect of polyunsaturated fatty acids in rats, using the cortical stimulation model. *Eur J Pharmacol* 1998;341:145–52.

Xiao Y, Li X. Polyunsaturated fatty acids modify mouse hippocampal neuronal excitability during excitotoxic or convulsant stimulation. *Brain Res* 1999;846:112–21.

Yehuda S, Carasso RL, Mostofsky DI. Essential fatty acid preparation (SR-3) raises the seizure threshold in rats. *Eur J Pharmacol* 1994;254:193–8.

Yuen AW, Sander JW. Is omega-3 fatty acid deficiency a factor contributing to refractory seizures and SUDEP? A hypothesis. *Seizure* 2004;13:104–07.

Yuen AW, Sander JW, Fluegel D, Patsalos PN, Bell GS, Johnson T, Koepp MJ. Omega-3 fatty acid supplementation in patients with chronic epilepsy: A randomized trial. *Epilepsy Behav* 2005;7:253–8.

Yuen AW, Flugel D, Poepel A, Bell GS, Peacock JL, Sander JW. Non-randomized open trial of eicosapentaenoic acid (EPA), an omega-3 fatty acid, in ten people with chronic epilepsy. *Epilepsy Behav* 2012;23:370–2.

# 28 Sudden Death in Epilepsy
## Relationship to the Sleep–Wake Circadian Cycle and Fractal Physiology

*John D. Hughes and Susumu Sato*

## CONTENTS

## INTRODUCTION

Most case series of patients experiencing sudden death in the setting of epilepsy document a significant preponderance of cases occurring during sleep, especially nocturnal sleep (Kloster and Engelskjøn 1999; Langan et al. 2005). However, the mechanisms underlying this strong tendency have gone relatively unexplored when considering the etiology of sudden unexpected death in epilepsy (SUDEP). In general, three main mechanisms have been proposed to explain SUDEP: (1) a seizure poses an insurmountable autonomic stress to the heart resulting in an arrhythmia, (2) the epileptogenic process itself deranges central autonomic network function substantially, thus rendering the heart more vulnerable to arrhythmogenesis, and (3) a prolonged postictal apnea results in death. Of course, these are not mutually exclusive explanations, and they may all play a role in SUDEP, with potentially additive effects in a given patient. The first two mechanisms appear to be potentially highly synergistic. In this chapter, we will review aspects of the sleep–wake cycle and other circadian factors that are potentially relevant to the pathogenesis of SUDEP, with emphasis on the role of dysfunctional central autonomic cardiac regulation. Additionally, we will propose a unifying theory of the pathogenesis of SUDEP based on the reviewed evidence. Unfortunately, because of the very limited research in this area, much of our discussion will be speculative, but we hope it may stimulate much needed research.

## CIRCADIAN PHYSIOLOGY

The central nervous system generates an endogenous circadian rhythm of approximately 24 hours that originates from the suprachiasmatic nucleus (SCN) of the hypothalamus (Moore 2007) and affects virtually every organ in the body; as a result, many physiological phenomena exhibit circadian fluctuations to some degree. These rhythms tend to be entrained to the environmental light–dark cycle, moderated via the retinohypothalamic tract, which projects information about environmental light to the SCN. The sleep–wake cycle is generally entrained to this SCN-generated circadian cycle but may have a 24-hour circadian cycle of its own, independent of the SCN-generated cycle, but rather determined by various social and professional factors (i.e., shift work) or due to a pathological "phase shift." Significant changes in diverse physiological systems take place during the three different components of the sleep–wake cycle: wakefulness, nonrapid eye movement (NREM) sleep, and rapid eye movement (REM) sleep. Of particular interest with regard to SUDEP are the sleep-related changes that take place in the brain that play a role in the occurrence of seizures, as well as changes that take place in the autonomic nervous system that might play a role in cardiac arrhythmogenesis. These will be highlighted in the discussion that follows.

## THE SLEEP–WAKE CIRCADIAN CYCLE

Sleep consists of a series of cycles within the circadian cycle, called ultradian cycles. Each cycle lasts approximately 90 minutes and starts with a series of deepening NREM stages culminating in slow-wave sleep (stages 1 to 3). NREM sleep consists of relatively synchronized brain activity (including sleep spindles, K-complexes, and delta activity) and relatively regular, invariant activity of respiratory and other organ systems. NREM sleep may also be characterized by the presence or absence of a "cyclic alternating pattern" characterized by periodic (approximately every 20–40 seconds), brief "microarousals" (cyclic alternating pattern phase A) associated with increased autonomic activity, interspersed with periods free of microarousals (cyclic alternating pattern phase B) (Terzano and Parinno 2000; Halasz et al. 2004). Each ultradian cycle, of which there are normally four to six per night, theoretically ends with a period of REM sleep, which consists of tonic periods of "desynchronized" cortical activity and muscle atonia (except extraocular and respiratory muscles), and phasic periods of REMs, muscle twitches, and blood pressure variations. In general, NREM periods are longer with greater quantity of slow-wave sleep during ultradian cycles early in the night and REM periods become longer with little or no slow-wave sleep in cycles later in the night. In practice, there is significant individual variability in the number of cycles and occurrence and duration of stages within a cycle. Overall, NREM sleep comprises about 80% of sleep time, although it may comprise a greater percentage in various epileptic populations, who experience reduced REM sleep.

## SEIZURES AND THE SLEEP–WAKE CYCLE

An awareness of a relationship between the sleep–wake cycle and the occurrence of seizures dates back to antiquity and has been the subject of intense research in the past several decades and of several recent reviews (Malow 2005; Foldvary-Schaefer and Grigg-Damberger 2006). Sleep has traditionally been viewed as an epileptogenic state, due in general to the thalamocortical synchrony that may predispose to seizure generation. A number of early studies (Janz 1962) divided seizures into those occurring during sleep (nocturnal), those occurring while awake (diurnal), and those occurring randomly (diffuse). One early formulation was that idiopathic generalized seizures (of genetic origin) tended to occur while waking (often within a short time of waking from sleep, during a presumed period of sleep inertia with some relative retained cortical synchrony), acquired partial seizures occurred predominantly while asleep, and generalized seizures in the setting of diffuse brain pathologies occurred rather randomly. Numerous studies in recent years have demonstrated that the relationship is not quite so straightforward, and while there are some epilepsy syndromes that demonstrate a profound sleep or waking predominance (such as juvenile myoclonic epilepsy with seizures shortly after awakening or autosomal dominant frontal lobe epilepsy with seizures exclusively during sleep), many seizure types defy strict sleep–wake cycle component occurrence categorization. Of particular interest with regard to SUDEP is the relationship of partial seizures that exhibit pathology in central (cortical) autonomic structures (medial temporal lobe, orbitofrontal cortex, cingulate gyrus, insular cortex). All of these structures may be implicated in the epileptogenic network involved with complex partial seizures in the setting of medial temporal lobe epilepsy, though they certainly may be the origin of partial seizures independently. In fact, diffuse

cortical and subcortical limbic and autonomic centers tend to be involved in focal seizures originating in the limbic system (Mraovitch and Calando 1999). All of these structures not only tend to produce autonomic phenomena when stimulated exogenously and during seizures, but have been potentially implicated in cardiac arrhythmogenicity related to seizures (Lathers 2008). This topic is the subject of other comprehensive reviews in this book.

Studies attempting to address the pattern of occurrence of partial complex seizures of medial temporal lobe origin in terms of the sleep–wake cycle have demonstrated conflicting results. Despite the conventional wisdom dating back to and before Janz (1962) that partial seizures and in particular complex partial seizures have a significant sleep state predominance, studies by Quigg (2000) have demonstrated just the opposite, namely, that complex partial seizures in temporal lobe epilepsy are concentrated during late afternoon wakefulness and occur in the same circadian phase in human and experimental rat models. Although other studies have confirmed the conventional wisdom (Herman et al. 2001) demonstrating a nocturnal sleep predominance, the preponderance of evidence seems to be accumulating for a late afternoon predominance for complex partial seizure occurrence (Durazzo et al. 2008). However, one aspect of the circadian timing of medial temporal lobe epilepsy which is clear is that secondary generalization tends to occur almost exclusively during nocturnal sleep (Jobst et al. 2001). Quigg (2000) has discussed the possible seizure-protecting effect of melatonin during the night (though the data on the role of melatonin as a proconvulsant vs. an anticonvulsant is somewhat conflicting). Additionally, varying circadian sleep–wake cycle levels of neurotransmitters may play a role. A recent study reported significantly increased receptor sensitivity to the neuropeptide orexin (important for the maintenance of arousal and with minimal brain activity during sleep) in the epileptic hippocampus. The authors speculated on the potential epileptogenicity of orexin in medial temporal lobe seizures (Morales et al. 2008). Even if there is a circadian protective effect on the occurrence of nocturnal partial complex seizures, it seems that if a seizure does occur during nocturnal sleep, it tends to propagate more extensively and often secondarily generalizes.

We previously alluded to the profound synchronizing effect of NREM sleep on cortical activity as measured with the electroencephalography (EEG). Specifically, NREM sleep consists of highly synchronous activity in the form of sleep spindles (12–14 Hz) and K-complexes (which represent the particularly synchronized activity of diffuse cortical regions in producing a transient 0.5- to 2-s biphasic potential) on a background of theta and delta activity. During slow-wave sleep, the delta activity may intermittently appear be quite regular and rhythmic. However, it is well accepted that even in the absence of obvious synchronicity or rhythmicity to visual inspection, cortical activity of lower frequencies (theta, delta) requires significantly greater synchronization over significantly larger areas of cortex than faster frequencies (Buzsaki and Draguhn 2004). Niedermeyer (2008) and others have written about the potential of K-complexes in particular to induce interictal or even ictal activity as a result of its profound synchronizing effect. Sleep spindles, which represent highly synchronized activity in thalamocortical systems, are theorized to be "transformed" into generalized 3-per-second spike–wave complexes in models of absence epilepsy (Kostopoulos 2000). More recently, Steriade et al. (1993) have described a slow (<1 Hz) oscillation throughout NREM sleep, which becomes more rhythmic as sleep deepens and which consists of a rhythmic alternation of membrane potential (membrane "bistability"). A period of significant membrane depolarization, highly synchronized throughout much of cortex and involving both cortical pyramidal cells and interneurons, alternates with a period of cellular quiescence that they have referred to as a period of "disfacilitation," consisting of a hyperpolarized membrane potential with increased membrane resistance and an absence of cortical synaptic activity. Although, like spindles, the slow oscillation is present diffusely in corticothalamic systems, the slow oscillation is believed to be intrinsically generated in cortex with coherence across large areas of cortex, as the slow oscillation occurs in deafferented cortical slabs. The highly synchronous and precipitous onset of the depolarized state from a state of diffuse cellular quiescence of the hyperpolarized state creates the K-complex of the surface EEG and presents an unprecedented epileptogenetic potential (Steriade and Amzica 1998). Indeed, it has demonstrated in a model of seizures occurring in a thalamically deafferented region of cat neocortex during NREM sleep that spike–wave activity emerges with cellular evidence of a paroxysmal depolarzing shift directly from the activity of the slow oscillation (Steriade and Contreras 1998; Steriade et al. 1998). The generation and propagation of epileptiform activity has also been shown to be lowered in the hippocampus during the slow oscillation (Nazer and Dickson 2009). Additionally, the physiological ripple rhythm (150–250 Hz), which originates in the hippocampus during NREM sleep (Buzsaki 1998; Sirota et al. 2003;) with involvement of neocortex as well during that sleep state (Grenier et al. 2001) and is postulated to be involved in memory consolidation, appears to be the forerunner of the pathological fast ripple (250–500 Hz) activity that is instrumental in the initiation of partial seizures (Foffani et al. 2007; Engel et al. 2009). Finally, Terzano and Parinno (2000) have emphasized the propensity for epileptiform activity to occur during the synchronized activity of the cyclic alternating pattern phase A, which may consist of serial K-complexes and bursts of "hypersynchronous" delta activity, among other patterns. This group describes a tremendous preponderance of interictal and ictal activity beginning during the cyclic alternating pattern phase A microarousals in a wide variety of seizure types (Parino et al. 2006). Finally, infraslow oscillations in the frequency range of 0.02 to 0.2 Hz, a frequency range not detected with standard alternating current EEG instrumentation, have been described during NREM sleep. This slow cyclic modulation of cortical excitability appears to be associated with the production of interictal epileptic activity (Vanhatalo et al. 2004).

The physiological basis of infraslow oscillations has not been well characterized and whether infraslow oscillations and the cyclic alternating pattern are a manifestation of the same underlying physiological mechanism is unclear.

With this discussion as a background, it is not surprising that interictal discharges are significantly more frequent in the relatively synchronized states of drowsiness and NREM sleep in most seizure types and partial complex seizures of medial temporal lobe origin are no exception (Clemens et al. 2005). Although temporal lobe seizures appear to have a late afternoon predominance, there is nonetheless an overwhelming preponderance of interictal discharges during NREM sleep as opposed to the waking state. Furthermore, interictal discharges propagate to a much wider territory of cortex during NREM sleep, often with contralateral involvement of discharges that are strictly unilateral during wakefulness (Nita et al. 2007). Also, as mentioned, seizures are much more likely to secondarily generalize during NREM sleep. It may be that the extensive interareal hypersynchrony present during NREM sleep is particularly conducive to the development of interictal discharges regardless of seizure type, to the development of certain types of generalized ictal activity, such as with 3-per-second spike–wave activity, and to secondary generalization of partial seizures, but not to the development of some types of partial seizures. Such profound synchrony may not be as crucial for the interictal–ictal transformation that may take place at a much more focal level in temporal lobe epilepsy.

REM sleep, with its desynchronized cortical activity, is felt to be relatively suppressive with regard to epileptiform activity. When interictal discharges do occur, they tend to be more focal with less propagation than during NREM sleep or even during wakefulness. Ictal transformation is much less frequent during REM than NREM sleep, though it can occur (Malow 2005).

## CARDIOVASCULAR PHYSIOLOGICAL ACTIVITY DURING SLEEP

In general, NREM sleep is characterized by an increase in parasympathetic cardiac activity (vagal dominance) with little or no change in sympathetic activity (Parmeggiani and Morrison 1990). As a result, NREM sleep is characterized by a reduced heart rate and reduced blood pressure as compared with wakefulness. A decrease in the gain or responsiveness of the sinoatrial baroreflex, which normally counteracts an increase in blood pressure with a decrease in heart rate, is felt to account for the paradoxical simultaneous fall in blood pressure and heart rate. This resetting of the baroreflex is potentially relevant given the role of this reflex in buffering abrupt increases in blood pressure related to surges in sympathetic activity. There is little overall change in stroke volume or peripheral vascular resistance during NREM sleep; the reduced blood pressure is primarily related to the fall in heart rate. Additionally, NREM sleep can be characterized by transient increases in blood pressure and heart rate associated with the microarousals of the cyclic alternating pattern

(Ferri et al. 2000; Ferini-Strambi et al. 2000). These changes are generally felt to be related to surges in sympathetic outflow related to overall heightened somatic and autonomic system activity with the arousal. Such surges rely on buffering by the baroreflex to limit their magnitude. However, the baroreflex, which has a decreased gain in NREM sleep, is felt to be rapidly reset or even "overwhelmed" by the arousal effect of the cyclic alternating pattern phase A (Murali et al. 2003; Iellamo et al. 2004). Interestingly, a recent report demonstrated decreased baroreflex function in chronic temporal lobe epilepsy patients (Dutsch et al. 2006).

Tonic REM sleep is also characterized by a vagal, parasympathetic predominance, apparently associated with a mild decrease in sympathetic activity compared with NREM sleep, resulting in an even more profound vagal dominance. As a result, the heart rate and blood pressure fall below NREM sleep levels during tonic REM sleep. REM sleep generally is characterized by the lowest blood pressures during the 24-hour circadian cycle (Coote 1982). Additionally, sinus pauses may accompany the bradycardia of REM sleep. Indeed, otherwise healthy adults may experience periods of asystole during REM sleep requiring the use of a pacemaker (Guilleminault et al. 1984). However, the phasic component of REM sleep is characterized by significant surges in sympathetic activity that may be accompanied by a decrease in parasympathetic activity. This results in significant transient increases in blood pressure and heart rate. Peripheral vascular resistance is overall relatively unchanged, with vasoconstriction in muscle vasculature offset by vasodilatation in renal and mesenteric vasculature. This autonomic pattern of relative lability or "instability" seems to be mediated predominantly by higher central nervous system structures, which tend to "override" local and medullary reflexes (Silvani and Lenzi 2005; Silvani 2008). This surge in sympathetic activity in the setting of tonic low parasympathetic activity predisposes REM sleep to the occurrence of ventricular ectopy (Garcia-Touchard et al. 2007).

An additional aspect of autonomic function, heart rate variability, is of particular relevance to the topic of sudden death. Heart rate variability refers to the relative constancy or "variability" in the R–R interval from one QRS complex to the next in the cardiac cycle (De Jong and Randall 2005). Conventional (stochastic) heart rate variability analysis can be performed in the time or the frequency domain. Time domain analysis basically determines the standard deviation of the R–R intervals in a period of time (or related measures); frequency analysis is performed with a fast Fourier transform to determine the range and power of frequency components of the R–R intervals. This analysis generally involves separate analyses of low-frequency and high-frequency components. The high-frequency band is felt to reflect predominantly parasympathetic influences, which are more rapid, including the vagally dominated baroreflex. The low-frequency band reflects both sympathetic and parasympathetic activity, perhaps with a modest sympathetic predominance. The high frequency/low frequency ratio therefore approximates the parasympathetic/sympathetic ratio of activities. A sympathetic predominance

is felt to predispose to ventricular arrhythmias, which many authorities feel to be commonly implicated in sudden death. A significant parasympathetic predominance, however, can also predispose to bradyarrhythmias or sinus arrest, which can occur in REM sleep (Janssens et al. 2007). It has been suggested that "sympathovagal balance" is important for cardiac health. However, Skinner (1993) has emphasized that sympathovagal balance can also be pathological and can predispose to arrhythmias if the tone of both systems is high. He has described this scenario in NREM sleep in cats with an increase in ventricular premature contractions (although in general, the vagal predominance of NREM sleep has been felt to suppress premature ventricular contractions and ventricular arrhythmias). Skinner (1993) has also described heightened tone in both components of the autonomic nervous system in the setting of stress with minimal change in heart rate leading to an increase in premature ventricular contractions.

It is now well known that a decrease in the various measures of heart rate variability are indicative of impaired cardiac health in congestive heart failure patients and are predictive of negative outcomes. Decreased heart rate variability has also been shown to be predictive of poor cardiac outcomes in other patient populations as well, including those with several neurological disorders (Korpelainen et al. 1997). Furthermore, heart rate variability has been demonstrated to be significantly decreased in temporal lobe epilepsy patients (Ansakorpi et al. 2002), with this effect more pronounced nocturnally "reflecting a suppression of circadian heart rate variability dynamics" (Ronkainen et al. 2005; Persson et al. 2007). One study in children with partial seizures showed that heart rate variability is especially impaired at night (Ferri et al. 2002). Finally, a recent study showed that patients with frontal lobe epilepsy, in whom seizures occur almost exclusively at night, have a unique pattern of decreased heart rate variability, with lower parasympathetic drive (Harnod et al. 2009).

## HEART RATE VARIABILITY AND FRACTAL PHYSIOLOGY

Recent years have seen an increasing interest in the application of techniques of fractal physiology to heart rate variability data (see Goldberger et al. 1990 or West and Goldberger 1987 for an introduction to fractal physiology). Fractal phenomena tend to demonstrate the phenomenon of self-similarity. Structures that demonstrate fractal qualities in the spatial domain tend to look similar no matter what the scale (i.e., the same spatial patterns occur across all spatial scales). They are said to be "scale-free." Phenomena that change over time can also exhibit fractal qualities in the temporal domain. The patterns of change from interval to interval are independent of the time scale. Such systems tend to obey a power law in the temporal domain, such that a relationship between two variables ($a$ and $f$) that change over time can be characterized by the equation $a = Af^\alpha$, wherein $a$ is proportional to $f$ raised to some particular power, $\alpha$ (power law). When $\alpha$ approaches a value of $-1$, so that the relationship approximates $1/f$

(inverse power law), the system is said to be governed by $1/f$ statistics (Shlesinger 1987). This $1/f$ activity is the defining feature of mathematically defined "complex systems," which are systems made up of many interacting parts and the system as a whole is organized to optimize adaptation to changing environmental influences. Complex systems are not functioning at equilibrium and are not designed to maintain some specific "set" point. In fact, such systems are said to operate "far from equilibrium" (Peng et al. 1994). The traditional notion that the ultimate goal of biological systems is the maintenance of homeostasis appears in need of some modification. In fact, true homeostasis is eschewed by healthy biological systems. Deviations from baseline function in a scale-invariant manner appear to be the sign of a healthy biological system (Goldberger et al. 2002a,b; Lipsitz 2002). To casual visual inspection, temporal data characterized by scale-invariant $1/f$ dynamics generally looks like nothing but random "noise." The data generated by such a system has been referred to as "pink noise" to differentiate it from truly random "white noise" and from Brownian motion or "brown noise." Closer examination of such data is revealing. Although data comprising typical white noise exhibits continuous relatively small but variable fluctuations from some baseline level (preserving homeostasis in the traditional sense), brown noise demonstrates only large relatively persistent deviations from a baseline over time. Pink noise characterized by $1/f$ dynamics demonstrates both types of temporal fluctuations. Therefore, its time series is temporally scale-invariant. Fluctuations on a small time scale (seconds) are approximately mirrored by proportional fluctuations on longer time scales (hours or days). Heart rate data exhibit such $1/f$ temporal dynamics (Perkiomaki et al. 2005). A 10-s fluctuation in heart rate observed every few minutes might be magnified by a similar 10-min fluctuation every several hours (with the 10-s fluctuations superimposed). For a comprehensive review of $1/f$ dynamics in biological systems, see Gisiger (2001).

Although not all of the variability of heart rate data can be attributed to fractal physiological mechanisms, clearly a substantial component of it can be. Indeed, heart rate variability in a healthy heart exhibits temporal self-similarity over a time scale of seconds to many hours (Saul et al. 1988). Additionally, the fractal component of heart rate variability appears to be mediated primarily if not exclusively by the central autonomic system as opposed to the intrinsic cardiac nervous system. Indeed, the SCN has been implicated in regulation of fractal cardiac physiology; bilateral lesions of SCN eliminate fractal heart rate regulation (Hu et al. 1988a, 1988b). Although a transplanted heart exhibits intrinsic rhythmicity and even some minimal degree of nonfractal heart rate variability, true fractal heart rate variability does not develop for approximately 6 months, following adequate reinnervation with host autonomic fibers to impart an influence from the central autonomic system. Some disease processes with significant systemic cardiovascular pathology may lose their heart rate variability due to impaired effector function such as blood vessel wall compliance (Malpas

2002), but that would not apply to the fractal component of heart rate variability.

What is the significance of fractal physiology? As we alluded to above, systems that exhibit $1/f$ dynamics seem especially suited to adapt to physiological challenges on many time scales. An optimized ability of the neurocardiac system to meet physiological challenges while maintaining the normal coordinated activity of its electrical conduction system seems to be conferred by fractal dynamics. Congestive heart failure patients and several other patient groups demonstrate a loss of fractal physiology in heart rate variability data that predicts poor cardiac outcomes including death secondary to cardiac arrhythmias. In fact, recent evidence has shown that impoverished fractal physiology is a far better predictor of future ventricular arrhythmias in patients with left ventricular dysfunction than analysis of traditional heart rate variability data (Makikallio et al. 2001).

With regard to SUDEP, it has now been demonstrated that refractory temporal lobe epilepsy patients, a group of patients at particular risk of SUDEP in association with secondarily generalized seizures, demonstrate not only reduced heart rate variability by conventional measures but also a significantly reduced component of fractal heart rate variation dynamics. Additionally, the fractal component of heart rate variability demonstrates a clear circadian variation, such that there is a decrease in the magnitude of fractal dynamics of heart rate variability during NREM sleep, with preservation in REM sleep (Ivanov 2007; Bunde et al. 2000; Togo and Yamamoto 2001; Aoyagi et al. 2007). Interestingly, the "normal" departure from $1/f$ dynamics in NREM sleep deviates toward white noise whereas it deviates toward brown noise in waking patients with primary autonomic failure, a disorder, which like NREM sleep, is characterized by a parasympathetic predominance (Aoyagi et al. 2007).

## A PROPOSED PATHOPHYSIOLOGY OF SUDEP

We synthesize the information discussed so far in the chapter in the following way. The epileptic network in temporal lobe epilepsy patients, especially chronic refractory temporal lobe epilepsy patients at higher risk for SUDEP, induces changes in the central cortical autonomic function necessary to impart fractal dynamics on the heart, disturbing or eliminating this fractal phenomenon. Preliminary evidence suggests this derangement is more pronounced at night, in the setting of a preexisting physiological reduction in fractal dynamics during NREM sleep. Fractal autonomic dynamics are felt to be necessary to protect the heart in the setting of physiological challenges on various time scales (e.g., rapid intense surges as well as sustained increases in sympathetic activity). A seizure, especially a generalized tonic–clonic event, with its associated rapid increase in sympathetic activity, is one such challenge (most witnessed events of SUDEP have been associated with generalized tonic–clonic seizures). The sympathetic activity seen in the lockstep phenomenon, which refers to an increase in sympathetic activity time-locked to interictal discharges

(Lathers et al. 1987; Stauffer et al. 1989, 1990; Dodd-O and Lathers 1990; O'Rourke and Lathers 1990; Lathers and Schraeder 2010a, ch. 28), is another. As we described, due to its multiphenomenal synchronizing affects, NREM sleep results in a significant increase in interictal discharges in temporal lobe epilepsy (as well as most other seizure types) and produces almost all secondarily generalized seizures in patients with temporal lobe epilepsy. Additionally, although partial complex seizures have a diurnal rather than nocturnal predominance, 60% of such seizures associated with electrocardiographic abnormalities actually occurred during NREM sleep (Nei et al. 2000). Of course, not all patients succumb to SUDEP at night and while asleep. We propose that the reduced or absent fractal physiology of temporal lobe epilepsy patients will render them more vulnerable to an arrhythmia throughout the circadian cycle, though with a significantly greater propensity during nocturnal sleep, with its inherent autonomic instability, and with even greater likelihood in the setting of the poorly "buffered" heart rate surge associated with a generalized tonic–clonic seizure.

Carbamazepine discontinuation has been associated with SUDEP. A recent study demonstrated that sudden carbamazepine withdrawal leads to an increase in nocturnal sympathetic activity (Hennessy et al. 2001), which may be ineffectively buffered in SUDEP patients. Nei et al. (2004) reviewed heart rate data from seizure patients including a subset that ultimately succumbed to SUDEP. They observed greater blood pressure fluctuations during seizures occurring in nocturnal sleep than daytime seizures with significantly greater fluctuations in SUDEP versus non-SUDEP patients. Therefore, the neurocardiac system is less capable of buffering these rapid changes at night, with the SUDEP patients apparently even less adept at this buffering mechanism. This deranged physiology will also render such patients more susceptible to the development of a ventricular arrhythmia or even a serious bradyarrhythmia due to the more modest autonomic effects of a partial complex seizure (as opposed to a generalized tonic–clonic seizure) during the day or simply due to various autonomic challenges that patients will face during their daily lives. Stress is one such challenge. Recently, the role of emotional stress in the etiology of SUDEP has been emphasized (Lathers and Schraeder 2006; 2010b, ch. 17). Even mild stress has been noted to decrease fractal heart rate variability to some degree (Hoshikawa and Yamamoto 1997). Therefore, theoretically, stress could simultaneously increase sympathetic tone and decrease the fractal dynamics necessary to adapt to this change in tone and could have an additive effect on the preexisting heart rate variability pathophysiology in temporal lobe epilepsy patients. Furthermore, chronic stress and anxiety may increase the percentage of time that patients experience the cyclic alternating pattern during NREM sleep (Terzano and Parrino 2000). This alteration will increase the number of transient sympathetic challenges (to up to several hundred per night), or at another time scale, it simply increases their repetitive distribution throughout the night (persistence of recurrent challenges) or the average level of

sympathetic activity throughout the night. Additionally, these arousals are much more likely to simultaneously activate an epileptiform discharge (Niedermeyer 2008) that may add its own deleterious autonomic effect via the lockstep or related phenomena. For the same reason, REM sleep, with its significant autonomic instability, would also pose a significant autonomic challenge to such patients, and, despite its relative epileptiform suppressing effect could potentially be an especially arrhythmogenic period in patients with impaired fractal physiology. Interestingly, one recent study found that the interictal spike rate was significantly higher during REM sleep in patients with localized epilepsy who had a history of secondary generalization, a population at higher risk for SUDEP (Clemens et al. 2005).

## CONCLUSION

We regard the preceding discussion as a unifying theory for SUDEP occurrence in patients who have a deranged central autonomic system due to structural or functional changes in their epileptic networks or perhaps even due to nonepileptic central autonomic nervous system functional changes in association with more widespread cerebral pathology that gives rise to partial or symptomatic generalized seizures. The majority of SUDEP victims have structural brain pathology, usually nonprogressive, of some sort. Patients with idiopathic generalized epilepsies appear less likely to develop SUDEP. Of note, newly diagnosed epileptic patients were found not to demonstrate a difference in heart rate variability versus controls. This finding suggests that chronic lesions, especially evolving plastic epileptic networks, experience a gradual reorganization in the central autonomic network over time with loss of complexity and the fractal dynamics it produces. Such a mechanism, with resultant reduced buffering of autonomic fluctuations especially in sleep, in combination with a dramatically increased quantity and field of distribution of interictal epileptiform discharges and secondarily generalized seizures in medial temporal lobe epilepsy patients due to the profound synchronizing effects of NREM sleep, could account for or certainly contribute to the nocturnal sleep state predominance of SUDEP cases. Current research is attempting to address mechanisms to induce or restore nonlinear fractal dynamics in biological systems lacking such characteristics to increase adaptability and resilience in the face of environmental challenges (Schiff et al. 1994; In et al. 1995). Such research may prove critical to the development of future strategies to prevent sudden death in the setting of epilepsy.

## REFERENCES

Ansakorpi H, Korpelainen JT, Huikuri HV, et al. Heart rate dynamics in refractory and well controlled temporal lobe epilepsy. *J Neurol Neurosurg Psychiatr* 2002;72:26–30.

Aoyagi N, Struzik Z, Kiyaon K, et al. Autonomic imbalance and breakdown of long-range dependence in healthy heart rate. *Methods Inf Med* 2007;46:174–8.

Bunde A, Havlin S, Kantelhardt JW, et al. Correlated and uncorrelated regions in heart-rate fluctuations during sleep. *Phys Rev Lett* 2000;85:3736–9.

Buzsaki G. Memory consolidation during sleep: A neurophysiological perspective. *J Sleep Res* 1998;7(Suppl 1):17–23.

Buzsaki G, Draguhn A. Neuronal oscillations in cortical networks. *Science* 2004;304(5679):1926–9.

Clemens Z, Jansky J, Clemens B, et al. Factors affecting spiking related to sleep and wake states in temporal lobe epilepsy. *Seizure* 2005;14:52–7.

Coote JH. Respiratory and circulatory control during sleep. *J Exp Biol* 1982;100:223–44.

De Jong MJ, Randall DC. Heart rate variability analysis in the assessment of autonomic function in heart failure. *J Cardiovasc Nurs* 2005;20(3):186–95.

Dodd-O JM, Lathers CM. A characterization of the lockstep phenomenon in phenobarbitol-pretreated cats. In: Lathers CM, Schraeder PL, eds. *Epilepsy and Sudden Death.* New York, NY: Marcel Dekker; 1990, pp. 199–220.

Durazzo TS, Spencer SS, Duckrow RB, et al. Temporal distributions of seizure occurrence from various epileptogenic regions. *Neurology* 2008;70:1265–71.

Dutsch M, Hilz MJ, Devinsky O. Impaired baroreflex function in temporal lobe epilepsy. *J Neurol* 2006;253:1300–8.

Engel Jr. J, Bragin A, Staba R, et al. High-frequency oscillations: What is normal and what is not? *Epilepsia* 2009;50(4):598–604.

Ferini-Strambi L, Bianchi A, Zucconi M, et al. The impact of the cyclic alternating pattern on heart rate variability during sleep in healthy adults. *Clin Neurophysiol* 2000;111:99–101.

Ferri R, Curzi-Dascalova L, Arzimanoglou A, et al. Heart rate variability during sleep in children with partial epilepsy. *J Sleep Res* 2002;11:153–60.

Ferri R, Parrino L, Smerieri A, et al. Cyclic alternating pattern and spectral analysis of heart rate variability during normal sleep. *J Sleep Res* 2000;9:13–8.

Foldvary-Schaefer N, Grigg-Damberger M. Sleep and epilepsy: What we know, don't know and need to know. *J Clin Neurophysiol* 2006;23(1):4–20.

Foffani G, Uzcategui YG, Gal B, et al. Reduced spike-timing reliability correlates with the emergence of fast ripples in the rat epileptic hippocampus. *Neuron* 2007;55(6):930–41.

Garcia-Touchard A, Somers VK, Kara T. Ventricular ectopy during REM sleep: Implications for nocturnal sudden cardiac death. *Nat Clin Pract Card* 2007;4(5):284–8.

Gisiger T. Scale invariance in biology: Coincidence or footprint of a universal mechanism? *Biol Rev* 2001;76:161–209.

Goldberger AL, Amaral LAN, Hausdorff JM, et al. Fractal dynamics in physiology: Alterations with disease and aging. *Proc Natl Acad Sci USA* 2002a;99(Suppl 1):2466–72.

Goldberger AL, Peng CK, Lipsitz LA. What is physiologic complexity and how does it change with aging and disease? *Neurobiol Aging* 2002b;23:23–6.

Goldberger AL, Rigney DR, West BJ. Chaos and fractals in human physiology. *Sci Am* 1990; 262(2):43–9.

Grenier F, Timofeev I, Steriade M. Focal synchronization of ripples (80–200 Hz) in neocortex and their neuronal correlates. *J Neurophysiol* 2001;86(4):1884–98.

Guilleminault C, Pool P, Motta J, et al. Sinus arrest during REM sleep in young adults. *New Engl J Med* 1984;311:1006–10.

Halasz P, Terzano M, Parrino L, et al. The nature of arousal in sleep. *J Sleep Res* 2004;13:1–23.

Harnod T, Yang CCH, Hsin YL, et al. Heart rate variability in patients with frontal lobe epilepsy. *Seizure* 2009;18:21–5.

Hennessy MJ, Tighe GM, Binnie CD, et al. Sudden withdrawal of carbamazepine increases sudden cardiac sympathetic activity in sleep. *Neurology* 2001;57:1650–4.

Herman ST, Walczak TS, Bazil CW. Distribution of partial seizures during the sleep–wake cycle: Differences by seizure onset site. *Neurology* 2001;56(11):1453–9.

Hoshikawa Y, Yamamoto Y. Effects of Stroop color–word conflict on autonomic motor system responses. *Am J Physiol–Heart C* 1997;272:H1113–21.

Hu K, Scheer FAJL, Buijs RM, et al. The circadian pacemaker generates similar circadian rhythms in the fractal structure of heart rate in humans and rats. *Cardiovasc Res* 2008a;80:62–8.

Hu K, Scheer FAJL, Buijs RM, et al. The endogenous circadian pacemaker imparts a scale-invariant pattern of heart of heart rate fluctuations across time scales spanning minutes to 24 hours. *J Biol Rhythm* 2008b;23:265–73.

Janssens W, Willems R, Pevernagie D, et al. REM sleep-related brady-arrhythmia syndrome. *Sleep Breath* 2007;11(3):195–9.

Iellamo F, Placidi F, Marciani MG, et al. Baroreflex buffering of sympathetic activation during sleep: Evidence from autonomic assessment of sleep macroarchitecture and microarchitecture. *Hypertension* 2004;43:814–9.

In VV, Mahan SE, Ditto WL, et al. Experimental maintenance of chaos. *Phys Rev Lett* 1995;74(22):4420–3.

Ivanov PC. Scale-invariant aspects of cardiac dynamics: Observing sleep stages and circadian phases. *IEEE Eng Med Biol Mag* 2007;26(6):33–7.

Janz D. The grand mal epilepsies and the sleeping–waking cycle. *Epilepsia* 1962;3:69–109.

Jobst BC, Williamson PD, Neuschwander TB, et al. Secondarily generalized seizures in mesial temporal epilepsy: Clinical characteristics, lateralizing signs and association with the sleep–wake cycle. *Epilepsia* 2001;42(1):1279–87.

Kloster R, Engelskjøn T. Sudden unexpected death in epilepsy (SUDEP): A clinical perspective and a search for risk factors. *J Neurol Neurosurg* 1999;67:439–44.

Korpelainen JT, Sotaniemi KA, Huikuri HV, et al. Circadian rhythm of heart rate variability is reversibly abolished in ischemic stroke. *Stroke* 1997;28:2150–4.

Kostopoulos GK. Spike-and-wave discharges of absence seizures as a transformation of sleep spindles: The continuing development of a hypothesis. *Clin Neurophysiol* 2000;111(Suppl 2): S27–38.

Langan Y, Nashef L, Sander JW. Case control study of SUDEP. *Neurology* 2005;64:1131–3.

Lathers CM. The mystery of sudden death: Mechanisms for risks. *Epilepsy Behav* 2008;12:3–24.

Lathers CM, Schraeder PL. Stress and sudden death. *Epilepsy Behav* 2006;9 (2):236–42.

Lathers CM, Schraeder PL. Animal model for sudden unexpected death in persons with epilepsy. Chapter 28 In: Lathers CM, Schraeder PL, Bungo MW, Leestma JE, eds. *Sudden Death in Epilepsy: Forensic and Clinical Issues.* Boca Raton, FL: CRC Press/Taylor & Francis Group; 2010a.

Lathers CM, Schraeder PL. Stress and SUDEP. Chapter 17 In: Lathers CM, Schraeder PL, Bungo MW, Leestma JE, editors. *Sudden Death in Epilepsy: Forensic and Clinical Issues.* Boca Raton, FL: CRC Press/Taylor & Francis Group; 2010b.

Lathers CM, Schraeder PL, Weiner FW. Synchronization of cardiac autonomic neural discharge with epileptogenic activity: The lockstep phenomenon. *Electroencephalogr Clin Neurophysiol* 1987;67:247–59.

Lipsitz LA. Dynamics of stability: The physiological basis of functional health and frailty. *J Gerontol* 2002;57A:B115–25.

Makikallio TH, Huikuri HV, Makikallio A, et al. Prediction of sudden cardiac death by fractal analysis of heart rate variability in elderly subjects. *J Am Coll Cardiol* 2001;37:1395–402.

Malow BA. Sleep and epilepsy. *Neurol Clin* 2005;23(4):1127–47.

Malpas SC. Neural influences on cardiovascular variability: Possibilities and pitfalls. *Am J Physiol–Heart C* 2002;282:H6–20.

Morales A, Bonnet C, Bourgoin N. Unexpected expression of orexin-B in basal conditions and increased levels in the rat hippocampus during pilocarpine-induced epileptogenesis. *Brain Res* 2006;1109:164–75.

Moore RY. Suprachiasmatic nucleus in sleep–wake regulation. *Sleep Med* 2007;8:S27–33.

Mraovitch S, Calando Y. Interactions between limbic, thalamo-striatal-cortical and central autonomic pathways during epileptic seizure progression. *J Comp Neurol* 1999;411:145–61.

Murali NS, Svatikova A, Somers VK. Cardiovascular physiology and sleep. *Front Biosci* 2003;8:s636–52.

Nazer F, Dickson FN. The slow oscillation facilitates epileptiform events in the hippocampus. *J Neurophysiol* 2009;102(3):1880–9.

Nei M, Ho RT, Abou-Khalil BW. EEG and ECG in sudden unexplained death in epilepsy. *Epilepsia* 2004;45(4):338–45.

Nei M, Ho RT, Sperling MR. EKG abnormalities during partial seizures in refractory epilepsy. *Epilepsia* 2000;41(5):542–8.

Niedermeyer E. Epileptiform K complexes. *Am J Electroneurodiagnostic Technol* 2008;48(1):48–51.

Nita DA, Cisse Y, Timofeev I, et al. Waking-sleep modulation of paroxysmal activities induced by partial cortical deafferentation. *Cerebr Cortex* 2007;17:272–83.

O'Rourke DK, Lathers CM. Interspike interval histogram characterization of synchronized cardiac sympathetic neural discharge and epileptogenic activity in the electrocortogram of the cat. In: Lathers CM, Schraeder PL, eds. *Epilepsy and Sudden Death*. New York, NY: Marcel Dekker; 1990, pp. 239–60.

Parino L, Halasz P, Tassinari CA, et al. CAP, epilepsy and motor events during sleep: The unifying role of arousal. *Sleep Med Rev* 2006;10:267–85.

Parmeggiani PL, Morrison AR. Alterations in autonomic function during sleep. In: Lowey AD, Spyer KM, eds. *Central Regulation of Autonomic Functions*. New York, NY: Oxford University Press; 1990, pp. 367–90.

Peng CK, Buldyrev SV, Hausdorff JM, et al. Non-equilibrium dynamics as an indispensable characteristic of a healthy biological system. *Integr Phys Behav Sci* 1994;29:283–93.

Perkiomaki JS, Makikallio TH, Huikuri HV, et al. Fractal and complexity measures of heart rate variability. *Clin Exp Hypertens* 2005;2–3:149–58.

Persson H, Kumlien E, Ericson M, et al. Circadian variation in heart-rate variability in localization-related epilepsy. *Epilepsia* 2007;48(5):917–22.

Quigg M. Circadian rhythms: Interactions with seizures and epilepsy. *Epilepsy Res* 2000;42:43–55.

Ronkainen E, Ansakorpi H, Huikuri HV, et al. Suppressed circadian heart rate dynamics in temporal lobe epilepsy. *J Neuro Neurosurg Psychiatr* 2005;76:1382–6.

Saul JP, Albrecht P, Berger RD, et al. Analysis of long term heart rate variability: Methods, 1/f scaling and implications. *Comput Cardiol* 1988;14:419–22.

Schiff SL, Jerger K, Duong DH, et al. Controlling chaos in the brain. *Nature* 1994;370(6491):615–20.

Shlesinger MF. Fractal time and 1/f noise in complex systems. *Ann N Y Acad Sci* 1987;504:214–28.

Silvani A. Physiological sleep-dependent changes in arterial blood pressure: Central autonomic commands and baroreflex control. *Clin Exp Pharmacol Physiol* 2008;35:987–94.

Silvani A, Lenzi P. Reflex cardiovascular control in sleep. In: Parmeggiani PL, Velluti RA, eds. *The Physiologic Nature of Sleep*. London: Imperial College Press; 2005; pp. 323–50.

Sirota A, Csicsvari J, Buhl D, et al. Communication between neocortex and hippocampus during sleep in rodents. *Proc Natl Acad Sci USA* 2003;100(4):2065–9.

Skinner JE. Neurocardiology: Brain mechanisms underlying fatal cardiac arrhythmias. *Neurol Clinics* 1993;11(2):325–51.

Stauffer AZ, Dodd-O J, Lathers CM. The relationship of the lockstep phenomenon and precipitous changes in mean arterial blood pressure. *Electroenphalogr Clin Neurophysiol* 1989;72(4):340–5.

Stauffer AZ, Dodd-O JM, Lathers CM. Relationship of the lockstep phenomenon and precipitous changes in blood pressure. In: Lathers CM, Schraeder PL, eds. *Epilepsy and Sudden Death*. New York, NY: Marcel Dekker; 1990, pp. 221–38.

Steriade M, Amzica F. Slow sleep oscillation, rhythmic K-complexes, and their paroxysmal developments. *J Sleep Res* 1998;7(Suppl 1):30–5.

Steriade M, Amzica F, Neckelman D, et al. Spike-wave complexes and fast components of cortically generated seizures: II. Extra- and intracellular patterns. *J Neurophysiol* 1998;80(3):1456–79.

Steriade M, Contreras D. Spike-wave complexes and fast components of cortically generated seizures. I. Role of the neocortex and thalamus. *J Neurophysiol* 1998;80(3):1439–55.

Steriade M, Nunez A, Amzica F. A novel slow (<1 Hz) oscillation of neocortical neurons in vivo: Depolarizing and hyperpolarizing components. *J Neurosci* 1993;13(8):3252–65.

Terzano MG, Parrino L. Origin and significance of the cyclic alternating pattern (CAP). *Sleep Med Rev* 2000;4(1):101–23.

Togo F, Yamamoto Y. Decreased fractal component of human heart rate variability during non-REM sleep. *Am J Physiol Heart C* 2001;280:H17–21.

Vanhatalo S, Palva JM, Holmes MD, et al. Infraslow oscillations modulate excitability and interictal epileptic activity in the human cortex during sleep. *Proc Natl Acad Sci USA* 2004;101(14):5053–7.

West BJ, Goldberger AL. Physiology in fractal dimensions. *Am Sci* 1987;75:354–64.

# 29 Lockstep in Humans
## *Bridging the Gap*

*Jeremy D. Slater*

## CONTENTS

## CHALLENGE

The exact pathophysiology of sudden unexplained death in epilepsy (SUDEP) remains unknown, but a growing body of evidence points to peri-ictal (occurring concurrently with a seizure) respiratory, cardiac, or autonomic dysfunction. Not every case of SUDEP necessarily has the same cause; these causes are also not mutually exclusive. Proposed causes for SUDEP fall into three primary categories: cardiovascular, including ictal arrhythmias or asystole; neurogenic pulmonary edema; or ictal respiratory suppression (Leung et al. 2006; Sowers et al. 2013; Zhao et al. 2014). A retrospective review of data from multiple epilepsy monitoring units examined patients who died from SUDEP. The data suggest that the patients had postictal centrally mediated cardiorespiratory dysfunction, especially associated with antiepileptic drug (AED) withdrawal (Ryvlin et al. 2013). The "lockstep phenomenon" (LSP), which has been identified in animal models, is one potential mechanism for seizures triggering cardiac arrhythmias to cause SUDEP. In LSP, abnormal cardiac sympathetic neural discharges and cardiac arrhythmias are linked temporally to interictal and ictal epileptic activity (Lathers et al. 1987; Stauffer et al. 1989). The mechanism by which this association occurs has not been fully delineated.

There is only indirect evidence to support the hypothesis that the LSP occurs in humans with epilepsy. Several cortical areas commonly involved in refractory epilepsy have been implicated in central control of autonomic function. The central autonomic network includes cortical limbic areas, including the amygdala, anterior insula, anterior cingulate cortex, ventromedial prefrontal cortex, and posterior orbitofrontal cortex (Devinsky 2004; Nagai et al. 2004). Both spontaneous and provoked seizure activities involving these regions have been associated with a broad variety of autonomic manifestations including tachy- and bradyarrhythmias and blood pressure changes. These heart rate and blood pressure alterations frequently occur in a sequential progression, suggestive of spatially separated mapping of function (Van Buren 1958; Van Buren and Ajmone-Marsan 1960; Van Buren et al. 1961; Oppenheimer et al. 1992). These autonomic manifestations are similar to the ictal and interictal findings in animal models of LSP.

Published work examining subtle variations in heart rate has provided an additional line of evidence for the LSP. Heart rate variability (HRV) is a broad term encompassing a number of different metrics derived from the cardiac RR interval. Studies using time-domain, spectral, and nonlinear analyses have all to varying degrees demonstrated a relationship between HRV and risk of both sudden and nonsudden cardiac death (Camm et al. 1996; Huikuri and Stein 2013; Lombardi et al. 2001). Low-frequency HRV values indicate relative sympathetic nerve tone dominance, and high HRV values indicate greater vagal nerve tone (Ansakorpi et al. 2002; Xhyheri et al. 2012). Evidence suggestive of LSP reflected as an increase or a reduction in RR intervals concurrent with interictal discharges has been published, but the mechanism for this is unknown. Clear links between changes to HRV and interictal discharges, as well as those between changes to HRV and SUDEP, remain controversial, with published evidence both for and against (DeGiorgio and DeGiorgio 2010; DeGiorgio et al. 2010; Rauscher et al. 2011; Surges et al. 2009; Zaatreh et al. 2003). Reduced cardiac fractal physiology (the presence of fractal scaling, long-range correlations responsible for part of HRV) has been identified as a better predictor of ventricular arrhythmias than traditional HRV and has been detected in patients with refractory temporal lobe epilepsy, a group at high risk for SUDEP (Makikallio et al. 2001; Ansakorpi et al. 2002; Penttilä et al. 2003). This reduction is most prominent during sleep, specifically non–rapid eye movement stage. SUDEP most commonly occurs at night, and patients with nocturnal seizures are at higher risk (Nobili et al. 2011; Lamberts et al. 2012). This temporal link suggests that these findings could be related.

Integrating this work to date, Hughes and Sato (2011) proposed the following hypothesis:

> The epileptic network in temporal lobe epilepsy patients, especially chronic refractory temporal lobe epilepsy patients at higher risk for SUDEP, induces changes in the central cortical autonomic function necessary to impart fractal

dynamics on the heart, disturbing or eliminating this fractal phenomenon. Preliminary evidence suggests this derangement is more pronounced at night, in the setting of a pre-existing physiological reduction in fractal dynamics during non rapid eye movement sleep. Fractal autonomic dynamics are felt to be necessary to protect the heart in the setting of physiological challenges on various time scales, e.g., rapid intense surges as well as sustained increases in sympathetic activity. A seizure, especially a generalized tonic-clonic event, with its associated rapid increase in sympathetic activity, is one such challenge (most witnessed events of SUDEP have been associated with generalized tonic-clonic seizures). The sympathetic activity seen in the lock-step phenomenon, which refers to an increase in sympathetic activity time-locked to interictal discharges, is another.

This theory, if true, would support the use of metrics of cardiac autonomic function as biomarkers of SUDEP risk. One gap in the evidence needed to test this hypothesis is confirmation of the occurrence (and consistency if there is such an occurrence) of the LSP in human subjects with epilepsy. Studies examining the relationship of epileptic activity to autonomic change have, for the most part, been limited by the use of scalp recordings for spike and seizure detection (Zaatreh et al. 2003). One demonstration of the limitation of scalp recordings is evidence of changes to HRV detected up to 5 minutes prior to electrographic seizure onset (Behbahani et al. 2013); the changes to HRV were associated with seizures but were occurring prior to evidence of the seizure on scalp recording. This observation highlights the fact that the accuracy with which one can assess synchronization between bursts in cardiac autonomic activity and epileptic discharges is dependent on the degree to which all such discharges are detected.

Methods with potentially greater sensitivity for spike detection include magnetoencephalography (MEG) and electrocorticography (ECog). While MEG has been demonstrated under specific circumstances to detect a greater number of epileptic discharges than scalp electroencephalogram (EEG), the comparison is complex; MEG is sensitive primarily to the tangential component of the spike dipole, whereas EEG is sensitive to both the radial and tangential components. In cases of superficial sources, MEG may provide a higher degree of spatial localization than EEG, but spike number detection is variable. Depending on the source, MEG may detect more spikes, fewer spikes, the same number, or none at all (Ahlfors et al. 2010; Kakisaka et al. 2013). Invasive recordings using ECog have a sensitivity to epileptic spikes 10- to 20-fold greater than scalp recordings (Tao et al. 2005). The difficulty with using ECog for such an investigation is that the subdural grid and strip placements needed for the clinical investigation only infrequently target some of the cortical regions involved in autonomic control.

Stereoelectroencephalography (sEEG) would seem the optimal method for investigating the relationship between cortical activity and autonomic function. This technology utilizes from 8 to 12 depth electrodes placed at various locations in one or both hemispheres (the locations being determined by the epilepsy team as most effective for testing the preimplant hypothesis regarding location of the seizure onset zone) as part of the presurgical workup. One possibility is that the occurrence of the LSP may be dependent on the area of cortex involved with the epileptic discharge. The sEEG target locations frequently include the amygdala, anterior insula, anterior cingulate cortex, ventromedial prefrontal cortex, and posterior orbitofrontal cortex—All critical areas for central autonomic control.

An additional gap in current knowledge is whether neocortical temporal and extratemporal epilepsies are associated with the same changes to heart rate dynamics as those seen with temporal lobe epilepsy. Patients with frontal lobe epilepsy have demonstrated faster average interictal heart rates and increased high-frequency power in HRV compared to healthy controls, but whether this response is a direct effect of the epilepsy or a consequence of the autonomic activation occurring with the physiologic arousal that precedes the motor manifestation of these seizures is not entirely clear (Harnod et al. 2009; Calandra-Buonaura et al. 2012). Even in those patients with medically refractory temporal lobe epilepsy, whose heart rate dynamics are greater than in those whose seizures are well controlled, the impact of AEDs and that of successful epilepsy surgery is unknown. There is a trend for higher sympathetic or lower parasympathetic tone in patients receiving pharmacotherapy (Ansakorpi et al. 2002; Calandra-Buonaura et al. 2012; Lotufo et al. 2012). An optimal experimental design would include a means by which these questions could be addressed as well.

The root cause of circadian variability of SUDEP risk has not been established. In contrast with sudden cardiac death in the general population, which is more frequent in the morning than at night (Muller et al. 1987; Willich et al. 1987), the risk for sudden death in patients with epilepsy in general increases at night (Langan et al. 2005). In healthy subjects, cardiac fractal complexity decreases during the night compared to daytime; the magnitude of the change is comparable to the difference between healthy and diseased subjects (Ivanov et al. 1999). This relationship was originally thought to be due to differences between the sleep and wake states, but subsequent work has demonstrated evidence for circadian variability of cardiac fractal complexity at shorter time scales of up to 1 hour, with a 24-hour peak occurring at approximately 10 a.m. (Hu et al. 2004). Central nervous system (CNS) influence has been revealed by lesion experiments in animal models showing that destruction of the suprachiasmatic nucleus (SCN) eliminates cardiac fractal complexity circadian rhythms (Hu et al. 2008); the mechanism by which the SCN exerts its influence remains unknown. Although interactions between sleep and epilepsy have been long known, the effects of seizures on SCN, if any, have not been established (Tallavajhula and Slater 2012). If, however, the "transfer function" per se between SCN and heart is a product of the areas of cortex responsible for central autonomic control, the circadian effect on SUDEP risk may simply be the result of the seizure activity itself, which is in turn subject to circadian influence.

Cardiac fractal complexity appears to have its origins in CNS autonomic controls. HRV is attenuated with pharmacologic blockade of parasympathetic input and enhanced with sympathetic blockade; local modulators of blood vessels (nitric oxide synthase inhibitors, or agonist/antagonists of α-adrenergic receptors) do not produce these effects (Sharma 2009). If the two systems, the EEG activity generated by the CNS and the heart rate generated as the result of autonomic activity, are viewed as linked oscillators, reduced fractal complexity of CNS electrical activity could then result in reduced fractal complexity of heart rate. Two lines of evidence support this concept. First, fractal complexity has been detected in brain electrical activity, and changes to various metrics of nonlinear dynamics have been identified before, during, and after seizures, as well as other neurologic disorders including Alzheimer's disease and autism spectrum disorder (Chaovalitwongse et al. 2005; Abasolo et al. 2007; Abasolo et al. 2008; Ahmadlou et al. 2010; Xiaodong et al. 2010). Second, a study of healthy volunteers demonstrated a significant central autonomic fractal correlation between scalp EEG recordings and HRV (Lin and Sharif 2011). Taken together, this represents an extension of the Hughes–Sato hypothesis in providing a mechanism for the causal link between epileptic activity and risk of cardiac sudden death. In short, a seizure (or an epileptic spike or sharp wave) triggers a decrease in fractal complexity of the cortical electrical activity. This makes sense from the standpoint that a seizure is the result of hypersynchronous neuronal activity with too many neurons engaged in an identical firing pattern. By definition, this is a system of reduced complexity. If the cortical electrical activity in turn drives the cardiac autonomic activity, the reduced fractal complexity of the cortical electrical activity potentially results in reduced fractal complexity of cardiac autonomic activity, which has been linked to increased risk of sudden cardiac death.

## PROPOSED EXPERIMENTAL PARADIGM

To address effectively many of the outstanding issues related to clarifying the effects of epileptic activity on CNS control of cardiac autonomic function, and in particular to try to demonstrate the LSP in humans, investigators could take advantage of the prolonged recording of intracranial ECog that takes place during sEEG recordings of patients with refractory epilepsy prior to resective surgery. Such patients are at the highest risk for SUDEP. Patients undergoing invasive recording have extensive workups preceding the intervention with detailed histories; imaging; neuropsychological testing; and, commonly, additional ancillary testing including positron emission tomography and MEG. Those who undergo surgery and achieve seizure freedom can be studied to determine if proposed biomarkers that were elevated prior to surgery have now normalized.

After the implantation of sEEG electrodes, the patient routinely undergoes progressive reduction and in many cases elimination of AEDs. Once a sufficient number of seizures are recorded, the electrodes are removed, medications are restarted, and patient is sent home, with the majority eventually returning for a resective surgery. If high-resolution ECG monitoring were performed at baseline prior to sEEG implantation, then continued throughout the hospitalization, and again performed at 6- and 12-month intervals post resection, the proposed Holter-based metrics of SUDEP risk (including T-wave alternans, HRV, and heart rate turbulence—See Chapter 16) could be repeatedly derived and compared. As previously noted, invasive recording of brain electrical activity has a much greater sensitivity to both spikes and seizures than scalp recordings. Demonstration of the presence or absence of a link between epileptic activity and changes to cardiac fractal complexity can be accomplished with a high degree of statistical certainty, effectively testing for the LSP.

With a sufficiently large cohort and follow-up of at least 1 year post resection, the impact of AED withdrawal, and the impact of seizure freedom on these metrics could be determined. Depending on the patient cohort and the sEEG electrode placement, determining which epileptic brain networks have the highest association with changes in cardiac autonomic function might be possible. Successful completion of such a study could have a number of significant benefits. Identification of the brain regions with the highest association with autonomic impact would help stratify SUDEP risk, allowing targeted intervention for specific epilepsy syndromes. Finally, demonstration of reduced risk of SUDEP with AEDs as well as epilepsy surgery would positively impact the risk/benefit ratio of both the medical and surgical therapies; identification of specific AEDs associated with lower risk would help guide drug choice. Successful completion of such a study would advance the capacity to test potential interventions to reduce SUDEP risk, consequently improving the quality of life of patients suffering from epilepsy.

## CONCLUSIONS

The challenge facing all investigators with respect to SUDEP predictors and evaluation of interventions is that the time necessary to assess accurately a change in the rate of sudden death can be daunting. One way to address such a problem is to find surrogate biomarkers that can be used to demonstrate a reduced risk of sudden death in the absence of waiting for death itself to occur. The discovery of the LSP in animal models creates one possible path toward this end. If one can convincingly demonstrate in humans that a similar change to cardiac autonomic state takes place with spikes and seizures as seen in animal models, the case for using cardiac autonomic markers as biomarkers for SUDEP would be bolstered. If an additional link between brain and heart in the form of linked fractal dimensional complexity could be demonstrated, the case would be even stronger.

The optimal means to test these possibilities would be to perform recordings in humans with epilepsy that have the greatest sensitivity and specificity for spike and seizure detection, that is, recordings using intracranial electrodes. By utilizing sEEG, many of the cortical regions thought responsible for central control of autonomic function can be monitored. As this population is undergoing workup and testing prior to resective brain surgery to treat medically refractory epilepsy, monitoring of cardiac autonomic biomarkers before and after surgical intervention would also comprise an assessment of the impact of successful epilepsy surgery on SUDEP risk.

An additional potential impact of the completion of such a study may be on the goal of epilepsy therapy. The current goal is the suppression of clinical seizures, not the total suppression of interictal discharges. The classic reasoning for this approach is as follows:

1. The clinical seizures are what matter—They are what interfere with quality of life.
2. Aggressive treatment to suppress spikes is impossible, given that it would require so much medication that the patient would suffer significant adverse effects.
3. Epileptic spikes do not actually do any harm.

Several areas of research challenge this view:

1. Multiple studies have demonstrated the occurrence of cognitive deficits concurrent with spikes (not seizures) (Aarts et al. 1984; Kasteleijn-NolstTrenite 1995).
2. Increasing recognition that the cognitive deficits associated with seizures are due to some degree to abnormal electrical activity disrupting normal cortical network function outside of clinical seizures (Binnie 2003; Aldenkamp and Arends 2004).

We do not yet have enough evidence to determine when the goal of therapy should be the elimination of spikes rather than the suppression of clinical seizures, but if a study clearly demonstrated that both spikes and seizures trigger an increased risk of SUDEP in humans, the ultimate goal of therapy would change to maximally reducing SUDEP risk by suppressing interictal epileptiform discharges, in addition to the suppression of clinical seizures.

## REFERENCES

Aarts JH, Binnie CD, Smit AM, Wilkins AJ. Selective cognitive impairment during focal and generalized epileptiform EEG activity. *Brain* 1984;107(Pt1):293–308.

Abasolo D, Hornero R, Escudero J, Espino P. A study on the possible usefulness of detrended fluctuation analysis of the electroencephalogram background activity in Alzheimer's disease. *IEEE Trans Biomed Eng* 2008;55(9):2171–9.

Abasolo D, James CJ, Hornero R. Non-linear analysis of intracranial electroencephalogram recordings with approximate entropy and Lempel-Ziv complexity for epileptic seizure detection. *Conf Proc IEEE Eng Med Biol Soc* 2007;1953–6.

Ahlfors SP, Han J, Belliveau JW, Hamalainen MS. Sensitivity of MEG and EEG to source orientation. *Brain Topogr* 2010; 23(3):227–32.

Ahmadlou M, Adeli H, Adeli A. Fractality and a wavelet-chaos-neural network methodology for EEG-based diagnosis of autistic spectrum disorder. *J Clin Neurophysiol* 2010;27(5):328–33.

Aldenkamp AP, Arends J. Effects of epileptiform EEG discharges on cognitive function: Is the concept of "transient cognitive impairment" still valid? *Epilepsy Behav* 2004;5(Suppl 1):S25–34.

Ansakorpi H, Korpelainen JT, Huikuri HV, Tolonen U, Myllyla VV, Isojarvi JI. Heart rate dynamics in refractory and well controlled temporal lobe epilepsy. *J Neurol Neurosurg Psychiatry* 2002;72(1):26–30.

Behbahani S, Dabanloo NJ, Nasrabadi AM, Teixeira CA, Dourado A. Pre-ictal heartrate variability assessment of epileptic seizures by means of linear and non-linear analyses. *Anadolu Kardiyol Derg* 2013;13(8):797–803.

Binnie C D. Cognitive impairment during epileptiform discharges: Is it ever justifiable to treat the EEG? *Lancet Neurol* 2003;2(12): 725–30.

Calandra-Buonaura G, Toschi N, Provini F, Corazza I, Bisulli F, Barletta G, Cortelli P. Physiologic autonomic arousal heralds motor manifestations of seizures in nocturnal frontal lobe epilepsy: Implications for pathophysiology. *Sleep Med* 2012;13(3):252–62.

Camm AJ, Malik M, Bigger JT, Breithardt G, Cerutti S, Cohen RJ, Singer DH. Heart rate variability: Standards of measurement, physiological interpretation and clinical use. Task Force of the European Society of Cardiology and the North American Society of Pacing and Electrophysiology. *Circulation* 1996; 93(5):1043–65.

Chaovalitwongse W, Iasemidis LD, Pardalos PM, Carney PR, Shiau DS, Sackellares JC. Performance of a seizure warning algorithm based on the dynamics of intracranial EEG. *Epilepsy Res* 2005;64(3):93–113.

DeGiorgio CM, DeGiorgio AC. SUDEP and heart rate variability. *Epilepsy Res* 2010;90(3):309–10;author reply311–2.

DeGiorgio CM, Miller P, Meymandi S, Chin A, Epps J, Gordon S, Harper RM. RMSSD, a measure of vagus-mediated heartrate variability, is associated with risk factors for SUDEP: The SUDEP-7 inventory. *Epilepsy Behav* 2010;19(1):78–81.

Devinsky O. Effects of seizures on autonomic and cardiovascular function. *Epilepsy Curr* 2004;4(2):43–6.

Harnod T, Yang CC, Hsin YL, Wang PJ, Shieh KR, Kuo TB. Heart rate variability in patients with frontal lobe epilepsy. *Seizure* 2009;18(1):21–5.

Hu, K, Ivanov P, Hilton MF, Chen Z, Ayers RT, Stanley HE, Shea SA. Endogenous circadian rhythm in an index of cardiac vulnerability independent of changes in behavior. *Proc Natl Acad Sci USA* 2004;101(52):18223–7.

Hu K, Scheer FA, Buijs RM, Shea SA. The circadian pacemaker generates similar circadian rhythms in the fractal structure of heartrate in humans and rats. *Cardiovasc Res* 2008;80(1):62–8.

Hughes JD, Sato S. Sudden death in epilepsy: Relationship to sleep-wake circadian cycle and fractal physiology. In: Lathers CM, Schraeder PL, Bungo MW, Leestma JE, eds. *Sudden Death in Epilepsy: Forensic and Clinical Issues.* Boca Raton, FL: CRC Press/Taylor & Francis Group; 2011, pp. 333–46.

Huikuri HV, Stein PK. Heart rate variability in risk stratification of cardiac patients. *Prog Cardiovasc Dis* 2013;56(2):153–9.

Ivanov P, Bunde A, Amaral LA, Havlin S, Fritsch-Yelle J, Baevsky RM, Goldberger AL. Sleep-wake differences in scaling behavior of the human heartbeat: Analysis of terrestrial and long-term space flight data. *Europhys Lett* 1999;48(5):594–600.

Kakisaka Y, Alkawadri R, Wang ZI, Enatsu R, Mosher JC, Dubarry AS, Burgess RC. Sensitivity of scalp 10-20 EEG and magnetoencephalography. *Epileptic Disord* 2013;15(1): 27–31.

Kasteleijn-Nolst Trenite DG. Transient cognitive impairment during subclinical epileptiform electroencephalographic discharges. *Semin Pediatr Neurol* 1995;2(4):246–53.

Lamberts RJ, Thijs RD, Laffan A, Langan Y, Sander JW. Sudden unexpected death in epilepsy: People with nocturnal seizures maybe at highest risk. *Epilepsia* 2012;53(2):253–7.

Langan,Y, Nashef L, Sander JW. Case-control study of SUDEP. *Neurology* 2005;64(7):1131–3.

Lathers CM, Schraeder PL, Weiner FL. Synchronization of cardiac autonomic neural discharge with epileptogenic activity: The lock step phenomenon. *Electroencephalogr Clin Neurophysiol* 1987;67(3):247–59.

Leung H , Kwan P, Elger CE. Finding the missing link between ictalbradyarrhythmia, ictalasystole, and sudden unexpected death in epilepsy. *Epilepsy Behav* 2006;9(1):19–30.

Lin DC, Sharif A. Integrated central-autonomic multifractal complexity in the heartrate variability of healthy humans. *Front Physiol* 2011;2:123.

Lombardi F, Makikallio TH, Myerburg RJ, Huikuri HV. Sudden cardiac death: Role of heartrate variability to identify patients at risk. *Cardiovasc Res* 2001;50(2):210–7.

Lotufo PA, Valiengo L, Bensenor IM, Brunoni AR. A systematic review and meta-analysis of heart rate variability in epilepsy and antiepileptic drugs. *Epilepsia* 2012;53(2):272–82.

Makikallio TH, Huikuri HV, Makikallio A, Sourander LB, Mitrani RD, Castellanos A, Myerburg RJ. Prediction of sudden cardiac death by fractal analysis of heartrate variability in elderly subjects. *J Am Coll Cardiol* 2001;37(5):1395–402.

Muller JE, Ludmer PL, Willich SN, Tofler GH, Aylmer G, Klangos I, Stone PH. Circadian variation in the frequency of sudden cardiac death. *Circulation* 1987;75(1):131–8.

Nagai Y, Critchley HD, Featherstone E, Trimble MR, Dolan RJ. Activity in ventromedial prefrontal cortex covaries with sympathetic skin conductance level: A physiological account of a "default mode" of brain function. *Neuroimage* 2004;22(1):243–51.

Nobili L, Proserpio P, Rubboli G, Montano N, Didato G, Tassinari CA. Sudden unexpected death in epilepsy (SUDEP) and sleep. *Sleep Med Rev* 2011;15(4):237–46.

Oppenheimer SM, Gelb A, Girvin JP, Hachinski VC. Cardiovascular effects of human insular cortex stimulation. *Neurology* 1992; 42(9):1727–32.

Penttilä J, Helminen A, Jartti T, Kuusela T, Huikuri HV, Tulppo MP, Scheinin H. Effect of cardiac vagal outflow on complexity and fractal correlation properties of heart rate dynamics. *Auton and Autacoid Pharmacol* 2003;23(3):173–9.

Rauscher G, DeGiorgio AC, Miller PR, DeGiorgio CM. Sudden unexpected death in epilepsy associated with progressive deterioration in heart rate variability. *Epilepsy Behav* 2011;21(1): 103–5.

Ryvlin P, Nashef L, Lhatoo SD, Bateman LM, Bird J, Bleasel A, Tomson T. Incidence and mechanisms of cardiorespiratory arrests in epilepsy monitoring units (MORTEMUS): A retrospective study. *Lancet Neurol* 2013;12(10):966–77.

Sharma V. Deterministic chaos and fractal complexity in the dynamics of cardiovascular behavior: Perspectives on a new frontier. *Open Cardiovasc Med J* 2009;3:110–23.

Sowers LP, Massey CA, Gehlbach BK, Granner MA, Richerson GB. Sudden unexpected death in epilepsy: Fatal post-ictal respiratory and arousal mechanisms. *Respir Physiol Neurobiol* 2013;189(2):315–23.

Stauffer AZ, Dodd-O J, Lathers CM. The relationship of the lock-step phenomenon and precipitous changes in mean arterial blood pressure. *Electro encephalogr Clin Neurophysiol* 1989; 72(4):340–5.

Surges R, Henneberger C, Adjei P, Scott CA, Sander JW, Walker MC. Do alterations in inter-ictal heart rate variability predict sudden unexpected death in epilepsy? *Epilepsy Res* 2009;87(2–3): 277–80.

Tallavajhula SS, Slater JD. Sleep and Epilepsy. *Sleep Med Clin* 2012;7(4):619–30.

Tao JX, Ray A, Hawes-Ebersole S, Ebersole JS. Intra cranial EEG substrates of scalp EEG interictal spikes. *Epilepsia* 2005;46(5):669–76.

Van Buren JM. Some autonomic concomitants of ictalautomatism; A study of temporal lobe attacks. *Brain* 1958;81(4):505–28.

Van Buren JM, Ajmone-Marsan C. A correlation of autonomic and EEG components in temporal lobe epilepsy. *Arch Neurol* 1960;3:683–703.

VanBuren JM, Bucknam CA, Pritchard WL. Autonomic representation in the human orbitotemporal cortex. *Neurology* 1961;11:214–24.

Willich SN, Levy D, Rocco MB, Tofler GH, Stone PH, Muller, JE. Circadian variation in the incidence of sudden cardiac death in the Framingham Heart Study population. *Am J Cardiol* 1987;60(10):801–6.

Xhyheri B, Manfrini O, Mazzolini M, Pizzi C, Bugiardini R. Heart rate variability today. *Prog Cardiovasc Dis* 2012;55(3):321–31.

Xiaodong Y, Wei C, Shanshan M, Tongfeng S. Research of complex physiological signals based on nonlinear theory. Paper presented at the Biomedical Engineering and Informatics (BMEI), 20103rd International Conferenceon, October 16–18, 2010.

Zaatreh MM, Quint SR, Tennison MB, D'CruzO, Vaughn BB. Heart rate variability during interictal epileptiform discharges. *Epilepsy Res* 2003;54(2–3):85–90.

Zhao H, Lin G, Shi M, Gao J, Wang Y, Wang H, Cao Y. The mechanism of neurogenic pulmonary edemain epilepsy. *J Physiol Sci* 2014;64(1):65–72.

# 30 Postictal Generalized EEG Suppression and Sudden Unexpected Death in Epilepsy

*Joon Kang and Maromi Nei*

## CONTENTS

## INTRODUCTION

Since the initial reports of the electroencephalogram (EEG) recordings in sudden unexpected death in epilepsy (SUDEP), there has been tremendous effort in the field to determine if there are specific EEG patterns that correlate with SUDEP. Identification of such patterns may (1) shed light on the pathophysiology behind SUDEP, (2) potentially aid in identifying those at high risk for SUDEP, and (3) further the development of potentially life-saving interventions to prevent SUDEP. Postictal generalized EEG suppression (PGES) has been reported in several monitored SUDEP and near-SUDEP cases. Although there is some evidence to suggest that prolonged PGES may be a risk factor for SUDEP, the data are conflicting at this time. Many questions regarding the etiology and role of PGES remain unanswered, but data are emerging regarding its potential significance in SUDEP.

## CASE REPORTS OF POSTICTAL GENERALIZED EEG SUPPRESSION IN SUDEP

Bird et al. (1997) reported SUDEP recorded during intracranial EEG and video monitoring of a 47-year-old man with intractable focal epilepsy. Depths and subdural electrodes were placed in the bilateral temporal lobes without any immediate peri- and postoperative complications. His antiepileptic medications were tapered rapidly over the 6 days following intracranial electrode implantation. The patient subsequently had a cluster of five seizures within a 24-hour period and died on the sixth day postoperatively. Of note, seizure clusters do not reliably precede SUDEP, but some data suggest seizure clusters might elevate SUDEP risk (Nei et al. 2004). His fifth and final seizure occurred after a 2.5-minute secondarily generalized tonic-clonic seizure (GTCS) during sleep.

There was no evidence of obvious respiratory distress, including asphyxia. The EEG recording demonstrated right mesial temporal onset, with spread to the left hemisphere within 15 seconds. Postictally, there was initially right and then left hemisphere suppression of the EEG without recovery. Notably, EKG artifact continued at a regular rate of 46 beats per minute for 2 minutes after generalized attenuation before gradually decreasing in amplitude until asystole occurred. The postmortem examination did not demonstrate an obvious cause of death, consistent with SUDEP.

Subsequently, McLean and Wilmalaratna (2007) also reported postictal diffuse suppression after a GTCS during an ambulatory EEG recording of SUDEP in a woman in her fifties. Similarly, near-SUDEP cases have reported postictal diffuse slowing, at times followed by diffuse attenuation (So et al. 2000; Tavee and Morris 2008; Espinosa et al. 2009).

## SEIZURES, POSTICTAL GENERALIZED EEG SUPPRESSION, AND SUDEP

There are very strong data indicating that SUDEP is a seizure-related event. Poor seizure control is a significant major risk factor for SUDEP, with increasing risk correlating with greater seizure frequency (Nilsson et al. 1999; Langan et al. 2000). GTCSs confer the highest risk for SUDEP. The majority of witnessed SUDEP cases are associated with a seizure at the time of sudden death, most commonly GTCSs (Langan et al. 2000; Tomson et al. 2005). A final generalized convulsive seizure immediately precedes any evidence of respiratory and/or cardiovascular compromise in several video-EEG-recorded reported cases of SUDEP (Lee 1998; McLean and Wilmalaratna 2007; Tao et al. 2010; Bateman et al. 2010; Lhatoo et al. 2010). It is highly probable that GTCSs trigger a cascade of events resulting in autonomic dysfunction, respiratory compromise, and cardiac arrhythmias, which ultimately culminates in SUDEP.

The observation of prolonged PGES occurring after the final generalized convulsive seizure, seen in many of the recorded SUDEP cases, gave rise to the hypothesis of "electrocerebral shutdown" (McLean and Wilmalaratna 2007). In this model, SUDEP is thought to be a centrally mediated process whereby the mechanisms involved in seizure suppression result in brain stem autonomic dysfunction and subsequent loss of protective reflexes that would normally prevent death when breathing is impaired or the airway is obstructed, such as the cough and gag reflex. γ-Aminobutyric acid, endocannabinoids (Deshpande et al. 2007), neuropeptide Y (Baraban et al. 1997), and adenosine (Dragunow et al. 1985; During et al. 1992) have been identified as potential neurotransmitters and neuromodulators that play a role in seizure termination (Lado and Moshe 2008). Pharmacologically induced seizures in mice with impaired clearance of adenosine and neuropeptide Y deficient mice have been shown to result in uncontrolled seizures and ultimately death (Baraban et al. 1997; Shen et al. 2010). Endocannabinoids have been shown to dampen seizure activity via activation of the presynaptic cannabinoid receptor 1 (Wallace et al. 2002), and application of the receptor antagonist has shown to result in electrographic status

epilepticus (Deshpande et al. 2007). Intrinsic defects in the mechanism of seizure termination may be involved in the pathophysiology of epilepsy-related death.

Peri-ictal cardiopulmonary dysfunction, such as bradycardia and apnea, occurs commonly. What is not understood is why and how, in a vast majority of seizures, people spontaneously recover. Thus, several questions arise: Is PGES the EEG representation of electrocerebral shutdown? Is there a correlation between PGES duration and increased risk of SUDEP? Can we use PGES as a marker for intervention and to prevent SUDEP?

## DATA ON POSTICTAL GENERALIZED EEG SUPPRESSION AND SUDEP

At least two studies have looked at the association of PGES and SUDEP, with conflicting results. Lhatoo et al. (2010) conducted a case-control study of 10 definite SUDEP cases with at least one recorded seizure in the video-EEG monitoring unit and 30 consecutively monitored controls, who were living patients with medically refractory epilepsy with at least one epileptic seizure around the time that the controls were monitored (Table 30.1). PGES was defined as the immediate postictal (within 30 seconds) generalized absence of EEG activity >10 uV in amplitude. PGES occurred in almost half (14/30) of the seizures in SUDEP

## TABLE 30.1
## Studies on PGES and SUDEP

| Study | Study Design | Number of Subjects/Sample | Frequency of PGES | Role of PGES in SUDEP |
|---|---|---|---|---|
| Lhatoo et al. 2010 | Retrospective Case control SUDEP study | 10 SUDEP cases, 30 controls | SUDEP: 50% Controls: 38% (of seizures) | Duration PGES and odds of SUDEP is directly related PGES >50 seconds is a marker of individuals at risk for SUDEP |
| Surges et al. 2011 | Retrospective Case control SUDEP study | 17 SUDEP cases, 17 controls | SUDEP: 4/17 Controls: 3/19 (of patients) 15% in all seizures 26% of all patients | No association between risk of SUDEP and duration/presence of PGES PGES associated with GTCS |
| Semmelroch et al. 2012 | Retrospective Case control Refractory focal epilepsy | 13 cases (+PGES), 12 controls (−PGES) | 27% of patients with GTCSs | PGES associated with immobility and nursing intervention |
| Tao et al. 2013 | Retrospective Review Refractory focal epilepsy | 151 CS | 65% of CS 58.7% of all patients | PGES associated with unresponsiveness/ immobility Tonic phase of CS predictor of PGES |
| Lamberts et al. 2013 | Retrospective review Refractory focal epilepsy | 154 CS | 37%[a] of CS 63%[a] of all patients | PGES is an inconsistent finding, thus not likely to be a reliable predictor for SUDEP PGES >20 seconds associated with nocturnal seizures, tapering of AEDs |

*Note:* CS, convulsive seizure; AED, antiepileptic drug.

[a] For PGES >20 seconds.

cases compared to 38% (35/92) of the seizures in controls. Although no significant difference in duration of PGES was detected across all seizure types, PGES with generalized motor seizures was significantly longer in SUDEP cases compared to control subjects (91.5 vs. 15.57 seconds). Age, gender, and the age at onset of seizures were identified as variables correlating with PGES duration. After adjusting for variables such as age, gender, and age of onset, the odds ratio (OR) for SUDEP for PGES >50 seconds for all seizure types was 5.22, and this value increased exponentially with PGES >80 seconds (OR, 23.46; confidence interval [CI], 2.92–188.54). A similarly increased risk was seen when only generalized motor seizures were analyzed, with a duration of PGES >20 seconds (OR, 12.99; CI, 1.24–135.78) associated with increased risk. For each 1-second increase in the duration of PGES, the odds of SUDEP increased by 1.7%. However, a similar larger study with 17 SUDEP cases and matched controls did not detect such significant differences in the presence or duration of PGES (Surges et al. 2011). The mean PGES duration in those who died from SUDEP was not significantly different from that of the matched living controls with epilepsy and was shorter than the mean duration of PGES reported in the Lhatoo et al. (2010) study.

Such discrepancies between the two studies may be partially due to clinical factors, including differences in the selection of control patients, number of seizures recorded, anticonvulsant use, and small sample sizes. In the Surges et al. (2011) study, both the controls and cases consisted of patients with temporal lobe epilepsy who had undergone evaluation for epilepsy surgery. The controls were living patients matched for admission date for video-EEG telemetry, age, and gender. This raises a potential built-in bias in the control patients. Successful epilepsy surgery resulting in postoperative seizure freedom has been shown to significantly reduce mortality rates, especially epilepsy-associated death (Sperling et al. 2005). The controls may have reduced their risk of SUDEP by undergoing surgery, but otherwise they have the same inherent biological risk and electrographical finding as the SUDEP patients (Bozorgi and Lhatoo 2013). Furthermore, the duration of PGES is not necessarily a consistent finding among seizures occurring in the same individual. Lamberts et al. (2013) demonstrated that PGES lasting longer than 20 seconds in patients with greater than two seizures was consistently present in 63% of the individuals overall and 37% of the patients with convulsive seizures. The consistency in presence or absence of PGES was dependent on the number of seizures recorded; the more seizures recorded, the less likely that the presence or absence of PGES was consistent within an individual. Medication may also influence the presence and duration of PGES, and medication reduction may affect the duration of postictal EEG recovery. In one study, Tilz et al. (2006) compared the postictal EEG recovery time (back to baseline EEG pattern) in 23 patients undergoing video-EEG monitoring randomized to either levetiracetam (11 patients) or placebo (12 patients). Whereas the placebo group's recovery

times remained at 90 seconds before and after randomization, they decreased in those randomized to levetiracetam from 130 (prior to levetiracetam) to 4 seconds (after levetiracetam was initiated). The investigation also revealed that there was a corresponding shorter recovery in level of consciousness in those who received levetiracetam. Although this was a limited sample and no PGES data are available, this study suggests that antiepileptic drugs may affect postictal EEG findings. Further studies with large numbers of controls and broader epilepsy types controlled for clinical variables, including medication taper, are needed to understand the significance of PGES and its potential correlation with SUDEP.

## PREVALENCE AND PREDICTORS OF POSTICTAL GENERALIZED EEG SUPPRESSION

PGES is commonly seen after convulsive seizures in adults but at highly variable prevalence rates. The prevalence of PGES after convulsive seizures in adults is as low as 15% (Surges et al. 2011) and as high as 65% (Tao et al. 2013). In contrast to adults, PGES appears to be less common in children, occurring in only 2 (8%) of 200 seizures in one study (Kim et al. 2006) and 16.1% in another (Moseley et al. 2013). This discrepancy in prevalence rates between children and adults suggests that PGES may not be only a phenomenon of cerebral metabolic exhaustion but an active process requiring a certain degree of cerebral maturity. This hypothesis is further supported by results from a study by Pavlova et al. (2013) in which the duration of PGES was longer in adults than children (189 vs. 36.5 seconds). If PGES is indeed associated with increased risk for SUDEP, these lower pediatric rates of PGES might correlate with the known lower risk for SUDEP in children (Tomson et al. 2005).

There are several factors that predict the presence of PGES. PGES is more likely to occur after secondarily GTCSs (Surges et al. 2011) and in the presence of a longer tonic phase (Tao et al. 2013). PGES greater than 20 seconds has been associated with convulsive seizures starting from sleep and in convulsive seizures after anticonvulsants reduction (Lamberts et al. 2013).

## POSSIBLE MECHANISMS UNDERLYING POSTICTAL GENERALIZED EEG SUPPRESSION

The mechanisms underlying PGES and its possible relation to SUDEP are not clear at this time. One possibility is that PGES represents a profound cortical neuronal inhibitory mechanism of abrupt onset, possibly with associated inhibition of the brain stem respiratory centers (Lhatoo et al. 2010). Postictal central apnea was reported to be the initiating event in one near-SUDEP case (So et al. 2000). Additionally, respiratory changes (such as central apnea, obstructive apnea, hypercarbia, and hypoxia) are frequently seen during and after seizures (Nashef et al. 1996; Blum et al. 2000; So et al. 2000; Swallow et al. 2002; O'Regan and Brown 2005; Seyal et al. 2010), and the degree of postictal hypercarbia and hypoxia is also much more than expected from the brief ictal apnea (Seyal et al. 2010). This raises the possibility that PGES reflects centrally mediated prolonged apnea. However, using formal respiratory monitoring, Seyal and colleagues (Seyal et al. 2012) demonstrated that PGES was not associated with postictal central apnea. In this study, the investigators found that apnea is not initiated during PGES in the postictal period and in all but three cases ceased before the onset of PGES. Notably, the rate and amplitude of airflow increased in the postictal period and in the setting of PGES (Seyal et al. 2010). These findings do not support the hypothesis that PGES correlates with the inhibition of brain stem respiratory centers. They did not focus on cardiac telemetry data. Additionally, Pavlova et al. found that while PGES was longer in adults, apnea and bradycardia were more common in children, also suggesting that PGES might not directly cause autonomic dysfunction.

An alternative explanation for PGES is that it is the result, not the cause, of the severity of seizure-induced pulmonary dysfunction. Seyal et al. (2012) found that seizures with PGES or bilateral attenuation had significantly longer periods of oxygen desaturation, lower nadirs of hypoxemia, and higher rises in end-tidal $CO_2$ relative to generalized convulsions without PGES or bilateral attenuation. In rats and monkeys, hypoxia and hypercarbia can suppress neuronal activity (Balestrino and Somjen 1988; Fano et al. 2007; Zappe et al. 2008), and a similar process might occur in humans, explaining the association of greater oxygen desaturation with PGES or bilateral attenuation. Hypoventilation occurs in one-third of partial-onset seizures in patients undergoing video-EEG telemetry (Bateman et al. 2008). Such hypoventilation may be due to abnormalities in the medullary arousal system involving the neurotransmitter serotonin, similar to that seen in sudden infant death syndrome (Kinney et al. 2003) and/or a defect in seizure termination, possibly involving a neurotransmitter such as adenosine.

Serotonin receptors are found in brain stem and are thought to be critical in arousal and stimulating respiratory response to hypercarbia. The risk for seizure-related sudden death appears to be minimized by serotonin agonists in animal models. Limited data in humans similarly link the use of serotonin-reuptake inhibitors with reduced ictal hypoxemia, suggesting that serotonin activity may also be important in modulating respiratory centers in patients with epilepsy (Bateman et al. 2010). Respiratory dysfunction might also arise from a defect in seizure termination via net overstimulation with adenosine. Adenosine, a product of energy metabolism, is a powerful endogenous anticonvulsant released by astrocytes after a seizure (Dragunow et al. 1985). Overstimulation of adenosine receptors, which are located in the brain stem, hippocampus and neocortex, can result in severe cardiopulmonary dysfunction (Thomas et al. 2000; Barraco et al. 1990). Studies have suggested that abnormal concentration of adenosine receptors (Faingold 2012) and/or impairment of adenosine clearance (Shen et al. 2010) in some epilepsy patients can increase the likelihood of sudden death via profound respiratory suppression.

PGES could represent the direct effect of seizure-induced autonomic dysfunction, which might also contribute to cardiac dysregulation. GTCSs with prolonged PGES (>20 seconds) have been associated with higher sympathetic activation and greater reduction in vagal tone than GTCSs with shorter PGES (Poh et al. 2012). Such decreased vagal modulation has been linked to risk for malignant arrhythmias and sudden cardiac death in nonepilepsy populations and might have the same relation in epilepsy (Molgaard et al. 1991). It is possible that such a mechanism may have been involved in a case of near-SUDEP caused by seizure-induced ventricular tachycardia, which occurred almost simultaneously with the onset of PGES (Espinosa et al. 2009), and in cases of SUDEP and near-SUDEP associated with ventricular tachyarrhythmias (Nei 2009; Ferlisi et al. 2013).

## POSTICTAL GENERALIZED EEG SUPPRESSION AND STIMULATION

Patients with PGES are significantly more likely to be motionless or unresponsive than those without PGES (Tao et al. 2013; Semmelroch et al. 2012). Increased supervision and relatively unskilled intervention (such as airway protection, repositioning, or light tactile stimulation) after a seizure have been postulated to exert a possible protective effect on preventing SUDEP (Langan et al. 2005; Lamberts et al. 2012). If PGES is indeed a marker of severe pulmonary dysfunction, there may be potential for its use in identifying those who will benefit from increased supervision and intervention. Earlier nursing intervention after seizure onset appears to decrease the duration of PGES as well as ictal hypoxemia (Seyal et al. 2013).

## CONCLUSIONS

The significance of PGES and its potential relationship to SUDEP remains uncertain, though several lines of animal and human data suggest that it may be a marker in patients at risk for SUDEP. However, although PGES occurs consistently in EEG-recorded cases of SUDEP, it is also commonly observed after convulsive seizures not resulting in death, especially in adults. PGES may be a marker of global cerebral depression, including deeper subcortical and brain stem structures such as the brain stem reticular formation, which might impair recovery from seizure-induced cardiopulmonary dysfunction (Lado and Moshe 2008; Lhatoo et al. 2010). It is possible that patients with PGES are at a higher risk of postictal autonomic dysfunction and that earlier clinical intervention, such as administration of supplemental oxygen, oropharyngeal suction, and patient repositioning, may reduce the risk for prolonged postictal cardiorespiratory dysfunction, possibly reducing the risk for SUDEP. Clearly, additional large-scale studies are needed to evaluate concurrent physiological parameters (including EEG, respiratory, and cardiac data) during seizures to better understand the clinical significance of PGES and its possible relation to SUDEP.

# REFERENCES

Balestrino M, Somjen GG. Concentration of carbon dioxide, interstitial pH and synaptic transmission in hippocampal formation of the rat. *J Physiol* 1988;396:247–66.

Baraban SC, Hollopeter G, Erickson JC, Schwartzkroin PA, Palmiter RD. Knock-out mice reveal a critical antiepileptic role for neuropeptide Y. *J Neurosci* 1997;17(23):8927–36.

Barraco RA, Janusz CA, Schoener EP, Simpson LL Cardiorespiratory function is altered by picomole injections of 5'-N-ethylcarboxamidoadenosine into the nucleus tractus solitarius of rats. *Brain Res* 1990;507:234–46.

Bateman LM, Li CS, Lin TC, Seyal M. Serotonin reuptake inhibitors are associated with reduced severity of ictal hypoxemia in medically refractory partial epilepsy. *Epilepsia* 2010;51(10): 2211–4.

Bateman LM, Li CS, Seyal M. Ictal hypoxemia in localization-related epilepsy: Analysis of incidence, severity and risk factors. *Brain* 2008;131(Pt 12):3239–45.

Bird JM, Dembny KT, Sandeman D, Butler S. Sudden unexplained death in epilepsy: An intracranially monitored case. *Epilepsia* 1997;38(s11):S52–6.

Blum AS, Ives JR, Goldberger AL, Al-Aweel IC, Krishnamurthy KB, Drislane FW, Schomer DL. Oxygen desaturations triggered by partial seizures: Implications for cardiopulmonary instability in epilepsy. *Epilepsia* 2000;41(5):536–41.

Bozorgi A, Lhatoo SD. Seizures, cerebral shut down, and SUDEP. *Epilepsy Curr* 2013;13(5):236–40.

Deshpande LS, Blair RE, Ziobro JM, Sombati S, Martin BR, DeLorenzo RJ. Endocannabinoids block status epilepticus in cultured hippocampal neurons. *Eur J Pharmacol* 2007; 558(1–3):52–9.

Dragunow M, Goddard GV, Laverty R. Is adenosine an endogenous anticonvulsant? *Epilepsia* 1985;26(5):480–7.

During MJ, Spencer DD. Adenosine: A potential mediator of seizure arrest and post-ictal refractoriness. *Anal Neuro* 1992;32(5):619–24.

Espinosa PS, Lee JW, Tedrow UB, Bromfield E, Dworetzky BA. Sudden unexpected near death in Epilepsy (SUNDEP): Malignant ventricular arrhythmia from a partial seizure. *Neurology* 2009;72:1702–3.

Faingold C. Lecture on Respiration, Seizures and SUDEP-Possible Prevention Approaches. Partners against Mortality in Epilepsy Conference, June 21–24; 2012.

Fano S, Behrens CJ, Heinemann U. Hypoxia suppresses kainate-induced gamma-oscillations in rat hippocampal slices. *Neuroreport* 2007;18(17):1827–31.

Ferlisi M, Tomei R, Carletti M, Moretto G, Zanoni T. Seizure induced ventricular fibrillation: A case of near-SUDEP. *Seizure* 2013;22(3):249–51.

Kim AJ, Kuroda MM, Nordli DR Jr. Abruptly attenuated terminal ictal pattern in pediatrics. *J Clin Neurophysiol.* 2006;23(6):532–50.

Kinney HC, Randall LL, Sleeper LA, Willinger M, Belliveau RA, Zec N, Rava LA et al. Serotonergic brainstem abnormalities in Northern Plains Indians with the sudden infant death syndrome. *J Neuropathol Exp Neurol* 2003;62(11):1178–91.

Lado FA, Moshe SL. How do seizures stop? *Epilepsia* 2008;49(10): 1651–64.

Lamberts RJ, Gaitatzis A, Sander JW, Elger CE, Surges R, Thijs RD. Postictal generalized EEG suppression: An inconsistent finding in people with multiple seizures. *Neurology* 2013; 81(14):1252–6.

Lamberts RJ, Thijs RD, Laffan A, Langan Y, Sander JW. Sudden unexpected death in epilepsy: People with nocturnal seizures may be at highest risk. *Epilepsia* 2012;53(2):253–7.

Langan Y, Nashef L, Sander JWAS. Sudden unexpected death in epilepsy: A series of witnessed deaths. *J Neurol Neurosurg Psychiatry* 2000;68:211–3.

Langan Y, Nashef L, Sander JW. Case-control study of SUDEP. *Neurology* 2005;64(7):1131–3.

Lee MA. EEG video recording of sudden unexpected death in epilepsy. *Epilepsia* 1998;39(Suppl 6):120–121.

Lhatoo SD, Faulkner HJ, Dembny K, Trippick K, Johnson C, Bird JM. An electroclinical case-control study of sudden unexpected death in epilepsy. *Ann Neurol* 2010;68(6):787–96.

McLean BN, Wimalaratna S. Sudden death in epilepsy recorded in ambulatory EEG. *J Neurol Neurosurg Psychiatry* 2007;78(12): 1395–7.

Molgaard H, Sorensen KE, Bjerregaard P. Attenuated 24-h heart rate variability in apparently healthy subjects, subsequently suffering sudden cardiac death. *Clin Auton Res* 1991;1(3): 233–7.

Moseley BD, So E, Wirrell EC, Nelson C, Lee RW, Mandrekar J, Britton JW. Characteristics of postictal generalized EEG suppression in children. *Epilepsy Res* 2013;106(1–2):123–7.

Nashef L, Walker F, Allen P, Sander JW, Shorvon SD, Fish DR. Apnoea and bradycardia during epileptic seizures: Relation to sudden death in epilepsy. *J Neurol Neurosurg Psychiatry* 1996;60(3):297–300.

Nei M. Cardiac effects of seizures. *Epilepsy Curr* 2009;9(4):91–5.

Nei M, Ho RT, Abou-Khalil BW, Drislane FW, Liporace J, Romeo A, Sperling MR. EEG and ECG in sudden unexplained death in epilepsy. *Epilepsia* 2004;45(4):338–45.

Nilsson L, Farahmand BY, Persson PG, Thiblin I, Tomson T. Risk factors for sudden death in epilepsy: A case control study. *Lancet* 1999;353:888–93.

O'Regan ME, Brown JK. Abnormalities in cardiac and respiratory functions observed during seizures in childhood. *Dev Med Child Neurol* 2005;47(1):4–9.

Pavlova M, Singh K, Abdennadher M, Katz ES, Dworetzky BA, White DP, Llewellyn N, Kothare SV. Comparison of cardiorespiratory and EEG abnormalities with seizures in adults and children. *Epilepsy Behav* 2013;29(3):537–41.

Poh MZ, Loddenkemper T, Reinsberger C, Swenson NC, Goyal S, Madsen JR, Picard RW. Autonomic changes with seizures correlate with postictal EEG suppression. *Neurology* 2012;78(23):1868–76.

Semmelroch M, Elwes RD, Lozsadi DA, Nashef L. Retrospective audit of postictal generalized EEG suppression in telemetry. *Epilepsia* 2012; 53:e21–4.

Seyal M, Bateman LM, Albertson TE, Lin TC, Li CS. Respiratory changes with seizures in localization-related epilepsy: Analysis of peri-ictal hypercapnia and airflow patterns. *Epilepsia* 2010; 51(8):1359–64.

Seyal M, Hardin KA, Bateman LM Postictal generalized EEG suppression is linked to seizure-associated respiratory dysfunction but not postictal apnea. *Epilepsia* 2012;53:825–31.

Seyal M, Bateman LM, Li CS. Impact of periictal interventions on respiratory dysfunction, postictal EEG suppression, and postictal immobility. *Epilepsia* 2013;54(2):377–82.

Shen HY, Li T, Boison D. A novel mouse model for sudden unexpected death in epilepsy (SUDEP): Role of impaired adenosine clearance. *Epilepsia* 2010;51(3):465–8.

So EL, Sam MC, Lagerlund TL. Postictal central apnea as a cause of SUDEP: Evidence from near-SUDEP incident. *Epilepsia* 2000;41(11):1494–7.

Sperling MR, Harris A, Nei M, Liporace JD, O'Connor MJ. Mortality after epilepsy surgery. *Epilepsia* 2005;46:49–53.

Surges R, Strzelczyk A, Scott CA, Walker MC, Sander JW. Post-ictal generalized electroencephalographic suppression is associated with generalized seizures. *Epilepsy Behav* 2011; 21(3):271–4.

Swallow RA, Hillier CE, Smith PE. Sudden unexplained death in epilepsy (SUDEP) following previous seizure-related pulmonary oedema: Case report and review of possible preventative treatment. *Seizure* 2002;11(7):446–8.

Tao JX, Qian S, Baldwin M, Chen XJ, Rose S, Ebersole SH, Ebersole JS. SUDEP, suspected positional airway obstruction, and hypoventilation in postictal coma. *Epilepsia* 2010;51(11): 2344–7.

Tao JX, Yung I, Lee A, Rose S, Jacobsen J, Ebersole JS. Tonic phase of generalized convulsive seizure is an independent predictor of postictal generalized EEG suppression. *Epilepsia* 2013;54(5):858–65.

Tavee J, Morris H. Severe postictal laryngospasm as a potential mechanism for sudden unexpected death in epilepsy: A near miss in an EMU. *Epilepsia* 2008;49(12):2113–7.

Thomas T, St Lambert JH, Dashwood MR, Spyer KM. Localization and action of adenosine A2a receptors in regions of the brainstem important in cardiovascular control. *Neuroscience* 2000;95(2):513–8.

Tilz C, Stefan H, Hopfengaertner R, Kerling F, Genow A, Wang-Tilz Y. Influence of levetiracetam on ictal and postictal EEG in patients with partial seizures. *Eur J Neurol* 2006;13(12):1352–8.

Tomson T, Walczak T, Sillanpaa M, Sander JW. Sudden unexpected death in epilepsy: A review of incidence and risk factors. *Epilepsia* 2005;46(Suppl 11):54–61.

Wallace MJ, Martin BR, DeLorenzo RJ. Evidence for a physiological role of endocannabinoids in the modulation of seizure threshold and severity. *Eur J Pharmacol* 2002;452:295–301.

Zappe AC, Uludağ K, Oeltermann A, Uğurbil K, Logothetis NK. The influence of moderate hypercapnia on neural activity in the anesthetized nonhuman primate. *Cereb Cortex* 2008; 18(11):2666–73.

# 31 Mechanisms of SUDEP
## *Lessons from Cases Occurring in the Epilepsy Monitoring Unit*

*Torbjörn Tomson, Lina Nashef, and Philippe Ryvlin*

## CONTENTS

## INTRODUCTION

The mechanisms underlying sudden unexpected death in epilepsy (SUDEP) are unclear and so is our understanding of the final events leading up to SUDEP, although a number of theories have been proposed. These include ictal or postictal respiratory distress, such as central or obstructive apnea or pulmonary edema; ictal cardiac arrhythmias or other ictal or postictal cardiac effects; and ictal cerebral electrical shutdown with generalized electroencephalogram (EEG) suppression (Tomson et al. 2008). A better understanding of the pathophysiology of SUDEP is essential as it can guide the development of preventive strategies as well as effective interventions. Direct observations of SUDEP cases can help us better understand these mechanisms, and the best opportunities for the study of informative cases are those that happen while the patient is in the epilepsy monitoring unit (EMU). This was the incentive for the Mortality in the Epilepsy Monitoring Unit Study (MORTEMUS), which aimed at collecting and reviewing as many cases as possible of cardiorespiratory arrest to identify SUDEP and near-SUDEP cases (Nashef et al. 2012) that have occurred during video-EEG monitoring (Ryvlin et al. 2013). This chapter summarizes the main findings of MORTEMUS.

## MORTEMUS METHODOLOGY

The MORTEMUS had two arms, one to estimate death rates in EMUs and the second to focus on mechanisms of death. To achieve the latter, the study aimed to provide a comprehensive and uniform review of recorded and available data on all SUDEP and near-SUDEP cases from EMUs to gain further insight into mechanisms as well as circumstances around SUDEP. Hence, 5 previously published SUDEP cases were reviewed (Bird et al. 1997; Bateman et al. 2010; Lhatoo et al. 2010; Tao et al. 2010) along with 11 new SUDEP cases identified mainly through a systematic retrospective survey of EMUs in Europe, Israel, Australia, and New Zealand. A further nine near-SUDEP cases, of which three had been reported previously (So et al. 2000; Espinosa et al. 2009; Lanz et al. 2011), were identified and included in the analysis. Available video-EEG and electrocardiogram recordings from all cases were analyzed by a panel (the authors of this chapter) to establish the sequence of events leading to SUDEP or near-SUDEP and the immediate circumstances in which these deaths occurred.

## LESSONS LEARNED

### PATIENT CHARACTERISTICS AND CIRCUMSTANCES SURROUNDING THE EVENT

Of 16 SUDEP and 9 near-SUDEP cases identified as having occurred on an EMU, 11 and 4, respectively, were monitored at the time of cardiorespiratory arrest. All patients who died were adults. Antiepileptic drugs (AEDs) had been reduced by >50% in 12 of the 15 SUDEP cases where such information was available. The same was true for five of the nine near-SUDEP cases. Of the 16 SUDEP cases, 14 occurred at night, corroborating previous observations of nocturnal seizures as a risk factor for SUDEP (Lamberts et al. 2012). Suboptimal supervision during the night could be a contributing explanation for the specific risks associated with nocturnal seizures. Resuscitation was initiated with a delay exceeding 10 minutes from the initially observed apnea in all SUDEP cases. In contrast, resuscitation was started within 3 minutes in all near-SUDEP cases.

Body position was possible to assess from the video recordings in 15 SUDEP cases. The position was found to be prone in 13, in accordance with previous observations of preponderance of the prone position at the time of death

**TABLE 31.1**

**Summary of Key Findings and Conclusions in MORTEMUS**

1. SUDEP was triggered by a GTCS in almost all cases
2. SUDEP preceded by a significant reduction in AED treatment
3. Postictal neurovegetative breakdown with initial rapid breathing replaced followed by transient or terminal cardiorespiratory dysfunction most common sequence of events
4. Prone position in 13 out of 15 SUDEP cases
5. Significant delay in starting resuscitation in most SUDEPs
6. Results highlight need to improve monitoring and supervision including pulse oximetry in EMUs

among SUDEP cases occurring in environments other than the EMU (Kloster and Engelskjøn 1999).

## SEQUENCE OF EVENTS

Every monitored case of SUDEP or near-SUDEP was preceded by a seizure. In all of the 11 monitored SUDEP cases where such information was available, and in all but 2 of the 9 near-SUDEP cases, the event occurred after a generalized tonic-clonic seizure (GTCS). Two of the near-SUDEP cases were triggered by a complex partial seizure. In SUDEP cases, GTCS was followed by an early postictal neurovegetative breakdown (i.e., breakdown of central autonomic control) characterized by initial rapid breathing (18–50 breaths per minute) replaced within 3 minutes by transient or terminal cardiorespiratory dysfunction. Terminal apnea always preceded terminal asystole. Ictal cardiac arrhythmias, occurring as the main cause of cardiorespiratory arrest, were not observed in the SUDEP cases, whereas this was observed in two of the near-SUDEP cases (ictal ventricular fibrillation and ictal asystole, respectively). EEG assessment in the immediate postictal phase was hampered by respiratory artifacts. However, postictal generalized EEG suppression was observed in all monitored SUDEP cases once the EEG was possible to interpret (Table 31.1).

## CONCLUSIONS

In the particular subpopulation of people with refractory epilepsy who are investigated in EMUs, the MORTEMUS has confirmed that SUDEP is triggered by seizures, and in particular GTCS, and revealed that the predominant sequence of events is an early postictal neurovegetative breakdown ending in terminal apnea followed by asystole. Previous reports of witnessed SUDEP cases outside the hospital have also suggested respiratory distress as a frequent and prominent finding. Although we did not find ictal cardiac arrhythmia to be the primary event in any of the monitored SUDEP cases, it cannot be excluded that this could play a role in SUDEP considering the limited number of cases in MORTEMUS. Of note is the delay in resuscitation exceeding 10 minutes from the initially observed apnea in all SUDEP cases, raising the possibility that early resuscitation may be protective in

this setting. The nocturnal preponderance supports the view that nighttime supervision of high-risk patients might reduce SUDEP risk in general. The observations suggest a need for reassessment of safety protocols in EMUs where AED withdrawal might pose additional risk to patients. This should include respiratory monitoring with pulse oximetry. This would enhance patient safety and at the same time facilitate the assessment of the role of respiratory distress in SUDEP.

## REFERENCES

Bateman LM, Spitz M, Seyal M. Ictal hypoventilation contributes to cardiac arrhythmia and SUDEP: Report on two deaths in video-EEG-monitored patients. *Epilepsia* 2010;51:916–20.

Bird JM, Dembny AT, Sandeman D, Butler S. Sudden unexplained death in epilepsy: An intracranially monitored case. *Epilepsia* 1997;38(Suppl 11):S52–6.

Espinosa PS, Lee JW, Tedrow UB, Bromfield EB, Dworetzky BA. Sudden unexpected near death in epilepsy: Malignant arrhythmia from a partial seizure. *Neurology* 2009;72:1702–3.

Kloster R, Engelskjøn T. Sudden unexpected death in epilepsy (SUDEP): A clinical perspective and a search for risk factors. *J Neurol Neurosurg Psychiatry* 1999;67(4):439–44.

Lamberts RJ, Thijs RD, Laffan A, Langan Y, Sander JW. Sudden unexpected death in epilepsy: People with nocturnal seizures may be at highest risk. *Epilepsia* 2012;53:253–7.

Lanz M, Oehl B, Brandt A, Schulze-Bonhage A. seizure induced cardiac asystole in epilepsy patients undergoing video-EEG monitoring. *Seizure* 2011;20:167–72.

Lhatoo SD, Faulkner HJ, Dembny K, Trippick K, Johnson C, Bird JM. An electroclinical case-control study of sudden unexpected death in epilepsy. *Ann Neurol* 2010;68:787–96.

Nashef L, So EL, Ryvlin P, Tomson T. Unifying the definitions of sudden unexpected death in epilepsy. *Epilepsia* 2012;53:227–33.

Ryvlin P, Nashef L, Lhatoo SD, Bateman LM, Bird J, Bleasel A, Boon P. et al. Incidence and mechanisms of cardiorespiratory arrests in epilepsy monitoring units (MORTEMUS): A retrospective study. *Lancet Neurol* 2013;12:966–77.

So EL, Sam MC, Lagerlund TL. Postictal central apnea as a cause of SUDEP: Evidence from near-SUDEP incident. *Epilepsia* 2000;41:1494–7.

Tao JX, Qian S, Baldwin M, Chen XJ, Rose S, Ebersole SH, Ebersole JS. SUDEP, suspected positional airway obstruction, and hypoventilation in postictal coma. *Epilepsia* 2010;51:2344–7.

Tomson T, Nashef L, Ryvlin P. Sudden unexpected death in epilepsy: Current knowledge and future directions. *Lancet Neurol* 2008;7:1021–31.

# 32 Compliance with Antiepileptic Drug Treatment and the Risk of SUDEP

*Torbjörn Tomson*

## CONTENTS

The ultimate goal of all research on sudden unexpected death in epilepsy (SUDEP) is to find methods to reduce its risk, the most devastating consequence of epilepsy. As poorly controlled epilepsy appears to be associated with a particularly high risk of SUDEP (Tomson et al. 2008), and as drug treatment is the mainstay in epilepsy therapy, much attention has been paid to the management of the pharmacotherapy in epilepsy. Among the drug-related risk factors investigated are polytherapy with antiepileptic drugs, use of specific anticonvulsants, and adherence to prescribed antiepileptic drug regimen (Tomson et al. 2008).

Such treatment-related risk factors are of particular interest as they may be amenable to changes that eventually prevent or reduce the risk of SUDEP. Poor compliance with antiepileptic drug treatment has been of special interest as this is a common cause of treatment failure (Cramer et al. 2002) and is manifested in increased frequency of hospitalizations and emergency room admissions (Davis et al. 2008). Poor compliance has frequently been suggested as a risk factor for SUDEP (Téllez-Zenteno et al. 2005; Tomson et al. 2005; Monté et al. 2007). This chapter discusses nonadherence with drug treatment and evidence that it may play a role in SUDEP.

## WHAT IS COMPLIANCE AND NONCOMPLIANCE?

Compliance can be defined as "the extent to which a person's behavior (in terms of medications, following diet, or executing life style changes) coincides with medical or health advice" (Haynes 1979). Even confining the discussion to noncompliance with drug therapy, noncompliance remains a major issue in medicine in general. It has been estimated that half of patients for whom appropriate therapy is prescribed fail to receive full benefit because of inadequate adherence to treatment (Haynes 1979). Epilepsy is no exception. A consensus document published following the First International Workshop on Compliance in Epilepsy (Leppik and Schmidt 1988) suggested that compliance can be categorized into three dimensions: (1) type of behavior (consistent overcompliers, consistent undercompliers, or those who are irregular in behavior), (2) extent of compliance (ranging from those who do not take the medication at all to those who take every dose as prescribed), and (3) whether the patient is intentionally or unintentionally noncompliant. Cramer and collaborators (Cramer et al. 2008) stress the importance of distinguishing between medication compliance and medication persistence; the latter refers to the act of continuing treatment for the prescribed duration.

Depending on methods used, criteria and definitions, and type of population, estimates of noncompliance among epilepsy patients range from 20% to 65% (Leppik 1988; Tomson 1995; Davis et al. 2008). However, as suggested by the consensus document from the workshop, it is better to describe the extent of noncompliance using continuous variables rather than an oversimplified either/or dichotomy.

## HOW CAN COMPLIANCE BE ASSESSED?

Many different methods have been used to assess compliance in different epilepsy populations. These have been grouped into two categories, direct and indirect (Paschal et al. 2008). Direct measures involve determination of drug concentrations in plasma, saliva, and hair, whereas indirect methods utilize manual or electronic pill counts, self-reports, and medication refills. All methods have their merits and limitations, although plasma drug level monitoring is more standard.

## HOW DOES POOR COMPLIANCE RELATE TO THE RISK OF SUDEP?

Nonadherence to the prescribed antiepileptic drug treatment, i.e., noncompliance, has been claimed to be a major cause of treatment failure in epilepsy. Some early small-scale studies have indicated that unreliable drug intake and poor compliance could explain the majority of seizures in selected populations of patients with poor seizure control (Kutt et al. 1966; Cramer and Mattson 1991). A more recent questionnaire-based survey of 670 epilepsy patients in the United States found that 45% of patients reported a seizure after a missed dose (Cramer et al. 2002). Thus, nonadherence to anticonvulsant treatment is associated with poor seizure control. It is therefore reasonable to assume that poor medication compliance also increases the risk of SUDEP as SUDEP in most instances occurs in the context of a seizure (Langan et al. 2000). Poor control of generalized tonic-clonic seizures has also been the strongest and most consistent risk factor in case-control studies (Tomson et al. 2008; Hesdorffer et al. 2012).

In a retrospective cohort study, Faught and colleagues (Faught et al. 2008) used Medicaid claims data to evaluate adherence to treatment in more than 33,000 patients with antiepileptic drug prescriptions. Nonadherence was associated with a more than threefold increase in mortality compared to adherence with a hazard ratio of 3.32 (95% confidence interval, 3.11–3.54). Ridsdale and coworkers (Ridsdale et al. 2011) carried out a nested case-control study utilizing data from the UK General Practice Research Database from 1993 to 2007. In this study, mortality was associated with having collected the last antiepileptic drug prescription 91–182 days previously, rather than within 90 days (odds ratio, 1.72; confidence interval, 1.47–2.01). This late collection of the prescription was interpreted as missed prescription or poor compliance. Unfortunately, both studies analyzed all causes of mortality but not SUDEP specifically.

Noncompliance could theoretically increase the risk of SUDEP through mechanisms other than increasing the risk of seizures. The role of autonomic cardiac control has been much discussed in relation to SUDEP. Decreased heart rate variability is used as a marker of autonomic function and is associated with risk of sudden death in clinical conditions other than epilepsy (Bigger et al. 1993). People with chronic epilepsy have also been shown to have decreased heart rate variability, and it has been speculated that decreased heart

rate variability could be associated with increased risk of cardiac arrhythmias in relation to seizures and thus to SUDEP (Persson et al. 2007).

Two studies have analyzed the effects of rapid withdrawal of antiepileptic drugs on heart rate variability (Kennebäck et al. 1997; Hennessy et al. 2001). In the first study, 10 patients on carbamazepine or phenytoin were studied in conjunction with abrupt drug withdrawal due to adverse effects (Kennebäck et al. 1997). A significant reduction in both time and frequency domains of heart rate variability was observed. In addition, 3 of the 10 patients had a 10-fold increase in ventricular premature beats. The second study noted increased sympathetic activity in sleep when carbamazepine was withdrawn during monitoring for epilepsy surgery workup (Hennessy et al. 2001). Although the antiepileptic drug withdrawal in these studies was planned, it may mimic the situation in noncompliant patients and indicate that cardiac or autonomic effects can follow rapid changes in plasma levels of at least some antiepileptic drugs.

## POSTMORTEM DRUG LEVELS

The notion that poor compliance is a major risk factor for SUDEP largely stems from reports of postmortem concentrations of antiepileptic drugs in SUDEP victims. Subtherapeutic or even undetectable drug levels were frequently found in SUDEP cases from coroners' offices. The results of such studies are presented in Table 32.1. The proportion found to have such low or undetectable drug concentrations ranged from 65% to almost all cases in uncontrolled studies (Terrence et al. 1975; Leestma et al. 1984; Leestma et al. 1989; Earnest et al. 1992; Langan et al. 1998; Ficker et al. 1998; Lear-Kaul et al. 2005, Table 1). However, such results are difficult to interpret. First, postmortem drug concentrations may not be readily comparable to plasma concentrations obtained in live patients. The postmortem analysis is often made on whole blood rather than plasma. Additionally, the concentration of an anticonvulsant may change after death, e.g., by redistribution to other tissues than blood. It has been

## TABLE 32.1

### Studies of Postmortem Concentrations of Antiepileptic Drugs in SUDEP

| Reference | SUDEP Cases (*n*) | Observation Antiepileptic Drug Levels in SUDEP | Controls |
|---|---|---|---|
| Terrence (1975) | 37 | 19/37 Not therapeutic 15/37 undetectable | None |
| Leestma (1984) | 66 | 46/66 Subtherapeutic or undetectable | None |
| Leestma (1989) | 54 | 51/54 Subtherapeutic or undetectable | None |
| Earnest (1992) | 39 | 34/39 Subtherapeutic or undetectable | None |
| Langan (1998) | 6 | 4/6 Subtherapeutic or absent | None |
| Ficker (1998) | 4 | 4/4 Subtherapeutic or absent | None |
| Kloster (1999) | 23 | 13/23 Subtherapeutic | 0/7 Subtherapeutic in non-SUDEP deaths |
| Opeskin (1999) | 44 | 10/44 Subtherapeutic 13/44 undetectable | 13/44 Subtherapeutic 11/44 Undetectable among non-SUDEP deaths |
| George (2000) | 52 | 36/52 Subtherapeutic | 15/44 Subtherapeutic in non-SUDEP deaths |
| Lear-Kaul (2005) | 67 | 51/67 Subtherapeutic or absent | None |

shown that such alterations can substantially reduce phenytoin concentrations after death (Tomson et al. 1998). Similar changes are likely to occur with some other antiepileptic drugs. Second, findings of "subtherapeutic" postmortem plasma concentrations do not necessarily indicate that the patient had been noncompliant or that he or she was undertreated. The often-quoted therapeutic ranges are in general poorly defined for antiepileptic drugs, and it is well established that seizures in a large proportion of patients with epilepsy are well controlled at drug concentrations below these ranges (Patsalos et al. 2008).

A more meaningful interpretation of postmortem drug levels in SUDEP victims, therefore, requires an appropriate control group in addition to taking into account the possible postmortem changes in concentrations. Few studies have included control populations, and the results are somewhat conflicting. In a retrospective study from the United States, George and Davies (1998) examined postmortem antiepileptic drug levels in 52 SUDEP cases and 44 deceased epilepsy controls whose deaths were considered to be unrelated to their epilepsy (ischemic heart disease, accidents including drowning, suicide, and homicide). Antiepileptic drug levels were found to be subtherapeutic in 69% of the SUDEP cases compared to 34% of the control population. Another retrospective study from the National Epilepsy Centre in Norway analyzed postmortem serum concentrations of antiepileptic drugs in 23 SUDEP cases and 7 epilepsy control cases who had died due to other reasons than SUDEP (e.g., pneumonia, cardiac disease, status epilepticus, trauma, suicide, and drowning) (Kloster et al. 1999). Subtherapeutic concentrations were noted in 57% of SUDEP victims compared with none among the non-SUDEP deaths. A third retrospective controlled study analyzed coroner's cases from Australia (Opeskin et al. 1999). There were 44 SUDEP cases and 1 control per SUDEP case. Controls were epilepsy patients who died of causes other than epilepsy (e.g., ischemic heart disease, accidents that could be due to poor seizure control, and suicide). Compared with the controls, the SUDEP cases showed no difference in the number with undetectable or subtherapeutic levels. The number with therapeutic concentrations was the same (21) in both groups.

Hence, while the studies from the United States and Norway found low postmortem antiepileptic drug concentrations to be more common among SUDEP cases than controls, this was not the case in the study from Australia. Differences among the control groups could contribute to these apparently conflicting observations. In this comparison, controls are meant to represent drug concentrations in the average non-SUDEP epilepsy population. However, as the controls are patients who died due to various reasons, it may well be that depending on the cause of death antiepileptic drug levels differ from those of the general epilepsy population. As examples, patients who die in status epilepticus or seizure-related accidents may do so because of low drug levels. Even with the inclusion of a control group, it is difficult to assess the level of compliance with the prescribed treatment regimen using postmortem drug levels.

## OTHER METHODS TO ASSESS NONADHERENCE

The level of adherence to antiepileptic drug treatment in SUDEP cases has been assessed by methods other than measuring postmortem drug levels. In a case-control study from Minnesota, compliance was assessed by anticonvulsant levels at the last visit in 17 SUDEP cases and 67 living epilepsy controls (Walczak et al. 2001). Very few of the cases (6%) and controls (15%) had none of their anticonvulsant levels within the therapeutic range. Levels were therapeutic in 59% of the cases and 40% of the controls. Hence, compliance appeared to be high among SUDEP cases judging from drug levels at the last visit, but this was based on a spot check on one single occasion per patient. Instead, a Swedish case-control study analyzed the within-patient variation in antiepileptic drug plasma concentrations during the last year before death in 57 SUDEP cases or the comparison period in 171 living epilepsy controls (Nilsson et al. 2001). Fluctuations in drug levels over time have been considered to reflect the level of noncompliance (Leppik 1988). No significant association was found between SUDEP risk and degree of within-patient variation in drug levels over time. Thus, none of these studies indicate that noncompliance is more frequent among SUDEP cases than in living epilepsy controls.

Williams et al. (2006) compared concentrations of antiepileptic drugs in hair in 16 SUDEP patients, 9 non-SUDEP epilepsy-related deaths, 31 epilepsy outpatients, and 38 epilepsy inpatients. Drug concentrations were measured in 1-cm hair segments, with 1 cm assumed to represent 1 month's growth. The coefficient of variation of the corrected mean hair concentration was used as the index of variability of antiepileptic drug compliance in an individual. The observed variability of hair concentrations was greater in SUDEP cases than in epilepsy outpatients or inpatients, suggesting more variable antiepileptic drug ingestion over time.

In a controlled prospective study from Australia, compliance was assessed by questionnaires completed by the patients' physicians (Opeskin and Berkovic 2003). Doctors were asked to indicate whether compliance with antiepileptic drug treatment was good or poor, based on detail in medication usage and antemortem drug levels. Poor compliance was not considered to be more common among the 50 SUDEP cases than among the 50 epilepsy controls who died from other causes.

## CONCLUSIONS

The available data on the level of adherence to prescribed anticonvulsant medication among SUDEP cases are conflicting, irrespective of the method used to assess compliance. In particular, there is no consistent evidence from controlled studies that SUDEP victims are less compliant than epilepsy patients in general. However, it is incorrect to conclude from this finding that noncompliance cannot play a role in SUDEP. Medication compliance is likely to improve seizure control and thus probably reduces the risk of SUDEP, although firm evidence is lacking.

# REFERENCES

Bigger JT, Fleiss JL, Rolnitzky LM et al. Frequency domain measures of heart period variability to assess risk late after myocardial infarction. *J Am Coll Cardiol* 1993;21(3):729–36.

Cramer JA, Glassman M, Rienzi V. The relationship between poor medication compliance and seizures. *Epilepsy Behav* 2002; 3(4):338–42.

Cramer JA. Mattson RH. Monitoring compliance with antiepileptic drug therapy. In: Cramer JA, Spilker B, eds. *Patient Compliance in Medical Practice and Clinical Trial*. New York, NY: Raven Press; 1991, pp. 123–27.

Cramer JA, Roy A, Burrell A et al. Medication compliance and persistence: Terminology and definitions. *Value Health* 2008;11:44–7.

Davis KL, Candrilli SD, Edin HM. Prevalence and cost of non-adherence with antiepileptic drugs in an adult managed care population. *Epilepsia* 2008;49:446–54.

Earnest MP, Thomas GE, Eden RA, Hossack KF. The sudden unexplained death syndrome in epilepsy: Demographic, clinical and post-mortem features. *Epilepsia* 1992;33(2):310–6.

Faught E, Duh MS, Weiner JR, Guérin A, Cunnington M. Nonadherence to antiepileptic drugs and increased mortality: Findings from the RANSOM Study. *Neurology* 2008;71(20):1572–8.

Ficker DM, So EL, Annegers JF, O'Brien PC, Cascino GD, Belau PG. Population-based study of the incidence of sudden unexplained death in epilepsy. *Neurology* 1998;51:1270–74.

George JR, Davis GG. Comparison of anti-epileptic drug levels in different cases of sudden death. *J Forensic Sci* 1998;43:598–603.

Haynes, RB. Introduction. In: Haynes RB, Taylor DW, Sacket DL, eds. *Compliance in Health Care*. Baltimore: Johns Hopkins University Press; 1979, pp. 1–7.

Hennessy MJ, Tighe MG, Binnie CD, Nashef L. Sudden withdrawal of carbamazepine increases cardiac sympathetic activity in sleep. *Neurology* 2001;57(9):1650–4.

Hesdorffer DC, Tomson T, Benn E, Sander JW, Nilsson L, Langan Y et al. ILAE Commission on Epidemiology (Subcommission on Mortality). Do antiepileptic drugs or generalized tonic-clonic seizure frequency increase SUDEP risk? A combined analysis. *Epilepsia* 2012;53(2):249–52.

Kennebäck G, Ericson M, Tomson T, Bergfeldt L. Changes in arrhythmia profile and heart rate variability during abrupt withdrawal of antiepileptic drugs. Implications for sudden death. *Seizure* 1997;6:369–75.

Kloster R., Engelskjon T. Sudden unexpected death in epilepsy: A clinical perspective and a search for risk factors. *J Neurol Neurosurg Psychiatry* 1999;67:439–44.

Kutt H, Haynes J, McDowell F. Some causes of ineffectiveness of diphenylhydantoin. *Arch Neurol* 1966;14:489–92.

Langan Y, Nashef L, Sander JW. Sudden unexpected death in epilepsy: A series of witnessed deaths. *J Neurol Neurosurg Psychiatry* 2000;68:211–3.

Langan Y, Nolan N, Hutchinson M. The incidence of sudden unexpected death in epilepsy (SUDEP) in South Dublin and Wicklow. *Seizure* 1998 Oct;7(5):355–8.

Lear-Kaul KC, Coughlin L, Dobersen MJ. Sudden unexpected death in epilepsy, a retrospective study. *Am J Forensic Med Pathol* 2005;26:11–7.

Leestma JE, Kalelkar MB, Teas SS, Jay GW, Hughes JR. Sudden unexpected death associated with seizures: Analysis of 66 cases. *Epilepsia* 1984;25:84–8.

Leestma JE, Walczak T, Hughes JR, Kalelkar MB, Teas SS. A prospective study on sudden unexpected death in epilepsy. *Ann Neurol* 1989;26:195–203.

Leppik IE, Schmidt D. Consensus statement on compliance in epilepsy. In: Schmidt D, Leppik IE, eds. *Compliance in Epilepsy* (*Epilepsy Res* Suppl. 1). Amsterdam, the Netherlands: Elsevier Science Publishers; 1988, pp. 179–82.

Leppik, IE. Variability of phenytoin, carbamazepine, and valproate concentrations in a clinical population. In: Schmidt D, Leppik IE, eds. *Compliance in Epilepsy* (*Epilepsy Res* Suppl. 1). Amsterdam, the Netherlands: Elsevier Science Publishers; 1988, pp. 85–90.

Monté CP, Arends JB, Tan IY, Aldenkamp AP, Limburg M, de Krom MD. Sudden unexpected death in epilepsy patients: Risk factors. A systematic review. *Seizure* 2007;16(1):1–7.

Nilsson L, Bergman U, Diwan VK, Farahmand BY, Persson PG, Tomson T. Antiepileptic drug therapy and its management in sudden unexpected death in epilepsy: A case-control study. *Epilepsia* 2001;42:667–73.

Opeskin K, Berkovic SF. Risk factors for sudden unexpected death in epilepsy: A controlled prospective study based on coroners cases. *Seizure* 2003;12:456–64.

Opeskin K, Burke MP, Cordner SM, Berkovic SF. Comparison of antiepileptic drug levels in sudden unexpected death in epilepsy with death from other causes. *Epilepsia* 1999;40: 1795–8.

Paschal AM, Hawley SR, St Romain T, Ablah E. Measures of adherence to epilepsy treatment: Review of present practices and recommendations for future directions. *Epilepsia* 2008; 49(7):1115–22.

Patsalos PN, Berry DJ, Bourgeois BF et al. Antiepileptic drugs—Best practice guidelines for therapeutic drug monitoring: A position paper by the subcommission on therapeutic drug monitoring, ILAE Commission on Therapeutic Strategies. *Epilepsia* 2008;49(7):1239–76.

Persson H, Kumlien E, EricsonM. Tomson T. Circadian variation in heart-rate variability in localization-related epilepsy. *Epilepsia* 2007;48(5):917–22.

Ridsdale L, Charlton J, Asworth M, Richardson MP, Gulliford MC. Epilepsy mortality and risk factors for death in epilepsy: A population-based study. *Br J Gen Pract* 2011 May;61(586):e271–8.

Téllez-Zenteno JF, Ronquillo LH, Wiebe S. Sudden unexpected death in epilepsy: Evidence-based analysis of incidence and risk factors. *Epilepsy Res* 2005;65:101–15.

Terrence Jr. CF, Wisotzkey HW, Perper JA. Unexpected, unexplained death in epileptic patients. *Neurology* 1975;25:594–8.

Tomson T, Nashef L, Ryvlin P. Sudden unexpected death in epilepsy: Current knowledge and future directions. *Lancet Neurol* 2008;7(11):1021–31.

Tomson T, Skold AC, Holmgen P, Nilsson L, Danielsson B. Postmortem changes in blood concentrations of phenytoin and carbamazepine: An experimental study. *Ther Drug Monit* 1998;20:309–12.

Tomson T, Walczak T, Sillanpää Sander JWAS. Sudden unexpected death in epilepsy: A review of incidence and risk factors. *Epilepsia* 2005;46(S11):54–61.

Tomson T. Non-compliance and intractability of epilepsy. In: Johannessen SI, Gram L, Sillanpää M, Tomson T, eds. *Intractable Epilepsy*. Petersfield, UK: Wrightson Biomedical Publ; 1995, pp. 93–103.

Walczak TS, Leppik IE, D'Amelio M. et al. Incidence and risk factors in sudden unexpected death in epilepsy: A prospective cohort study. *Neurology* 2001;56:519–25.

Williams J, Lawthom C, Dunstan F et al. Variability of antiepileptic medication taking behaviour in sudden unexplained death in epilepsy: Hair analysis at autopsy. *J Neurol Neurosurg Psychiatry* 2006;77:481–4.

# 33 Providing Information about SUDEP
## *The Benefits and Challenges*

*Rosemary Panelli, W. Henry Smithson, and Jane Hanna*

## CONTENTS

## INTRODUCTION

Sudden unexpected death in people with epilepsy was recognized in the early twentieth century (Spratling 1904), along with identified risks and recommendations for its prevention; however, by the 1960s a myth had gained hold in the medical literature that epilepsy was not fatal. "Patients with epilepsy had moved from asylums into the community and there was much less opportunity for observation. Risks from epilepsy were minimized then denied; that seizures could not be fatal became 'common knowledge' despite evidence to the contrary" (Nashef 1995). The development of effective pharmacotherapies gave added reassurance to the community that the condition would be controlled. However, deaths continued to occur and it became clear that there was no medical explanation. In the United Kingdom, bereaved families, shocked by the lack of scientific knowledge, began working to provide mutual support and to seek answers. A charity was formed in 1995 (originally known as Epilepsy Bereaved and now known as SUDEP Action), and the phenomenon defined as sudden unexpected death in epilepsy (SUDEP) rapidly became a specific focus for research and action in clinical practice.

There is much about SUDEP that remains unknown, and this complicates the assessment of risk and communication of advice to patients. The goal of SUDEP information provision is to assist informed patient decision making and to reduce risk, while avoiding any negative impact on quality of life. However, opinions differ on how best to facilitate such outcomes. This chapter explores that challenge and considers options for the timing and method of providing information to patients and families.

## SUDDEN UNEXPECTED DEATH IN EPILEPSY: OUT OF THE SHADOWS

The nature of the scientific uncertainty on SUDEP has changed. Although there is no known cause, research has made significant advances in the understanding of risk factors associated with SUDEP. As a result, SUDEP awareness campaigns have multiplied with international networking as the key to effective use of experience and resources.

The first ever international workshop on SUDEP in 1996 identified the need for comprehensive research (Nashef et al. 1997) and led to a government-funded nationwide audit of epilepsy-related deaths in the United Kingdom. This National Sentinel Clinical Audit of Epilepsy-Related Death (Hanna et al. 2002) found significant problems of access to specialist epilepsy services, reviews, and problems with medication use, concluding that there was significant potential for reduction of death if these risk factors were addressed. The audit motivated policy makers in the United Kingdom to develop government action plans on epilepsy (Department of Health 2003; Welsh Assembly Government 2009) and to develop national clinical guidelines that included SUDEP.

When SUDEP occurs in families who are unaware of the phenomenon, the distress to the bereaved and the wider community is multiplied. A qualitative study found that the bereaved reported positively when the medical team offered condolences, support, and information and negatively when contact was not offered, delayed, or was defensive in nature (Kennelly and Riesel 2002; Bellon et al. 2014). Families were grateful for the offer regardless of whether it was taken up. As a result of this evidence, epilepsy guidelines in the United Kingdom recommend that health professionals contact families to offer their condolences, invite them to discuss the death, and offer referral to bereavement counseling and SUDEP support groups (Kennelly and Riesel 2002; Stokes et al. 2004; Cook 2005).

Community-based SUDEP support services are gradually appearing internationally. The first service was developed in the United Kingdom by the charity Epilepsy Bereaved (www .sudep.org) in 1995, which is known today as SUDEP Action. The service is not dissimilar to the sudden infant death syndrome (SIDS) program (Woodward et al. 1985) and offers bespoke support to the bereaved through a dedicated helpline; collaborative meetings of families, researchers, and clinicians; a biennial memorial service; and information, education, and research services.

In Australia, epilepsy agencies support and link SUDEP families, organize biennial memorial services, and develop resource materials. A SUDEP-related research fund has also been established (www.epilepsyaustralia.net/).

In 2005, Epilepsy Australia and SUDEP Action initiated an international global conversation on SUDEP (www.sudep globalconversation.com) and disseminated an all-encompassing book filled with a combination of scientific research and family stories, which has been used by epilepsy agencies worldwide on SUDEP campaigns (Chapman et al. 2005). In 2010, SUDEP Aware from Canada (Jeffs and Elizabeth 2014) joined the collaboration for a second edition titled *SUDEP–Continuing the Global Conversation* (Chapman et al. 2011). SUDEP Aware provides support for bereaved families and funding for research (www.sudepaware.org/). SUDEP Aware's *Making Sense of SUDEP* information brochures are widely used by epilepsy agencies across North America and Canada.

In 2013, SUDEP Action launched the first online registration of epilepsy deaths (www.epilepsydeathsregister.org), and it is currently working with partner organizations to support register development in other countries using this web platform. Cases can be registered by families and friends, health professionals, or coroners/medical examiners to provide a better understanding of why individuals die and how the deaths are investigated. It will also raise public awareness of SUDEP as well as strengthen the campaign for more effective clinical and coronial epilepsy services.

In France, families have been involved in the French Epilepsy Mortality Surveillance Network, a network of neurologists who systematically report deaths of people with epilepsy and case details, following family consent, to a central registry. This is in parallel with the Mortality in Epilepsy Monitoring Unit Study (MORTEMUS), which collects detailed information about deaths in hospital video-EEG monitoring units across France and worldwide.

Following the first national workshop on SUDEP in the Netherlands during 2013, epilepsy agencies, including bereaved families, are collaborating on a series of initiatives aimed at developing SUDEP awareness and research.

In the United States, bereaved families have supported the development of a SUDEP-targeted research program through CURE (www.cureepilepsy.org/home.asp) and participated in the 2008 SUDEP symposium sponsored by the National

Institute of Health and the National Institute of Neurological Disorders and Stroke (NINDS). Today, in North America federal agencies are providing significant funding opportunities to gain a better understanding of risk factors, mechanisms, and management of individuals who die from SUDEP. Initiatives include the development of a Sudden Death in the Young Registry funded by the National Heart, Lung, and Blood Institute; NINDS; and Center for Disease Control (CDC) (http://www.cdc.gov/sids/CaseRegistry.htm). Recent efforts by organizations such as the Epilepsy Foundation's SUDEP Institute, events such as the Partners Against Mortality in Epilepsy educational conferences (www.aesnet .org/pame/epilepsy currents), and data collection through the North American SUDEP Registry (www.sudep-registry .org) have resulted in increased knowledge and awareness of SUDEP.

## RISK COMMUNICATION: CURRENT PRACTICE

A number of risk factors for SUDEP have been put forward, including suboptimal seizure control, young adult, early onset of epilepsy, absence of treatment or nonadherence to antiepileptic drugs (AEDs), polytherapy, sudden and frequent changes to AEDs, the prone position, being in the bedroom, sleeping, being alone, and being male (Monte et al. 2007; Tomson et al. 2008; Hughes 2009; Shankar et al. 2013). The effect of nocturnal supervision was examined in only one case–control study but was found protective (Langan et al. 2005). Overall, a high frequency of seizures (particularly generalized tonic-clonic seizures) is the strongest risk factor for SUDEP (Hesdorffer et al. 2011). A recent study of deaths in a 9-year study population in Cornwall found that the majority did not have an epilepsy specialist review in the year before death, mirroring the earlier national audit that a significant number of deaths may be in people not engaged with epilepsy services (Shankar et al. 2014). The UK National Sentinel audit identified some 45 individuals who were never referred to secondary care or who died waiting for referral (Hanna et al. 2002).

Despite some contradictory voices, the body of medical opinion has been building that some SUDEP deaths are potentially avoidable (Hanna et al. 2002; Opeskin and Berkovic 2003; So 2006; Hitiris et al. 2007; Monte et al. 2007; Faught et al. 2008; Tomson et al. 2008; Hughes 2009; Surges et al. 2009; So et al. 2009). A report of the American Epilepsy Society and the Epilepsy Foundation Joint Task Force on SUDEP supports the view that certain risk factors associated with SUDEP may be modifiable, namely, uncontrolled seizures, subtherapeutic drug levels, and number of AEDs used. The report supported optimization of seizure control as a treatment goal. It also noted the need to raise awareness of SUDEP in both medical and lay communities (So et al. 2009).

It has been suggested that the precautionary approach of the SIDS risk reduction campaign is a suitable model for SUDEP (So et al. 2009) (Table 33.1). SIDS is a rare event with no one cause identified, yet during the past two decades many

## TABLE 33.1
### Risk Factors and Preventative Strategies

| Risk Factors | Strategies | Comment |
|---|---|---|
| Young age, early onset of epilepsy and IQ | Nonmodifiable | Individual risk assessment information provision |
| Seizure activity (especially GTCS) | Optimal diagnosis, treatment, and review | |
| Long duration of epilepsy | Consider surgery | |
| Polytherapy | Medication review | Patients should use the smallest number of AEDs to control seizures |
| Subtherapeutic levels AED | Medication review and assess adherence | |
| Nocturnal seizures | Nocturnal supervision but no recommendation about seizure detectors | Limited evidence on efficacy of seizure detectors |

*Source:* So, EL et al., *Epilepsia*, 50(4), 917–22, 2009.
*Note:* GTCS, generalized tonic-clonic seizure; IQ refers to Learning Disabilities.

countries around the world have launched successful campaigns informing the public about the risk factors for SIDS (Moon et al. 2007; Ryvlin et al. 2013). A precautionary approach for SUDEP would support prevention strategies based on optimization of seizure control, effective AED treatment, supervision in appropriate cases, and information to patients and caregivers. This precautionary approach is supported by a reasonable body of policy makers (Department of Health 2003; Stokes et al. 2004; Welsh Assembly Government 2009) and expert opinion in North America (Institute of Medicine 2012).

For more than 10 years, clinical guidelines in Scotland and those produced by the National Institute of Health and Clinical Excellence (NICE) for England and Wales have recommended discussion of SUDEP as part of general epilepsy information (Scottish Intercollegiate Guidelines Network 2003; Stokes et al. 2004). The NICE guideline sets out information to show why preventing seizures is important. It is based on the view that SUDEP risk can be minimized by optimizing seizure control and by families being aware of the potential consequences of nocturnal seizures. It also recommends tailored information on the individual's risk of SUDEP as part of any counseling checklist for people with epilepsy, and their families and/or caregivers. This advice is also given by the American Epilepsy Society, which recommends disclosure but, in keeping with the Scottish and English guidance, does not give specific advice about how and when SUDEP should be discussed and by whom (Vegni et al. 2011; Mendonça et al. 2011).

The first survey of clinical practice related to risk communication and SUDEP asked neurologists in the United Kingdom if they told patients about SUDEP (Morton et al. 2006). The neurologists who replied reported a wide variation in practice. Whereas 30.3% of respondents reported that they discussed SUDEP with the majority or all of their patients, 68.7% discussed the issue with very few or none of their patients. Interestingly, clinicians with a special interest in epilepsy were significantly more likely to discuss SUDEP. A more recent hospital audit in Scotland of documented SUDEP discussion found that routine discussion was noted in only 4% of cases (Waddell et al. 2013).

A survey of Italian epileptologists reported similar findings. The survey found that physicians reported a wide variation of practice, with 28% discussing SUDEP with all or the majority of their patients and 62% discussing SUDEP with only a few (Vegni et al. 2011). This lack of consensus has been explored in the United States using a focus group study of neurologists, epileptologists, and advanced practice nurses (Miller et al. 2014). The findings mirrored the U.K. experience. Disclosure was supported by all professional groups, driven by practical and moral accountability to ensure that patients and families had accurate information on which to form their decisions about epilepsy. However, there was also a moral concern not to cause fear in patients by giving this information and all groups expressed a wish for standardized information delivery.

Specialist nurses have been shown to be more likely than clinicians to discuss SUDEP. A survey in the United Kingdom found that 56% of specialist nurses discussed SUDEP with the majority of their patients. Most combined SUDEP with discussion of general and specific risks of epilepsy (Lewis et al. 2008). No specialist nurse supported nondisclosure.

Research with parents in Wales found that 52% were aware of SUDEP. Only 16% of patients had been informed by a healthcare professional, with 70% reporting that they found the information via alternative sources. It concluded that parents of children with epilepsy should receive tailored information about SUDEP as this could help minimize risk factors and help reassure the parents. It also concluded that providing parents with tailored information could prevent the use of less reliable information sources (Jones and Naude 2013).

## ETHICAL AND LEGAL ARGUMENTS FOR DISCLOSURE

The main arguments for disclosure are that it supports patient autonomy, informs choices on adherence and self-management, reduces fear by managing natural anxieties, and avoids the harm of false assurance. Research repeatedly tells us that people with epilepsy feel they receive insufficient information about their condition (Couldridge et al. 2001). A qualitative study found that patients felt a pressing need for information, including "… more concrete answers on SUDEP" to discuss treatment options and medication in detail (Prinjha et al. 2005). This suggests that clinicians need to check regularly with patients how much information they would like about their condition. The perspective of caregivers is also a consideration. Research shows that patient decision making involves an extended social context (Fraenkel and McGraw 2007); however, in any event caregivers may need accurate information in their own right. Families affected by SUDEP described a variety of roles associated with care such as keeping records of seizures and responding to seizures. Many considered that they needed more information on SUDEP as it pertains to these roles (Kennelly and Riesel 2002). One study found that parents expected this (Gayatri et al. 2010). Research in Canada that included parents of children with epilepsy and families who had lost children found that all participants wanted information about SUDEP and generally wanted this early at the time of diagnosis. Knowing the actual risk of SUDEP was relieving especially to the parents who overestimated the risk (Ramachandran Nair et al. 2013).

The ethical principle of patient autonomy involves the patient's right to know about their own medical condition and prognosis. The American Epilepsy Society and the Epilepsy Foundation Joint Task Force on SUDEP considered discussion of SUDEP consistent with the ethical principles of patient autonomy and consistent with the need to accept that some persons with epilepsy have increased risks of morbidity and death (So et al. 2009). Examples of professional guidance based on the autonomy principle fully support the patient's right to information about his or her condition. The amount of information given on a condition should depend on the patient's wishes and need for information. This should be determined by discussion with a patient and not be based on assumptions of what patients require (General Medical Council 2008). Provision of information is also important to the relationship of trust between doctor and patient. Where information on risks is withheld and risks later materialize, it is natural that those affected by the consequences will seek to understand why information was not shared. They may experience the harm of false assurance. There is some limited evidence on the negative impact of false assurance in the context of medical screening, including public confidence and legal action (Petticrew et al. 2001); however, the impact of most seizures being presented as benign (apart from accidents and status epilepticus) has not been researched. Relatives bereaved through SUDEP frequently report, however, that their grief is exacerbated because epilepsy was presented in this way and it proved to be false (Kennelly and Riesel 2002). Further, the relationship of trust between the bereaved and the medical professional is more likely to be maintained where information withholding is patient centered and withstands scrutiny.

A common assumption is that discussing the risk of SUDEP will create anxieties. The only research on epilepsy and death anxiety comprises studies looking at the death anxiety associated with epilepsy generally. A study of 373 epilepsy patients found that approximately two-thirds harbored fears of death from their next seizure (Mittan 1986). In a more recent cross-sectional study of 92 patients having epilepsy for a minimum of 5 years, 56.52% of patients had either moderate or high death anxiety (Otoom et al. 2007). Not surprisingly, death anxiety was likely to be higher in patients with generalized epilepsy. Otoom et al. (2007) emphasize the importance of counseling patients to reduce anxiety. Anecdotal reports from clinicians who regularly talk about SUDEP mention the potential for reduction of fear by putting fears into perspective. Indeed, there is some evidence to support this logic. A case–control study on the benefits of a weekend educational program (SEE, known then as the Sepulveda Epilepsy Education program but known more recently as Seizures and Epilepsy Education), which included discussion of risk of mortality, found subsequent decrease in anxiety (Helgeson et al. 1990). The experience of this program was that lack of discussion of mortality led to adverse suppression of natural anxiety. Fear was also associated with overprotection and overcontrol of the person with epilepsy (Mittan 2005).

SUDEP is now in the public domain, and use of the Internet to access health information is common (Fox and Duggan 2013). Not all websites provide clear and accurate information, and there is the potential for anxiety founded on inappropriate advice (Jones and Naude 2013; Tonsaker et al. 2014). In addition, patients who discover SUDEP themselves may be disappointed or angry that their doctor did not discuss it. Trust between patient and physician may be so damaged that any future attempts to put the issue in context may no longer be well received or followed. Personal discussion with their own doctor is the best way for people to hear about, and appraise, their own unique epilepsy-related risk. Frank discussion can build trust in the therapeutic relationship.

A legal duty to discuss a risk prima facie arises where there is a significant risk that would affect the judgment of the reasonable patient (*Bolitho v. City and Hackney Health Authority* 1998; *Pearce v. United Bristol Healthcare NHS Trust* 1999). Risks that are only remote possibilities can be regarded as material if the severity of the risk materializing is very serious. In the context of a SUDEP, it could be argued that there is a material risk to be addressed where discussion might influence behavior, improve compliance, or be relevant to issues of supervision or where optimum treatment is not in place (Beran et al. 2004). The courts in many countries will test the medical evidence offered by parties in litigation to reach their own conclusions on the magnitude and severity of risk, and the ease by which the risk might be avoided (*Videto v. Kennedy* 1981; *Rogers v. Whitaker* 1992; *Bolitho v. City and Hackney Health Authority* 1998). The existence of guidelines, although not predictive of negligence, would be a relevant consideration in examining the rationality of withholding information. It has been argued that a claim would fail in a SUDEP case because of the need to prove causation between the actions of the physician and the death (Beran 2006). However, the more recent authority of *Chester v. Afshar* (2005) has extended the law of causation to include the scenario in which risk is inherent in a condition and not caused by medical intervention. This would be a helpful legal authority in a SUDEP case. There are also two Scottish judicial determinations (Taylor 2002; Duff 2011) as well as recorded cases of out-of-court settlements and related judicial proceedings in the United States, all of which support the need for disclosure (Wannamaker 2011).

The Scottish determinations were the outcome of Fatal Accident Inquiries. This type of inquiry is held in Scotland by a judicial officer called a sheriff where a death concerns public interest. The purpose is to make recommendations to prevent future deaths. In the case of Collette Findlay, the deceased's mother had died from epilepsy in 1988. The deceased presented with seizures in 1991. The family was reassured that she suffered from benign focal seizures of childhood and she was discharged by the specialist to general practice on AEDs. Beginning in1991, she had four to five seizures yearly; varying in frequency and severity, but there was no annual review or rereferral for specialist care. The court found a catalog of failures to look after the deceased in a proper manner. These included a failure on the part of specialists to alert the general practitioner as to what circumstances required rereferral; a failure on the part of the general practice to prescribe appropriate levels of medication; a failure to rerefer the deceased when the seizures did not stop after 2 years; a failure to rerefer the deceased when the intensity, form, and duration of her seizures altered as the deceased matured; and a failure by the medical team to discuss with the deceased's family the diagnosis, the attendant risks, and how these risks might be properly managed. The sheriff stated that given the association between seizures and SUDEP and the potential for control it was a "short step" to the view that if the deceased had been referred for review she might not have died. He determined that the family ought to have been informed that the deceased was

suffering from epilepsy, the risks of SUDEP explained, and a discussion held on how her condition might be managed. The most important recommendation was considered to be the need for a personal care plan. The sheriff suggested that all the key issues would have been addressed if a care plan, "… shared or otherwise" had been produced, and "… it might have saved her life" (Taylor 2002). The sheriff was clear that for the purposes of the public inquiry it was not necessary for there to be any scientific certainty. Any legal judgment is determined by balance of probabilities, and in this case the concern was whether preventative measures "might" have saved a life. The sheriff was clear that information on SUDEP could be relevant to how proactive a family might be in probing decisions about treatment as well as informing discussions on how risks might be reduced. The sheriff accepted that the question of informing about SUDEP must be left to the discretion of the medical profession to form a view. In particular, he accepted that there might be people of "an extreme disposition" where discussion might cause harm. Nevertheless, he said, "I do, however, accept that in the vast majority of cases there should be such a discussion" (Taylor 2002).

Nine years later, a second Fatal Accident Inquiry was convened to investigate the deaths of two young women with epilepsy (Erin Casey and Christina Ilia), taking evidence from 29 witnesses over 30 days (Duff 2011). It concluded that SUDEP is normally associated with a seizure; the risk of SUDEP occurring is reduced if the frequency of seizures is reduced; the frequency and incidence of seizures can be reduced by a number of factors, some related to lifestyle but the most important related to adherence to antiepileptic medication; and if a seizure occurs intervention by another person might prevent SUDEP from taking place (Table 33.2).

The inquiry into the death of Erin Casey focused on the relationship between communication of risk and medicines management. Erin had been considered at low risk of

## TABLE 33.2
### Recommendations from the Fatal Accident Inquiry Scotland 2011

| | |
|---|---|
| Clinicians | The vast majority of patients with epilepsy, or their parents or carers where appropriate, should be advised on SUDEP on first diagnosis or shortly thereafter. |
| | A decision may be made not to inform or to delay informing where there is an assessment that there is a risk of serious harm to a particular patient from the information or that the person lacks capacity. The decision should be recorded. |
| | Consideration should be given of support needs of patients on diagnosis and in managing medicines especially where the medication regime is complex. Consideration should be given to monitoring the uptake of repeat prescriptions. |
| | A letter should be sent to the patient and any referring general physician summarizing any consultation and treatment decisions. |
| | Written information should be reviewed to check if it is adequate. |
| Health services | Consider the adequacy of existing guidelines including clarifying the status of guidelines. |
| | Consider training needs to include communication with particular emphasis on supporting teenagers or young adults moving toward independence, engaging in risky activities, or beginning to take responsibility for them. |
| Investigation of death | Review practice in relation to the scene of death of a sudden unexpected death and the practice of, ab initio, describing it as a "crime scene." |

*Source:* Duff, AJM, Determination of Sheriff Alistair Duff, Sheriff of Tayside Central and Fife at Dundee. Inquiry held under the Fatal Accidents and Sudden Death Inquiry (Scotland) Act 1976 into the deaths of Erin Casey and Christina Fiorre Ilia, at http://www.scotcourts.gov.uk/opinions/2011FAI40.html, 2011.

SUDEP, was considered compliant with medication, and was not informed about her risk. There was no medical record of nonadherence, but evidence at the inquiry was presented that Erin was not picking up her prescriptions and not taking her medication as prescribed.

> Had Erin been referred to an epilepsy specialist nurse service (had one existed in Fife) there is, in my view, a real possibility that she would have been provided with more advice and information, informed about the risk of SUDEP and that her seizure frequency and compliance with medication would have been monitored. She might have complied better with taking her medication. Seizures might have been eliminated. She might not have succumbed to SUDEP (Duff 2011).

Both judicial determinations from Scotland recommend that SUDEP should be discussed early on with the vast majority of patients. The judges recognized the importance of clinical discretion to withhold discussion, but the most recent determination recommends that the reason for withholding, such as serious harm to the patient or incapacity, should be recorded (Duff 2011). It is worth noting, however, that no actions for negligence have yet been reported in cases involving SUDEP deaths and, instead, systems for investigation in public interest have been activated by some families affected by SUDEP. The two aforementioned Scottish cases both led to changes in service provision. Following the 2002 Fatal Accident Inquiry, an epilepsy clinic to review patients with epilepsy was established by the general practice and the 2009 Ombudsman's Report makes reference to the creation of a new epilepsy specialist nurse post.

## ARGUMENTS FOR NONDISCLOSURE

The main arguments against disclosure are that (1) telling patients will cause anxiety for no benefit, (2) there is no research on patient wishes in this area and that patients may not want to hear about SUDEP, and (3) a clinician may be successfully sued for denying a patient "the right not to know" the risks associated with a condition.

It is understood that patients vary in personality and coping styles and therefore in their attitude to information and how they use it to navigate health issues (Andrewes et al. 1999; Politi et al. 2007). Some may not want to be involved in aspects of discussion or decision making with their healthcare providers. In the SUDEP debate, those who argue for the right not to know highlight differing patient-information-seeking behavior such as active searching (seekers), conscious blocking (avoiders), and a combination of styles (weavers) (Morton et al. 2006; Pinder 1990), expressing concern that where broad requirements to discuss SUDEP with all patients are mandatory preference is therefore given to the needs of seekers above all others.

But this need not be so. Where guidelines do exist, there are options for variation. Patients' wishes are clearly highlighted in ethical literature on information giving, and clinical guidelines are always recognized as being subject to clinical discretion where there is good reason not to follow a guideline. The General Medical Council (2008) advises

doctors to provide patients with appropriate information, which should include an explanation of any risks to which they may attach significance. Doctors must not make assumptions about a patient's understanding of risk or the importance they attach to different outcomes. They should discuss these issues with their patient. A clinician who probed patient wishes on information provision would have good reason not to inform if the patients indicated that they did not want to have full information including risks of seizures; if the issue was regularly revisited; and if there was no material reason to override this, such as nonadherence to treatment. Pinder (1990) investigated information provision using Parkinson's disease as the case study. She found that clinical practice on information giving was rarely determined by an accurate assessment of what the patient wanted, but it was largely dictated by clinician's assumptions as to what patients did or did not want to know. Clinicians were broadly divided into three groups of information-giving style: Closed, open, or changing. Pinder concluded that identifying patient wishes necessitates proactive engagement by a clinician to discover what the patient wants to know, and ought to know, about their condition and its treatment. However, the medical literature suggests that many clinicians have taken specific positions on when to discuss SUDEP, such as only if a patient asks, at the time of prescribing AEDs, or only in cases with (Pinder 1990) recognized risk factors (Morton et al. 2006).

Outside the epilepsy field, there is some evidence in the literature from which to draw, including a systematic review and a meta-analysis that provide some general indication of the relationship between bad news and anxiety. The evidence suggests that anxiety is a common and adaptive initial response to an "at risk" notification, but it usually dissipates within a month (Shaw et al. 1999; Marteau 2008). Psychological theories of self-regulation describe the ways that humans maintain equilibrium while responding to threat (Taylor 1991). Clearly, fear unchecked can become negative and restrictive, but natural anxiety should not be assumed as harmful.

Some authors contributing to the SUDEP debate have put forward the argument for a patient's right not to know (Beran 2006; Black 2005), even suggesting that in some circumstances clinicians could be sued if they tell patients about SUDEP (Beran et al. 2004). Although therapeutic privilege provides a defense to the legal right to know where there is good reason that discussing SUDEP with a patient will cause harm, the concept of a legal right not to know, although recently mooted in the context of routine HIV testing and genetics, is not one that has rooted yet in any established legal concept or legal authority.

A therapeutic privilege exists in medical care to withhold information where it would cause harm to the patient. This concept is recognized by medical law as a defense to a legal action based on failure to disclose a material risk. Therapeutic privilege is normally confined to a psychiatric setting. What is clear from professional guidance and legal precedents is that therapeutic privilege does not mean unfettered discretion to decide one way or another, but instead it is conditional on a process of rational decision making. The General Medical

Council (2008) of the United Kingdom, for example, states that such information should not be withheld and that it is necessary for making decisions unless the clinician believes the patient would be caused serious harm beyond being upset or refusing treatment. Any decision to withhold information should be recorded, justified, and reviewed. The concern about the harm of raising patient anxiety is discussed regularly in the medical literature on SUDEP as the reason for not providing information. Temporary anxiety in a patient is not normally viewed by the courts or ethical bodies as being sufficient to constitute sensible medical grounds for withholding information (*Deriche v. Easling Hospital NHS Trust* 2003). The only epilepsy-related research on this subject is a survey of neurologists, some of whom report anxiety (Morton et al. 2006). One-third of respondents thought that information about SUDEP caused anxiety; but they were not asked how they assessed this, whether they followed up to check if anxieties were lasting and whether the patient was offered or responded well to further information and support. Interestingly, doctors who discussed SUDEP with the majority of their patients were less likely to report negative reactions, suggesting, as the author recognized, a practice effect. The lack of evidence on patient harm from discussion of SUDEP was highlighted in the recent Scottish investigation. The Scottish Public Services Ombudsman (2009) declared that "much of the evidence in this area is … at best anecdotal and any reliance on an assumption about patients' reactions must be tempered by the lack of actual hard evidence."

## SUDEP INFORMATION: WHEN AND HOW?

Epilepsy is a burden on all patients, with varied risks and impact depending on the type and control of the condition, associated comorbidity, and how each person manages their unique circumstances and treatment. The impact can be lessened, and it is now recommended practice to give advice tailored to the individual context (Stokes et al. 2004; Miller et al. 2014).

Where the decision is made to inform patients about SUDEP, the timing and method of communication continue to be points of debate with little standardization of approach and few recommendations. The question may arise in a consultation if the patient initiates the discussion, if the professional initiates the discussion, or if the consultation addresses potentially risky behavior such as poor adherence to treatment.

Should the question be answered if the patient asks? The literature on this question supports disclosure should a patient ask a question relevant to SUDEP (Beran et al. 2004; Black 2005; Morton et al. 2006; Brodie and Holmes 2008; So et al. 2009; Miller et al. 2014). However, this approach clearly places the onus of asking on patients, who may not know which questions to frame. Consequently, disclosure is likely to be restricted to those individuals who are already well informed and confident enough to seek information.

Should the question be addressed only in patients at high risk for SUDEP? It is generally agreed that SUDEP information should be provided to high-risk groups, such as those with poorly controlled seizures, allowing them the opportunity to participate in risk assessment (So 2006; Tomson et al. 2008; Brodie and Holmes 2008). This may include screening for cardiac interventions and discussion of options for supervision (Tomson et al. 2008, 2009; Finsterer and Stollberger 2009). Where patients have epilepsy and learning difficulties, professional guidelines recommend that health professionals be aware of the higher mortality risks and discuss these with the individuals affected, and their families and/or caregivers (Stokes et al. 2004). For people with newly diagnosed or mild epilepsy, the risk may be lower, but SUDEP deaths do occur in this group as noted by the Scottish Fatal Accident Inquiries (Taylor 2002; Duff 2011). Nevertheless, the assumption has prevailed that SUDEP is a risk for only those with intractable epilepsy (Tomson et al. 2008), which, to some extent, ignores "… the larger group of individuals with better but not fully controlled epilepsy who have a lower, but nevertheless real, risk of SUDEP" (Tomson et al. 2008). In the clinical audit of epilepsy-related death in the United Kingdom, a number of SUDEP cases were recorded in patients having only rare seizures. Looking at 158 adult patients who had attended specialist care, 5% were known to have had less than one seizure per year, 3% were people noted to have had a single seizure or the first in many years, and 4% were people considered to be seizure free. It was noted that 25% of the deaths were in people whose records did not record the frequency of seizures, and 22% were in people where the records were not clear. Six percent of the patients who died were not treated with AEDs (Hanna et al. 2002).

There is general agreement that SUDEP discussion should take place if circumstances warrant this. This is particularly important with the nonadherent patient (Black 2005; Morton et al. 2006; So et al. 2009; Miller et al. 2014). The challenge is timely identification of nonadherence. Research in other chronic conditions has shown that it is often difficult for a doctor to know who will comply with treatments as prescribed and why (Wertheimer and Santella 2003; Horne 2006). Further, during the consultation patients often overestimate adherence so as not to disappoint (Horne 2006). Waiting until the patient is known to be nonadherent may be too late, or it may be impossible to change their behavior.

The report of the Fatal Accident Inquiry into the death of Erin Casey is illustrative as the clinical team considered Erin low risk and adherent to treatment. The judge found that Erin, who died only 7 months following diagnosis, did not find her medication straightforward and without any support or effective monitoring was not in fact taking it as prescribed or indeed picking up her repeat prescriptions. She did not give any indication in appointments that she was failing to adhere to her medication regime but did express concerns about tiredness and weight gain and interaction with the contraceptive pill leading to a reduction in dose. The judge concluded there was a real possibility that had Erin been told about the risk of SUDEP she would have managed her condition differently. He recommended that the vast majority of people with epilepsy should be advised of the risk of SUDEP on or shortly after diagnosis unless a particular patient is judged to be at risk of serious harm by the provision of such information.

It may underline the need to comply with the regime of medication and it may reinforce the merit in adopting modes of lifestyle which could reduce the risk of seizure and therefore of succumbing to SUDEP. Finally it would give the clinician, the patient and their family the opportunity to consider issues of night supervision, the use of seizure alarms and the practice of resuscitation techniques all of which, on the evidence which I accepted, might reduce the risk of SUDEP (Duff 2011).

With evidence that maintenance of a stable AED regimen might reduce risk, it would be timely for discussion about risks and benefits of treatment to include the small risk of fatality from a seizure (Cook 2005; Faught et al. 2008; Tomson et al. 2008; Hughes 2009). In the words of a person with epilepsy, "for many, the decision to take medication is a huge one. If they are not aware of the dangers of seizures as well as the side-effects of medication I do not feel that their decisions are truly informed" (Kearton 2005).

## ADHERENCE, SELF-MANAGEMENT, AND SHARED DECISIONS

Nonadherence to prescribed medication regimens in epilepsy is associated with a more than threefold increased risk of mortality (Faught et al. 2008). However, the issue of adherence is not straightforward (Wertheimer and Santella 2003; Horne 2006; Chapman et al. 2014). When attempting to address this problem, it must be remembered that nonadherence is a variable and dynamic behavior and patients may not necessarily be consistently adherent or not adherent.

A guideline for the United Kingdom on shared decision making and medicines adherence suggests that medicine taking is "… a complex human behaviour …" and that unwanted and unused medicines "… reflect inadequate communication between professionals and patients …" (Nunes et al. 2009). Health professionals working with epilepsy patients recognize the complexities of risk communication and adherence reflected in a recurring troubling scenario, aspects of which are reflected in the stories of David, Celine, and Peter presented in *Sudden Unexpected Death in Epilepsy: A Global Conversation* (Chapman et al. 2005). A young person dies, and discussions with family and friends reveal the picture of a vibrant individual who did not want to have epilepsy. Seizures were embarrassing and a nuisance, but they believed coping well meant not to fuss and friends were told not to worry. It appears that their doctors may have considered them to be well controlled, adherent, and adequately informed patients. However, these patients and their families did not realize that epilepsy could be fatal and the bereaved families often indicate that adherence was likely to have been spasmodic. Frequently, bereaved families believe that the young adults would have handled their epilepsy differently if they had really understood the risks of their condition, and this possibility continues to haunt them. Driving, employment, and the adverse effects of medication are all issues for young people to navigate. They balance their lives with their epilepsy as they believe best. However, some coping and self-management styles, while apparently successful, if not adequately informed, may in fact lead to vulnerability.

Self-management of epilepsy (how people live with the condition) is a complex activity that can be measured by exploring various domains including control of seizures, provision and use of information, use of medicines, staying safe, and lifestyle (Dilorio et al. 1994). A study of adherence and self-management showed an association between nonadherence and low self-management scores. Patients at risk through low self-management scores were those people in employment, those living with others, and those with a high level of education (Smithson et al. 2012).

Research across chronic conditions has consistently found that lack of adherence is associated with patients' doubts about their need for medication and concerns about side effects (Horne 2006). Patients with asthma, for example, were significantly more likely to endorse the need for regular medication if they shared the "medical view" of asthma as an "acute or chronic condition" with potentially serious consequences. If, on the other hand, patients saw their condition as chronic only, they were more likely to doubt the need for regular medication. The implications for asthma treatment were that it is not sufficient to advise a patient to take medication but that a clear rationale is needed. A medicines Necessity Concerns Framework has been developed, and this postulates that adherence to treatments is the interplay between patients' belief in their personal need for treatment and their concerns about potential adverse consequences of treatment. Nonadherence is increased when patients express high concerns and low necessity (Horne et al. 2013). This framework was applied to a population with epilepsy, and it has been shown that people with strong concerns about AEDs were more likely to be nonadherent (Chapman et al. 2014).

Behavioral theory might help explain why patients who have a mind-set that seizures are benign may make poor decisions regarding the management of their condition because they are missing important information (Austin 2011). The severity of any potential harm is recognized as a key influence on health behavior and decision making (Weinstein 1999). If patients and caregivers do not appreciate that avoidance of fatality is one reason for treatment, it raises the question of whether this lack of information is significant to patient decisions about adherence and self-management. In people with epilepsy, there is some evidence that a discussion of the risks of the condition (including SUDEP) by specialist nurses can improve adherence (Lewis 2008) and that missed prescriptions are a risk factor in epilepsy death (Ridsdale et al. 2011). The risk of death following a seizure might be significant to some patients in balancing the risks and benefits of their behavior.

Some information on epilepsy routinely imparted to patients may create major disincentives for engagement with treatment. The concern over possible loss of a driver's license, or unpleasant side effects, for example, may inhibit reporting of seizures or attendance at appointments. It is logical to fully inform patients about risks soon after diagnosis when there is possibly the greatest potential to communicate the imperative of aiming for seizure freedom through appropriate treatment and lifestyle choices. As time passes, if few seizures are experienced with no apparent harmful effects, there is the potential for patients to become blasé about seizures and more concerned about the daily inconvenience of treatment and lifestyle adaptation.

Whether an individual patient is perceived to be at high or low risk for SUDEP, his or her behavior cannot be predicted. Private decisions take place outside the consulting room. Life changes occur, and people with epilepsy will make decisions based on the framework of knowledge that they have been given, with some choices leading to fatal outcomes. For example, when a young woman unexpectedly becomes pregnant she may decide to stop her epilepsy medication without consulting any doctor. National investigations of maternal deaths consistently raise concerns that many pregnant women with epilepsy are concerned about the side effects of medication, and there are a steady number of women who die each year that appear to have stopped medication, with and without the knowledge of their medical team. The importance of preconception counseling for women with epilepsy of childbearing age is a key recommendation of the report into all maternal deaths released in the United Kingdom (Lewis 2007). Because not all pregnancies are planned, it is imperative that such information must be given at the first opportunity, with frank two-way communication underpinning true physician–patient concordance (Horne 2006) and hopefully engendering informed patient adherence.

In the United Kingdom, detailed professional guidance has been developed to mark the shift toward patients and doctors making decisions together and reflects exchange of information between patients and doctors as being central to decision making (Nunes et al. 2009). This should include information on diagnosis, prognosis, and uncertainties, plus information on the potential benefits, risks, and burdens of treatment and of not treating (General Medical Council 2008).

Focusing on comprehensive epilepsy education as the framework for SUDEP discussions is a positive recommendation (So 2009), although models and evaluation of such programs have been limited (Institute of Medicine 2012). Fortunately, in recent years the Managing Epilepsy Well network of the CDC (http://www.cdc.gov/epilepsy/) in the United States has begun to provide leadership in the development and testing of innovative self-management programs.

## CONCLUSION

The cause of SUDEP is yet to be discovered; however, the identification of certain risk factors now provides a platform for preventative action. Strong campaigns by community-based epilepsy organizations have increased awareness of epilepsy-related risk in people with epilepsy, the broader community, health and forensic professionals, and policy makers. Guidelines in some countries now address the need for improved patient education regarding risk management as well as high-quality medical management. Unfortunately, many countries are yet to be influenced by these developments, so the future goal must be the development of global strategies through international networking. Scientific research into SUDEP is increasing, and the establishment of international epilepsy-related death registers will gradually bring together important data to assist in demystifying this tragic phenomenon.

For many years, there has been reluctance by some health professionals to talk openly about SUDEP. However, the weight of opinion is shifting to full disclosure. A call for openness on SUDEP, encouraging early discussion of risk, was backed by an international expert panel and 14 international epilepsy organizations at the 30th International Epilepsy Congress in Montreal during 2013 (www.sudep.org/article/sudepactionleadscallforopenness2013).

In response to calls for disclosure and discussion, many health professionals are unsure of how to respond. This suggests that the philosophy of self-management and informed decision making have not been universally adopted into epilepsy care. If this framework was in place, it would be a short and self-evident step to include SUDEP in usual risk communication. Consequently, the SUDEP debate has injected some urgency into the discussion on how epilepsy education generally should take place, something which is long overdue (Prinjha et al. 2005).

Risk assessment and communication should not stand alone from the general epilepsy information that is integral to patient decision making. We would therefore endorse the vision for optimal education in epilepsy as a foundation for patient self-management recently put forward by the Institute of Medicine.

> People who are informed, supported and actively engaged in productive interactions with "prepared, proactive, practice teams" (Wagner et al. 2005) should be at the center of a health care system that is designed to provide access to high-quality epilepsy care. To be consistent with this broad framework for the delivery of health care, appropriate educational programs and resources ought to be readily available to ensure that people with epilepsy (and their families and care-givers) are knowledgeable about the condition and have the requisite skills to engage in productive interactions with their health care team (Institute of Medicine 2012).

With this knowledge, the patient is better able to manage their condition and make informed choices about medicines and personal safety.

## REFERENCES

Andrewes D, Camp K, Kilpatrick C, Cook M. The assessment and treatment of concerns and anxiety in patients undergoing presurgical monitoring for epilepsy. *Epilepsia* 1999;40(11):1535–42.

Austin L. SUDEP: Risk perception and communication. In: Chapman D, Panelli R, Hanna J, Jeffs T, eds. *Sudden Unexpected Death in Epilepsy: Continuing the Global Conversation.* Camberwell: Epilepsy Australia, Epilpesy Bereaved & SUDEP Aware; 2011.

Bellon M, Panelli R, Rillotta F. 2014. Exploring the experiences and needs of people bereaved by epilepsy: Results from an online Australian survey (poster). 10th Asian and Oceanian Congress, Singapore.

Beran, RG. SUDEP—To discuss or not discuss: That is the question. *Lancet Neurol* 2006;5(6):464–5.

Beran R, Weber S, Sungaran R, Venn N, Hung. Review of the legal obligations of the doctor to discuss Sudden Unexplained Death in Epilepsy (SUDEP)—A cohort controlled comparative cross-matched study in an outpatient epilepsy clinic. *Seizure* 2004;13(7):523–8.

Black A. SUDEP—Whether to tell and when? *Medical Law* 2005;24(1):41–9.

Bolitho v. City and Hackney Health Authority. 1998. AC 232.

Brodie MJ and Holmes GL. Should all patients be told about sudden unexpected death in epilepsy (SUDEP)? Pros and cons. *Epilepsia* 2008;49 (S9):99–101.

Chapman SCE, Horne R, Chater A, Hukins D, Smithson WH. Patients' perspectives on antiepileptic medication: Relationships between beliefs about medicines and adherence among patients with epilepsy in UK primary care. *Epilepsy & Behavior* 2014; 31:312–20.

Chapman D, Moss B, Panelli R, Pollard R, eds. *Sudden Unexpected Death in Epilepsy: A Global Conversation*. Camberwell: Epilepsy Australia & Epilepsy Bereaved; 2005.

Chapman D, Panelli R, Hanna J, Jeffs T, eds. *Sudden Unexpected Death in Epilepsy: Continuing the Global Conversation*. Camberwell: Epilepsy Australia, Epilepsy Bereaved & SUDEP Aware; 2011.

Chester v. Afshar. 2005, 1 A.C. 134.

Cook M. Reflecting on my clinical experience. In: Chapman D, Moss B, Panelli R, Pollard R, eds. *Sudden Unexpected Death in Epilepsy: A Global Conversation*. Camberwell: Epilepsy Australia & Epilepsy Bereaved; 2005.

Couldridge L, Kendall S, March A. A systematic overview—A decade of research. The information and counselling needs of people with epilepsy. *Seizure* 2001;10(8):605–14.

Department of Health. *Improving Services for People with Epilepsy*. London: Department of Health; 2003.

Deriche v. Easling Hospital NHS Trust. 2003. EWHC 3104 (QB).

Dilorio C, Faherty B, Manteuffel B. Epilepsy self-management: Partial and extension. *Nursing & Health* 1994;173:167–74.

Duff AJM. Determination of Sheriff Alistair Duff, Sheriff of Tayside Central and Fife at Dundee. Inquiry held under fatal accidents and sudden deaths inquiry (Scotland) Act 1976 into the deaths of Erin Casey and Christina Fiorre Ilia; 2011.

Faught E, Duh MS, Weiner JR, Guerin A, Cunnington MC. Nonadherence to antiepileptic drugs and increased mortality: Findings from the RANSOM study. *Neurology* 2008;71(20):1572–8.

Finsterer, J., and C. Stollberger. 2009. Cardiopulmonary surveillance to prevent SUDEP. *Lancet Neurol* 8(2):131–2; author reply 132–3.

Fox S, Duggan M. 2013. Health Online 2013, Pew Research Center, Available at http://www.pewinternet.org/2013/01/15 /health-online-2013/.

Fraenkel L, McGraw S. Participation in medical decision making: The patients' perspective. *Med Decis Making* 2007;27(5):vs533–8.

Gayatri NA, Morrall MC, Jain V, Kashyape P, Pysden K, Ferrie C. Parental and physician beliefs regarding the provision and content of written sudden unexpected death in epilepsy (SUDEP) information. *Epilepsia* 2010;51(5):777–82.

General Medical Council. *Consent: Patients and Doctors Making Decisions Together*. London: General Medical Council; 2008.

Hanna NJ, Black M, Sander JWS, Smithson WS, Appleton R, Brown S, Fish DR. The national sentinel clinical audit of epilepsy related death: Epilepsy—Death in the shadows: The Stationary Office; 2002.

Helgeson DC., Mittan R, Tan SY, Chayasirisobhon S. Sepulveda Epilepsy Education: The efficacy of a psychoeducational treatment program in treating medical and psychosocial aspects of epilepsy. *Epilepsia* 1990;31(1):75–82.

Hesdorffer DC, T Tomson, Benn E, Sander JW, Nilsson L, Langan Y, Walczak TS, Beghi E, Brodie MJ, Hauser A. ILAE Commission on Epidemiology, and Subcommission on Mortality. Combined analysis of risk factors for SUDEP. *Epilepsia* 2011;52(6):1150–9.

Hitiris N, Suratman S, Kelly K, Stephen LJ, Sills GJ, Brodie MJ. Sudden unexpected death in epilepsy: A search for risk factors. *Epilepsy Behav* 2007;10(1):138–41.

Horne R. Compliance, adherence, and concordance: Implications for asthma treatment. *Chest* 2006;130(S1):65–72.

Horne R, Chapman SC, Parham R, Freemantle N, Forbes A, Cooper V. Understanding patients' adherence-related beliefs about medicines prescribed for long-term conditions: A meta-analytic review of the Necessity-Concerns Framework. *PLoS One* 2013;8(12):e80633.

Hughes JR. A review of sudden unexpected death in epilepsy: Prediction of patients at risk. *Epilepsy Behav* 2009;14(2):280–7.

Institute of Medicine. *Epilepsy across the Spectrum: Promoting Health and Understanding*. Washington, DC: Institute of Medicine; 2012.

Jeffs, TC, Elizabeth JD. Our epilepsy story: SUDEP Aware. *Epilepsia* 2014; http://dx.doi.org/10.1111/epi.12599.

Jones L, Naude JT. Sudden unexpected death in epilepsy information provision to parents of children with epilepsy-a service evaluation. *J Neurol Neurosurg Psychiatry* 2013;84(11):e2.

Kearton M. Living with the risks. In: Chapman D. Moss B, Panelli R, Pollard R, eds. *Sudden Unexpected Death in Epilepsy: A Global Conversation*. Camberwell, Australia: Epilepsy Australia & Epilepsy Bereaved; 2005, pp. 54–56.

Kennelly C, Riesel J. Sudden death and epilepsy: The views and experiences of bereaved relatives and carers [Report by College of Health] 2002. Available at https://www.sudep.org /sudden-death-and-epilepsy#.

Langan Y, Nashef L, Sander JW. Case-control study of SUDEP. *Neurology* 2005;64(7):1131–3.

Lewis G, ed. *The Confidential Enquiry into Maternal and Child Health (CEMACH)*. Saving mothers' lives: Reviewing maternal deaths to make motherhood safer—2003–2005 The seventh report on confidential enquiries into maternal death in the United Kingdom. London: CEMACH; 2007.

Lewis S, Higgins, Goodwin M. Informing patients about sudden unexpected death in epilepsy: A survey of specialist nurses. *Br J Neurosci Nurs* 2008;4(1):30–4.

Marteau TM. Screening for aortic aneurysm: Detection is not as harmful as it might seem. *Brit Med J* 2008;336(7651):973–4.

Mendonça PR, Arida RM, Cavalheiro EA, Scorza FA. Show and tell: Revelations about SUDEP from the Latin American Summer School on epilepsy. *Epilepsy Behav* 2011;22(4):813–4.

Miller WR, Young N, Friedman D, Buelow JM, Devinsky O. Discussing sudden unexpected death in epilepsy (SUDEP) with patients: Practices of health-care providers. *Epilepsy Behav* 2014;32:38–41.

Mittan R. Fear of seizures. In: Whitman S. Hermann B, eds. *Psychopathology in Epilepsy: Social Dimensions*, New York: Oxford University Press; 1986.

Mittan R. Managing fear. In: Chapman D, Panelli R, Hanna J, Jeffs T, eds. *Sudden Unexpected Death in Epilepsy: Continuing the Global Conversation*. Camberwell: Epilepsy Australia & Epilepsy Bereaved; 2005.

Monte CP, Arends JB, Tan IY, Aldenkamp AP, Limburg M, de Krom MC. Sudden unexpected death in epilepsy patients: Risk factors. A systematic review. *Seizure* 2007;16(1):1–7.

Moon RY, Horne RS, Hauck FR. Sudden infant death syndrome. *Lancet* 2007;370(9598):1578–87.

Morton B, Richardson A, Duncan S. Sudden unexpected death in epilepsy (SUDEP): Don't ask, don't tell? *J Neurol Neurosurg Psychiatry* 2006;77(2):199–202.

Nashef L. Sudden unexpected death in epilepsy: Incidence, circumstances and mechanisms. MD Thesis, University of Bristol; 1995.

Nashef L, Annegers JF, Brown SW. Introduction and overview. Sudden unexpected death in epilepsy. *Epilepsia* 1997; 38(S11):1–2.

Nunes V, Neilson J, O'Flynn J, Calvert N, Kuntze S, Smithson H, Benson J et al. *Clinical Guidelines and Evidence Review for Medicines Adherence: Involving Patients in Decisions about Prescribed Medicines and Supporting Adherence.* London: National Collaborating Centre for Primary Care and Royal College of General Practitioners; 2009.

Opeskin K, Berkovic SF. Risk factors for sudden unexpected death in epilepsy: A controlled prospective study based on coroners cases. *Seizure* 2003;12(7):45664.

Otoom S, Al-Jishi A, Montgomery A, Ghwanmeh M, Atoum A. Death anxiety in patients with epilepsy. *Seizure* 2007;16(2):142–6.

Pearce v. United Bristol Healthcare NHS Trust. 1999, 48 BMLR 118.

Petticrew M, Sowden A, Lister-Sharp D. False-negative results in screening programs. Medical, psychological, and other implications. *Int J Technol Assess* 2001;17(2):164–70.

Pinder R. What to expect: Information and the management of uncertainty in Parkinson's disease. *Disabil Handicap Soc* 1990;5(1):77–92.

Politi MC, Han PK, Col NF. Communicating the uncertainty of harms and benefits of medical interventions. *Med Decis Making* 2007;27(5):681–95.

Prinjha S, Chapple A, Herxheimer A, McPherson A. Many people with epilepsy want to know more: A qualitative study. *Fam Pract* 2005;22(4):435–41.

Ramachandran Nair R, Jack SM, Meaney BF, Ronen GM. SUDEP: What do parents want to know? *Epilepsy Behav* 2013;29(3):560–4.

Ridsdale L, Charlton J, Ashworth M, Richardson MP, Gulliford MC. Epilepsy mortality and risk factors for death in epilepsy: A population-based study. *Brit J Gen Pract* 2011;61(586):e271–8.

Rogers v. Whitaker. 1992. 175 CLR 479.

Ryvlin P, Nashef L, Tomson T. Prevention of sudden unexpected death in epilepsy: A realistic goal? *Epilepsia* 2013;54(S2):23–8.

Scottish Intercollegiate Guidelines Network. *Diagnosis and Management of Epilepsy in Adults.* Edinburgh: Scottish Intercollegiate Guidelines Network; 2003.

Scottish Public Services Ombudsman. Report 200700075. http://www.spso.org.uk/investigation-reports/2009/march/fife-nhs-board; March 2009.

Shankar R, Cox D, Jalihal V, Brown S, Hanna J, McLean B. Sudden unexpected death in epilepsy (SUDEP): Development of a safety checklist. *Seizure* 2013;22(10):812–7.

Shankar R, Jalihal V, Walker M, Laugharne R, McLean B, Carlyon E, Hanna J et al. A community study in Cornwall UK of sudden unexpected death in epilepsy (SUDEP) in a 9-year population sample. *Seizure* 2014;23(5):382–5.

Shaw C, Abrams K, Marteau TM. Psychological impact of predicting individuals' risks of illness: A systematic review. *Soc Sci Med* 1999;49(12):1571–98.

Smithson WH, Hukins D, Colwell B, Mathers N. Developing a method to identify medicines non-adherence in a community sample of adults with epilepsy. *Epilepsy Behav* 2012;24(1):49–53.

So EL. Demystifying sudden unexplained death in epilepsy—Are we close? *Epilepsia* 2006;47(S1):87–92.

So EL. Symposium on the neurophysiology of sudden unexpected death in epilepsy. *J Clin Neurophysiol* 2009;26(5):295–6.

So EL, Bainbridge J, Buchhalter JR, Donalty J, Donner EJ, Finucane A, Graves NM et al. Report of the American Epilepsy Society and the Epilepsy Foundation joint task force on sudden unexplained death in epilepsy. *Epilepsia* 2009;50(4):917–22.

Spratling WP. Prognosis. In: *Epilepsy and Its Treatment.* Philadelphia: WB Saunders; 1904.

Stokes T, Shaw EJ, Juarez-Garcia A, Camosso-Stefinovic J, Baker R. Clinical guidelines and evidence review for the epilepsies: Diagnosis and management in adults and children in primary and secondary care, CG20 full guideline: Royal College of General Practitioners (RCGP); 2004.

Surges R, Thijs RD, Tan HL, Sander JW. Sudden unexpected death in epilepsy: Risk factors and potential pathomechanisms. *Nat Rev Neurol* 2009;5(9):492–504.

Taylor JA. 2002. Determination of Sheriff James Taylor, Sheriff of the Sheriffdom of Glasgow and Strathkelvin at Glasgow. Inquiry held under fatal accidents and sudden death inquiry (Scotland) Act 1976 into the death of Colette Marie Findlay.

Taylor SE. Asymmetrical effects of positive and negative events: The mobilization-minimization hypothesis. *Psychol Bull* 1991;110(1):67–85.

Tomson T, Nashef L, Ryvlin P. Sudden unexpected death in epilepsy: Current knowledge and future directions. *Lancet Neurol* 2008;7(11):1021–31.

Tomson T, Nashef L, Ryvlin P. Cardiopulmonary surveillance to prevent SUDEP: Author's reply. *Lancet Neurol* 2009;8:132–3.

Tonsaker, T., Bartlett G, and Trpkov C. Health information on the Internet: Gold mine or minefield? *Can Fam Physician* 2014;60(5):407–8.

Vegni E, Leone D, Canevini M, Tinuper P, Moja E. Sudden unexpected death in epilepsy (SUDEP): A pilot study on truth telling among Italian epileptologists. *Neurol Sci* 2011;32(2):331–5.

Videto v. Kennedy. 1981. 125 DLR (3rd) 12.

Waddell B., McColl K, Turner C, Norman A, Coker A, White K, Roberts R, Heath CA. Are we discussing SUDEP? A retrospective case note analysis. *Seizure* 2013;22(1):74–6.

Wagner EH., Bennett SM, Austin BT, Greene SK, Vonkorff M. Finding common ground: Patient centredness and evidence-based chronic illness care. *J Altern Complem Med* 2005;11(S1):7–15.

Wannamaker BB. Medicolegal and clinical experiences In: Lathers CM, Schraeder PL, Bungo MW, Leestma JE, eds. *Sudden Death in Epilepsy: Forensic and Clinical Issues.* Boca Raton: CRC Press/Taylor & Francis Group; 2011.

Weinstein ND. What does it mean to understand a risk? Evaluating risk comprehension. *J Natl Cancer I Monogr* 1999;(25):15–20.

Welsh Assembly Government. *Service Development Directives for Epilepsy.* Wales: Welsh Assembly Government; 2009.

Wertheimer AI., Santella TM. Medication compliance research: Still so far to go. *Journal of Applied Research in Clinical and Experimental Therapeutics* 2003;3(3):254–61.

Woodward S, Pope A, Robson WJ, Hagan O. Bereavement counselling after sudden infant death. *Brit Med J (Clin Res Ed)* 1985;290(6465):363–5.

# 34 Mechanistic SUDEP Risk Factor Studies for Animals and Humans

*Claire M. Lathers, Steven C. Schachter, Braxton B. Wannamaker, Jan E. Leestma, and Paul L. Schraeder*

## CONTENTS

## DIFFERENT MECHANISMS OF SUDEP ARE INVOLVED IN DIFFERENT PATIENTS

Mechanisms of sudden unexpected death in epilepsy (SUDEP) are various and include changes in the central and peripheral autonomic nervous system, cardiac rhythm, i.e., arrhythmias, and pulmonary function including pulmonary edema, obstructive apnea, and larygospasm (Lathers 2011, ch. 44). A global focus is needed to resolve the *risk factors for* and *mechanisms of* epilepsy and sudden death (Lathers 2009). To this end, we have recently developed a new unique method of research for studying the risk factors and mechanism(s) underlying SUDEP based on a comprehensive and systems-based approach in Chapters 4 and 5.

## ROLE OF CENTRAL/PERIPHERAL AUTONOMIC NERVOUS SYSTEMS AND CARDIOPULMONARY SYSTEMS AND INTERACTION BETWEEN THE TWO SYSTEMS

This relationship is a very important research area that has yet to be explored with a definitive study. Seizure or interictally induced autonomic nervous system disturbances that lead to cardiac arrhythmias and pulmonary dysfunction are interrelated mechanisms contributing to the occurrence of SUDEP. An in-depth understanding of the risk factors for and mechanisms of SUDEP using different animal models to provide data allowing interrelated research conclusions will result

from animal studies. Dr. Alkadhi's laboratory (2011, ch. 26) has reported that in rat sympathetic ganglia the expression of ganglionic long-term potentiation (gLTP) may accentuate cardiac arrhythmias and that gLTP is triggered by a serotonin 5-HT3 receptor dependent mechanism. High rate of seizure occurrence may also induce LTP in autonomic ganglia and may lead to cardiopulmonary dysfunction including cardiac arrhythmias and increased risk for neurogenic pulmonary edema and respiratory depression, leading to SUDEP. The effect of psychosocial stress to accentuate seizure-induced synaptic plasticity in autonomic ganglia needs to be studied. Dr. Stewart's rat model (2011, ch. 39) defining seizure-associated autonomic activity and resulting cardiac arrhythmia that can be fatal has been extended to permit a full examination of laryngeal physiology during seizure activity. His group has shown seizure spread through the autonomic nervous system and need to establish mechanistic linkages between cardiac and respiratory derangements during seizures that can be lethal. Dr. Bealer (2011, ch. 38) has established sympathetic nervous system dysregulation of cardiac function and myocyte potassium channel remodeling in seizures and needs to extend his finding further. A strong relationship across basic science projects in time course from acute to chronic, ictal and interictal, and autonomic control of cardiopulmonary function is needed to define and link physiological details into a comprehensive picture of risks and mechanisms of SUDEP. Animal models and results will inform about essential preventative therapies for SUDEP.

The role the autonomic nervous system, cardiac arrhythmias, and respiratory changes, i.e., cardiopulmonary systems, occurring during seizure activities are interrelated mechanisms contributing to the occurrence of SUDEP need to be studied to provide an in-depth understanding of the risk factors for and mechanisms of SUDEP using a new distinctive research strategy. An overall research strategy should combine the following types of methodological approaches to integrate data from both animal and human studies in our unique, new SUDEP Cluster Classification and Identification (ID) method to further understanding of mechanisms and risk factors for SUDEP and preventive(s) tactics (Lathers et al. 2014). One research strategy is to use our new innovative method SUDEP Cluster ID method for victims of SUDEP, living people with epilepsy, and animal data, combining both mechanisms of and risk factors for SUDEP. Data from future studies will be used to fill in data gaps and to increase the numbers for each risk factor parameters and cases of SUDEP. In another research strategy, mechanisms of SUDEP will be examined in three different animal models and laboratories of brain, cardiac, and respiratory sites to explore mechanistic contributions of the central and peripheral autonomic nervous system and changes in adrenergic and serotonergic neurotransmitters using in vivo whole animal and in vitro techniques. In one of our research strategies, mechanistic and risk factor data obtained in living people with epilepsy and SUDEP autopsy data will be used in our new SUDEP Cluster ID method. Another research strategy uses data mining of existing databases: Normal humans NASA database and epilepsy patients in a private practice; autopsy reports and psychological postmortem studies, government registries or databases (NASA, Centers for Disease Control and Prevention), both international and national (Koehler et al. ch. 9, 2011; Lathers et al. 2011), genetic findings of SUDEP, and individual laboratory data of Terrence et al. (1981), Lathers (1980, 2009, ch. 25, 44, 2011), Lathers et al. (1977, 1978, 1982, 1986a,b, 1988a,b,c, 1989, 1990, 2008, ch. 1, 4 in 2011, Epi Behav 2011), Lathers and Schraeder (ch. 61, 2011), Schraeder and Lathers (1983), Lathers and Spivey (1987), Leestma (ch. 2, 2011), Leestma and Lathers (Chapter 9 in this book), Tomson (1998, 2011, Chapter 32 in this book) and others. An additional research strategy recognizes the need for a standardized SUDEP form for coroner's offices and medical examiner's offices and will address this need, including requesting genetic analysis postmortem in SUDEP cases. An exciting fifth research strategy will use an ambulatory electrocardiogram assessment of autonomic function and T-wave alternans study to evaluate SUDEP risk using Drs. Verrier and Schachter's unique method to analyze EKG morphology for risk prediction of potentially fatal cardiac arrhythmia in human studies (2011, ch. 43).

## CLARIFICATION: ROLE OF CARDIAC VERSUS RESPIRATORY IN ACTUAL DEATH EVENTS

It is evident that the occurrence of seizure-related apnea/pulmonary edema/hypoxia/acidosis may well have the potential to set the stage for acute cardiac rhythm disturbance and vice versa. It is not possible to say which single putative mechanism

or combination of mechanisms predominated in any given victim of SUDEP (Lathers and Schraeder 2011, ch. 61).

## ARRHYTHOMOGENESIS AND ACUTE HYPOXIA HAVE BEEN SHOWN TO INTERACT IN A NEGATIVE MANNER AND THE COMBINATION BECOMES RISK FACTORS FOR SUDEP

When an increased risk for arrhythmias is combined with acute hypoxemia associated with the occurrence of neurogenic pulmonary edema and/or associated central apnea, sudden death may be the outcome. For additional information about the role of arrhythmogenesis and acute hypoxia as risk factors for SUDEP, see the discussion in Chapter 1 of this book and in these references (Lathers et al. 2008; Mameli and Alessandro 2011, ch. 37; Lathers et al. 2011; Lathers et al. 2011, chs. 1 and 4). Future basic animal studies must address issues of seizures, cardiac arrhythmias, hypoxemia, and stress.

## APPROACHES FOR SUDEP SOLUTIONS

In general, no one animal model for disease completely mimics the symptoms and findings of the disease state in humans. When possible, risk factors and all supporting medical information must be obtained for people with epilepsy who are thought to be potential candidates for SUDEP (Lathers 2011, ch. 25). See discussion in Chapter 1, this book.

## SEIZURE MECHANISMS IN CARDIAC ELECTROPHYSIOLOGY AND THE LOCK STEP PHENOMENON (LSP)

When patients with generalized tonic–clonic seizures on no medications were compared with healthy controls, the patients exhibited higher standard deviation of all R–R intervals, higher standard deviation of mean R–R intervals in 5 minute recordings, and higher heart rate variability compared to the controls. Heart rate variability exhibited a reduction in high frequency parasympathetic activity and an increase of low frequency sympathetic values in patients with epilepsy when compared with people in the normal population. It was concluded that the increased sympathetic control of the heart rate in those with epilepsy who have generalized tonic–clonic seizures may play a role in development of ventricular tachyarrhythmias in these epileptics and may be associated with the higher incidence of sudden death when compared to controls (Everengul et al. 2005). Heart rate variability of epilepsy patients is lower at night than during daytime, indicating subtle autonomic dysfunction at night, when risk of SUDEP is greatest based on epidemiologic studies (Woodley et al. 1977). Control of the heart rate is perturbed by alterations in autonomic function in clinical syndromes of sudden cardiac death, congestive failure, space sickness, and physiologic aging. There is a loss of complex physiological variability in pathological conditions including heart rate dynamics before sudden death (Poon and Merrill 1997). Use of detrended fluctuation analysis of heart beat time series may distinguish healthy from pathologic data sets (Peng et al. 1995). Studies are needed to determine how to identify which patients with epilepsy are at risk for SUDEP (Lathers et al. 2011, ch. 4).

## POWER SPECTRAL ANALYSIS OF HEART RATE AS A TECHNIQUE TO ASSESS AUTONOMIC ACTIVITY RELATED TO RISK FACTORS FOR SUDEP

Epileptogenic activity is associated with cardiac rate and rhythm changes (Howell and Blumhardt 1990). Quint et al. (1990) discussed power spectral analysis of heart rate to assess autonomic activity related to risk factors for SUDEP. Goodman et al. (1990; 2011, ch. 40) found typical cardiovascular responses during a fully kindled generalized seizure in rats that consisted of a large increase in blood pressure accompanied by a profound bradycardia during the first 20–30 seconds of the seizure. Lathers and Schraeder (1982) reported bradycardia associated with interictal subconvulsant epileptiform discharges in cats that died in asystole, whereas an increase in heart rate occurred in animals dying in ventricular fibrillation. Gamma-aminobutyric acid (GABA) neurotransmission regulates, in part, the central control of cardiovascular function (Schwartz and Lathers 1990). Inhibition of central GABAergic tone using picrotoxin or bicuculline results in enhanced sympathetic outflow to the heart and increased coronary resistance and arrhythmias (Segal et al. 1984). $GABA_A$, administered into the cerebral ventricles prior to the agonist muscimol prevents these cardiac changes. Thus, central neuronal excitability/inhibitory states are important for development of seizures and cardiovascular abnormalities, including arrhythmias. In humans, drugs known to facilitate GABAergic neurotransmission are clinically effective anticonvulsants, i.e., benzodiazepines and barbiturates (Schwartz and Lathers 1990, ch. 17).

## NEW ANTIEPILEPTIC DRUGS: BETA BLOCKERS? OTHER DRUGS?

The cardiac arrhythmias that may trigger sudden death in patients originate from three primary sites of action, namely, directly in the heart, in the peripheral autonomic nervous system, or in the central autonomic nervous system or from combinations of some or all of these factors (Lathers et al. 1977; Lathers et al. 1978). The central and peripheral autonomic nervous systems are interconnected in patients without cardiac transplant. Pharmacological agents capable of suppressing epileptiform activity and the sympathetic component of cardiac arrhythmias are expected to prevent interictal activity and cardiac arrhythmias that contribute to SUDEP (Lathers and Schraeder 1982; Schraeder and Lathers 1983; Carnel et al. 1985; Lathers et al. 1988c). Timolol possesses components of both of these capabilities. Blockade of cardiac $beta_1$ receptors, a cardiac neurodepressant effect, and/or membrane

depressant actions of beta-blocking agents are thought to contribute, at least in part, to the antiarrhythmic actions of beta-blocking agents (Lathers et al. 1977; Lathers 1980; Spivey and Lathers 1985; Lathers et al. 1986a,b; Lathers and Spivey 1987; Lathers et al. 1988a,b; Lathers et al. 1990). Since pentylenetetrazol is an accepted convulsive model and since some drugs capable of suppressing pentylenetetrazol-induced epileptiform activity are anticonvulsants, the data suggest that timolol exhibits an anticonvulsant action. To determine whether timolol has intrinsic "anticonvulsant" properties separate from an ability to reverse the effects of pentylenetetrazol, studies are needed to determine whether timolol and other beta-blockers will protect against seizures induced in other experimental models of epilepsy and in people with epilepsy. The capability of timolol to suppress interictal discharges and cardiac arrhythmias elicited in other in vivo experimental models not involving pentylenetetrazol should be examined. If timolol also suppresses interictal discharges and arrhythmias in these experimental models, this would provide additional evidence to support the suggestion that timolol may be an effective agent for use in epileptic patients to prevent SUDEP. Other studies in Dr. Lathers' laboratory also established antiepileptic drug activity of propranolol and valium when given via the intraosseous route to suppress seizures in pigs (Jim et al. 1988, 1989; Lathers et al. 1989).

## CONCLUSION

Mechanisms of SUDEP include risk categories of brain seizure activity, cardiac arrhythmogenic factors, respiratory factors including increased lung weights, acute pulmonary edema, and hypoxia, and brain psychological factors including stress (Lathers et al. 2008). Clarification of risk factors and establishment of the mechanisms of SUDEP will help to develop preventative measures for SUDEP. Although it appears to be most important to attempt full seizure control, this goal is unobtainable in up to 1 in 3 people with epilepsy, and therefore other approaches to prevent SUDEP are urgently needed. Prospective studies of people with epilepsy are needed to determine how to identify which people with epilepsy are at risk for SUDEP (Lathers et al. 2008). We propose several prospective studies using people with epilepsy to develop their SUDEP Cluster Risk Factor ID and then to determine their risk for death and potential response to therapeutic agents. We propose several prospective studies using animals and humans to explore the role of central and peripheral autonomic nervous systems, the cardiac and pulmonary systems, and their interactions. Studies of multiple animal models using different species and contribute to understanding the interrelated different mechanisms of SUDEP and possible combinations thereof in different humans while delineating risk factors for SUDEP. Translational studies, i.e., whole animal experimental data leading to human studies will be performed to transition findings in animals to relevance for humans. Prospective studies in humans are needed. Retrospective human autopsy data studies will be performed to mine data for mechanisms of and risk factors for death.

## REFERENCES

Alkadhi KA, Alzoubi KH. Synaptic plasticity of autonomic ganglia: Role of chronic stress and implication in cardiovascular disease and sudden death. Chapter 26 In: Lathers CM, Schraeder PL, Bungo MW, Leestma JE, eds. *Sudden Death in Epilepsy: Forensic and Clinical Issues*. Boca Raton: CRC Press/Taylor & Francis Group; 2011, pp. 395–426.

Bealer SL, Metcalf CS, Little JG, Vatta M, Brewster A, Anderson AE. Chapter 38 In: Lathers CM, Schraeder PL, Bungo MW, Leestma JE, eds. *Sudden Death in Epilepsy: Forensic and Clinical Issues*. Boca Raton, FL: CRC Press/Taylor & Francis Group; 2011, pp. 333–46.

Carnel SB, Schaeder PL, Lathers CM. Effect of Phenobarbital pretreatment on cardiac neural discharge and pentylenetetrazol-induced epileptogenic activity in the cat. *Pharmacology* 1985; 30(4):225–40.

Evrengül H, Tanriverdi H, Dursunoglu D, Kaftan A, Kuru O, Unlu U, Kilic M. Time and frequency domain analyses of heart rate variability in patients with epilepsy. *Epilepsy Res* 2005;63(2–3): 131–9.

Goodman JH, Homan RW, Crawford IW. Acute cardiovascular response during kindled seizures. In: Lathers CM, Schraeder PL, eds. *Epilepsy and Sudden Death*. New York: Marcel Dekker; 1990, pp. 169–87.

Howell SJ, Blumhardt LD. The role of EEG monitoring in diagnosis of epilepsy related cardiac arrhythmias mimicking epilepsy. Chapter 7 In: Lathers CM, Schraeder PL, eds. *Epilepsy and Sudden Death*. New York: Marcel Dekker; 1990, pp. 101–20.

Jim KF, Lathers CM, Farris VL, Pratt LF, Spivey WH. Suppression of pentylenetetrazol-elicited seizure activity by intraosseous lorazepam in pigs. *Epilepsia* 1989;30(4):480–6.

Jim KF, Lathers CM, Spivey WH, Matthews WD, Kahn C, Dolce K. Suppression of pentylenetetrazol-elicited seizure activity by intraosseous propranolol in pigs. *J Clin Pharmacol* 1988;28(12): 1106–11.

Koehler SA, Schraeder PL, Lathers CM, Wecht CH. One-year postmortem forensic analysis of deaths in persons with epilepsy. Chapter 9 In: Lathers CM, Schraeder PL, Bungo MW, Leestma JE, eds. *Sudden Death in Epilepsy: Forensic and Clinical Issues*. Boca Raton, FL: CRC Press/Taylor & Francis Group; 2011, pp. 145–59.

Lathers CM. Effect of timolol on postganglionic cardiac and preganglionic splanchnic sympathetic neural discharge associated with ouabain-induced arrhythmia. *Eur J Pharmacol* 1980;64:95–106.

Lathers CM. Sudden death. Personal reflections global call for action. *Epilepsy Behav* 2009;15(3):269–77.

Lathers CM. Animal model for sudden cardiac death: Autonomic cardiac sympathetic nonuniform neural discharge. Chapter 25 In: Lathers CM, Schraeder PL, Bungo MW, Leestma JE, eds. *Sudden Death in Epilepsy: Forensic and Clinical Issues*. Boca Raton, FL: CRC Press/Taylor & Francis Group; 2011, pp. 427–36.

Lathers CM. Arrhythmogenic, respiratory, and psychological risk factors for sudden unexpected death and epilepsy: Case histories. Chapter 44 In: Lathers CM, Schraeder PL, Bungo MW, Leestma JE, eds. *Sudden Death in Epilepsy: Forensic and Clinical Issues*. Boca Raton, FL: CRC Press/Taylor & Francis Group; 2011, pp. 713–4.

Lathers CM, Jim KF, Spivey WH. A comparison of intraosseous and intravenous routes of administration for antiseizure agents. *Epilepsia* 1989;30(4):472–9.

Lathers CM, Kelliher GJ, Roberts J, Beasley AB. Nonuniform cardiac sympathetic nerve discharge: Mechanism for coronary occlusion and digitalis-induced arrhythmia. Young Investigator

Award, American College of Cardiology, February 24, 1976. *Circulation* 1978;57:1058–65.

Lathers CM, Koehler SA, Wecht CH, Schraeder PL. Forensic antiepileptic drug levels in autopsy cases of epilepsy. *Epilepsy Behav* 2011;22(4):778–85.

Lathers CM, Levin RM, Spivey WH. Regional distribution of myocardial beta receptors in the cat. *European J Pharmacol* 1986a;130:111–7.

Lathers CM, Roberts J, Kelliher GJ. Correlation of ouabain-induced arrhythmia and nonuniformity in the histamine-evoked discharge of cardiac sympathetic nerves. *J Pharmacol Exp Therap* 1977;203:467–79.

Lathers CM, Schraeder PL. Autonomic dysfunction in epilepsy: Characterization of autonomic cardiac neural discharge associated with pentylenetetrazol-induced epileptogenic activity. *Epilepsia* 1982;23(6):633–47.

Lathers CM, Schraeder PL. SUDEP: A mystery yet to be solved. Chapter 61 In: Lathers CM, Schraeder PL, Bungo, MW, Leestma JE, eds. *Sudden Death in Epilepsy: Forensic and Clinical Issues*. Boca Raton, FL: CRC Press/Taylor & Francis Group; 2011, pp. 967–72.

Lathers CM, Schraeder PL, Bungo MW. The mystery of sudden death: Mechanisms for risks. *Epilepsy Behav* 2008;12(1):3–24.

Lathers CM, Schraeder PL, Bungo MW. Neurocardiologic mechanistic risk factors in sudden unexpected death in epilepsy. Chapter 1 In: Lathers CM, Schraeder PL, Bungo MW, Leestma JE, eds. *Sudden Death in Epilepsy: Forensic and Clinical Issues*. Boca Raton, FL: CRC Press/Taylor & Francis Group; 2011, pp. 1–36.

Lathers CM, Schraeder PL, Bungo MW. Unanswered questions: SUDEP clinical studies needed. Chapter 4 In: Lathers CM, Schraeder PL, Bungo MW, Leestma JE, eds. *Sudden Death in Epilepsy: Forensic and Clinical Issues*. Boca Raton, FL: CRC Press/Taylor & Francis Group; 2011, pp. 67–76.

Lathers CM, Spivey WH. The effect of beta blockers on cardiac neural discharge associated with coronary occlusion in the cat. *J Clin Pharmacol* 1987;27(8):582–92.

Lathers CM, Spivey WH, Levin RM. The effect of chronic timolol in an animal model for myocardial infarction. *J Clin Pharmacol* 1988a;28(8)736–45.

Lathers CM, Spivey WH, Levin RM, Tumer N. The effect of dilevalol on cardiac autonomic neural discharge, plasma catecholamines, and myocardial beta receptor density associated with coronary occlusion. *J Clin Pharmacol* 1990;30(3):241–53.

Lathers CM, Spivey WH, Suter LE, Lerner JP, Tumer N, Levin RM. The effect of acute and chronic administration of timolol on cardiac sympathetic neural discharge, arrhythmia, and beta receptor density associated with coronary occlusion in the cat. *Life Sci* 1986b;39:2121–41.

Lathers CM, Spivey WH, Tumer N. The effect of timolol given five minutes post coronary occlusion on plasma catecholamines. *J Clin Pharmacol* 1988b;28(4):289–99.

Lathers CM, Tumer N, Kraras CM: The effect of intracerebroventricular D-Ala2-methionine enkephalinamide and naloxone on cardiovascular parameters in the cat. *Life Sci* 1988c;43: 2287–98.

Leestma JE. Forensic considerations and sudden unexpected death in epilepsy. Chapter 2 In: Lathers CM, Schraeder PL, Bungo MW, Leestma JE, eds. *Sudden Death in Epilepsy: Forensic and Clinical Iissues*. Boca Raton, FL: CRC Press/Taylor & Francis Group; 1990, pp. 37–56.

Mameli O, Alessandro CM. Sudden epileptic death n experimental animal models. Chapter 37 In: Lathers CM, Schraeder PL, Bungo MW, Leestma JE, eds. *Sudden Death in Epilepsy: Forensic and Clinical Issues*. Boca Raton, FL: CRC Press/Taylor & Francis Group; 2011, pp. 591–614.

Peng CK, Havlin S, Stanley HE, Goldberger AL. Quantification of scaling exponents and crossover phenomena in nonstationary heartbeat time series. *Chaos* 1995;5(1):82–7.

Poon CS, Merrill CK. Decrease of cardiac chaos in congestive heart failure. *Nature* 1997;389(6650):492–5.

Quint SR, Messinheimer JA, Tennison MB. Power spectral analysis: A procedure for assessing autonomic activity related to risk factors for sudden death in persons with epilepsy. In: Lathers CM, Schraeder PL, eds. *Epilepsy and Sudden Death.* New York: Marcel Dekker; 1990, pp. 261–92.

Schraeder PL, Lathers CM. Cardiac neural discharge and epileptogenic activity in the cat: An animal model for unexplained death. *Life Sci* 1983;32(12):1371–82.

Schwartz RD, Lathers CM. GABA neurotransmission, epileptogenic activity, and cardiac arrhythmias. Chapter 17 In: Lathers CM, Schraeder PL, eds. *Epilepsy and Sudden Death.* New York: Marcel Dekker; 1990, pp. 293–309.

Segal SA, Jacob T, Gillis RA. Blockade of central nervous system GABAergic tone causes sympathetic-mediated increases in coronary vascular resistance in cats. *Circ Res* 1984;5:404–15.

Spivey WH, Lathers CM. Effect of timolol on the sympathetic nervous system in coronary occlusion in cats. *Ann Emerg Med* 1985;14(10):939–44.

Stewart M. The urethane/kainate seizure model as a tool to explore physiology and death associates with seizures. Chapter 39 In: Lathers CM, Schraeder PL, Bungo MW, Leestma JE, eds. *Sudden Death in Epilepsy: Forensic and Clinical Issues.* Boca Raton, FL: CRC Press/Taylor & Francis Group; 2011, pp. 625–45.

Terrence CE, Rao GR, Perper JA. Neurogenic pulmonary edema in unexpected, unexplained death in epileptic patients. *Neurology* 1981;25:594–5.

Tomson T, Skold AC, Holmgen P, Nilsson L, Danielsson B. Postmortem changes in blood concentrations of phenytoin and carbamazepine: An experimental study. *The Drug Monitor* 1008;20:309–12.

Tomson T. Compliance with antiepileptic drug treatment and the risk of sudden unexpected death in epilepsy. Chapter 51 In: Lathers CM, Schraeder PL, Bungo MW, Leestma JE, eds. *Sudden Death in Epilepsy: Forensic and Clinical Issues.* Boca Raton, FL: CRC Press/Taylor & Francis Group; 2011, pp. 845–52.

Verrier RL, Schachter SC. Neurocardiac interactions in sudden unexpected death in epilepsy: Can ambulatory electrocardiogram-based assessment of autonomic function and T-wave alternans help to evaluate risk? Chapter 43 In: Lathers CM, Schraeder PL, Bungo MW, Leestma JE, eds. *Sudden Death in Epilepsy: Forensic and Clinical Issues.* Boca Raton, FL: CRC Press/Taylor & Francis Group; 2011, pp. 693–709.

Woodley D, Chambers W, Starke H, Dzindzio B, Forker AD. Intermittent complete atrioventricular block masquerading as epilepsy in the mitral valve prolapse syndrome. *Chest* 1977;72(3):369–72.

# Index

For Product Safety Concerns and Information please contact our EU
representative  GPSR@taylorandfrancis.com
Taylor & Francis Verlag GmbH, Kaufingerstraße 24, 80331 München, Germany

www.ingramcontent.com/pod-product-compliance
Lightning Source LLC
Chambersburg PA
CBHW082304210326
41598CB00028B/4441